MICROSURGICAL ANATOMY

MICROSURGICAL ANATOMY

Editors-in-Chief

Zhong Shizhen

Associate Professor of Anatomy
First PLA Medical College
Guangzhou, China

Han Yongjian

Associate Professor of Anatomy
Zhejiang Medical College
Hangzhou, China

and

Yen Wenchun

Senior Lecturer in Anatomy
The Sanitary School of Xian
Xian, China

MTP PRESS LIMITED
a member of the KLUWER ACADEMIC PUBLISHERS GROUP
LANCASTER / BOSTON / THE HAGUE / DORDRECHT

Published in the UK and Europe by
MTP Press Limited
Falcon House
Lancaster, England

British Library Cataloguing in Publication Data

Microsurgical anatomy.
1. Anatomy, Surgical and topographical
I. Zhong, Shizhen II. Han, Yongjian
III. Yen, Wenchun
611'.00246171 QM531

Published in the USA by
MTP Press
A division of Kluwer Boston Inc
190 Old Derby Street
Hingham, MA 02043, USA

Library of Congress Cataloging in Publication Data

Microsurgical anatomy.
Translated from the Chinese.
Bibliography: p.
Includes index.
1. Microsurgery. 2. Anatomy, Human. I. Zhong, Shizhen. II. Han, Yung-chien. III. Yen, Wenchun.
[DNLM: 1. Anatomy. 2. Microsurgery. WO 512 M627]
RD33.6.M48 1985 611 85-18243

ISBN-13: 978-94-010-8677-6 e-ISBN-13: 978-94-009-4914-0
DOI: 10.1007/978-94-009-4914-0

Softcover reprint of the hardcover 1st edition 1985

Typeset by Blackpool Typesetting Services Ltd., Blackpool
Printed by Dotesios Ltd., Bradford-on-Avon

Contents

Editors and Contributors

EDITORS-IN-CHIEF

Zhong Shizhen, Associate Professor of Anatomy, First PLA Medical College, Guangzhou, China

Han Yongjian, Associate Professor of Anatomy, Zhejiang Medical College, Hangzhou, China

Yen Wenchun, Senior Lecturer in Anatomy, The Sanitary School of Xian, Xian, China

EDITORIAL STAFF

Wang Qihua, Associate Professor of Anatomy, Guangzhou Medical and Pharmaceutical College, Guangzhou, China

Liu Muzhi, Lecturer of Anatomy, First PLA Medical College, Guangzhou, China

Zhu Jiakai, Associate Professor of Surgery, Zhongshan Medical College, Guangzhou, China

Zhang Weilong, Associate Professor of Anatomy, Norman Bethune Medical College, Changchun, China

Tao Yongsong, Lecturer of Anatomy, First PLA Medical College, Guangzhou, China

REVISERS

He Guangchi, Professor of Anatomy, Third PLA Medical College, Zhongqing, China

Zhao Minxue, Professor of Anatomy, Anhui Medical College, Hefei, China

Yang Dongyue, Late Professor of Surgery, Shanghai First Medical College, Shanghai, China

Feng Chengluo, Lecturer of English Language, Shanghai First Medical College, Shanghai, China

CONTRIBUTORS

Zhou Jiabao, Zhang Kequ, Zhang Ming, Zhejiang Medical College, Hangzhou, China

Chen Yaoliang, Chen Zhiyi, Shanghai First Medical College, Shanghai, China

Qin Dengyou, Zhang Shixing, Wu Renxia, Anhui Medical College, Hefei, China

Huang Gongkang, Miao Hua, Bengbu Medical College, Bengbu, China

Wu Yongmu, Nanjing Medical College, Nanjing, China

Zhang Mingxuan, Haerbin Medical College, Haerbin, China

Zheng Zhiliang, Norman Bethune Medical College, Changchun, China

Li Ji, Xu Enduo, Jiang Shuxue, Bai Shuling, Zhongguo Medical College, Shenyang, China

Yan Guofan, Military General Hospital, Shenyang, China

Chen Eryu, Liu Zhengjin, Third PLA Medical College, Zhongqing, China

Yu Guozhong, Zhongshan Medical College, Guangzhou, China

Zhong Ruchuan, Huang Hongjun, He Qinghua, Wang Zhinan, Huang Xiaying, Guangzhou Medical College, Guangzhou, China

Lin Zhengyan, Zeng Raoxiang, Zhang Guien, Xiao Xiangying, Liu Qinglin, Guangzhou Medical and Pharmaceutical College, Guangzhou, China

Xu Dachuan, Sun Bo, Zhou Changman, Luo Lisheng, Cheng Junping, First PLA Medical College, Guangzhou, China

Tao Xiangluo, Zhejiang Medical College, Hangzhou, China

Han Fengyue, Beijing Second Medical College, Beijing, China

Preface

Since the advent of microsurgery, there has always been a need for a systematic presentation of relevant anatomical biometry. In view of this urgent demand, this monograph has been compiled on the basis of recent research done by Chinese colleagues in the fields of microsurgery and related anatomical sciences from more than fourteen medical colleges in the hope of providing a complete set of anatomical data covering most areas of modern microsurgery.

This volume presents thirteen chapters dealing with the applied anatomy of free skin flap, muscle, bone and omental grafting and of intestinal and small organ transplantation including reconstruction of the thumb using toes. Space is also devoted to the microsurgical anatomy of the central and peripheral nervous systems, the lymphatic system and the middle ear. To help understanding, 212 illustrations, involving 21 photographic plates, are included.

The authors are particularly indebted to Professors He Guangchi and Zhao Minxue for their valuable suggestions and revision of the manuscript, and also to the late Professor Yang Dongyue for his personal contribution in the field of microsurgery and everlasting inspiration. The authors also wish to express their gratitude to the publishers for their great enthusiasm in producing this first edition.

ZHONG SHIZHEN
HAN YONGJIAN
YEN WENCHUN

1

The relationship between microsurgery and microsurgical anatomy

ZHONG SHIZHEN, HAN YONGJIAN AND ZHU JIAKAI

A BRIEF ACCOUNT OF THE DEVELOPMENT OF MICROSURGERY

Microsurgical technique is one of the most rapidly advancing surgical techniques in this decade. Surgical operations can be done under an operating microscope with fine instruments made for this purpose. Since the magnification of the object exceeds the limit of human sight, the operating field has been changed from macroscopic to microscopic, and many fine operations, which could not be performed previously with the naked eye, are now capable of being carried out successfully, thus increasing the extent of operative treatment and bringing about a profound change in surgical techniques.

Periods of development of microsurgery

The development of microsurgery can be divided into two periods.

The first period (1921–59)

In this period microsurgical techniques were mainly employed for rather simple otologic and ophthalmic operations such as fenestration and decompression of the inner ear, stapes mobilization and corneal suturing. The technique developed slowly and was not at first popularly accepted. However, there were still some important contributions: Nylen and Holmgren (1921) first used the operating microscope for performing the fenestration of the inner ear (see Nylen, 1972), and Perritt (1950) used it to accomplish corneal suturing.

The second period (from 1960 to date)

As an example of an important breakthrough in this period, the microvascular suture has laid the foundation for up-to-date microsurgery. Jacobson and Suarez (1960) anastomosed 20 blood vessels of 1.3–3.2 mm in diameter under the operating microscope, and all of them were well patent. This experiment attracted much attention in surgical circles. The skill of microvascular suture, with which a vessel of about 0.2 mm in diameter can now be sutured, marks the maturity of microsurgical technique. Modern microsurgery has developed from the anastomosis of blood vessels to anastomoses of the lymphatics, the lacrimal ducts, the genito-urinary and digestive tracts, nerve fascicles, etc., and it has also advanced from the free transplantation of a single tissue to that of composite ones or of small organs. At the same time, considerable progress has also been made in improving the operating microscope, microsurgical instruments and suture materials.

Significant achievements and progress in microsurgery

In 1966 Yang Dongyue *et al.* of the Shanghai First Medical College carried out the reconstruction of a thumb by means of the second toe transplantation, and in 1979, Cobbett reported the successful result in reconstruction of the thumb by toe transplantation.

In 1966 Green and others succeeded in replacing the cervical portion of the oesophagus by free intestinal segment grafting. In 1977, Zhang Disheng and others of the Shanghai Ninth People's Hospital reported the clinical application of intestinal segment grafting with good results.

Donaghy (1972) and Yasargil (1969) reported treatment of obliterated cerebrovascular diseases by means of extra–intracranial arterial bypass. In 1978, Zang Renho *et al.* of Xingjian Medical College performed the same operation.

In 1971 Thompson had free extensor digitorum brevis muscle transplantation to relieve facial paralysis by microneurovascular anastomosis, thus initiating the operation of free muscle transplantation. In 1978, Chen Zhongwei and others of the Shanghai Sixth People's Hospital succeeded in relieving Volkmann's ischaemic contracture of the forearm with free pectoralis major grafting.

In 1973 Harii and others first succeeded in transplanting free vascularized temporal skin flap. In 1973, Yang Dongyue and others (see Chen Zhongwei *et al.*, 1978) of Huashan Hospital in Shanghai used free skin flap in the groin region to repair postoperative buccofacial defect.

In 1972 McLean and Buncke repaired massive defect of the scalp by means of free great omentum. In 1977, Shen Zuyao and others of Ji Shui Tan Hospital in Beijing performed the same operation, and 2 years later Shen Zuyao and others modified the use of great omentum and introduced the omental axial skin flap technique (see Shen Zuyao *et al.*, 1979).

In 1972 Millesi and others used interfascicular grafting in repairing the peripheral nerve. In 1978 Zhu Jiakai and others carried out this operation in Zhongshan Medical College in Guangzhou and presented a survey on its long-term curative effect.

In 1974 O'Brien treated obstructive lymphoedema of the limbs by means of lymphaticovenous anastomosis, with good results. In 1979 Zhu Jiakai repeated the operation in Guangzhou.

In 1975 Taylor and others used free fibula grafting to repair massive bone defects of contralateral tibia by microvascular anastomosis. In 1977 Chen Zhongwei of the Shanghai Sixth People's Hospital carried out the same operation.

In 1976 Taylor was the first to repair a median nerve defect of 22 cm long in the contralateral upper limb with free vascularized radial nerve grafting.

In 1976 Baudet *et al.* proposed the method of free musculocutaneous flap transplantation, which was successfully performed by Yang Dongyue and others in the same year.

In 1977 Yang Dongyue used microsurgical technique in performing a homologous total knee joint transplantation by microneurovascular anastomosis. Earlier than this, Tamai made an experimental study of it on a dog in 1972.

In 1978 Taylor, using superficial circumflex iliac vessels, made a free composite tissue grafting of iliac bone with overlying skin. In 1980 Huang Gongkang and others of Bengbu Medical College transplanted a free iliac bone through anastomosis of the deep circumflex iliac artery (Huang Gongkang *et al.*, 1982).

In 1979 Zhu Jiakai treated a female patient suffering from an endocrine disturbance with homologous ovarian transplantation, with good results (Zhu Jiakai *et al.*, 1980).

In 1979 Zhang Zhaowu of the First PLA Medical College successfully repaired urethral defect with free autologous appendiceal transplantation (Zhang Zhaowu *et al.*, 1981).

APPLIED ANATOMY AS ONE OF THE IMPORTANT BASES OF MICROSURGERY

Microsurgical technique has been one of the achievements of modern surgery. In addition to the various basic knowledge and techniques of modern surgery, which bring about a noteworthy advance in microsurgery, there are two important factors, viz., the microsurgical equipment and skill on the one hand and the applied microsurgical anatomy on the other.

The developments of clinical and basic medicine are closely linked together and interact. The achievements of basic medicine provide a theoretical basis for the development of clinical medicine, and the latter will after all carry theoretical research forward to a higher standard. Surgery and surgical anatomy are interdependent and they interact as such. For example, as early as 1889, Manchot touched upon the dissection of cutaneous arteries in detail in his classical treatise 'Die Hautarterien des Menschlichen Koerpers', and introduced the concept of intradermal blood supply, which divided the whole body into 45 supplying areas. However, orthopaedics was not at that time sufficiently developed, and the significance of these basic anatomical theories was not fully recognized. As time passed, owing to developments in surgery, the anatomical basis soon became the guide to the clinical practice of many skin flaps with vascular pedicle. When orthopaedics developed to the stage requiring microsurgical technique, some traditional pedicular flaps were further substituted by vascularized free flaps following the success of microneurovascular anastomosis, thus widening the scope of operation. The improvement and design of various operations are all related to the applied anatomy of microarteries, veins and nerves, the previous data about which can no longer meet the need of recently designed operations. This will certainly ensure that surgeons and anatomists make a thorough study of this area.

In preparing a new microsurgical operation it is usually necessary to consider two aspects: one is the animal experiment, by which we can practise the various procedures of surgical manipulations to be carried out on fine structures under the microscope, and the other is the relevant knowledge of anatomy, which can help us to master the normal condition as well as possible variations in those main structures in the operating field so as to be able to draw up a corresponding plan of operation to increase the rate of success. Many accomplished surgeons used to pay close attention to the studies of animal experiments and cadaver dissections before operations. For instance, O'Brien had performed lymphaticovenous anastomosis experiments on nearly 100 dogs before he went into the treatment of obstructive lymphoedema. Taylor had also studied 100 cases of cadaver dissection relating to superficial vessels in the groin for the design of a free groin skin flap. Zhang Disheng and others had made experiments on dogs before they went on to repair the human oesophagus by means of free intestinal segment. When Yang Dongyue and his colleagues began to use the second toe for the reconstruction of the thumb the operation lasted 18–22 hours. When they later made use of the anatomical data derived from 50 cadavers, the time required for the operation was cut down to 4–6 hours. Zhu Jiakai and others made repeated studies on injected specimens of human lymphatics with a view to utilizing anatomical law before going into practical lymphaticovenous anastomosis. Based on the study of lymphatic distribution in the limbs, they were able to suggest a design of dividing the limb into four segments for operation, thus saving the procedure of lymphangiography prior to operation. Zhang Zhaowu and others made experiments on dogs and studied anatomical features of the blood vessels of the appendix and perineum on cadavers prior to the operation of replacement of the urethra by appendix.

A BRIEF ACCOUNT OF RESEARCH ON MICROSURGICAL ANATOMY

In the field of anatomy there existed a wide gap between macro- and microanatomy, which is understood to be macro–microanatomy, which was hardly touched upon by macroanatomy and even abandoned by microanatomy (histology). Though it had been claimed that this branch of anatomy might be a new field of scientific research, and there once even appeared some achievements, the practical value of macro–microanatomy remained obscure prior to the advent of microsurgery, which was entirely new and vital, and the desire to explore it was not strong enough to ensure that achievements were more than a trifle.

The development of microsurgical technique set new demands on anatomy and urgently demanded that macro–microanatomic data be used as a theoretical basis in making surgical designs. It turned out that microsurgical anatomy did eventually make further progress. Few anatomists abroad were engaged in research on microsurgical anatomy, and reports seldom appeared in journals other than clinical ones, which accounted for the urgent need of microanatomy data by the clinicians. Such scholars as Sunderland, Buncke, Taylor, Daniel, Smith, O'Brien, and Chater, however, presented some data on the application of anatomy to microsurgery in their clinical treatises or monographs.

Much of the research on microsurgical anatomy has been carried out by clinicians in China. Recently, anatomists have been keeping pace with them and have gone into the different fields of applying anatomy to microsurgery such as the anatomical study on the great omentum (Dept. of Anatomy Ningxia Medical College, 1977), the surgical anatomy of extra–intracranial arterial anastomosis (Zhong Shizhen *et al.*, 1981), the anatomical study on the reconstruction of the thumb by toe transplantation (Wu Jinbao *et al.*, 1980), the research on free fibula grafting (Guo Fen, 1978), the microsurgical anatomy of cerebral vessels (Zhang Weilong, 1984), the anatomical study on free skin flap (Li Fuzhuang, 1980), the microsurgical anatomy of peripheral nerve trunk (Zhong Shizhen *et al.*, 1980), the anatomical study on lymphaticovenous anastomosis (Liu Muzhi and Zhong Shizhen, 1979), the anatomical study on the replacement of oesophagus and vagina by intestinal segment (Tao Yongsong *et al.*, 1980), the anatomical study on transplantation of pancreas, thyroid and suprarenal glands (Xu Dachuan *et al.*, 1981a, b, 1982), the blood supply of the anterior part of iliac bone (Miao Hua *et al.*, 1981), the anatomy of the flaps with the intermuscular space and the intermuscular septum blood supply (Zhong Shizhen *et al.*, 1982b, c), the anatomy in relation to the renal grafting (Zhang Weilong *et al.*, 1981), the localization of recurrent laryngeal nerve within the vagus nerve trunk (Wang Qihua *et al.*, 1981c), and the microsurgical anatomy of the middle ear (Han Yongjian *et al.*, 1982a-c).

A comprehensive survey of the researches on microsurgical anatomy in China shows that it stepped a pace forward at the Annual Meeting of the Association of Chinese Anatomists in 1978, and during the meetings held in 1980 and 1982 a great many new achievements emerged and proved superior both in quality and quantity. We hope that the information about microsurgical anatomy hitherto collected might be well collated and edited in this book for the purpose of improving microsurgery further.

As mentioned above, Chinese anatomists engaged in research on microsurgical anatomy have made certain achievements, accumulated a lot of data and offered a reliable basis for the design and innovation of operations in recent years. Nevertheless, it seems that some of the basic theories of anatomy do not fit in with the clinical demand, and there are still some gaps to be filled. Moreover, there are some problems in which applied anatomy has not yet been involved, but which will definitely emerge in due course following the progress of science. For instance, the anastomosis of splanchnic nerves of viscera has not yet been placed on the work schedule by many surgeons. The applied anatomy of these nerves seems not to be in urgent need at present. It may be predicted, however, that once the problem of immunological rejection is well solved, the anastomosis of splanchnic nerves, which governs the functions of visceral organs, will certainly become an important topic. Therefore there will be a great number of problems in microsurgical anatomy to be investigated. It is hoped that anatomists and microsurgical clinicians will cordially cooperate to achieve greater success both in clinical practice and basic theories within a short time.

2

The anatomy and histology of small vessels

ZHONG RUCHUAN, ZHANG GUIEN, HE QINGHUA AND HUANG XIAYING

INTRODUCTION

It has been a long time since the arteries with a diameter of less than 1 mm were called the arterioles. In terms of morphological structures, arterioles belong to the muscular arteries just as the medium-sized arteries do, and they possess more than two layers of smooth muscles. The smallest precapillary arterioles, however, have only one layer of scattered smooth muscles. Not until the calibre of the arterioles is in excess of 60 μm do the three layers of their walls become complete, *viz.*, there exists a complete internal elastic lamina between the internal and middle tunics. The smooth muscles of the middle layer are arranged circularly or spirally and become continuous with those of larger muscular arteries (Figure 2.1). The external tunic is composed of a thin layer of connective

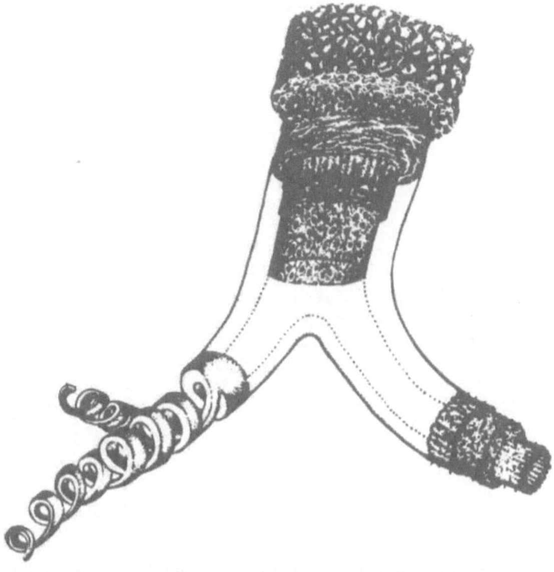

Figure 2.1 Diagram of the structure and muscular layers of the wall of medium-sized arteries and arterioles

tissue with many collagenous and reticular fibres. The venules also possess these three layers but, as compared with the companion arteries, their calibres are larger, and their walls are thinner and are provided with a smaller amount of smooth muscles and elastic fibres. Owing to the different locations and functions of the organs, the arterioles show some variations in their structure.

THE STRUCTURAL CHARACTERISTICS OF THE ARTERIOLES IN DIFFERENT PARTS OF THE BODY

ORDINARY ARTERIOLES

The calibres of the arterioles are smaller, but the tunicae intima, media and adventitia of the arterial wall are rather distinct. The outer and inner diameters and the thickness of the wall are regular, their ratio being 1 : 0.57 : 0.2 (Figure 2.2). The range of the calibre and the thickness of the wall may, however, vary with the functional activity of the corresponding organs and the vessels themselves, and some may differ considerably. Thus the walls of the arterioles in skeletal muscles, urinary organs and part of the reproductive tract, as well as the subcutaneous tissues of the limbs, are thicker, and those of the brain, the gastrointestinal tract and the lungs are relatively thinner. Seventy-five arterioles with a calibre less than 1 mm in different organs were measured. The thickness averages 104.1 μm, and the ratio of the thickness of the wall to the outer

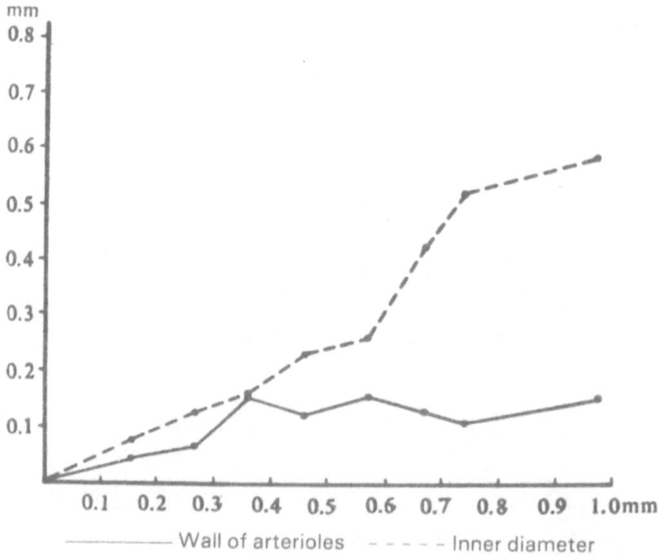

Figure 2.2 Relationship among the outer diameter, inner diameter and thickness of the wall of the arterioles, showing the outer diameter (abscissa), inner diameter and thickness (ordinate) in mm

diameter is 1 : 5. The three layers of the wall maintain a definite yet not absolute ratio (Figure 2.3) in accordance with the site where the arteriole is situated.

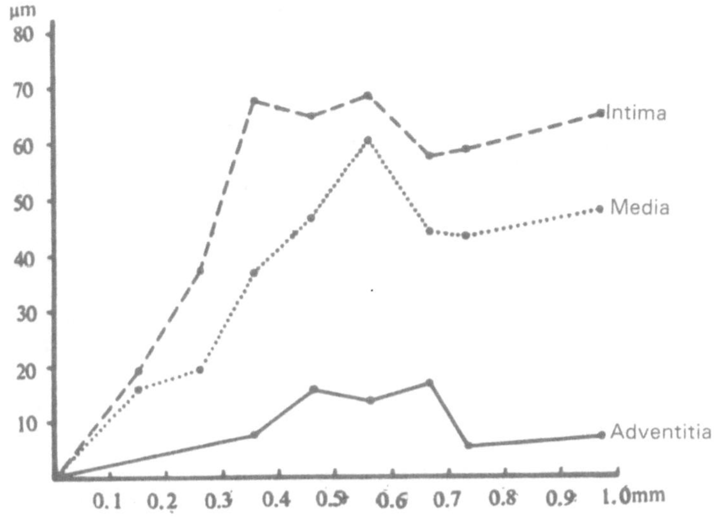

Figure 2.3 Relationship between the thickness of the layers of the arteriolar wall and the outer diameter of the vessel, showing the outer diameter (abscissa) and the thickness of the intima, media and adventitia (ordinate) in mm

Tunica intima

The tunica intima, being thin, is composed of endothelium and internal elastic limiting membrane. Its thickness is 2.5–25 μm, averaging 9.5 μm and representing 9% of the whole thickness of the wall. This thickness varies considerably in certain organs, e.g. the wall of the coronary arteries and that of the arterioles of the spermatic cord are thickened due to the increment in layers of the internal elastic limiting membrane.

Endothelium

The endothelial cells are spindle-shaped with a breadth of about 10 μm and a length of 20–50 μm. The longitudinal axis of the cell is parallel to that of the vessel (Figure 2.4). At the centre of the cell is a round or oval nucleus. After fixation the endothelium at the site of nucleus usually protrudes slightly toward the lumen of the vessel to a thickness of about 2–4 μm, the rest of the cytoplasm being very thin. Subjacent to the endothelium is a layer of extremely thin basal membrane, about 300–1500 Å in thickness.

We have observed under the electron microscope that the endothelial cells become connected with neighbouring cells by means of tight junctions, and such structures as microvilli and microfolds can be seen on the surface of the cell near

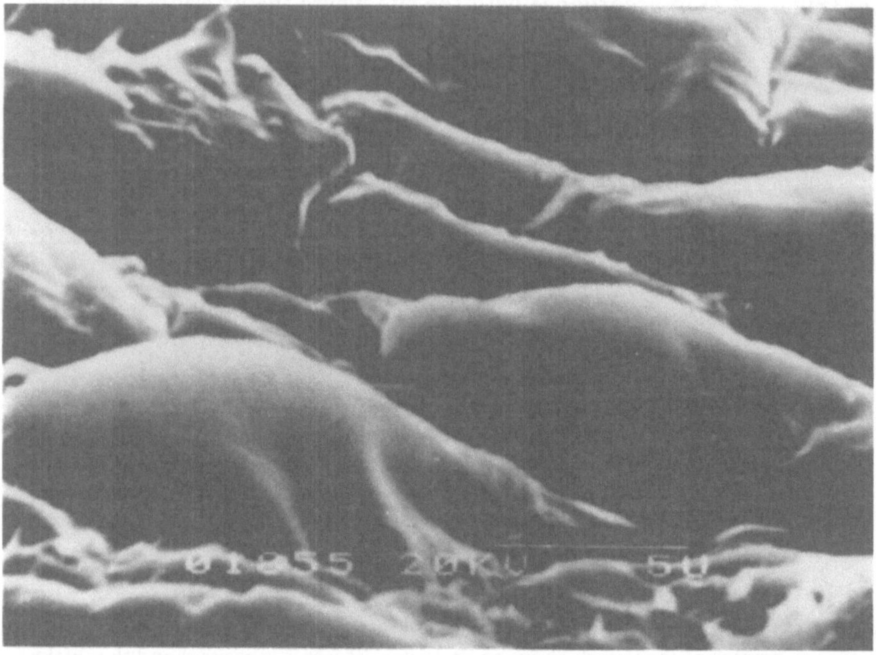

Figure 2.4 Scanning electron micrograph of the endothelial cells of an arteriole, ×3060

the junction. Using a scanning electron microscope it is observed that the presence or absence, the amount, and the morphology of the microvilli on the superficial surface of the endothelial cells vary with the site where the endothelial cells are situated. The microvilli on the surface of the endothelial cells of the arterioles of the greater omentum are relatively numerous (Figure 2.5). The ends of the microvilli swell slightly and appear in the form of drumsticks. The surfaces of the endothelial cells of the branches of the left gastric artery are provided with less, yet short and thick, microvilli (Figure 2.6), or there may appear some microfolds, but some, as shown in Figure 2.4, have smooth surfaces. Endothelial cells contain pinocytic vesicles with diameters of about 700Å as well as definite bundles of microfilaments. Sometimes these cells may send out processes, which get through the 'fenestrae' of the internal elastic limiting membrane and are connected with those of the smooth muscle cells on their deep surface, *viz*. forming 'synapses' with the processes of the muscle cells. The gap between the junctions is about 50Å wide.

Beneath the endothelial cells is the subendothelial layer which is, however, absent in smaller arterioles. Only in those larger arterioles may it be seen as an extremely thin layer, being mainly an amorphous matrix of acid mucoprotein. The matrix is connected with that of the tunica media through the fenestrae of the internal elastic limiting membrane. In the matrix of the endothelium, especially that of the arterioles of larger size, a small amount of elastic and collagenous fibres may sometimes be observed.

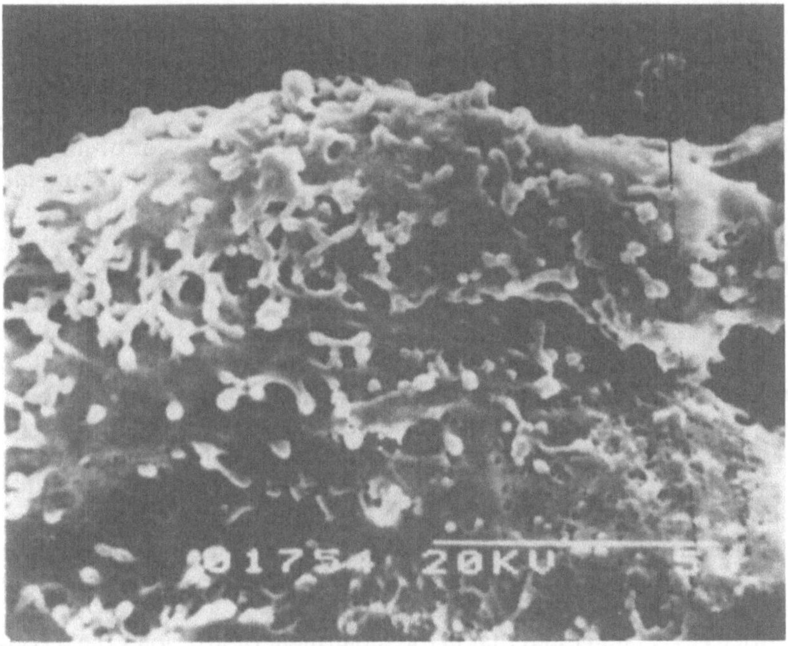

Figure 2.5 Scanning electron micrograph of microvilli on the surface of the endothelial cells of an arteriole in the greater omentum, ×4860

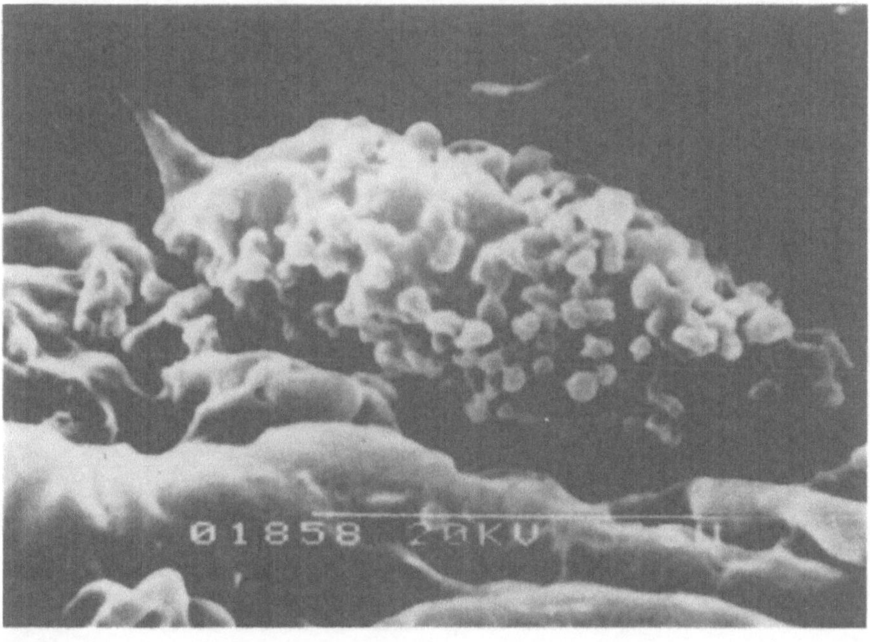

Figure 2.6 Scanning electron micrograph of the surface of endothelial cells of branches of the left gastric artery, ×6030

Internal elastic limiting membrane

The internal elastic limiting membranes of arterioles are usually well developed and clearly visible under the light microscope. It is a kind of membrane composed of many fine longitudinal elastic fibres, which often appear corrugated as waves after fixation. The membrane is provided with a lot of minute pores known as 'fenestrae', which can be seen clearly in oblique sections and measure 1–3 μm in diameter (Figure 2.7). Generally, arterioles have only one layer of internal elastic limiting membrane with a thickness of about 2–3 μm. The membrane may sometimes be composed of two or three layers, according to the organs supplied by the arterioles. The thickness and development of the internal elastic limiting membranes of the arterioles are subject to the particular functions and environment of the relevant organ. They are especially thickened in the arterioles of such organs as the cerebrum and lungs, where they bear little external pressure and tension, and the blood pressure within is comparatively low. The internal elastic limiting membranes of the coronary arteries are also well developed. The acceleration of normal senile change in vessels will lead to changes in arteries or arterioles. For example, the endothelium of the normal interlobular arteries of the kidney, having only one layer of internal elastic limiting membrane, usually increases in thickness in benign hypertension due to the fibrotic degeneration of the membrane.

O'Brien (1977) suggested that in the repairment of arterioles the reconstruction of the internal elastic membrane is due to the hypertrophy of the cells of the

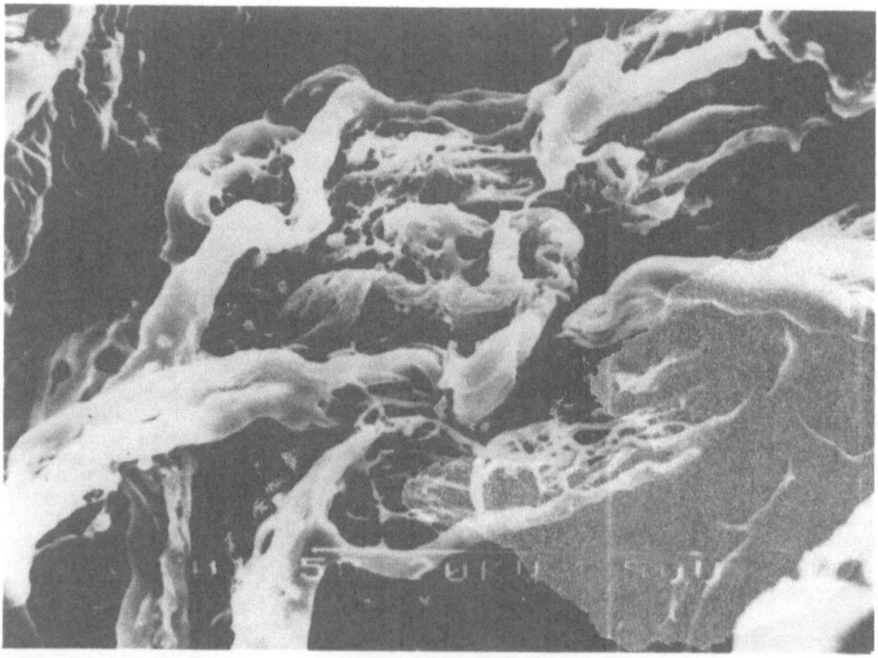

Figure 2.7 Scanning electron micrograph of the internal elastic limiting membrane of an arteriole, ×6030

tunica media as well as the formation of elastin fibrils. These hypertrophied cells may be smooth muscle cells which can pass through the internal elastic limiting membrane to reach the endothelium and produce the fine elastin fibrils, which are thereafter condensed tightly to form a renewed internal elastic limiting membrane. Severe breaks of the membrane and tunica media may lead to excessive hypertrophy of the internal tunic and constrictions of the lumen of the vessel, which is even divided into several compartments.

Tunica media

The chief elements constituting the middle tunic of arterioles are those circularly arranged smooth muscles and small amounts of collagenous, elastic and reticular fibres with matrix between the muscle fibres.

Arterioles with a calibre of less than 1 mm usually have a kind of tunica media of 20–70 μm in thickness, which averages 55 μm and accounts for 53% of the thickness of the arteriolar wall. The thickness of the tunica media of arterioles is mainly determined by the number of layers of smooth muscle, which may vary from two to ten with a mean of seven. The increasing number of layers of the smooth muscle is definitely connected with the increment in calibre of the arteriole. When the arteriole has an outer diameter of 0.2 mm there will be four layers of smooth muscle in the tunica media. When the outer diameter reaches 0.3 mm the number of smooth muscle layers becomes seven; as the outer diameter reaches 0.4 mm there will be ten layers, and as the diameter attains one mm the number of layers will be fourteen. Nevertheless, the number of layers of the smooth muscle varies again with the organ to which the arterioles belong, e.g. the tunica media is usually thick in those arterioles distributed to the subcutaneous tissue of the extremities, the muscles, the male and female reproductive canal, the parametrium, the broad ligament, the kidneys and ureters. The middle tunic of arterioles in the brain, lungs and the submucosa of the gastrointestinal tract is rather thin and is provided with lesser smooth muscles. Take for example the arterioles of the cerebrum (Figure 2.8a) and those of the kidney (Figure 2.8b); the tunica media is of the same thickness, yet the outer diameter of the former will double that of the latter. With the same

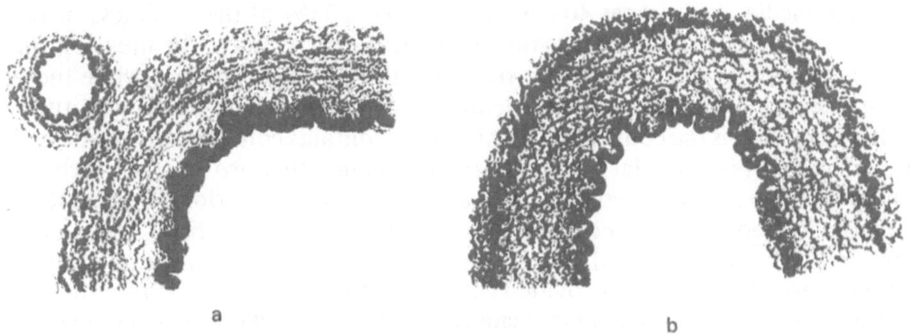

Figure 2.8 Comparison between arterioles of the cerebrum and those of the kidney. Weigert stain of elastic fibre. a: A renal arteriole; b: cerebral arteriole

calibre, the tunica media of the arterioles of the lower limb is thicker than that of the upper. The tunica media of some arterioles may attain great thickness, so do the afferent arterioles of the kidney, where the smooth muscles of the middle tunic are especially thick, and some even form longitudinally oriented cushions yet lack internal elastic limiting membrane. Again, the tunica media of the arterioles distributed to the adventitia of the ureter or to the spermatic cord is definitely thickened. Some other arterioles, such as those of the cerebrum, have in their sites of bifurcation extremely thin middle tunic which may, however, be entirely absent. There may be scattered longitudinal smooth muscles in the tunica intima, which have been thought to come from those of the media through the internal elastic limiting membrane.

The smooth muscle layer of the tunica media of arterioles is continuous with that of the larger muscular arteries, all of them being spirally arranged (Figure 2.1). Arterioles are able to regulate automatically the size of their lumen by means of elastic fibres and smooth muscles in order to control the amount of blood flow through the relevant organs. The smooth muscle cells are spindle-shaped, with a length of about 20 μm and a thickness of around 5 μm in the site of nucleus. They are provided with thin basement membrane and wrapped in extremely fine reticular fibres. Among the muscle cells are a small amount of matrix and fine elastic and collagenous fibres. The elastic fibres are wave-like in cross-section and their quantity varies with the artery of the organ. Thus, the media of the arterioles of the subcutaneous tissue of the extremities, the muscles, the kidney and ureter, and the ductus deferens are provided with more elastic fibres, while fibres are scanty in the arterioles of the cerebrum. No fibroblasts have been found in the media of the arterioles of all the organs, and the smooth muscle of the media has taken over the function of the fibroblasts. The matrix and the connective tissue fibres are all formed by the smooth muscle cells. This has been well confirmed by observation through the electron microscope, and has played the main role in the repair and regeneration of the intima and media of the arterioles.

Tunica adventitia

The adventitia of arterioles with a calibre of less than 1 mm is slightly thinner than the media. It averages 40 μm and represents 38% of the thickness of the wall. Arterioles of the subcutaneous tissue of the extremities, the muscles, the parametrium and the ureter are provided with thicker adventitia, while those of the cerebrum and the greater omentum are very thin. The main constituent of the adventitia is the connective tissue, which contains collagenous, elastic and a small amount of reticular fibres, the matrix being rather profuse, in which are found fibroblasts, histiocytes and fat cells. Some of the arterioles may contain separated smooth muscle cells and nerve fibres in the adventitia. These connective tissues are arranged loosely, while those subjacent to the media are rather dense, being usually provided with a layer of comparatively thin external elastic limiting membrane. This membrane gets thinner with the decrement in the calibre of the lumen and becomes an incomplete and broken layer, disappearing when the external calibre becomes less than 0.1 mm. Arterioles of the kidney and lung are provided with well-developed external elastic limiting membranes. Some of the arteries have characteristic structures for their walls due to differences in blood supply in accordance with their particular environment and physiological functions, and are thus called special arteries.

SPECIAL ARTERIOLES

Pulmonary arterioles

The characteristics of pulmonary arterioles are the largeness of their calibre and thinness of wall with profuse elastic fibres. The ratio of the internal to the external calibre is 0.48, and that of the thickness of the wall to the external calibre is 0.19. When the calibre is greater than 1000 μm and the elastic fibres of the wall become abundant, the arterioles may resemble an elastic artery structurally. Arterioles with a calibre of less than 1 mm are similar to the muscular arteries in structure, except for the thinness of media and scarcity of muscular fibres, yet there are more layers of internal elastic limiting membranes, and the adventitia is also provided with more elastic fibres. The media of pulmonary arterioles with a diameter of less than 100 μm is very thin and is provided with a layer of smooth muscle. What is peculiar is that the precapillary arterioles still have a layer of definite internal elastic limiting membrane, and that the elastic fibres of the adventitia are profuse and continuous with those of the alveolar wall. The structural characteristics of the pulmonary arterioles mentioned above are adaptable to the physiological functions of the lungs. The blood pressure of the pulmonary artery is lower than that of the systemic circulation, representing about one-sixth of the pressure of the aorta. Owing to the passage of the pulmonary arteries along the respiratory tract, the peripheral pressure exerted on them tends to be lower. This affords a greater possibility of expansion for the pulmonary arteries. All of these structural peculiarities fit in the functional demand of the pulmonary apparatus quite well.

Coronary arteries

In spite of their smaller calibre the walls of the coronary arteries are rather thick and the elastic fibres and membranes are all well developed. The characteristic features of the coronary arteries are the thickness of intima, profuseness of subendothelial elastic fibres and well-developed internal elastic limiting membranes, which usually consist of several layers, among which are a few longitudinal smooth muscles. The media contains, in addition to the circular smooth muscles, lots of longitudinal muscles which can even be separated into layers. The external elastic limiting membrane, however, is not well developed. In man the left coronary artery contains more profuse elastic fibres than the right one, and this is due to the greater burden of the left heart; hence the thicker wall of the ventricle and greater amount of blood flow in the left coronary. It may be established that the profuse amount of elastic fibres and the well-developed muscular layer of the coronary artery are related to the more laborious activities undertaken by the cardiac muscles, which lead to a greater need of blood supply. The quantity of blood flow usually increases by four to five times in exaggerated activity of the heart muscle. The structural characteristics of the coronary arteries mentioned above can alleviate the impact of the blood flow against the wall of the vessel, and regulate automatically the amount of blood flow to meet the need of cardiac activities.

Arterioles of brain

The cerebral arterioles belong to the muscular arteries. Because of the relative fixation of the cranial cavity, the arterioles of the meninges and the ventricles of the brain, the amplitude of vasocontraction and dilatation is lowered so that the pulsation of the cerebral arteries is barely visible to the naked eye. Though the amount of cerebral blood flow is plentiful, accounting for about 20% of that of the systemic circulation, it remains constant in capacity, the range of which is not wider than that of other organs, varying between ±30% and ±50%. (When the activity of the heart is enhanced, the cardiac flow increases by four to five times. The blood flow of the skeletal muscles can even increase by as much as 15 to 20 times.) As a result, the calibre of the cerebral arterioles is comparatively large with rather thin wall and thick internal elastic limiting membrane, while both the smooth muscles of the media and the adventitia are not very well developed. When the average value of the outer diameter is 0.53 mm that of the inner will be 0.36 mm. The ratio of the outer diameter to the inner is 0.68 (0.57 for ordinary arterioles). The thickness of the wall of the vessel is 78 mm, the ratio of it to the outer diameter being 0.15 (0.20 for ordinary arterioles). Hence the characteristic features of the cerebral arterioles are their large calibre and thin wall. The intima of the above-mentioned arteriole is 4.6 μm in thickness. The endothelium is thin, yet the internal elastic limiting membrane is quite thick and sometimes consists of two layers. The internal elastic limiting membrane plays an important role in buffering the impact of the blood flow against the wall. The membrane remains distinct and complete up to the arterioles with extremely minute calibre. As the capillaries are approached it appears as a very thin layer as well. The media is 40.5 μm thick with 2 to 12 layers of separately arranged smooth muscles. Between the muscle fibres may be seen very fine elastic fibres which may, however, be absent or replaced by many collagenous fibres. This has one of the distinguishing features between the cerebral vessels and those of other organs. The adventitia is 32 μm thick, which is thinner than the media. It is composed chiefly of collagenous fibres and a small amount of reticular and elastic fibres, so that it appears loose structurally. Cerebral arterioles with a diameter of less than 1 mm are not provided with external elastic limiting membranes. As the outer diameter reaches 1 mm the external elastic limiting membrane still appears as an incomplete, broken layer of very fine elastic fibres. It is especially true of the arterioles of the brain and the dura mater, where the adventitia may be extremely thin or even absent.

Arterioles of the male and female reproductive organs

Arterioles of the penis, after puberty, have thick intima with longitudinally directed smooth muscles which collect to form longitudinal ridges. The media is also thick, and there are longitudinal bundles of smooth muscles in adventitia. All of the arterioles of the uterus and ovaries and spermatic cord have rather profuse smooth muscles. The intima also has longitudinal smooth muscles forming endothelial cushions. Arterioles of the uterus and ovaries are peculiar in that the muscle layer of the media exhibits changes following menstrual cycles. During pregnancy muscles of the media of the uterine arterioles undergo degenerative changes which involve hyperplasia of the elastic and collagenous fibres of the intima, so that it appears thicker and gives rise to new smooth muscles, and a thin layer of connective tissue is formed around the degenerating media. Most of these arterioles are twisted spirally and hence known as the spiral arteries. This structural morphology keeps close pace with the particular physiological functions of the relevant organ.

Special arterioles, through having characteristics different from the ordinary ones, have to be taken into consideration in the course of vascular anastomosis in microsurgery.

VENULES

It is customary to call the veins following the capillaries the postcapillary veins, which are very similar to capillaries structurally, yet have a thin but dense and distinct layer of connective tissue in the wall. As the calibre reaches 50 μm there appear in the connective tissue a few scattered smooth muscle cells and a thin layer of adventitia. Not until the calibre reaches about 200 μm does the media begin to possess a continuous layer of smooth muscle. Venules are those small veins with a diameter of 0.2–1 mm. They are similar in structure to the accompanying arterioles, except for the following distinguishing features:

1. fewer elastic fibres with undeveloped internal and external elastic membranes, which may, however, be absent, the three basic layers being not clearly distinguished;
2. rather thin media with few smooth muscle cells but more collagenous fibres and fibroblastic cells;
3. the thickness of the adventitia keeps pace with that of the media or is slightly thinner (the adventitia of the veins larger than those medium-sized is thicker than the media).

The media of venules is generally provided with two to four layers of circular smooth muscle, among which are profuse loose connective tissues containing longitudinal elastic fibres. Venules with a calibre of less than 0.3 mm are almost devoid of the internal elastic limiting membrane which is not complete even in slightly larger venules. The internal calibres of venules are slightly larger than those of the companion arterioles. The ratio of the inner diameter to the outer of the venules we measured was 0.61 (that of the arterioles being 0.57). The ratio of the thickness of the wall to the outer diameter is 0.18 (that of the arterioles being 0.20). As a result, the lumen of venules is larger than that of the arterioles, and the walls are thinner. Judging from proportion, however, the wall of venules is still comparatively thicker (the ratio of the thickness of the wall of medium-sized veins to their outer calibre turns out to be 0.10; that for large veins is about 0.05 only). The thickness of the intima of venules accounts for about 5.2% of the whole thickness of the wall, the media 47.1% and the adventitia 47.7%.

In order to meet the particular need of the blood circulation of regional organs and to adapt the effect of the hydrodynamics of the blood, the structural differences of venules of different organs appear to be more distinct than those of the arterioles, and these differences are manifested especially in the amount, direction, and position of the smooth muscle fibres. Furthermore, changes in the external elastic fibres also remain more evident. The walls of venules of the limbs, the muscles, the spermatic cord, the suprarenal glands and the uterus in pregnancy, etc. are rather thick, and the muscle fibres, especially the longitudinal ones, are profuse. Which layer of the wall tends to be thicker depends on the type of relevant organ. Venules of the adrenal medulla usually possess more longitudinal muscles beneath the intima. In subcutaneous venules may be seen the prominences of the intima which lead to constrictions of the lumen. The longitudinal muscles of the adventitia are rather thick in the pampiniform plexus and renal venules, but thin in the venules of the brain, the retina, the bone and the corpus cavernosum penis, where the smooth muscles are scanty. There are more elastic fibres in the pulmonary venules and the pampiniform plexus. The muscle fibres and the longitudinal elastic and collagenous fibres surrounding them are regularly arranged in the venules of the subcutaneous tissue and the muscles of the extremities. That the walls of the venules become thickened quickly after being anastomosed with the arterioles indicates that there is a close relationship between the blood pressure and the structures of the vessel wall. This also proves that the blood vessels possess much more plasticity.

3

The applied anatomy of the free skin flap transplantation

LIU ZHENGJIN AND HE GUANGCHI

GENERAL CONSIDERATIONS

The free skin flap transplantation with vascular anastomosis is to transplant the flap with its vascular pedicle (sometimes together with a nerve, a muscle, or a bone, etc.) directly to the recipient area and by means of the microvascular anastomosis technique to re-establish the blood circulation. This technique was first brought successfully to clinical application by Harii, using a temporal flap in 1972. In 1973, Daniel and Yang Dongyue transplanted inguinal flaps to repair temporal and buccal defects. Later on, investigators both at home and abroad reported in succession similar clinical cases. Donor areas that have been used clinically are from all areas of the body, and the design of flaps is progressing. The design of a skin flap for transplantation with vascular anastomosis depends largely on the pattern of arterial supply of that flap. To the traditional direct cutaneous and musculocutaneous vessels, the anatomists of China have recently, according to their studies on cutaneous vessels, added some new patterns, i.e. the arterial truncal and reticular cutaneous vessel (Li Ji, 1980), the intermuscular septal cutaneous vessel (Zhong Shizhen, 1981) and the intermuscular space cutaneous vessel (Zhong Shizhen, 1982). Based on the cutaneous vessels investigated, some skin flap donors with good texture have been discovered. The fundamental requirement for the survival of a skin flap is a good circulation, and the recovery of the sensory function of a flap depends on the nerve anastomosis. Therefore, identification of the morphological patterns of the vessels and nerves of the skin is indispensable basic knowledge for the selection and design of the skin flap, and the operative procedure as well.

Blood supply of the skin flap

The arteries supplying the skin originate from the deep arterial trunk. They pierce through the deep fascia into the subcutaneous tissue, and then enter the reticular layer of the dermis. The arteries of the reticular layer are interlaced with each other, and send out ascending and descending branches. The ascending branches extend to the papillary layer of the dermis, while the terminals of the descending branches form vascular loops around the hair follicles and glands, and constitute glomeruli for the regulation of blood flow and storage of blood. The arteries of the reticular layer eventually form the reticular plexus. The branches of the arteries of the papillary layer can be divided into two groups: one proceeds to the deep layer and anastomoses with the arteries of the reticular layer, and the other goes to the superficial layer to form the papillary arterial plexus. In the most superficial part of the papillary layer of the dermis the plexus becomes a capillary network to supply the epidermis (Figure 3.1)

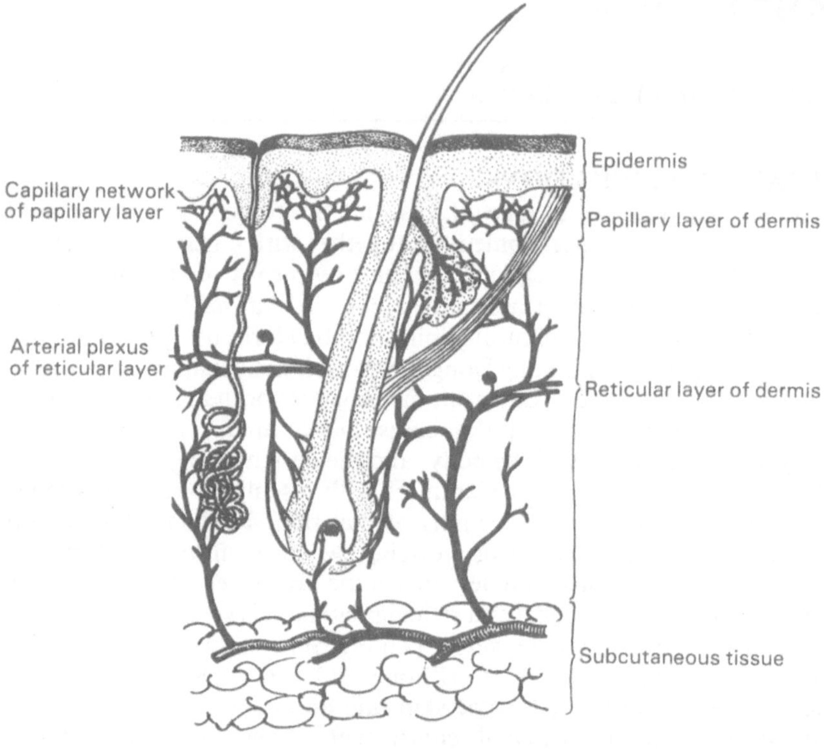

Figure 3.1 Blood supply of the skin

The venous blood from the interendothelial space of the papillary layer flows into the subpapillary venous plexus and thence to the subdermal venous plexus, whence the blood returns via the superficial and deep veins.

As the blood vessels of the skin are mainly found in the dermal layer, the whole thickness of the dermis must be considered in order to re-establish the blood circulation of the skin.

The vessels supplying the skin can be divided into two types, namely, the direct cutaneous vessel and the musculocutaneous vessel. The former can be further classified into three subtypes, i.e. the arterial truncal and reticular cutaneous vessel, the intermuscular septal cutaneous vessel, and the intermuscular space cutaneous vessel. The skin flaps are named after their supplying vessels.

Direct cutaneous vessels and the corresponding flap

The direct cutaneous artery arises from the deep arterial trunk. After piercing the deep fascia it takes a long course in the subcutaneous tissue, parallel to the skin surface, and gives off branches on the way to the skin and subcutaneous tissue (Figure 3.2). There is a definite rule regarding its origin but variations are

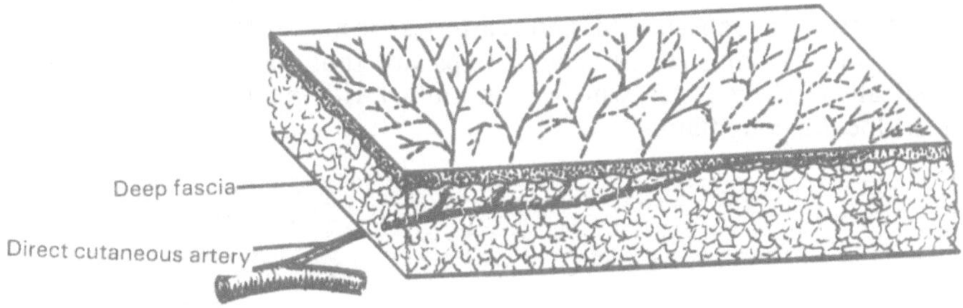

Figure 3.2 Direct cutaneous vessels

possible, such as the displacement of the artery itself, combination with neighbouring vessels to form a common trunk, or its absence. The direct cutaneous artery serves as the vascular axis of the flap it supplies, so that it is only necessary to anastomose it and the companion vein with the corresponding vessels of the recipient area in order to ensure the vitality of the flap. It follows that, in designing a flap of this type, the direct cutaneous artery is used as an axis to estimate the extent of the flap capable of being supplied by the artery. However, there are some anastomoses between the neighbouring arteries; hence the overlap of areas supplied. Generally, there is only one dominant vessel in a given area. If the area of arterial distribution diminishes for some reason, the neighbouring arteries will enlarge their distribution for the sake of compensation. The ratio of the width to length of the direct cutaneous arterial flap is relatively high. Smith proved it, in an experiment on rabbit, to be as high as 8 : 1. Yang Dongyue reported a successful case of thoracoabdominal flap transplantation by anastomosing the superficial epigastric vessels only, the area being 40 cm × 9 cm. This indicates that the area of a surviving vascular skin flap actually exceeds the distributing area of its vascular axis. This is due to the fact that the skin can tolerate anaemia to a high degree, and the communicating branches between two adjacent axial arteries are so abundant that the subcutaneous arterial network, which is invisible with the naked eye, can offer an adequate blood supply to the adjacent area.

According to clinical demands, an ideal direct cutaneous artery must be constant in its origin, position and distribution. It must also be convenient for operative manipulation; its calibre must be within the range of microsurgical technique. Venous drainage should be adequate in the environment and the company of sensory nerves would be advantageous. The direct cutaneous vascular flaps in recent clinical use are as follows: the temporal flap, the posterior auricular flap, the anterior and lateral thoracic flaps, the hypogastric flap, the inguinal flap, the posterior crural flap, the scrotal flap, the flap of the first toe web, etc.

Musculocutaneous vessels and the corresponding flap

The musculocutaneous arteries arise from those supplying the muscles. The arterial trunk, being stout, gives off numerous slender branches piercing the muscle and then the deep fascia perpendicularly forms a subcutaneous plexus to supply the tissue and skin overlying the muscle (Figure 3.3). The skin generally covers the muscles of the body. Since each muscle has adequate blood supply for itself, the musculocutaneous arteries are mainly the blood supply for the skin, and the musculocutaneous flaps are thus based on the arteries. Theoretically all the muscles, which are in contact with the skin, can be prepared as musculocutaneous flaps.

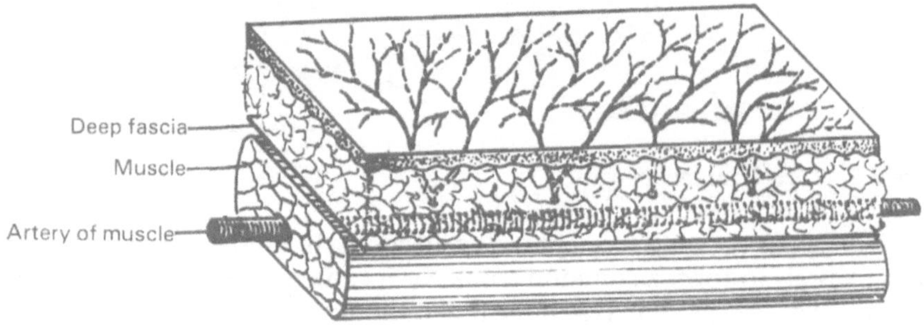

Figure 3.3 Musculocutaneous vessels

The musculocutaneous flap is a composite tissue flap consisting of skin, subcutaneous tissue and muscle, in which the skin is confined to the underlying muscle and supplied by perforating branches from the arterial trunk of the muscle. As long as the vascular pedicle is taken up and anastomosed the skin flap is able to survive. When the size of skin excised exceeds the extent of the muscle, the blood supply of the peripheral undermined portion of the skin, which is then supplied by the vessels of the fascia or the subcutaneous tissue, will possibly be inadequate. Nevertheless, this is not always true; Nahai pointed out that the size of the musculocutaneous flap involving the tensor fascia lata may be taken up to 14 cm × 40 cm, which is about three times as wide as the area of the muscle. The accordance of the musculocutaneous flap with the muscle in respect to their blood supply is to be discussed in Chapter Four.

Truncal–reticular cutaneous artery and the corresponding flap

Numerous fine cutaneous branches arising directly from the arterial trunk form an abundant cutaneous network to supply the overlying skin (Figure 3.4). This constitutes the basis for the truncal–reticular arterial flap. During operation the arterial trunk may be used as a pedicle, and the skin flap can be taken up along it. This type of flap offers a relatively large area of skin grafting. The arterial trunk has few variations, being constant in position but wider in calibre, and can be anastomosed at either end. The vascular pedicle may be taken long or short, within or beyond the extent of the flap. In the area of this flap there are superficial and deep groups of veins as well as the vascularized nerve, tendon and muscle, so that it is quite suitable for the recipient site. As both ends of the arterial trunk can be used for anastomosis the flap may serve as a bridge to connect other cutaneous or musculocutaneous flaps to make up a secondary flap or one of more grades. Flaps of this kind, which have recently been used clinically, are those of the forearm and the dorsum of foot.

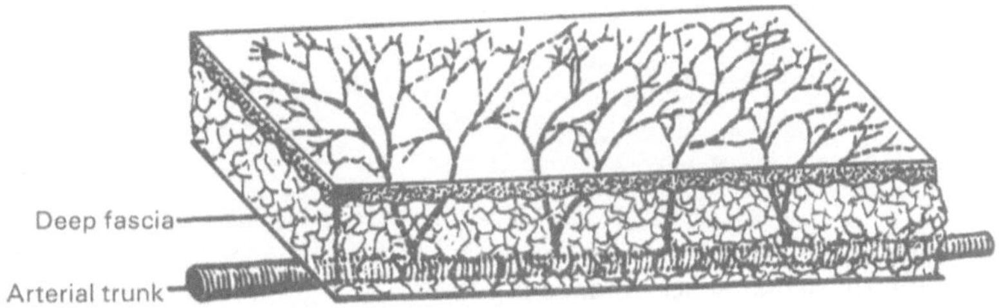

Figure 3.4 Truncal and reticular cutaneous artery

Intermuscular septal cutaneous vessels and the corresponding flap

The intermuscular septal artery arising from the arterial trunk of the limbs runs in the intermuscular septum and reaches the superficial layer to give off branches to the overlying skin (Figure 3.5). The arterial pedicle is relatively long and easy to expose and dissect. The artery forms extensive anastomoses with other cutaneous arteries and is accompanied by veins. In the area of the flap there exist large superficial veins and cutaneous nerves worth utilizing. If there is a need for longer and thicker arteries during operation, it is possible to take up a common stem of the intermuscular septal artery and any other muscular branch, or even the arterial trunk found by dissection upward along the intermuscular septum. Skin flaps with intermuscular septal vascular supply are as follows: the posterolateral femoral, the medial crural, and the medial and lateral brachial flaps, etc.

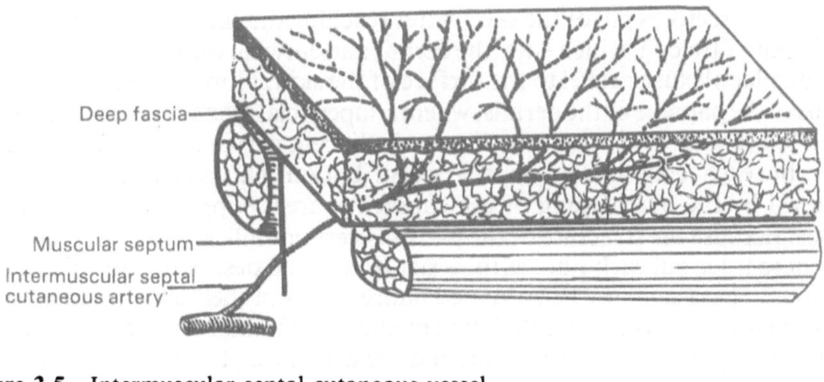

Figure 3.5 Intermuscular septal cutaneous vessel

Intermuscular space cutaneous vessels and the corresponding flap

The vessels passing through the intermuscular connective tissue space to reach the skin are called the intermuscular space cutaneous vessels (Figure 3.6).

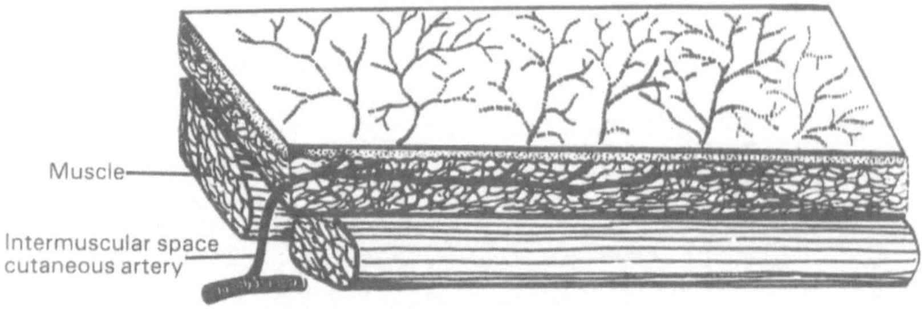

Figure 3.6 Intermuscular space cutaneous vessel

Generally speaking, the intermuscular septal cutaneous vessels mentioned above are also a part of the intermuscular space cutaneous vessels, but they run along the intermuscular septa of the limbs. The characteristic features of those two kinds of arteries are basically identical. Since the intermuscular spaces are more numerous than the intermuscular septa, the corresponding vessels of the former are more available. The calibre of this type of cutaneous vessels and the size of the flap are smaller. Flaps with intermuscular space vascular supply are as follows: the pectorodeltoid flap (pectorodeltoid muscular space), the infraspinatus flap (triangular space), the superior lateral brachial flap (quadrangular space), the middle lateral brachial flap (lateral bicipital space), the superior gluteal flap (lateral sacro-spinatous space), the superior posterior femoral flap (infragluteal space), the medial crural flap (medial intermuscular space of the leg), etc.

Innervation of the skin flap

The skin possesses many cutaneous nerves, which consist mainly of sensory and sympathetic nerve fibres. The latter fibres are distributed to the blood vessels, glands and erectores pili of the skin. After reaching the skin the cutaneous nerve divides into fasciculi, which enter the dermis and entwine with each other to form the reticular plexus parallel to the surface of the skin. Fibres arise from the deep plexus to the papillae of the dermis, where a superficial plexus of cutaneous nerve is formed (Figure 3.7). There the fibres of adjacent nerves interweave with each other, but each tends to reach its area of distribution. This pattern of distribution is shown by the overlapping of the cutaneous areas supplied by the adjacent nerves. Because the structure of the plexus is very complicated it is impossible at present to trace out each fibre as to its size, shape and destination by anatomical methods. These can only be estimated indirectly from their activities, i.e. those recorded with the electrical stimulation method, the animal experimental method after severing the dorsal nerve root, and the depiction of the cutaneous area of sensory loss of the patient with known spinal segmental injury.

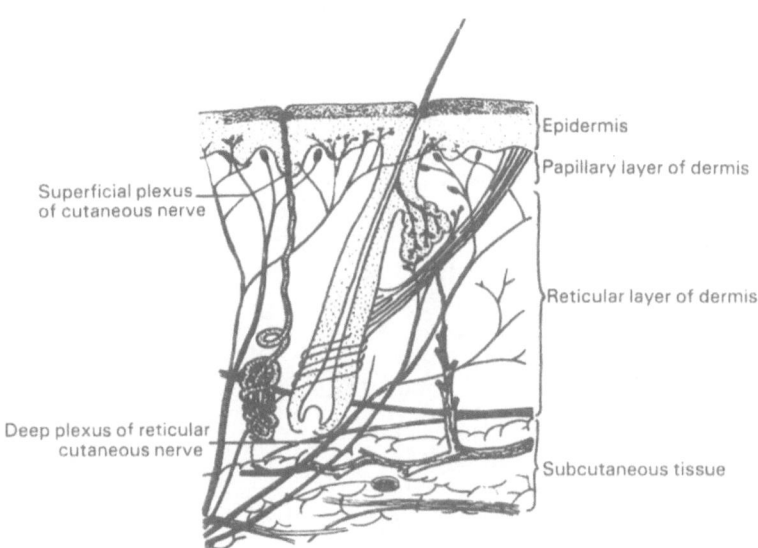

Figure 3.7 Innervation of the skin

The rule of distribution of cutaneous nerve

Cutaneous nerves mainly come from the sensory fibres of spinal nerves. The distribution of the spinal nerves displays rather distinct segmentation and overlapping.

In the embryonic stage, spinal nerves show very clear segmentation, and each nerve supplies the corresponding dermatome and myotome. After birth the dermatomes of the trunk are still arranged in the order of a series of girdles, but the breadth of each varies in its different parts. For example, the first cervical nerve is very small and lacks the dorsal root in 8% of the cases, hence the absence of cutaneous branches. The cutaneous areas supplied by the upper lumbar nerves are wide, while the fifth sacral and the coccygeal nerves supply only the skin of the perianal region. Owing to the appearance of limb bud, the segmental cutaneous distribution of spinal nerves on the trunk is discontinuous in some parts. As a result, the dermal segment of the fourth cervical nerve lies adjacent to that of the second thoracic nerve anteriorly, and that of the sixth cervical nerve is next to the dermatome of the first thoracic nerve on the back of the body. The fourth and fifth lumbar nerves do not supply the skin of the trunk, and the limbs are supplied by the branches of spinal plexuses. The cutaneous area of the extremity distributed by each spinal nerve is parallel to the long axis of the limb. When the cutaneous areas are analysed in terms of nerve origin and segmentation, it is found that they are arranged in order from the proximal to the distal ones on the anterolateral side of the upper limb, and in reverse order on the posteromedial side of it. In the case of lower limb they are arranged in order from the proximal to the distal ones on the anteromedial side and in reverse order on the posterolateral side. This rule may be used as a reference in designing sensory skin flaps (Figure 3.8).

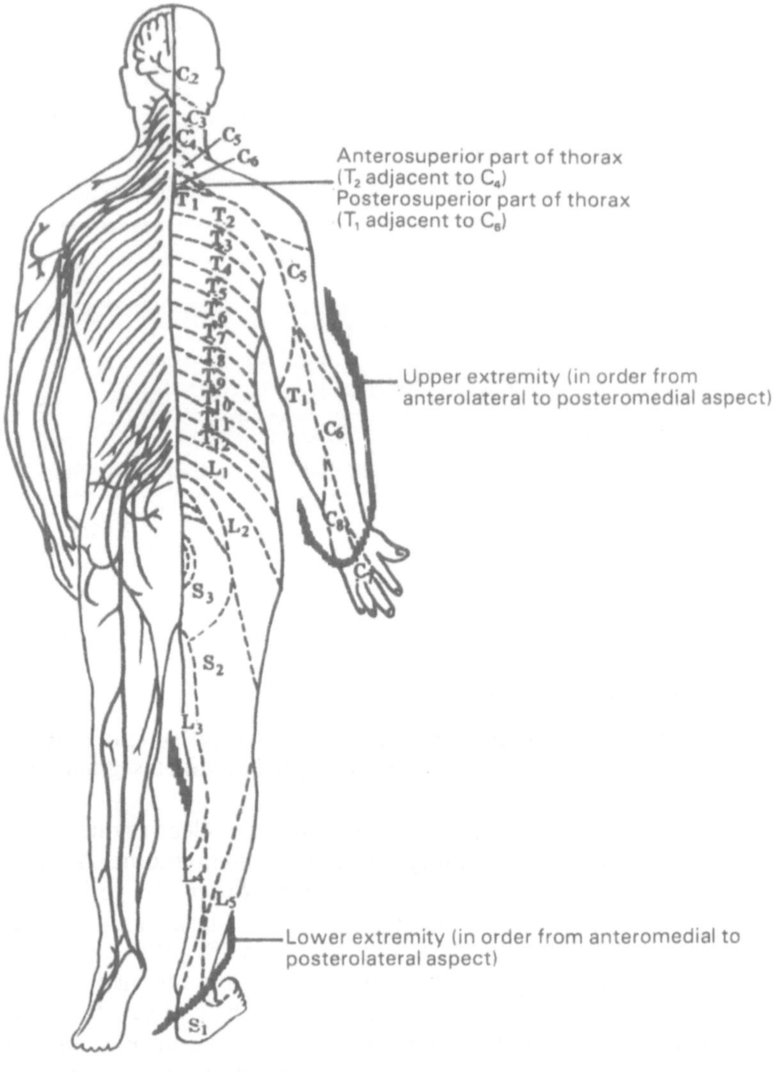

Figure 3.8 Rule of cutaneous innervation

The areas of adjacent cutaneous nerves overlap, and the overlapping is very extensive on the trunk. An intercostal nerve usually supplies the intercostal space of its own segment and one space above the segment and one below it as well. The area of distribution of a cutaneous nerve of the limb has a central autonomic zone, which is free from overlapping by other cutaneous nerves. Surrounding the autonomic zone is an irregular overlapping zone supplied by the nerve itself and its neighbours. When a certain cutaneous nerve is damaged, the sensation of the autonomic zone will be completely lost and that of the overlapping zone is only diminished. In order to save the flap from loss of sensation, attention should be paid to the management of the autonomic zone of the donor area in designing an innervated skin flap. The area of the autonomic or the overlapping zone, however, varies with different individuals and even with different sides of the same person.

Nerve distribution in different types of flap

According to the rule of distribution of cutaneous nerves and their relationship with the vessels, the nerve supply may be different in various types of flap.

Flaps with direct cutaneous vascular supply

In some of the flaps there may be found cutaneous nerves accompanying the axial vessels such as the anterior cutaneous branches of the intercostal nerve in the anterior pectoral flap, the popliteal cutaneous nerve in the posterior crural flap, and the deep peroneal nerve in the flap of the first toe web. In some of the flaps with direct cutaneous vascular supply, the longitudinal axial blood vessels ordinarily match with several non-accompanying segmental cutaneous nerves. Examples are the lateral cutaneous branches of the intercostal nerve in the lateral pectoral flap, and the eleventh thoracic, hypocostal and iliohypogastric nerves in the hypogastric flap.

Flaps with musculocutaneous vascular supply

The blood vessels and nerves which supply the muscle always get into the muscular substance together through its hilum. These nerves include mainly motor fibres and also some sensory ones, which are distributed to the overlying skin. During embryonic development some of the myotomes undergo the process of migration, so that they do not correspond to their dermatomes in the indistinctly segmented parts, and consequently the muscle and its overlying skin are not innervated by the same segmental nerve. Only in a small number of flaps may the cutaneous branches of the same origin be found as the muscular ones. For example, the nerve innervating the gracilis femoris has a sensory branch, which perforates the muscle and is distributed to the lower part of the musculocutaneous flap of gracilis. In the majority of cases the musculocutaneous vascular flaps are innervated by the cutaneous nerve of different origins with appropriate position. For example, the upper part of pectoralis major skin flap is innervated by the supraclavicular nerves, the rectus femoris flap by the intermediate femoral cutaneous nerve, the tensor fasciae latae skin flap by the lateral femoral cutaneous nerve, and the biceps femoris skin flap by the posterior femoral cutaneous nerve.

Flaps with truncal and reticular vascular supply

The arterial trunk is always accompanied by the nerve trunk, the branches of which are usually distributed to the area of this flap. Owing to its large size the flap is innervated by the other appropriate cutaneous nerve. For example, in the forearm flap, in addition to the superficial branch of radial nerve, there is also the lateral antebrachial cutaneous nerve; in the flap of dorsum pedis there is the medial cutaneous nerve of the dorsum of foot, except for the deep peroneal nerve.

Flaps with intermuscular septal vascular supply

Large cutaneous nerves are present in the anterior, posterior, medial and lateral aspects of limbs, and therefore in the neighbouring part of the intermuscular septum can usually be found a cutaneous nerve, which can be used for the grafting of this type of flap. For example, there is the posterior cutaneous nerve in the posterolateral femoral skin flap, the saphenous nerve in the medial crural skin flap, the medial brachial cutaneous skin flap, and the posterior antebrachial cutaneous nerve in the lateral brachial skin flap.

Flaps with intermuscular space vascular supply

Only parts of the intermuscular space vessels are accompanied by cutaneous nerves. For instance, the cutaneous vessels from the quadrangular space are accompanied by superolateral brachial cutaneous nerve, the cutaneous vessel from the lateral sacrospinal space by the supragluteal cutaneous nerve, and the cutaneous vessel from the infragluteal space by the posterior femoral cutaneous nerve. In other flaps, where cutaneous vessels are not accompanied by the cutaneous nerves, a large cutaneous nerve in the neighbourhood may be chosen for transplantation.

Principles for the selection of the donor and recipient areas

The aim of free skin flap transplantation lies in the satisfaction of the demand for filling the defect in the recipient area and, at the same time, in preventing the donor area from being disturbed in its function. Therefore, in designing and selecting the recipient area, the following principles should be taken into consideration.

Ensure the survival of transplanted skin flap

The key to the survival of the transplanted flap with vascular anastomosis is the successful re-establishment of blood circulation in the recipient area. For this reason one should first be familiar with the condition of the blood circulation of the donor and the recipient areas. In the donor area there must be at least one artery and one vein suitable for anastomosis, which are comparatively constant in course and convenient for exposure, and possess a sufficient length and a calibre fit for microanastomosis. The donor area should be so designed that ischaemia will not occur afterwards. In the recipient area the artery and veins for anastomosis must be healthy. Attention should also be paid to the collateral circulation available, which can prevent the recipient area from being deprived of blood supply after its blood vessels are anastomosed to those of the transplanted flap. The incision should be made in accordance with the position and course of the blood vessels and be convenient for operative manipulation. The artery and vein should not overlap each other to avoid compression of the vein and interference with its blood return. The vessels for anastomosis should be sufficiently long, lest breaks should ensue due to overtension. Nevertheless, excess in length will lead to tortuous course and will cause decrease in blood flow and even thrombosis.

Consider the function as well as the exterior appearance of the donor and recipient areas

In taking up a musculocutaneous flap we should consider whether the donor area is acceptable to the patient; whether it would cause any functional and sensory disturbances; how to make the suture of the donor area; and whether there is a need to make skin grafting for the donor site. In order to restore the indispensable functions of the recipient area and recover its external appearance, the skin of the donor area should be similar to the recipient area in colour and quality. For the re-establishment of the sensory function of the recipient area, a sensory nerve must be available.

Satisfy the demand for filling the defect of recipient site

Various defects in the recipient area are to be filled with appropriate grafts. The skin flap is used for the cutaneous defect. Defects consisting of both skin and muscle are to be repaired with musculocutaneous flaps, and the osteocutaneous flap is used for the cutaneous and skeletal defects. Some donor areas can supply more than one kind of graft according to the demand of the recipient area. For example, the dorsum pedis skin flap and its neighbouring structures can serve four purposes, viz., the skin as the skin graft; the vascularized skin flap with tendons of the dorsum of foot as the skin and tendon graft; the vascularized extensor digitorum brevis muscle and skin as the skin and muscle graft; and the composite vascularized skin and second toe for the reconstruction of toes.

THE TEMPOROPARIETAL AND FOREHEAD FLAPS

YAN GUOFAN AND XU ENDUO

The temporoparietal flap, also known as the scalp flap, is part of the scalp distributed by the parietal branches of the superficial temporal vessels. It is a peculiar hair-bearing donor, suitable for repairing the defects of hair, eyebrow and beard.

The forehead flap is a donor area supplied by the frontal branches of the superficial temporal vessels, which resembles the face in colour and thickness and may be used to repair the maxillofacial or nasal defect.

The temporoparietal and forehead flaps take the parietal or frontal branch respectively of the superficial temporal vessels as the trunk of the vascular pedicle, or these may be taken together with the main trunk of the superficial temporal vessels so as to make a long vascular pedicle.

Superficial temporal artery

The trunk of the superficial temporal artery arises perpendicularly from the maxillary artery behind the neck of the mandible. It is relatively constant in origin, whence it ascends in the substance of the parotid gland, anterior to the external auditory meatus and across the root of zygomatic arch, and finally reaches the subcutaneous tissue of the temporal region. At or slightly above the level of the zygomatic arch, the trunk of the superficial temporal artery is mostly of the straight or the slightly curved type, which accounts for 83.6%, while the curved or the sigmoid type accounts for 16.4%. Its length measured from the beginning to its bifurcation into the frontal and parietal branches averages 31.8 mm in adults. The outer diameter averages 2.6 mm (2.0–3.6 mm) at its commencement and 2.0 mm at the level of the zygomatic arch.

Branches of the superficial temporal artery

(1) Parotid branches are small and distributed to the parotid gland.

(2) Transverse facial artery is a large branch prior to the emergence of the superficial temporal artery from the parotid gland. Its outer diameter averages 1.7 mm in adults. After emerging from the substance of the parotid gland it passes anteriorly over the masseter between the zygomatic arch and parotid duct, and finally divides into several branches to the parotid gland and duct, the masseter and the neighbouring skin.

(3) Zygomatico-orbital artery mostly arises from the trunk of the superficial temporal artery above the zygomatic arch, a few being from its frontal branch. Its diameter averages 1.0 mm (0.5–1.8 mm) in adults. It proceeds along the superior border of the zygomatic arch between the two layers of the temporal fascia to the lateral portion of the orbit, where it supplies the orbicularis oculi and anastomoses with the ophthalmic and lacrimal arteries.

(4) Middle temporal artery mostly arises from the trunk of the superficial temporal artery. A small number of them may come from the maxillary artery or share a common trunk with the superior auricular artery. In the great majority of cases the origin of this artery is on the same level as, or slightly below, the zygomatic arch, but in individual cases it is above the zygomatic arch. The artery perforates the temporal fascia to enter the muscle, lying in the groove of the middle temporal artery against the squama of the temporal bone, where it gives off branches to the temporal muscle and anastomoses with the deep temporal branches of the maxillary artery.

(5) Anterior and superior auricular arteries are relatively numerous. They may arise from the trunk of the superficial temporal artery, the middle temporal artery, the transverse facial artery or the zygomatico-orbital artery. Most of them enter the auricle from the middle and upper parts of its anterior border to be distributed to the auricle and the external auditory meatus and anastomose

with the posterior auricular artery. Occasionally a relatively large superior auricular artery may be seen, with a diameter of about 0.8 mm. Since the anterior and superior auricular arteries are of great significance in the one-stage reconstruction of the auricle in total by means of the posterior auricular flap, they should be preserved as far as possible when the superficial temporal vascular pedicle is to be taken for repairing a defect of the external auricle.

(6) Frontal branch, one of the terminals of the superficial temporal artery, is always present. Its diameter is much greater than that of the parietal branch and averages 1.8 mm (0.9–2.7 mm). The direction of its course is obviously related to the level of bifurcation of the superficial temporal artery. When the bifurcation point is high the frontal branch remains horizontal; when the bifurcation is lowered the frontal branches tend to proceed perpendicularly, but most of them are below the margin of the hair on the forehead. The point of bifurcation of the superficial temporal artery above and below the supraorbital margin accounts for two-thirds and one-third of the cases respectively. The frontal branch gives off four to seven frontoparietal branches superioposteriorly to supply the frontal muscle and galea aponeurotica with the overlying skin. Of these there is usually one or more branches, whose outer diameters exceed 1 mm, which is of practical value in orthopaedic surgery and microsurgery. The frontal branch also gives rise to three to five fronto-orbital branches anterio-inferiorly, which are rather small. The frontal branch anastomoses freely with the supratrochlear, lacrimal and ophthalmic arteries and its fellow of the opposite side superficial temporal artery. Therefore the area of frontal skin flap which can be excised, involves the whole forehead. Though the forehead skin is rarely used as free flap, its application as island flap is very common.

(7) Parietal branch is also one of the terminal branches of the superficial temporal artery. It ascends backwards across the temporal fascia almost vertically and gives off many twigs all the way. The patterns of the parietal branch may be classified into the main stem type (55%), the bifurcation type (40%) and the radiant type (5%). In about one-third of the cases the parietal branch presents some special types, which include a small parietal branch with the frontal branch giving off an accessory parietal branch; a parietal branch replaced by the frontal or the postauricular arteries; and the anterior or downward shift of its origin. It is therefore necessary to look out for these possibilities. The outer diameter of the parietal branch averages 1.5 mm. There is a profuse anastomosis between the parietal branch and the ipsilateral frontal branch, the occipital and postauricular arteries and its fellow of the opposite side. It follows that a large temporal fascia flap can be obtained. Since there is frequently a large branch given off by the parietal 5 cm above the ear, which runs horizontally backward and lateralward to anastomose with the occipital artery, the temporoparietal flap can be extended toward the temporo-occipital region to make a longer flap.

Superficial temporal vein

The superficial temporal vein, formed by the anterior and posterior tributaries, is situated in the subcutaneous tissue. It ends into the posterior facial vein. The anterior tributary is joined by the supratrochlear and supraorbital veins, the posterior one by the the occipital and postauricular veins and its fellow of the opposite side.

(1) The stem of the superficial temporal vein averages 2.4 mm in diameter at the level of the zygomatic arch, being a little thicker than the corresponding artery. In about one-fifth of the cases it lies anterior to the superficial temporal artery. In the other one-fifth it lies posterior to it. Three-fifths of them intersect the artery, the vein lying mostly behind the artery in the upper portion and in front of it in its lower portion.

(2) The level of confluence of the anterior and posterior tributaries of the superficial temporal vein is higher than that of bifurcation of the corresponding artery in about three-fifths of the cases and lower in the other two-fifths. About four-fifths of the site of confluence lies behind the point of arterial bifurcation and in about one-fifth of the cases it remains anterior.

(3) The anterior tributary of the superficial temporal vein is inconstant. Its absence accounts for one-third of the cases. In about half of the cases it is parallel to the frontal branch of the temporal artery. In taking a forehead flap the middle temporal vein beneath the temporal fascia can be used for anastomosis in the absence of the anterior tributary of the vein.

(4) The posterior tributary of the superficial temporal vein is relatively constant and parallel to the parietal branch of the superficial temporal artery. None of them is absent. Most of them (about three-quarters) are situated 1 cm posterior to the parietal branch of the superficial temporal artery and in about one-quarter of the cases they remain 1 cm anterior to the artery.

Nerve

The frontal skin is innervated by the frontal nerve or the frontal branch of the supraorbital nerve. The temporoparietal skin is supplied by the superficial temporal branch of the auriculotemporal nerve, which accompanies the superficial temporal artery and its parietal branch. When a relatively large temporal fascia flap for free transplantation is needed, the auriculotemporal nerve may be selected for anastomosis.

THE PECTORODELTOID FLAP

ZHONG SHIZHEN AND XU DACHUAN

The skin flap of the pectorodeltoid region is soft and thin. Its colour matches that of the maxillofacial skin. Owing to its good quality the flap is suitable for repairing defects of the head and face. Since the cutaneous artery supplying the pectorodeltoid flap arises from the thoracoacromial artery and passes through the pectorodeltoid space to reach the skin, it belongs to the intermuscular space arterial flap.

Blood supply of pectorodeltoid flap

Thoracoacromial artery and its cutaneous branches

The blood supply of the pectorodeltoid flap arises from the relevant cutaneous branch of the thoracoacromial artery. The thoracoacromial artery, being a short trunk with an outer diameter averaging 3.3 mm and a length of 8.5 mm, originates from the second or the first part of the axillary artery. It pierces the clavipectoral fascia and divides, all the way, into the pectoral, clavicular, acromial and deltoid branches. Among these the pectoral branches are more numerous, averaging 3.4 branches, with relatively large calibre. The clavicular branch is small, and the acromial branch shares a common stem with the deltoid branch. The stem corresponds to the two terminals of the thoracoacromial artery (Figure 3.9). The cutaneous artery supplying the pectorodeltoid flap

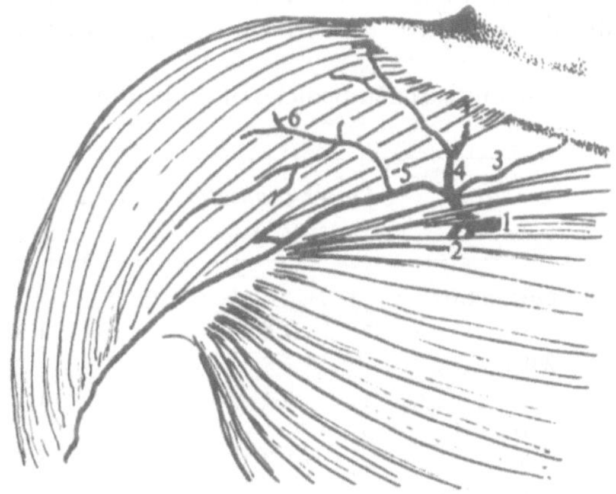

Figure 3.9 Arteries related to the pectorodeltoid flap. **1**: Thoracoacromial a.; **2**: pectoral branch; **3**: clavicular branch; **4**: acromial branch; **5**: deltoid branch; **6**: intermuscular space cutaneous a.

usually comes from the two terminals of the thoracoacromial artery. The larger cutaneous artery, which emerges from the pectorodeltoid space, may arise from the deltoid (23.7%), acromial (47.5%), clavicular (5%) and pectoral (3.8%) branches, and the acromiodeltoid trunk (20%). The diameter of the cutaneous artery averages 0.8 mm and its length within the intermuscular space is 8.0 mm.

Cephalic and thoracoacromial veins

Within the pectorodeltoid flap are the cephalic and thoracoacromial veins. The latter is not entirely accompanied by arteries. The tributaries from the deep portion of the pectoral muscle always end in the axillary vein and those from the acromion and deltoideus muscle end in the cephalic vein. The outer diameter of the cephalic vein is large, averaging 5.8 mm. In 3.8% of the specimens the cephalic vein is absent. The accompanying vein of the acromial branch and that of the deltoid branch are mostly single. Their outer diameters are large, averaging 1.8 mm and 1.9 mm respectively.

Applied anatomy of the pectorodeltoid flap

The cutaneous artery of the thoracoacromial trunk emerging from the pectorodeltoid space serves as the long axis of the pectorodeltoid flap and supplies the skin covering the lateral part of pectoralis muscle, the anterosuperior part of the deltoideus and the acromion. Its area is about 12 × 14 cm. The cutaneous branch of the thoracoacromial artery anastomoses with the branches of neighbouring suprascapular and posterior humeral circumflex arteries and the fine cutaneous arteries at the base of the neck to form a dense vascular network, thus enlarging the area of blood supply. As the outer diameter of the intermuscular space cutaneous branch of the thoracoacromial artery is rather small (0.8 mm) and the vascular pedicle is short (8.0 mm), which is inconvenient for surgical manipulation, Table 3.1 should be conferred with on the data for necessary adjustment.

Table 3.1 Data of cutaneous vascular pedicles of the pectorodeltoid region taken at different levels (mm)

Vessels taken	*Outer diameter of A*	*Outer diameter of V*	*Length of pedicle*
Intermuscular space cutaneous vessel	0.8	1.1	8.0
Cutaneous vessel with the acromial branch	1.1	1.6	18.3
Cutaneous vessel with the deltoid branch	1.2	1.6	25.4
Cutaneous vessel with the acromiodeltoid trunk	1.8	2.3	28.5
Cutaneous vessel with the last pectoral branch	2.1	2.8	35.4
Cutaneous vessel with the main trunk of thoracoacromial artery	3.4	3.8	42.1

It may be seen from this table that, in general, the nearer the site of taking to the proximal end of the arterial trunk, the longer the vascular pedicle and the greater the outer diameter of the vessels. As a matter of practice it is easy to separate the pectorodeltoid space in search for the acromiodeltoid trunk, the length and outer diameter of which are fairly ideal. If the arterial trunk proximal to the pectoral branch is dissected the clavipectoral fascia will have to be incised and this necessarily adds to the difficulty of surgical manoeuvre. It is therefore desirable to take the vascular pedicle at the site of the acromiodeltoid trunk. Measurements on the cadaver show that the point of bifurcation into the acromial and deltoid branches in 23.6 mm below the clavicle.

Within the flap there is a large cephalic vein, and in these specimens without a cephalic vein, a thick thoracoacromial vein can be found instead. As a result, the vein in the flap is much larger than that of the recipient area. In case of great disparity between the outer diameter of the vein in the donor area and that of the vein of the recipient area, an end-to-side venous anastomosis may be considered.

THE LATERAL THORACIC FLAP

JIANG SHUXUE AND LI JI

The skin of the lateral thoracic flap is characterized by its fine striations, thinness, having less subcutaneous tissue and its hairlessness. The flap is easy to take and is provided with a long vascular pedicle. The apposition of the anterior and posterior edges of the skin graft after taking the flap in the donor area can be done directly by suturing without skin grafting. The donor area is concealed, so that the operation is easily accepted by some patients. The blood supply of the lateral thoracic flap comes from various sources. The cutaneous arteries of the flap may arise from the brachial, lateral thoracic, axillary, dorsal thoracic, subscapular, and thoracoacromial arteries.

Arteries of the lateral flap

The lateral thoracic cutaneous arteries may be divided according to their diameters into two kinds; *viz.*, large and small arteries. The diameter of the former is 0.5 mm and that of the latter less than 0.5 mm.

Large cutaneous arteries

The large cutaneous arteries proceed in the subcutaneous tissue for a distance, averaging 120 mm. Their calibres are large, averaging 1.5 mm. They send out 8–18 branches all the way to supply the skin and subcutaneous tissue. According to the number of their branches, the cutaneous arteries can be divided into four types, listed in Table 3.2. For convenience, the cutaneous arteries from different sources are named, and their surface projections indicated as follows.

Humerothoracic cutaneous arteries

These arise from the superior end of the brachial or superficial brachial artery and pass through the tip of axilla to reach the flap. The incidence is 37%, and their calibre averages 1.6 mm. In most cases the artery runs along the inferior border of the pectoralis major forward to reach the mammillary line in the 5th–6th intercostal spaces. Sometimes it runs along the anterior or middle axillary line to the 5th and 6th intercostal spaces.

Lateral thoracic cutaneous arteries

These arise from the lateral thoracic artery. The incidence is 22%, and their calibre is 1.5 mm. They run along the middle or anterior axillary line to the 5th and 6th intercostal spaces.

Axillothoracic cutaneous arteries

These arise from the axillary artery and become superficial to the flap. The incidence is 15%, and their calibre is 1.4 mm. They run along the middle

Table 3.2 Type of cutaneous arteries of the lateral thoracic flap

Type	*Origin*	*Percentage (%)*
One-branched (52%)	Brachial or superficial brachial arteries	25
	Axillary arteries	12
	Lateral thoracic arteries	9
	Dorsal thoracic arteries	3
	Thoracoacromial arteries	3
Two-branched (27%)	Lateral thoracic arteries	9
	Brachial and lateral thoracic arteries	6
	Brachial and subscapular arteries	3
	Axillary arteries	3
	Dorsal thoracic and brachial arteries	3
	Dorsal thoracic and subscapular arteries	3
Three-branched (15%)	Two branches from brachial arteries, one from lateral thoracic arteries	6
	Brachial, axillary and dorsal thoracic arteries	6
	Brachial, subscapular and dorsal thoracic arteries	3
Four-branched (6%)	Superficial brachial, lateral thoracic, thoracoacromial and dorsal thoracic arteries	3
	Brachial, lateral thoracic, subscapular and dorsal thoracic arteries	3

axillary line to the 5th–6th intercostal spaces in most cases and a few run along the inferior border of the pectoralis major to the 5th and 6th intercostal spaces.

Dorsal thoracic cutaneous arteries

These arise from the thoracodorsal artery. The incidence is 15%, and their calibre is 1.2 mm. They run along the middle or posterior axillary line to the 5th and 6th intercostal spaces.

Subscapular cutaneous arteries

These arise from the subscapular artery. The incidence is 7%, and their calibre is 1.5 mm. They run along the middle axillary line to the 5th and 6th intercostal spaces.

Thoracoacromial cutaneous arteries

These arise from the thoracoacromial artery. The incidence is 3.7%, and their calibre is 1.8 mm. They run along the 5th and 6th intercostal spaces.

Small cutaneous arteries

Besides the large arteries mentioned above, the lateral thoracic flap is supplied by some small ones. These have short course and supply only a small area. They arise from the 3rd–9th intercostal arteries and the lateral thoracic and thoraco-dorsal arteries. They anastomose with the branches of the large cutaneous arteries.

The microvascular network of the lateral thoracic flap

Fresh specimens are injected with latex mixed with red lead into arteries for arteriography. The arteriograms show that each cutaneous artery sends out many branches anastomosing with one another to form a microvascular network over the whole flap (Figure 3.10). When the lateral thoracic flap is to be transplanted a larger cutaneous artery with greater outer diameter is used as the artery of the vascular pedicle, while those with smaller outer diameter may be ligated. Owing to the presence of a profuse microvascular network, there will be good circulation in the whole flap provided one artery and another vein both with larger calibres are well anastomosed with the corresponding vessels in the recipient area.

The appropriate site for the taking of lateral thoracic flap is a matter of great concern of the clinician but there is a difference in opinion. Taylor held that the lateral thoracic flap is a long narrow area with the anterior border of the latissimus dorsi as its longitudinal axis. Harii maintained that the flap is a quadrangular area, the anterior and posterior boundaries of which are the opposite borders of the pectoralis major and the latissimus dorsi, the upper and lower borders of which are the axillary artery and the eighth rib respectively. It has been proved that the size of the flap to be taken is based not only on the extent of distribution of the large cutaneous arteries but also on that of the small ones and the cutaneous microvascular network, so that the flap might be lengthened and widened considerably, viz., its anterior, posterior, upper, and lower limits may be extended to the midclavicular line, the region between the posterior axillary and scapular lines, the border of the hairy part of the axillary skin, and the tenth rib respectively. Within the boundaries mentioned above, a longitudinal oblique, or transverse flap may be designed at will (Figure 3.11, A, C).

Veins of the lateral thoracic flap

All of the large cutaneous arteries have accompanying veins, the outer diameter of which is larger than that of the artery. In addition, there are thoracoepigastric and costoaxillary veins and mammary venous plexus.

The thoracoepigastric vein is the main cutaneous vein of the lateral thoracic flap, which drains most of the venous blood courses upward along the middle axillary line in the superficial fascia. In most cases it ends in the lateral thoracic vein; a few directly join the axillary vein. In rare cases it may join the basilic vein. The outer diameter at its termination averages 3.4 mm. Owing to its large calibre and slight variation, the vein can be used for anastomosis. Since it possesses valves concave upward, attention should be paid during operation to the direction of the valves to ensure free return of blood.

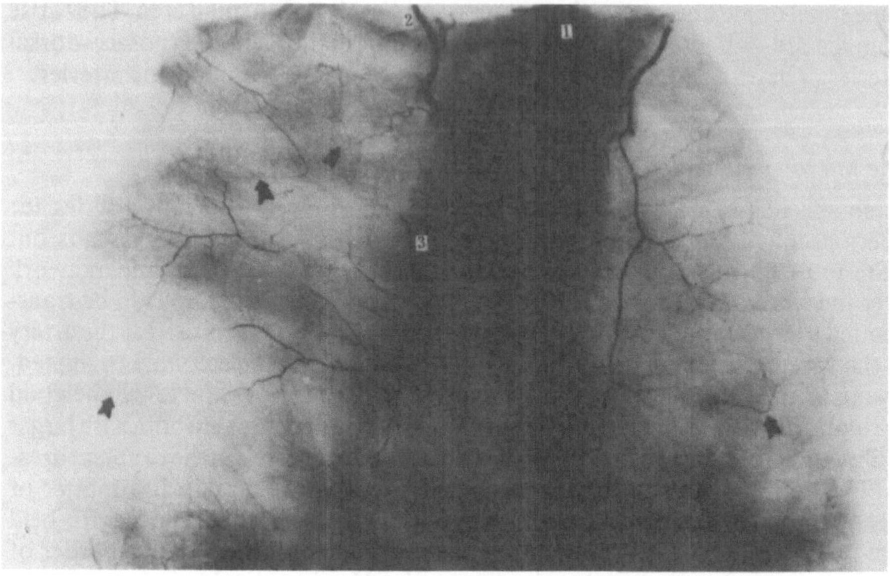

Figure 3.10A Arteriogram of the lateral thoracic flap (three-branched type). **1**: Humerothoracic cutaneous artery; **2**: axillothoracic cutaneous artery; **3**: dorsal thoracic cutaneous artery. The arrow indicates anatomoses between cutaneous arteries

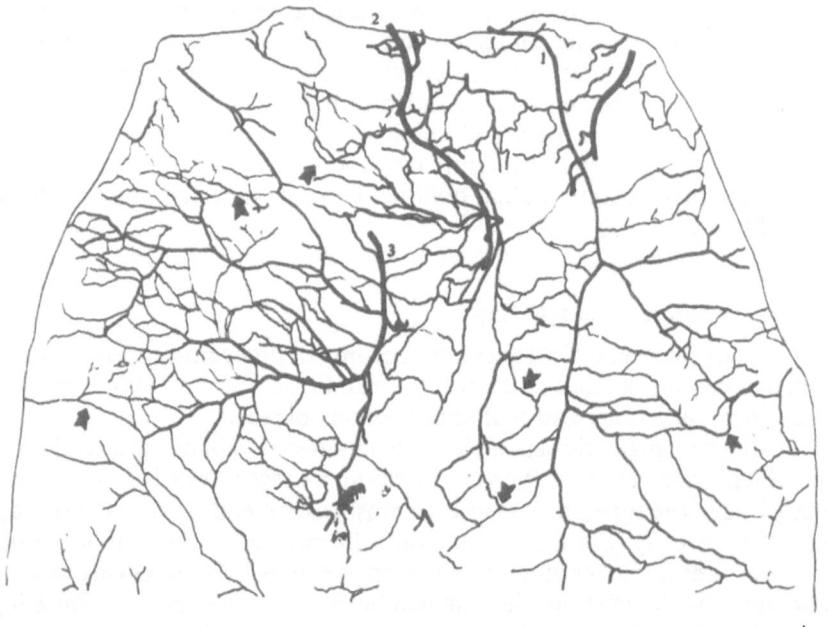

Figure 3.10B Key to the arteriogram of the lateral thoracic flap (three-branched type)

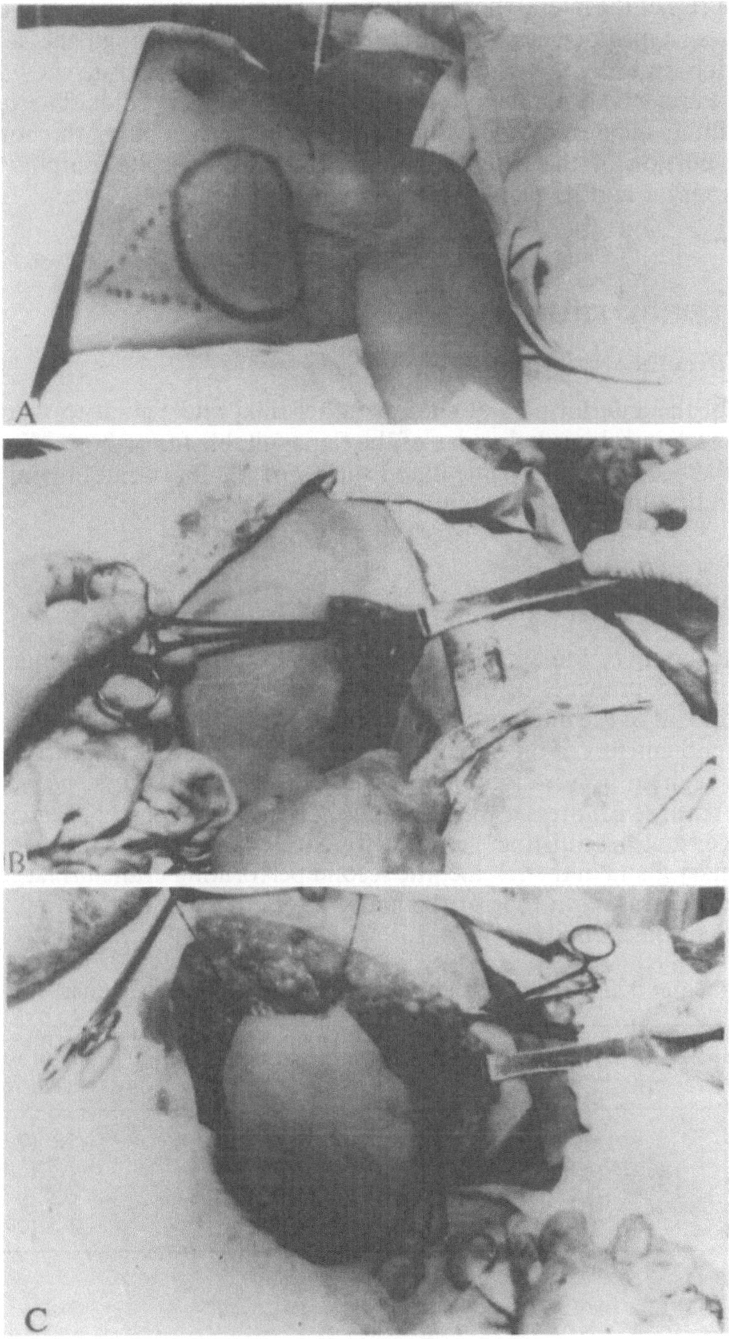

Figure 3.11 Operative photographs of the transplantation of the lateral thoracic flap. **A**: The extent of the flap; **B**: making a transverse incision in search of the vascular pedicle; **C**: skin flap detached with its vascular pedicle being connected

The vessels of the lateral thoracic flap vary greatly in their origin and course. However, all types of cutaneous arteries have to pass through the so-called vascular door in order to get to the flap. The door corresponds to the line connecting the upper ends of the posterior and anterior axillary folds. The vascular pedicle will be uncovered by making a transverse incision along the border of the hairy portion of the axillary skin between the opposite margins of the pectoralis major and latissimus dorsi (Figure 3.11 B,C).

THE ANTERIOR THORACIC FLAP

ZHONG SHIZHEN AND LIU MUZHI

The skin of the anterior part of chest is rather thin, and similar to that of the head and neck in colour, being one of the flaps suitable for orthopaedic operations on the head and neck. The blood supply of the flap comes mainly from the perforating branches of the internal thoracic artery.

Blood supply of anterior thoracic flap

The blood supply of the anterior thoracic flap exhibits distinct segmentation. The perforating branches of the internal thoracic artery, after emerging from the anterior end of the intercostal space, run downward and laterally. The data of the outer diameters of the upper four perforating branches measured at their course through the pectoralis major are shown in Table 3.3. It may be seen from this table that the calibres of the first and the second perforating branches are much larger and bear distinct sexual differences. Owing to its distribution to the mammary gland in the female, the second perforating branch is larger than the first in contrast with that of the male, where the first perforating branch is larger than the second.

Table 3.3 Outer diameter of the first to fourth perforating vessels (mm)

Ordinal number of perforating vessels	*Mean value for artery (range)*	*Mean value for vein (range)*
1	1.2 (0.4–1.7)	1.5 (0.6–2.8)
2	1.2 (0.4–1.8)	1.5 (0.6–2.9)
3	0.8 (0.3–1.5)	0.9 (0.3–1.6)
4	0.8 (0.4–1.5)	1.1 (0.4–2.5)

Applied anatomy of the anterior thoracic flap

After originating from the internal thoracic artery and during its passage through the anterior end of the intercostal space, the outer diameter of the perforating branch becomes much larger. Thereafter it gets narrower again, being usually less than 1 mm in diameter after piercing through the deep fascia. It follows that the pectoralis major should be separated in order to take the thick portion of the perforating vessel from the deep surface of the pectoralis major, and at the same time it is necessary to preserve the deep fascia with the flap.

The anterior thoracic flap may be taken medially as far as 1 cm lateral to the margin of the sternum and laterally to the deltopectoral groove and anterior axillary fold. A large perforating vessel may be distributed, all the way, over two (78%) or even three (60%) intercostal spaces. Table 3.3 also shows a great disparity between the minimal and maximal values of the outer diameters of the perforating vessels. It is, however, possible to encounter a perforating branch with small outer diameter and limited distribution, which adds difficulties to anastomosis. Therefore, in designing an operation, a flap involving several perforating vessels can be taken into consideration. It is possible to excise the corresponding costal cartilages and take the perforating vessels together with internal thoracic vessels. The outer diameter of the internal thoracic artery at the level of the second and third intercostal spaces averages 2.7 mm, the internal thoracic veins being one or two in number and the outer diameter, 2.3-3.1 mm.

THE INFRASPINATOUS FLAP

ZHONG SHIZHEN AND XU DACHUAN

The infraspinatous flap refers to the skin which covers the area corresponding to the infraspinatous fossa and the closely related regions. The flap lies concealed, yet it is not suitable for repairing facial defects because it is thick and not tender enough. Nevertheless, it is quite suitable for mending the parts of the foot which are subject to considerable pressure and friction. The flap takes as its axis the cutaneous branch of the circumflex scapular artery, which passes through the triangular space and belongs to the flaps with intermuscular space vascular supply.

Blood supply of the infraspinatous flap

The blood supply of this flap comes from the cutaneous branches of the circumflex scapular artery, which arises mostly from the subscapular artery (80%) and a few (5%) directly from the brachial artery. There are also 15% of the circumflex scapular arteries springing from a stem common to the posterior and anterior humeral circumflex, lateral thoracic or deep brachial artery.

The circumflex scapular artery passes through the triangular space (triangular foramen) near the lateral margin of the scapular. The triangular space is bounded by teres minor above, teres major below and long head of triceps brachii laterally. In the space the circumflex scapular artery is divided into two terminals: an infraspinatous fossa branch ascending underneath the deep surface of the teres minor and infraspinatous into the infraspinatous fossa to anastomose with the suprascapular artery and the deep branch of the transverse cervical artery, and an inferior angle branch descending along the lateral margin

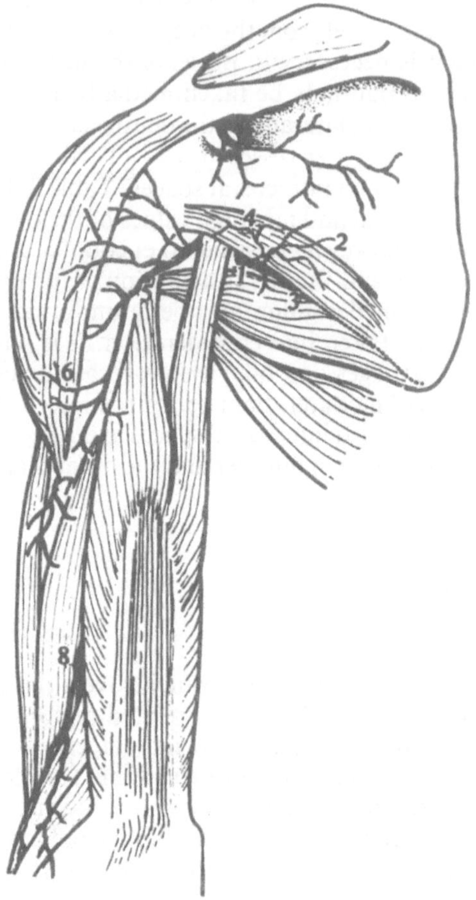

Figure 3.12 Arteries of the infraspinatous and lateral brachial flaps. **1**: Circumflex scapular artery; **2**: infraspinatous fossa; **3**: inferior angle branch; **4**: cutaneous branch in triangular space; **5**: posterior humeral circumflex artery; **6**: cutaneous branches from posterior humeral circumflex artery in intermuscular space; **7**: lateral humeral cutaneous artery; **8**: posterior branch of radial collateral artery

of scapula between the teres major and minor to get to the inferior angle of scapula, where it anastomoses with the deep branch of the transverse cervical artery (Figure 3.12).

The cutaneous branches of the circumflex scapular artery, one or two in number, have large outer diameter, averaging 1.2 mm. They may arise from the arterial trunk of the circumflex scapular (47%), inferior angle branch (47%) or infraspinatous fossa branch (6%). In the triangular space the cutaneous branch measures 23 mm in length. The two accompanying veins have outer diameters averaging 1.7 mm.

Applied anatomy of the infraspinatous flap

The infraspinatous flap takes as its axis the cutaneous branch of the circumflex scapular artery and covers the area over the infraspinatous fossa and neighbouring regions, so that its size reaches 12 cm × 18 cm. Owing to the fact that the subcutaneous vascular anastomoses with the vascular network around the scapula are fairly profuse, the size of the flap may be considerably enlarged. If the donor area is about 10 cm in breadth the cut edges of the skin in the excised part may be pulled together by suturing. If the excised area is much wider it can still be covered by means of infra-axillary flap transference or free skin grafting.

The triangular space is a guide for identifying the vascular pedicle of the flap. The surface projection of the space is 17 cm below the mid-point of the spine of scapula. It is easy to separate. The vascular pedicle of the flap can be traced back to the inferior angle branch, infraspinatous fossa branch or the trunk of the circumflex scapular vessels in order to get a longer and larger vascular pedicle necessary for the operation. Data in Table 3.4 may be referred to in designing and taking the vascular pedicle.

Table 3.4 Data of vascular pedicle of infraspinatous flaps taken at different levels (mm)

Vessels	*Outer diameter of artery*	*Outer diameter of vein*	*Length of pedicle*
Cutaneous branch of circumflex scapular artery	1.2	1.7	18
Cutaneous branch with inferior angle branch	1.8	2.2	24
Cutaneous branch with infraspinatous fossa branch	2.1	2.3	30
Cutaneous branch with the trunk of circumflex scapular artery	3.2	3.7	36

THE LATERAL BRACHIAL FLAP

LI JI AND JIANG SHUXUE

The lateral brachial flap is of better quality and belongs to the type with intermuscular space or intermuscular septal vascular supply. It has a long vascular pedicle, which is easy to dissect. Though the skin in its upper part is thicker, it remains a fairly good donor for free flap transplantation. According to the anatomy of the vascular pedicle, the lateral brachial flap can be divided into the following parts: the upper, middle, and lower lateral brachial flaps.

Upper lateral brachial flap

The artery of the vascular pedicle is the cutaneous branch of the posterior circumflex humeral artery, belonging to the intermuscular space arteries. It passes through the quadrangular space, emerging from the posterior border of the deltoid muscle, and is distributed to the skin of the deltoid region (Figure 3.12, 5,6). The outer diameter of the cutaneous artery measured at the site where it pierces into the deep fascia is 0.8–1.0 mm. If a larger portion of the vessel is needed for anastomosis, it can be traced back to the stem common to it and the posterior circumflex humeral artery, where the outer diameter may be 1.5–2.5 mm. The upper lateral brachial cutaneous nerve accompanying the cutaneous artery in the skin flap may be utilized. The companion vein is somewhat thicker than the artery.

Middle lateral brachial flap

The artery of the vascular pedicle is the lateral brachial cutaneous artery, belonging to the intermuscular space arteries. The incidence is 88%. It arises from the brachial artery about 22 mm below the anterior axillary fold and

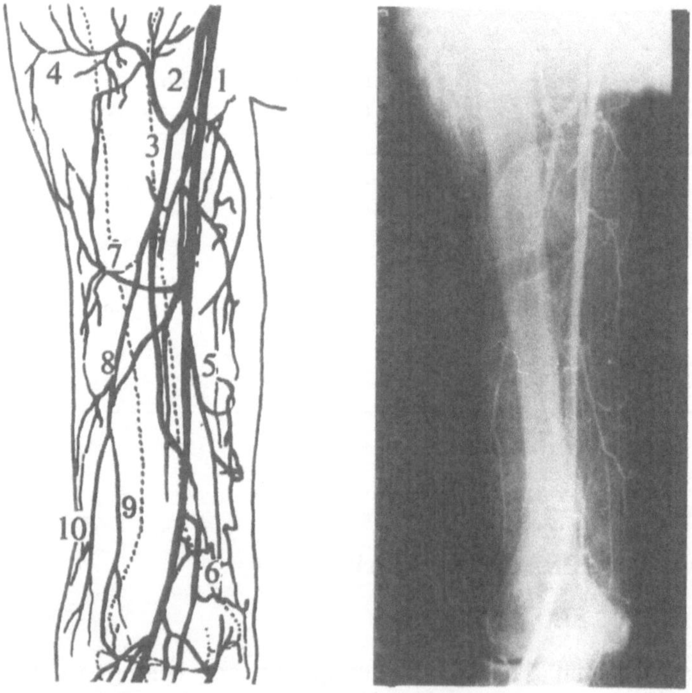

Figure 3.13 Arteriogram of the arm. **1**: Brachial artery; **2**: posterior circumflex humeral artery; **3**: arteria profunda brachii; **4**: cutaneous branch of posterior circumflex humeral artery; **5**: superior ulnar collateral artery; **6**: inferior ulnar collateral artery; **7**: lateral brachial cutaneous artery; **8**: radial collateral artery; **9**: anterior branch of radial collateral artery; **10**: posterior branch of radial collateral artery

course between the biceps brachii and the brachialis to be distributed to the region near the insertion of the deltoid. The outer diameter of the cutaneous artery measures from 0.8 to 1.2 mm where it penetrates the deep fascia, and 1.6 mm near its origin. The cephalic vein, which is large and superficial, may be used as the vein of the flap. This flap may be selected as the donor site for small skin grafting.

Lower lateral brachial flap

The artery of the vascular pedicle is the posterior branch of the radial collateral of the profunda brachii artery, belonging to the intermuscular septum arteries (Figure 3.14). The profunda brachii artery arises as a common stem (60%),

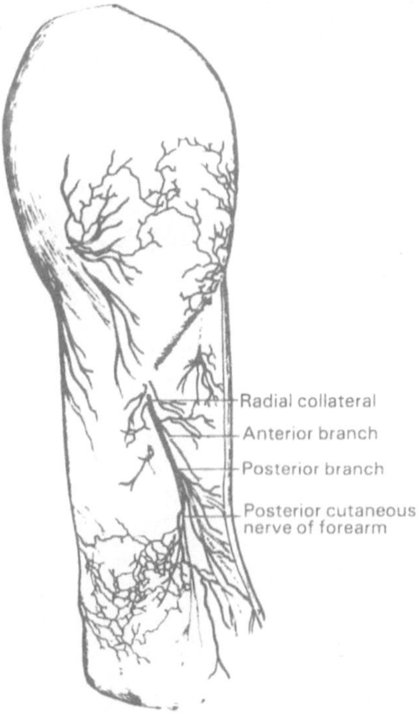

Figure 3.14 Neurovascular pedicle of the lower lateral brachial flap

or as the radial or middle collateral arteries (40%), from the brachial artery. The radial collateral artery accompanies the radial nerve in the radial sulcus of humerus and divides into anterior and posterior branches about 4 cm below the level of the insertion of the deltoid. The anterior branch penetrates the lateral intermuscular septum to reach the anterior part of the arm deeply and accompanies the radial nerve between the brachialis and brachioradialis.

Its outer diameter averages 0.8 mm, and its branches are mainly muscular and articular in nature and bear no relation to the blood supply of the flap. The posterior branch of the radial collateral artery attaches itself to the posterior aspect of the lateral intermuscular septum, descends between the brachioradial and triceps brachii, and gradually becomes superficial. Despite the large terminal branches supplying the brachioradial and extensor carpi radialis longus, most of the branches enter the subcutaneous tissue successively. The posterior branch is the main vascular pedicle of the lower lateral brachial flap, distributed to the skin of the lower and lateral parts of the arm and the upper part of the forearm. The average length, measured from the insertion of the deltoid, of the radial collateral artery together with its posterior branch in the lateral intermuscular septum is 61 mm. The outer diameter of the upper portion of the artery is 1.3 mm and that of the companion vein, one (25%) or two (75%) in number, averages 1.9 mm.

In the lower lateral brachial flap there is also the superficial and large cephalic vein, which can be used for venous anastomosis. Its outer diameter is 3.2 mm. The sensory nerve in the flap is the posterior cutaneous nerve of the forearm, which accompanies the posterior branch of the radial collateral artery or pierces the triceps brachii to get to the subcutaneous tissue. Its breadth is 2 mm.

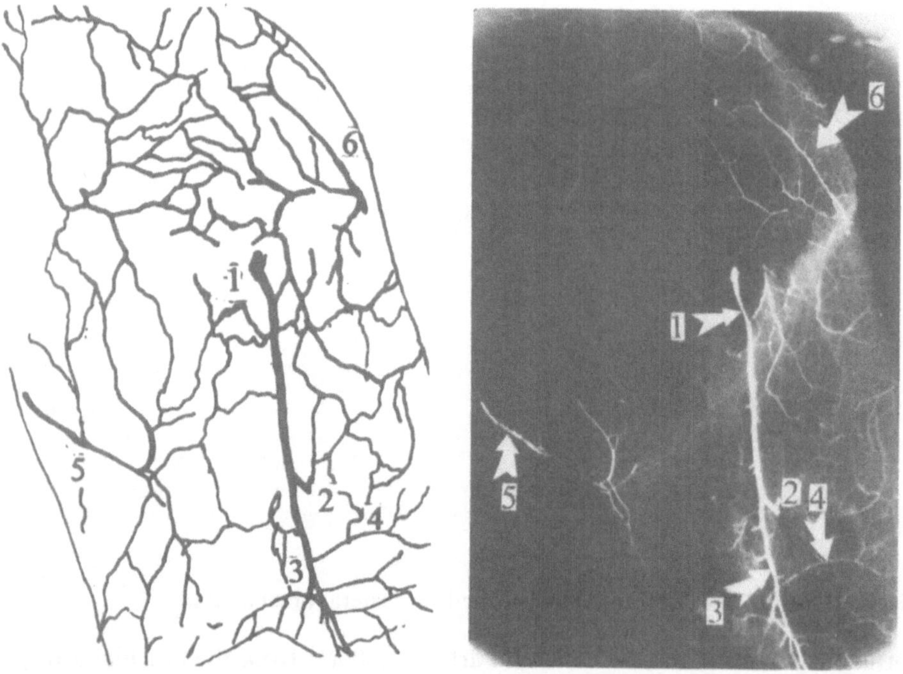

Figure 3.15 Arteriogram of the lateral brachial flap. **1**: Radial collateral artery; **2**: anterior branch of radial collateral artery; **3**: posterior branch of radial collateral artery; **4**: cutaneous branches of posterior branch of radial collateral artery; **5**: lateral brachial cutaneous artery; **6**: cutaneous branch of posterior circumflex humeral artery

Owing to the presence of profuse anastomoses among the cutaneous artery of the upper, middle and lower lateral brachial flaps mentioned above (Figure 3.15), the blood circulation of the flap can be well set up, as long as the radial collateral artery, the chief cutaneous artery, is anastomosed, and the flap can be taken further up to the middle part of the deltoid, or down to the antecubital region, and even over the anterior or posterior midline of the arm. If a large artery is needed for anastomosis the lateral head of triceps brachii may be divided in order to trace upward to approach the stem of the profunda brachii artery, the outer diameter of which averages 1.7 mm.

THE MEDIAL BRACHIAL FLAP

JIANG SHUXUE AND LI JI

The boundaries of the medial brachial flap are the brim of the hairy skin of the armpit above, the line connecting the medial and lateral epicondyles of the humerus below, and the midlines of the arm both anteriorly and posteriorly. The skin over the medial brachial region is characterized by its slender striations, thinness, elasticity, concealment and by having less subcutaneous tissue, and is an ideal donor for the repair of maxillofacial defect.

Arteries of the medial brachial flap

The cutaneous arteries of the medial brachial flap may arise from the superior ulnar collateral, the brachial, the profunda brachii, the axillary, the inferior ulnar collateral, the subscapular, or the posterior circumflex humeral artery (Figure 3.16).

The superior ulnar collateral artery is the chief vascular pedicle. It arises mostly from the brachial artery (89%), and a few from the arteria profunda brachii, the subscapular, or the circumflex scapular artery. Immediately after arising from the parent artery it keeps close to the ulnar nerve and remains medial to it. The proximal part of the artery is deeply situated. At the junction of the middle and lower one-third of the arm it pierces the medial intermuscular septum to the posterior part of the arm where it remains superficial. It gives off a lot of muscular branches all the way.

The superior ulnar collateral artery mostly (89%) sends out one to four cutaneous branches, which join the vascular network of the medial brachial flap. In a few cases (13%) it has no cutaneous branches. Under such circumstances other cutaneous arteries of the medial brachial flap become larger and serve as the arteries of the vascular pedicle. The calibre of the superior ulnar collateral artery at its commencement is large, averaging 1.7 (1.0–2.5) mm. The length of its vascular pedicle is comparatively long (80–140 mm).

According to their sources, the cutaneous arteries of the flap can be divided into four types: one-source type, in which the cutaneous arteries arise from only one artery, 10%; two-source type, 53%; three-source type, 32%; and four-source (or more) type, 5%.

By means of molybdenum target radiography it has been shown that there are rich anastomoses among the cutaneous arteries of the medial brachial flap (Figure 3.13).

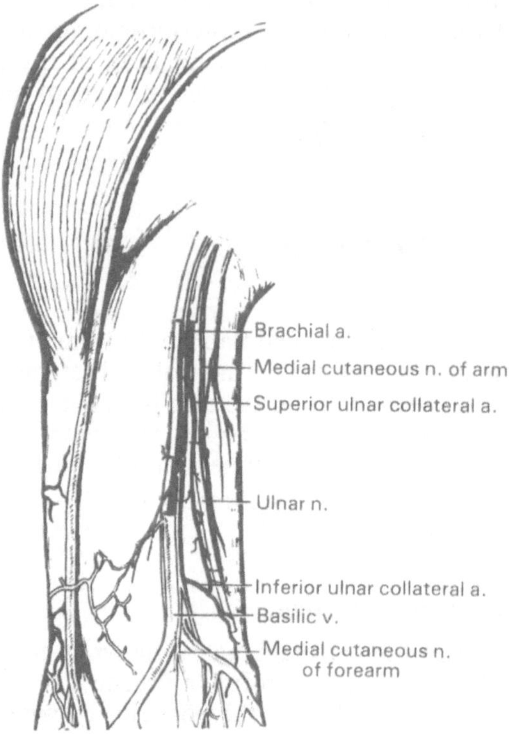

Figure 3.16 Arteries and nerves related to the medial brachial flap

Veins of the medial brachial flap

All of the cutaneous arteries possess accompanying veins, which have their corresponding endings. The chief cutaneous vein of the medial brachial flap is the basilic vein with its tributaries, which have large calibres and extensive draining areas. Most of the venous blood is drained by the basilic vein, which is, therefore, used as the vein of the vascular pedicle of the flap.

The basilic vein courses in the superficial fascia in front of the antecubital fossa. It passes through the branches of the medial antebrachial cutaneous nerve, ascending along the medial border of the biceps brachii. At the middle point of the arm, or a little below, it penetrates the deep fascia, ascends along the medial side of the brachial vein and finally joins the brachial vein about 63 mm below the upper end of the brachial artery.

The outer diameter of the basilic vein at its termination is 4.8 mm. Before ending in the brachial vein it receives one to six tributaries, which anastomose with one another to form venous arches or networks within the subcutaneous tissue. There are some communicating branches between the cephalic and basilic veins.

Nerves of the medial brachial flap

(1) The medial cutaneous nerve of the arm arises from the medial cord of the brachial plexus and passes between the axillary artery and vein to get to the medial side of the vein. It descends along the medial side of the brachial and basilic veins to the middle of the arm where it pierces the deep fascia to be distributed to the skin of the medial side of the arm. Its breadth at the level of the upper end of the brachial artery is 1.2 mm.

(2) The medial cutaneous nerve of the forearm arises from the medial cord of the brachial plexus. It passes between the axillary artery and vein to enter the arm. It then crosses in front of the brachial artery to its medial side, where it is accompanied by the basilic vein. The nerve pierces the deep fascia with the basilic vein a little below the middle of the arm and divides into two branches descending on either side of the basilic vein to be distributed to the medial aspect of the forearm. From its proximal segment the medial cutaneous nerve of the forearm sends out one to three branches, which are distributed to the skin over the lower half of the biceps brachii. Its transverse dimension at the level of the upper end of the brachial artery is 2.3 mm. The two cutaneous nerves mentioned above can be anastomosed with the nerves of the recipient area in order to make an innervated flap.

The process of taking the medial brachial flap

The flap is first cut along its posterior limit and then dissected forward together with the deep fascia to the medial intermuscular septum, which is incised to protect the underlying neurovascular bundle. A longitudinal incision is next made along the anterior border of the flap, which is dissected backward and medially to the medial intermuscular septum. Finally, the lower limit of the flap is incised and dissected proximally in search for the neurovascular bundle. It is noted that, in the course of taking the flap, over-traction of the ulnar and median nerves should be avoided, and in anastomosis of the veins the direction of the valves in the basilic vein should not be reversed, thus ensuring good circulation in the flap.

THE FOREARM FLAP

LI JI AND JIANG SHUXUE

The forearm flap has the following advantages such as better quality and larger area of the skin available, greater calibre and less variation in the vessels, and greater facility in taking, all of which are suitable for the repair of deformities after burns in the facial and cervical regions or of large areas of skin defect in other locations. It has also some disadvantages; viz., the donor site does not lie concealed and cannot be sutured directly by apposition of the cut edges, so that a full-thickness skin graft is needed, which often leaves a visible scar after operation. Nevertheless, it may still be regarded as a better donor of vascularized free flap.

The forearm flap belongs to those with truncal and reticular arterial supply. The trunk of radial artery and cephalic vein (or the radial vein) are usually taken as the vascular pedicle of the flap.

Arteries of the forearm flap

The radial artery is the main arterial trunk of the forearm flap. According to its topographical relation with the brachioradialis it is divided into covered and exposed parts. The former is situated in the upper part of the forearm and is covered by the brachioradialis, averaging 117 mm in length, while the latter is situated in the lower part of the forearm and lies superficially beneath the skin, being covered by superficial and deep fasciae only and averaging 101 mm in length. The outer diameter of the radial artery averages 2.7 mm measured at the upper portion of the forearm and 2.3 mm at the middle and lower portions. Either end of the radial artery can be anastomosed with the artery in the recipient area.

Some cutaneous and muscular branches are given off from either side of the radial artery (Figure 3.17) and are termed the radial cutaneous and muscular branches and the ulnar cutaneous and muscular branches respectively. The cutaneous branches of the exposed part of radial artery are more numerous, averaging 9.6 (4–18) in number, and those of the covered part are rather few, averaging 4.2 (0–10). The number of muscular branches of the two parts of radial artery is nearly equal. The outer diameters of the cutaneous and muscular branches are both much smaller, viz., from 0.1 to 1.1 mm, among which 0.5 mm is the most common.

There are extensive anastomoses among the cutaneous branches of the radial, ulnar, dorsal interosseous, and the lower end of the brachial arteries (Figure 3.17), which form a profuse subcutaneous network of minute arteries. The flap to be taken may extend as far as the lowest third of the forearm. The size of flap, which is 35 × 15 cm at most, far exceeds the area supplied by the cutaneous branches of the radial artery (Figure 3.18). This is due to the extensive anastomoses between the cutaneous branches of the radial and the neighbouring arteries, so that good circulation within the flap is ensured after transplantation.

There are also some cutaneous branches of smaller calibre given off from either side of the lower portion of the ulnar artery (Figure 3.17). The radial cutaneous branches of the ulnar artery average 4.8 in number, while the ulnar ones average 2.3 in number. These branches anastomose freely with those of the radial and dorsal interosseous arteries. Though they are divided in the course of transplantation, the parts left in the flap form the subcutaneous microarterial network of the forearm and serve to induce the blood from the radial cutaneous branches to the ulnar side of the flap.

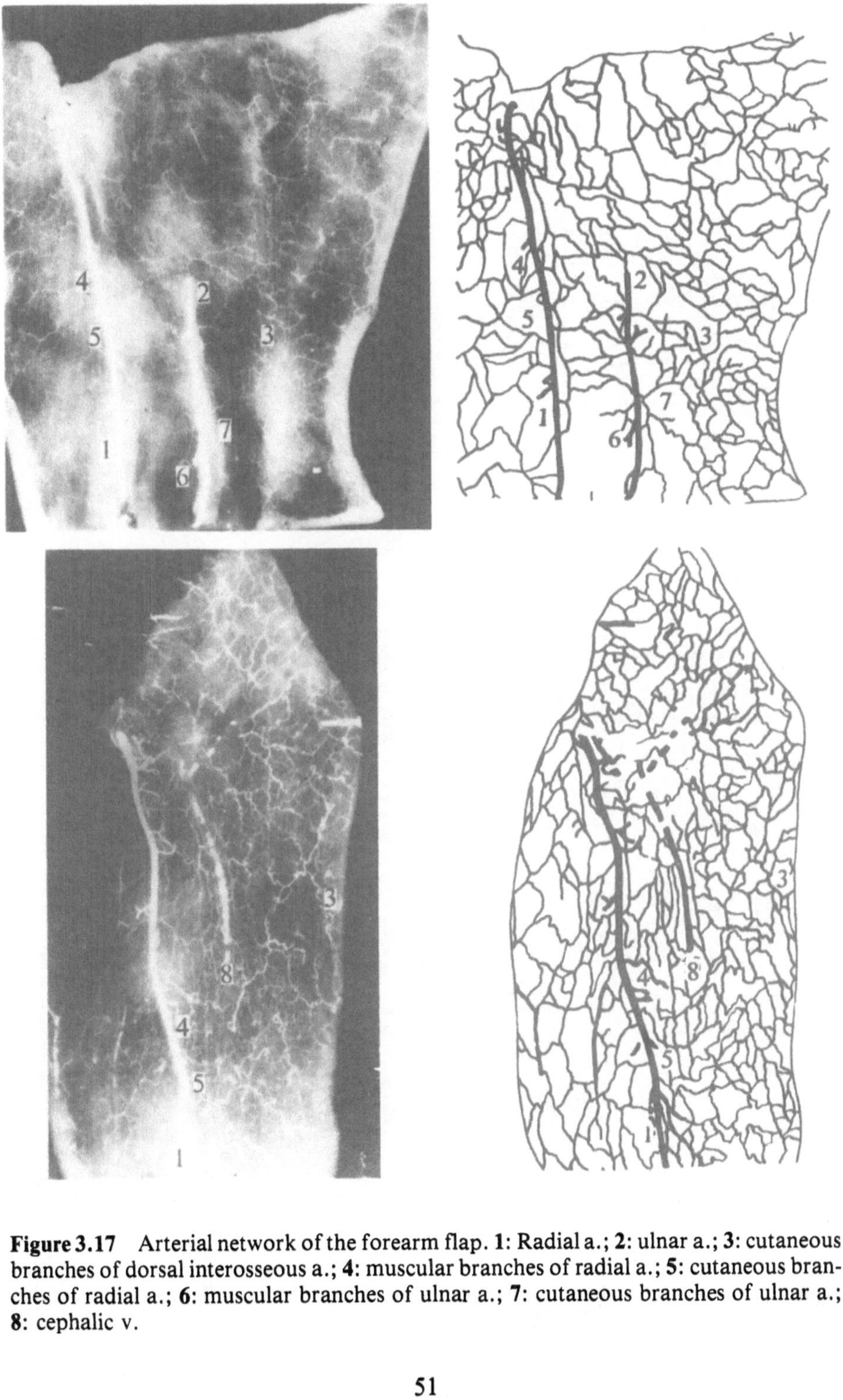

Figure 3.17 Arterial network of the forearm flap. **1**: Radial a.; **2**: ulnar a.; **3**: cutaneous branches of dorsal interosseous a.; **4**: muscular branches of radial a.; **5**: cutaneous branches of radial a.; **6**: muscular branches of ulnar a.; **7**: cutaneous branches of ulnar a.; **8**: cephalic v.

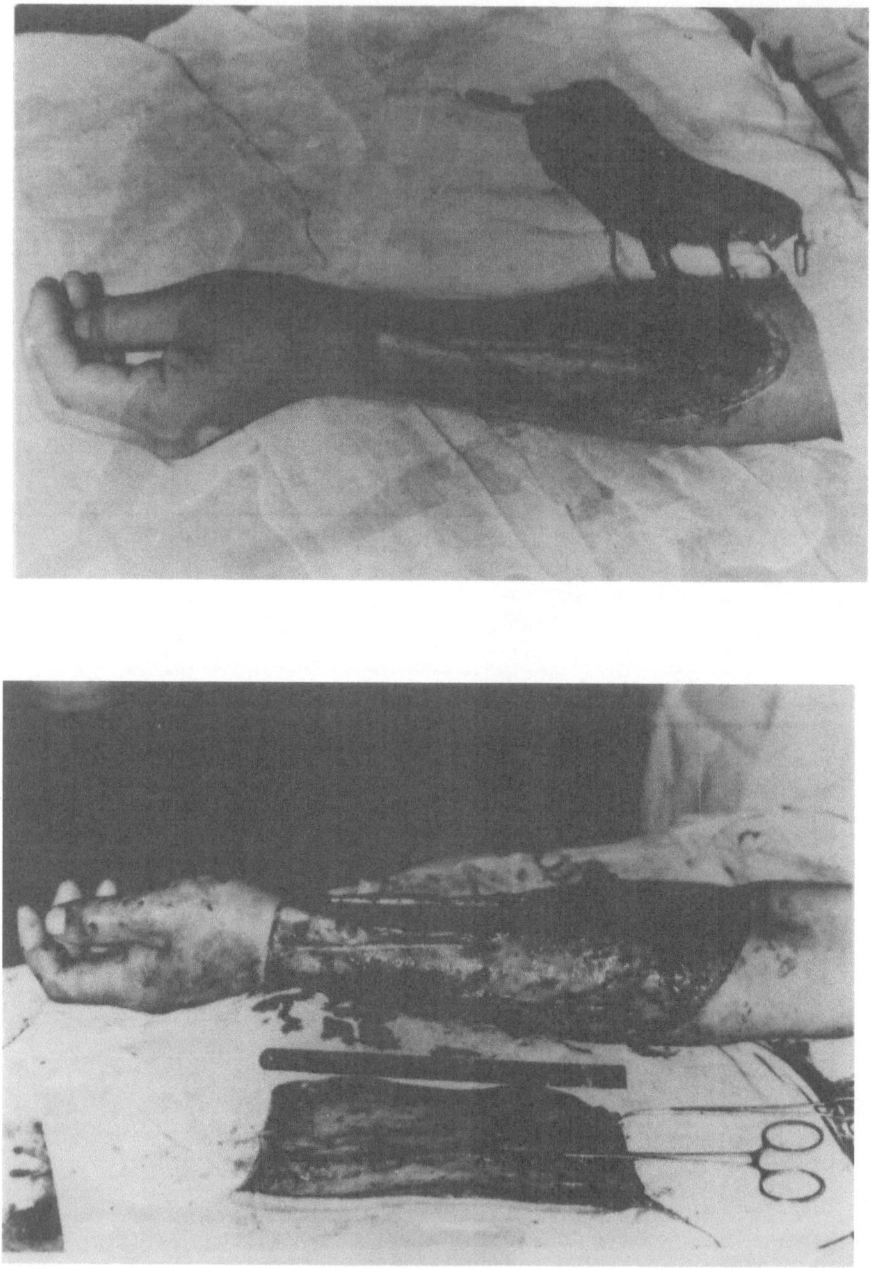

Figure 3.18 Operative photograph in course of taking of forearm flap. *Above:* vascular pedicle; *Below:* extent of the flap

Veins of the forearm flap

The cephalic vein arises from the radial side of the back of hand, ascending along the radial side of the forearm, and joins the medial cubital vein in the cubital fossa.

The mean outer diameter of the cephalic vein at the middle of the forearm is 2.8 mm. This vein is commonly used as the main channel for venous return in forearm skin grafting. In case of need, the vascular pedicle can be lengthened upward by excising the cephalic vein together with the median cubital as far as the communicating branches between the superficial and the deep veins. The communicating branch connecting the median cubital vein and the upper end of the radial vein should be preserved in order to facilitate blood return from the deep veins. The basilic vein in the forearm has to be preserved as far as possible so as to allow a full venous return from the back of the hand and the forearm.

There are two radial veins, namely the radial and the ulnar radial veins. Anastomotic branches, varying in number, exist between them. The mean outer diameter of either vein is 1.3 mm in the middle of forearm. Some of their cutaneous tributaries are in company with the corresponding branches of the radial artery. The radial veins sometimes anastomose with the tributaries of the cephalic vein in the forearm and carpal region, so that in free flap transplantation the radial veins can also be anastomosed with the veins in the recipient area to increase venous blood return.

Nerves of the forearm flap

The lateral cutaneous nerve of the forearm is one of the terminal branches of the musculocutaneous nerve. It pierces the deep fascia of the cubital fossa, lateral to the biceps tendon, and lies deep to the cephalic vein. This nerve is to be distributed to the lateral part of the forearm flap. The transverse dimension of its upper end averages 2.4 mm.

The anterior branch of the medial cutaneous nerve of the forearm accompanies the basilic vein and descends to the forearm, distributing to the medial part of the forearm flap. The transverse dimension of its upper end averages 2.1 mm.

The above-mentioned nerves are rather thick and can be used for anastomosis in the transplantation of sensory flap.

Taking the radial artery

According to the anatomical peculiarities of the radial artery and its cutaneous branches, it is enough to take the exposed part of the radial artery for a free flap grafting of small dimension. If a large flap is needed the covered part of the radial artery must also be included up to the commencement of the radial recurrent artery. In taking the vascular pedicle, the cutaneous branches arising from either side of the radial artery must not be damaged. The cutaneous branches of the covered part of the radial artery are less than those of the exposed part and lie close to the deep surface of the brachioradialis. They emerge from the ulnar border of the muscle to the subcutaneous tissue, so that dissection during operation has to be as close to the muscle fibres as possible in order to separate the epimyosium together with the subcutaneous tissue from the muscle, or to separate the subcutaneous tissue only but leave the epimyosium (deep fascia) in the donor site. The deep fascia near the radial artery should be taken off together with the arterial trunk and its cutaneous branches, otherwise the cutaneous branches will inevitably be damaged. As long as the cutaneous branches of the exposed part of the radial artery and the whole vascular network in the superficial fascia of the flap are perfectly intact, the blood supply of the flap will not be interfered with. Therefore, in taking the vascular pedicle there is no need to pay too much attention to the integrity of the cutaneous branches of the covered part of the radial artery. The length of the vascular pedicle depends mainly on the need of the free flap grafting but not on the size of the flap.

The muscular branches arising from either side of the radial artery should be cut and ligated. The blood supply of the flap will then be offered by the ulnar artery and its branches through their anastomoses with the muscular branches of the radial artery.

THE TRANSVERSE LUMBODORSAL FLAP

Wu Renxiu

The lumbodorsal region is the small part of the back between the posterior part of the iliac crest and the lower ribs. The arteries of this region retain the characteristics of segmental distribution and come from: (1) the subcostal arteries in the upper part passing through the latissimus dorsi, (2) the posterior branches of the first to fourth pairs of the lumbar arteries in the middle, and (3) the muscular and cutaneous branches of the superior gluteal artery passing through the gluteus maximus inferiorly to make a moderate supplement. They form a subdermal vascular network and anastomose freely with their fellows of the opposite side.

The lumbar arteries arise at right angles from the posterolateral wall of the abdominal aorta. They pass laterally across the anterior aspect of the first to fourth lumbar vertebrae and give off posterior branches between the transverse processes to supply muscles and skin of the region. The terminals of the lumbar arteries anastomose anteriorly with the inferior epigastric artery, superiorly with the intercostal arteries, and inferiorly with the superior gluteal, the iliolumbar and the deep circumflex iliac arteries. The third lumbar artery is rather constant in position and incidence. It runs obliquely across the lumbar triangle to the iliac crest and the gluteal region to anastomose with arteries such as the superior gluteal. The outer diameter of the lumbar artery, on emerging from the lateral margin of the erector spinalis, is 1.9 mm and that of the venae comitae is 2.3 mm. The length of the artery from the lateral margin of the erector spinalis to the iliac crest is 43 mm.

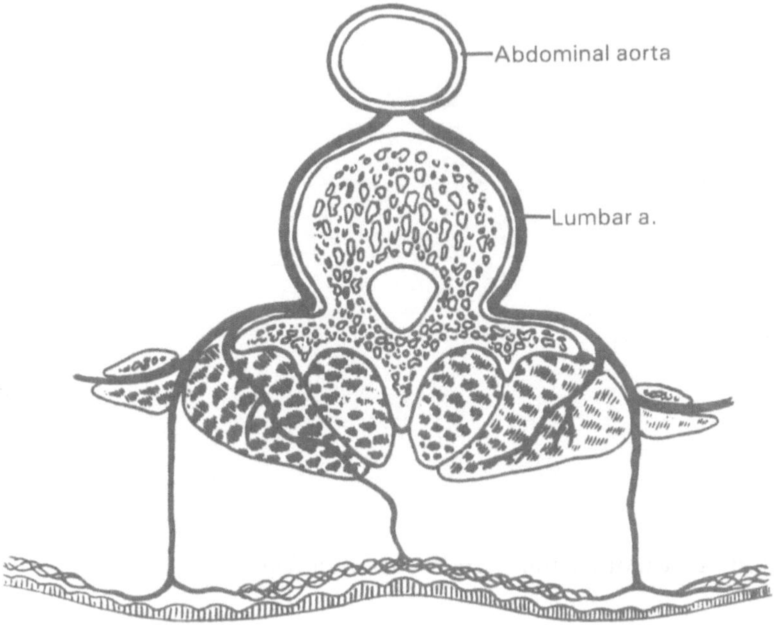

Figure 3.19 Course and distribution of the posterior branches of lumbar arteries

Hill *et al.* (1978) succeeded in treating a pressure sore in the sacral region with the transverse lumbosacral flap taken across the midline. The flap may generally be extended to the contralateral lumbar and lower intercostal arteries, and superiorly to the level of the twelfth thoracic or the first lumbar vertebra. The length-to-breadth ratio is 1.5 : 1. Its proximal one-third is the axial portion, while the distal two-thirds can be extended at will. According to the vascular distribution of the lumbodorsal region, we conclude that if a flap is desired, it is proper to take the middle one-third of the lumbodorsal skin as the axis, so that it can be shifted upward or downward with the perforating branches of the lumbar as the pedicle. If the third lumbar artery is to be used as the pedicle the flap can be taken in accordance with the course and direction of this artery.

THE SUPERIOR GLUTEAL FLAP

SUN BO AND CHENG JUNPING

The superior gluteal region lies concealed. The skin is rather thick and the superficial fascia plentiful. Therefore the superior gluteal flap is suitable for the repair of defects in those places with thick skin and for packing purposes. The flap receives its blood supply mainly from the posterior branch of the fourth lumbar artery and belongs to those with the intermuscular space vascular supply.

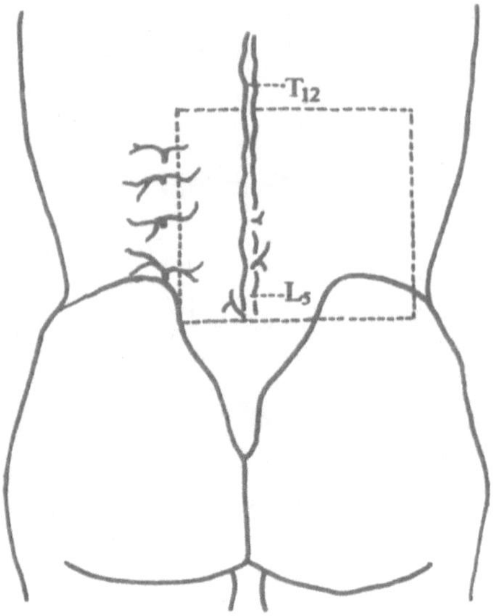

Figure 3.20 Extent of the transverse lumbodorsal flap

Blood supply of the flap

The artery supplying the flap is the posterior branch of the fourth lumbar artery. The lumbar arteries are four in number on either side. They arise from the abdominal aorta, pass across the body of the lumbar vertebrae backward and laterally to reach the posterior aspect of the psoas major and quadratus lumborum. The anterior branches of the lumbar arteries are distributed to the abdominal muscles, while the posterior branches arise in the intervals between the adjacent transverse processes, passing through the space between the sacrospinalis and quadratus lumborum and piercing the deep fascia at the lateral border of the sacrospinalis to be distributed to the skin of the lumbar and superior gluteal regions. The posterior branches of the upper three lumbar arteries pierce the deep fascia and the latissimus dorsi to be distributed to the overlying skin in belt fashion. However, they are not constant. Of these, only the posterior branch of the fourth lumbar artery, after piercing the deep fascia, is distributed directly to the skin, and its calibre and position are both fairly constant (Figure 3.21).

The posterior branch of the fourth lumbar artery runs obliquely downwards in the intermediate layer of thoracolumbar fascia between the sacrospinalis and quadratus lumborum. Its outer diameter measured at the commencement averages 1.3 mm (0.5–2.0 mm) and ranges between 0.5 mm and 1.3 mm after piercing the deep fascia. In 60% of the cases it appears as a single trunk, which measures about 25 mm (10–55 mm) in length from the tip of the transverse process to the lateral border of sacrospinalis. In the other 40% of the cases the posterior branch divides again into two or three small branches prior to its penetration through the deep fascia. The length of the posterior branch and its ramus

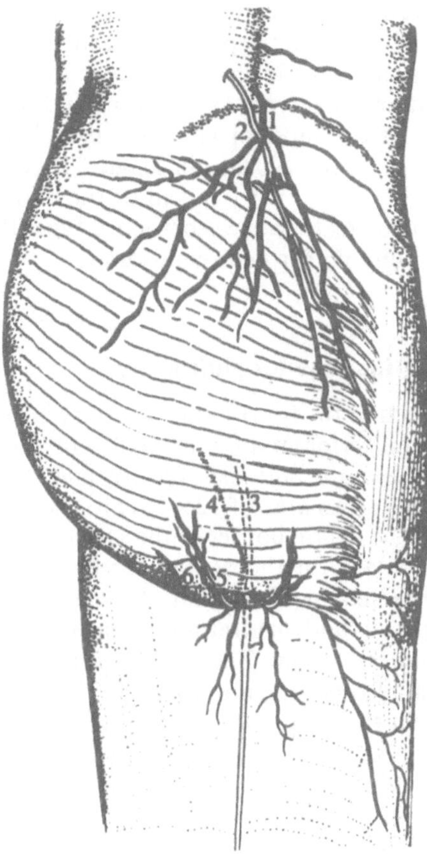

Figure 3.21 Neurovascular pedicle of the gluteal flap. **1**: Posterior branch of fourth lumbar a.;**2**: middle branch of superior gluteal cutaneous n.; **3**: posterior cutaneous n. of thigh; **4**: inferior gluteal a.; **5**: inferior gluteal cutaneous nerve; **6**: cutaneous branch of inferior gluteal a.

measured together totals about 33 mm (18–66 mm). In addition to the posterior branch of the fourth lumbar artery, the musculocutaneous branch of the superior gluteal artery also supplies the superior gluteal flap.

The posterior branch of the fourth lumbar artery emerges from the deep fascia at the angle formed by the lateral border of the sacrospinalis and the iliac crest, or a little higher, but not beyond 10 mm.

The superior gluteal flap is drained by the companion vein of the posterior branch of the fourth lumbar artery, which is always single. Its outer diameter is larger than that of the artery.

Nerve innervation of the flap

The superior gluteal flap is innervated by the superior gluteal cutaneous nerve, which usually gives off the anterior, middle and posterior branches. The points where they pierce the deep fascia are inconstant, but always remain in the neighbourhood of the point of exit of the posterior branch of the fourth lumbar artery through the deep fascia. This is especially true, for the middle branch of the superior gluteal cutaneous nerve is rather short and distributed to the anterior and posterior parts of the superior gluteal region. The middle branch, being longer than others, is about 140 mm in length. It is distributed to the intermediate part of the buttock. Fifty per cent of the middle branches have single trunk; 40% of them belong to the two-branched type. Its outer diameter ranges from 1 to 3.5 mm, suitable for neuroanastomosis.

Applied anatomy of the superior gluteal flap

If the posterior branch of the fourth lumbar artery is taken as the axis, the flap may extend to the posterior midline medially, to the posterior axillary fold laterally, to the middle of the buttock inferiorly and to 2 cm above the iliac crest superiorly, amounting to an area of 12 × 16 cm. The landmark for the vascular pedicle of the flap is the lateral border of the sacrospinalis, along which a longitudinal incision is made in the thoracolumbar fascia above the iliac crest. The sacrospinalis is retracted medially and the vascular pedicle can be found between the sacrospinalis and quadratus lumborum, i.e. within the intermediate layer of thoracolumbar fascia. The middle branch of the superior gluteal cutaneous nerve can also be found in the superficial fascia where the vascular pedicle emerges from the deep.

THE SCROTAL FLAP

ZHONG SHIZHEN AND TAO YONGSONG

The skin of the scrotum lying concealed is thin, tender and quite elastic. Although there are some pigmentation and thinly scattered crisp hairs, it can still serve as a kind of skin flap donor. Because of the small possibility of scrotal injury in extensive burns, there is greater chance for the scrotum to offer its skin. Owing to the looseness of the subcutaneous tissue, the donor area, after the flap is taken, may be sutured directly without skin grafting.

Blood supply of the scrotal flap

The blood supply of the scrotum has multiple sources, namely, the posterior scrotal artery (from the internal pudendal artery), the anterior scrotal artery (from the external pudendal artery) and the external spermatic artery (from the hypogastric artery), of which the posterior scrotal artery is the chief one.

The posterior scrotal artery is a branch of the perineal artery and appears as a single trunk on either side of the central perineal point, where its outer diameter averages 1.3 mm. When the artery reaches the root of the scrotum it divides into several small branches supplying most of the scrotal skin (see Figure 7.3).

The posterior scrotal vein, accompanying the artery, is mostly (82%) single, but a few have two branches (18%). Its outer diameter averages 1.7 mm.

Nerves of the scrotal flap

The posterior scrotal nerve is the chief sensory nerve of the scrotum. It is a branch of the perineal nerve, which arises from the pudendal nerve and gives off several fine muscular branches and a thick posterior scrotal nerve in the urogenital triangle. The posterior scrotal nerves are usually two in number, a medial and a lateral, measuring about 1.2 mm and 1.0 mm in breadth respectively.

There are, in addition, some nerve endings reaching the skin of the scrotum but innervating a very small area. These belong to the ilioinguinal nerve, the genital branch of the genitofemoral nerve and the perineal branch of the posterior femoral cutaneous nerve.

Neurovascular pedicle of the scrotal flap

The scrotal flap has a constant neurovascular pedicle. The posterior scrotal artery is a direct cutaneous artery, which supplies nearly all of the scrotal skin and accompanies the vein with very little variations. The medial branch of the posterior scrotal nerve is closely attached to the superficial surface of the posterior scrotal vessels and the lateral branch is situated lateral to the vessels. The breadth of the nerve and the calibre of the vessel are fit for microsurgical anastomosis. Neuroanastomosis is most important for the restoration of sensation of the flap.

The level of taking of the neurovascular pedicle is better chosen between the root of the scrotum and the central perineal point. On either side of the latter, the neurovascular pedicle remains 15 mm on the average from the midline and 13 mm from the surface of the skin. It lies in the superficial perineal pouch, close to the deep surface of the superficial perineal fascia (Colles' fascia) between the bulbocavernosus and ischiocavernosus. There is a distinct depression between the two muscles, which can be felt by palpation.

Deep to the scrotal skin is a thin layer of dartos muscle, which is innervated by sympathetic nerves and is capable of contraction and relaxation to adjust the rate of heat dissipation. When the vessels are divided during operation, the sympathetic nerves around them may be involved and the skin of the scrotum will finally relax. The flap taken from half of the scrotal skin in a relaxed condition of a living adult is estimated to reach a maximal area of 5×7 cm.

SKIN FLAP AT THE INGUINAL REGION

CHEN ERYU AND HE GUANGCHI

The arteries of the skin flaps in the inguinal region are the largest direct cutaneous arteries in the body. Since the successful transplantation of free inguinal flap with microvascular anastomosis by Daniel in 1973, studies on inguinal cutaneous arteries have notably increased. The first report was presented by Smith in 1972. Later, Taylor and O'Brien observed a maximum of 100 cases. Zhu Shengxiu *et al.* of China studied the arteries in the inguinal region in 19 clinical cases, and Li Fuzhuang made a survey of 100 cases of the superficial iliac and hypogastric arteries. Recently, Chen Eryu and her colleagues made a comprehensive study on the origin, course, branching, and distribution of the three superficial arteries in the groin based on the dissection of 50 adult cadavers.

Superficial arteries

The three superficial arteries in the inguinal groin are the superficial circumflex iliac, the superficial epigastric and the superficial external pudendal arteries, each possessing two main branches (Figure 3.22). The percentage of incidence is quite different in each of these branches. In designing a skin flap using any of these branches as an axis, the extent of the flap is positively related to the calibre of the main branches at their commencement.

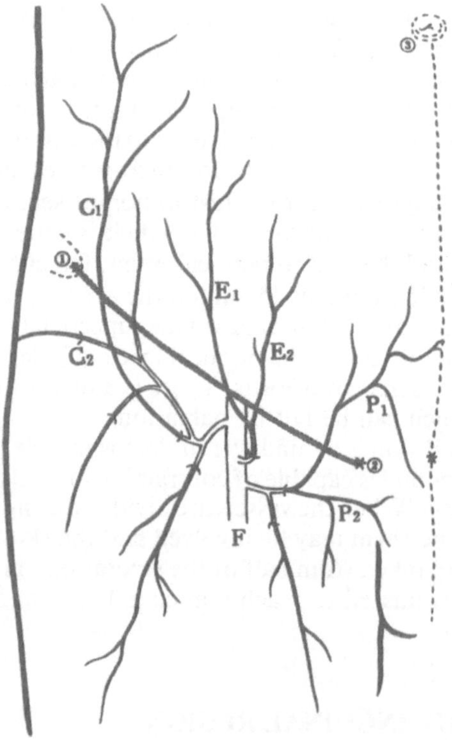

Figure 3.22 Superficial arteries in the inguinal region and their main branches. **1**: Anterior superior iliac spine; **2**: pubic tubercle; **3**: umbilicus; **F**: femoral a.; $\mathbf{C_1}$ & $\mathbf{C_2}$: SMB and DMB of SCIA; $\mathbf{E_1}$ & $\mathbf{E_2}$: LMB and MMB of SEA; $\mathbf{P_1}$ & $\mathbf{P_2}$: UMB and Low MB of SEPA

Superficial circumflex iliac artery (SCIA)

The SCIA possesses two main branches - superficial and deep. They are present simultaneously in 86% of cases, of which 56% originate from a common trunk. The trunk of SCIA is short, averaging less than 1.5 mm.

Superficial main branch (SMB)

The SMB is present in 86% of cases, its mean calibre being 0.8 mm. Before penetrating through the fascia lata, the SMB pursues a short course of about 5 mm in the deep layer. The site of penetration into the superficial fascia of the artery determines the thickness of the flap taken. That of the SMB is found concentrated in the circle with a radius of 15 mm, the centre of which is 15 mm lateral and 10 mm distal to the origin of the femoral artery. The course of a superficial artery usually indicates the axis of a free skin flap. The SMB frequently takes a course within 10 mm above or below a line drawn from a point 15 mm distal to the origin of the femoral artery to the anterior superior iliac spine. The SMB mostly turns upwards after having passed the anterior superior iliac spine to reach a level as high as about 100 mm above the spine and the umbilicus. It supplies the skin over the lateral half of the inguinal region (Figure 3.22).

Deep main branch (DMB)

The DMB is constantly present, its mean calibre being 1 mm. It is underneath the deep fascia and courses within 19 mm above or below a line kept parallel for 15 mm to the inguinal ligament. The DMB penetrates the fascia lata near the anterior superior iliac spine. The point of exit is found concentrated in a circle with a radius of 15 mm, the centre of which is 20 mm directly distal to the anterior superior iliac spine. Sometimes the DMB is crossed by the lateral cutaneous nerve of the thigh before it penetrates the deep fascia. After penetrating the deep fascia it turns laterally and downward, and then enters the gluteal region. Though the course of the DMB is rather deep, its branches and terminals are mostly distributed to the superficial fascia. Therefore, it is still considered a cutaneous artery. The DMB mainly supplies the upper lateral femoral and gluteal regions. The total area of distribution of SCIA determined by Li Fuzhuang *et al.* was 1.9-60 cm. A skin flap designed on the DMB pedicle will be very thick both in the skin and subcutaneous layers. Since the two main branches originating from a common trunk amount to 56% of the cases, the size of the flap may be enlarged provided both of them are taken into consideration.

Superficial epigastric artery (SEA)

The SEA also possesses two main branches, i.e. the medial and the lateral. They are present simultaneously in 34% of the cases, of which 20% originate from a common trunk.

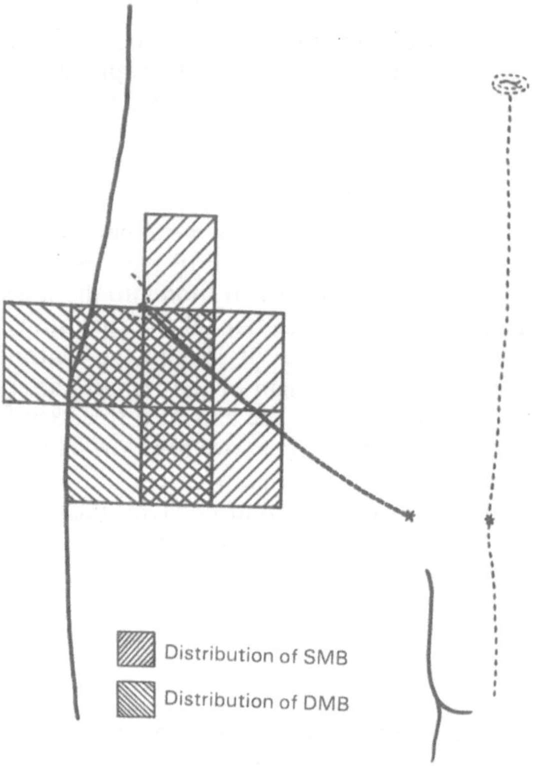

Figure 3.23 Central distributing areas of SCIA. The width of each small area equals one-quarter of the horizontal distance between the anterior superior iliac spine and the pubic tubercle. The length of each small area equals one-half of the perpendicular distance between the anterior superior iliac spine and the pubic tubercle

Medial main branch (MMB)

The MMB is present in 86% of the cases, its mean calibre being 1 mm. The MMB courses about 10 mm under the deep fascia before penetrating the cribriform fascia or the fascia lata. The points of exit are found concentrated in a circle with a radius of 10 mm, the centre of which is located 25 mm distal to the origin of the femoral artery. After getting into the superficial fascia, the MMB enters the abdominal wall about 10 mm medial to the origin of the femoral artery where it passes over the inguinal ligament and then courses almost perpendicularly upward. The MMB may reach as far as about 150 mm above the level of the origin of the femoral artery and so above that of the umbilicus. It frequently pursues a course within 10 mm on either side of a perpendicular line drawn 10 mm medial to the origin of the femoral artery. The MMB mainly supplies the medial half of the lower abdominal wall of the same side (Figure 3.24). The extended area of the MMB on the abdominal wall is about 78×38 mm on average.

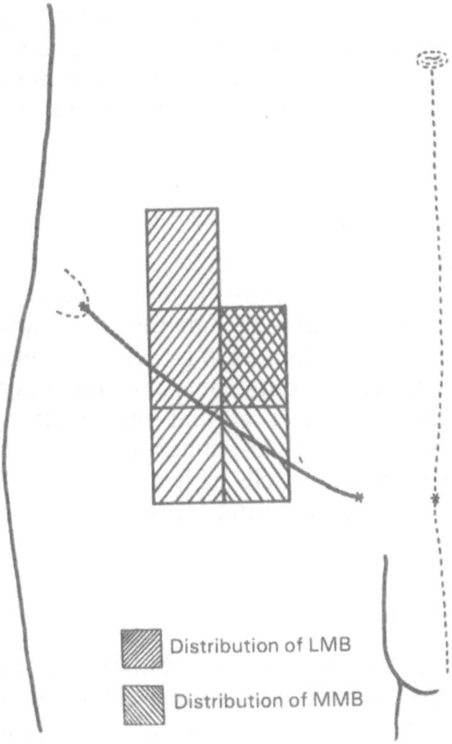

Figure 3.24 Central distributing area of SEA

Lateral main branch (LMB)

The LMB is present in 66% of cases, its mean calibre being 0.9 mm. After coursing for about 5 mm under the deep fascia, the LMB penetrates the fascia lata into the superficial fascia. The penetrating points are found concentrated in a circle with a radius of 10 mm, the centre of which is 5 mm lateral and 15 mm distal to the origin of the femoral artery. After getting into the superficial fascia, the LMB enters the abdominal wall about 10 mm lateral to the origin of the femoral artery by passing almost perpendicularly upward over the inguinal ligament. The LMB may reach as far as 150 mm above the level of the origin of the femoral artery and so above that of the umbilicus. The LMB frequently pursues a course within 10 mm on either side of a perpendicular line drawn 10 mm lateral to the origin of the femoral artery. The LMB mainly supplies the lateral half of the lower abdominal wall of the same side. Its territory on the abdominal wall is about 91 × 47 mm on average, being greater than that of the MMB. The total distributing area of SEA determined by Li Fuzhuang amounts to 40–100 cm.

Though the penetrating points of MMB and LMB are both near their origin, they course in the deep part of the superficial fascia, so that the skin flap involving either branch should include the whole layer of subcutaneous tissue. Because of much variety in the origin of SEA, it is suggested that the MMB or the LMB can be searched for on the surface of the inguinal ligament, 10 mm medial or lateral to the origin of the femoral artery, and the abdominal skin flap is to be adopted. Thus the arterial pedicle can be picked up more easily and interference due to lymph nodes below the inguinal ligament may be avoided.

Superficial external pudendal artery (SEPA)

The SEPA usually possesses two main branches, i.e. the upper and the lower. They are present simultaneously in 82% of cases, of which 6% originate from the common trunk. On approaching the great saphenous vein, the trunk of the SEPA and the lower main branch usually pass behind the vein, while the upper main branch passes in front of it. All of them penetrate the cribriform fascia into the superficial layer around the medial or lateral border of the terminal segment of the great saphenous vein. The penetrating points are found concentrated in a circle with a radius of 15 mm, the centre of which is 10 mm medial and 50 mm distal to the origin of the femoral artery.

The upper main branch (UMB)

The UMB is present in 88% of cases, its mean calibre being 1.0 mm. The UMB runs medially and upward, mostly crossing the inguinal ligament near the pubic tubercle. Few pass over the pubic crest to enter the suprapubic region. If a line is drawn from a point 51 mm distal to the origin of the femoral artery to the pubic tubercle, the UMB is frequently found within 10 mm on either side of the line. After entering the suprapubic region the UMB usually anastomoses with its fellow of the opposite side and frequently gives a downward branch to supply the penis or clitoris. Besides the external genitalia, the UMB mainly supplies the medial inguinal and suprapubic regions (Figures 3.25).

The low main branch (LowMB)

The LowMB is present in 95% of cases, its mean calibre being 1.1 mm. The LowMB runs medially almost in a horizontal direction and enters the prepubic region. If a line is drawn 50 mm distal to the origin of the femoral artery and parallel to the pubic crest, the LowMB frequently courses within 10 mm on either side of the line.

In addition to the upper part of the medial femoral region, all terminal branches of LowMB supply the external genitalia, chiefly the scrotum or the labium majus.

The SEPA is relatively constant. The UMB and the LowMB often come from a common trunk. Their calibres are large. They are intimately related to the terminal segment of the great saphenous vein. Their distributing area is constant and is always found in the medial upper femoral region. All of these become advantageous in using SEPA or its main branches as a vascular pedicle of the skin flap.

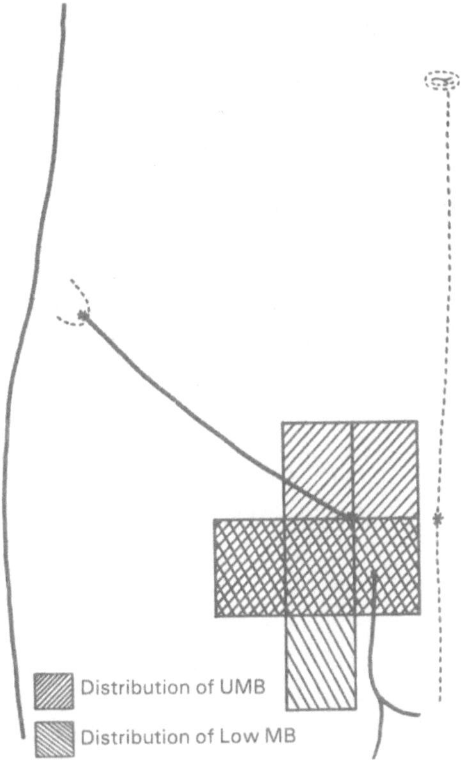

Figure 3.25 Central distributing area of SEPA

General survey of the superficial arteries

The three superficial arteries and their main branches may originate separately or from a common trunk with other arteries. They, however, may be absent. As a result, five types of arterial trunk are formed, i.e. superficial circumflex iliac artery, superficial circumflex iliacoepigastricopudendal arterial trunk, superficial epigastric artery, superficial epigastric external pudendal artery, and superficial external pudendal artery. Their average calibres are 1.3, 1.5, 1.3, 1.8 and 1.5 mm, respectively. In short, the calibre of the common trunk is larger than that of the artery arising separately.

These superficial arterial trunks mainly arise from the femoral artery. Their origins are arranged in order from lateral medialward (3–26). More than half of the superficial circumflex iliac arteries arise from the deep femoral artery and its branches, or from the deep circumflex iliac artery. Those originating from the femoral artery mostly arise from the lateral half of its wall. The superficial epigastric artery generally arises from the medial half of the wall of the femoral artery. The superficial external pudendal artery mainly arises from the medial wall of the femoral artery. The origin of the common trunk depends on the branch which is predominant. There is also a regular sequence in the vertical arrangement from above downward of the origins of the superficial arteries. Thus, the sequence of the origin of these five superficial arterial trunks on the femoral artery in most of the specimens, from above downward and from the posterolateral wall of the femoral artery via its anterior aspect to the posteromedial wall, is as follows: the superficial circumflex iliac artery, the superficial circumflex iliacoepigastric arterial trunk, the superficial epigastric artery, the superficial epigastricopudendal arterial trunk, and the superficial external pudendal artery. Any one of them might be absent but the order of arrangement will never be changed. The above regularity may be helpful in search for the root of any of the superficial arterial trunks during operation. By virtue of the location and calibre of the root of a superficial artery, the course and distribution of it and the size of the flap to be taken may also be estimated.

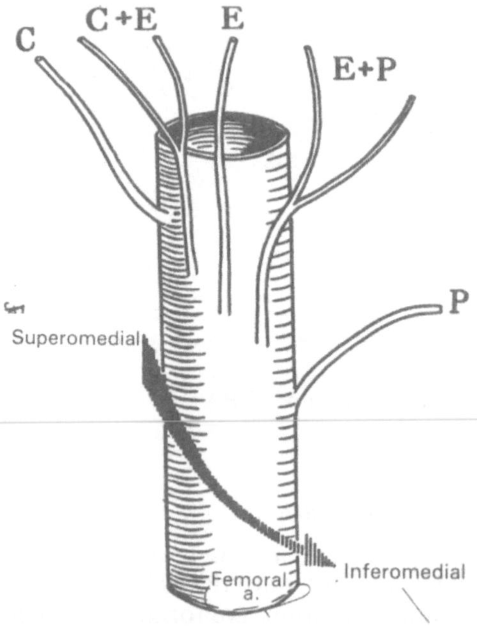

Figure 3.26 Origins of superficial arteries on the wall of the femoral artery. **C**: Superficial circumflex iliac artery; **C + E**: superficial circumflex iliacoepigastric arterial trunk; **E**: superficial epigastric artery; **E + P**: superficial epigastricopudendal arterial trunk; **P**: superficial external pudendal artery

Of the five superficial arteries arising separately, the superficial circumflex iliacoepigastric arterial trunk shows the highest incidence (66%). This varies greatly in different reports, probably owing to the differences in definition given to the arteries by different authors. The lowest rate (15.7%) was reported by Zhu Shengxiu *et al.*, the highest (66%) being ours, and in Li Fuzhuang's series it appeared to be 40%. The calibre of this trunk is large, being 1.5 mm on average. Its area of supply is relatively large and concentrated. Therefore, this arterial trunk is suggested as the first choice for the vascular pedicle of the inguinal flap.

Superficial veins

There are two groups of superficial veins in the inguinal region, i.e. the superficial and the deep veins. The superficial veins are comparatively large but usually do not accompany the corresponding arteries. They are located in the superficial layer of the subcutaneous tissue and have different patterns of confluence, of which separated drainage is the most common. They generally empty into the great saphenous vein or its tributaries in the femoral region, except for individual ones which join the femoral vein. The mean calibres of the superficial circumflex iliac, the superficial epigastric and the superficial external pudendal veins are 2.1, 2.1, and 2.0 mm respectively, being much larger than those of the corresponding arteries. Though the superficial circumflex iliac and superficial epigastric veins do not accompany the corresponding arteries, their course is usually similar to one of the two main branches of the corresponding artery or they may pursue between these branches. Therefore, the superficial veins can be used as a guide in the search for arteries. Li Fuzhuang also held that the course of the superficial veins is parallel to the arteries, the SCIV being usually within 20 mm below the corresponding artery and the SEV within 10 mm medial to the synonymous artery. In four-fifths of cases the superficial external pudendal vein is the companion vein of the SEPA and there do not exist two sets of superficial external pudendal veins.

Veins of the deep group are the companion veins of the superficial arteries. That of the superficial circumflex iliac artery usually ends in veins. However, those of the superficial epigastric and the superficial external pudendal arteries usually join the superficial veins.

THE POSTERIOR FEMORAL FLAP

ZHONG SHIZHEN AND LIU MUZHI

The posterior femoral flap consists of the posterosuperior and posterolateral femoral flaps. The former belongs to those with intermuscular space vascular supply and the latter to those with intermuscular septum vascular supply. Although flaps in this region are quite thick so that they have not yet been applied clinically, they might possibly be adopted as flap donors in the light of their concealed positions and other anatomical reasons.

Posterosuperior femoral flap

The vascular pedicle of the flap is formed by the cutaneous branches of the inferior gluteal vessels, one to four in number. The outer diameters of the cutaneous arteries measure 0.4–1.0 mm, those of the companion veins being slightly greater. The cutaneous vessels emerge from the subgluteal space (space under the gluteus maximus) and descend to the back of the thigh to be distributed to the skin of its upper portion and that over the lower part of the gluteal region. The skin with the subcutaneous tissue appears quite thick yet not so tender as to be suitable for the repair of deep defects. According to the distribution of the cutaneous vessels, the donor area measures about 10 × 15 cm, of which about one-third is situated above the gluteal fold and the other two-thirds below it. If a relatively large artery is needed for anastomosis, the cutaneous branch of the inferior gluteal artery can be traced back through the subgluteal space to the stem common to it and the muscular branches, where the outer diameter of the artery may reach 1.0–1.5 mm.

As to the sensory nerve of the flap, the posterior cutaneous nerve of the thigh may be adopted. The breadth of its trunk measures 2–3 mm where it passes from the subgluteal space to the back of the thigh over which it descends in the midline under cover of the deep fascia. The posterior cutaneous nerve of the thigh gives off in the subgluteal space gluteal and perineal branches which, after emerging from the subgluteal space and piercing the deep fascia, run upward and medialward to be distributed to the skin of the lower gluteal and perineal regions respectively. Therefore the posterior cutaneous nerve of the thigh must be taken 30 mm above the lower border of the gluteus maximus in order to preserve the gluteal branches.

Posterolateral femoral flap

For the convenience of description, the length of the thigh is divided, from the apex of greater trochanter to the lateral epicondyle of the femur, into four equal sections which are termed femoral 1/4, 2/4, 3/4 and 4/4 respectively. The vutaneous vessels of each section in the lateral intermuscular septum are introduced as follows (Figure 3.27).

(1) The vessels in the intermuscular septum of section femoral 1/4 are numerous, usually three to five in number, and of small calibre. One of them may have an outer diameter of more than 0.8 mm. This accounts for 71% of cases. They come from the first perforating artery and run horizontally to the lateral side. They then pass between the insertion of the gluteus maximus and the vastus lateralis, piercing the aponeurosis of the gluteus maximus and adhering so closely to the surrounding tissues that it is inconvenient to separate them during operation. The flap supplied by the intermuscular septum artery of this segment is lateral to the junction between the inferior gluteal and superior femoral regions and is estimated to be 10 × 10 cm in size.

(2) The vessels in the intermuscular septum of section femoral 2/4 are mostly branches of the first perforating artery. The vascular pedicle in this section is more ideal because of the constant position by which the intermuscular septum artery enters the skin. The latter pierces the lower border of the insertion of gluteus maximus in 97% of cases and possesses a large calibre averaging 1.6 mm, and a longer vascular pedicle averaging 47 mm. If a longer and larger artery is needed for operation, the stem common to the intermuscular septum artery and another muscular branch can be taken by dissecting upward along the intermuscular septum so as to double the length and calibre of the artery to facilitate the performance of operation. The companion veins are mostly two in number and slightly larger than the artery. The sensation of the flap can be recovered by means of the neighbouring posterior cutaneous nerve of the thigh,

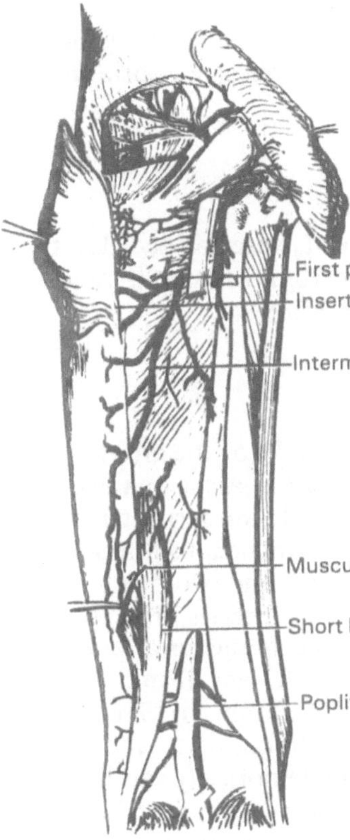

Figure 3.27 Vessels of the posterolateral femoral flap

which is situated in the midline of the back of the thigh, 20–25 mm from the lateral intermuscular septum under cover of the deep fascia. The intermuscular septum artery in this section supplies the skin of the posterolateral aspect of the thigh of sections 2/4–4/4, which is estimated to be about 10×20 cm in size.

(3) The intermuscular septum arteries of the section femoral 3/4 are rather few in number and represent only 23% of cases. The outer diameter averages 1.0 mm. The artery supplying the skin in this section is not the intermuscular septum artery but is mostly the musculo-cutaneous one penetrating the short head of biceps femoris perpendicularly to reach the skin. Its outer diameter is mostly 0.5–1.0 mm. It is suitable for vascular anastomosis but lacks the advantage of the intermuscular septum artery as long vascular pedicle.

(4) The intermuscular septum artery of the section femoral 4/4 mostly arises from the popliteal artery representing 97% of cases. Its outer diameter averages 1.1 mm. The skin nourished by the artery is over the back of the knee joint. It is generally unsuitable as a flap donor.

THE POSTERIOR CRURAL FLAP

BAI SHULING AND LI JI

The posterior crural flap has many advantages, viz., good quality, large area as a donor site, rich blood supply and concealed position, all of which make it suitable for flap grafting.

Arteries of the posterior crural flap

With the direct cutaneous arteries as its vascular pedicles, the posterior crural flap derives its blood supply mainly from the lateral, intermediate and medial popliteal cutaneous arteries (Figure 3.28).

Lateral popliteal cutaneous artery

The incidence rate is 100%, of which 65% of the arteries come independently from the stem of popliteal artery, 17.5% share a common stem from the popliteal with other cutaneous arteries or the posterior cutaneous arteries of the thigh, and 15% originate from the gastrocnemius arteries, of which one-third are from the medial gastrocnemius artery and two-thirds from the lateral. Only 2.5% of the lateral popliteal cutaneous arteries arise from its medial fellow. More than 50% of the lateral popliteal cutaneous arteries lie 11 mm lateral to the posterior median line (line C) of the leg and 18 mm above the intercondylar line (line A). Its mean outer diameter is 1.5 mm. In 13% of cases the artery gives off from its stem a fine muscular branch, less than 1 mm in calibre, to be distributed to the lower end of the biceps femoris. It can be ligated in taking the arterial pedicle. In 90% of cases the lateral popliteal cutaneous artery pierces the deep fascia 18 mm lateral to line C and sends off the ascending, lateral and descending branches. The latter may reach as far as 14 mm below line A.

After piercing the deep fascia, the lateral popliteal cutaneous artery is often in company with and deep to the lateral sural cutaneous nerve, and gives off numerous twigs to the skin and subcutaneous tissue.

Intermediate popliteal cutaneous artery

The artery arises from the popliteal (47%) and gastrocnemius (13%) arteries, making a total incidence rate of 60%. Its outer diameter averages 1.5 mm. In more than half of the cases the intermediate popliteal cutaneous artery pierces the deep fascia 13 mm lateral to line C and gives off all the way the ascending, lateral and descending branches. The descending branches may reach as far as 100 mm below line A.

Medial popliteal cutaneous artery

The artery, being always present, arises from the popliteal without exception. It is mostly single; a few (5%) remain double. It runs along the medial wall of the popliteal fossa under cover of the semitendinosus and semimembranosus.

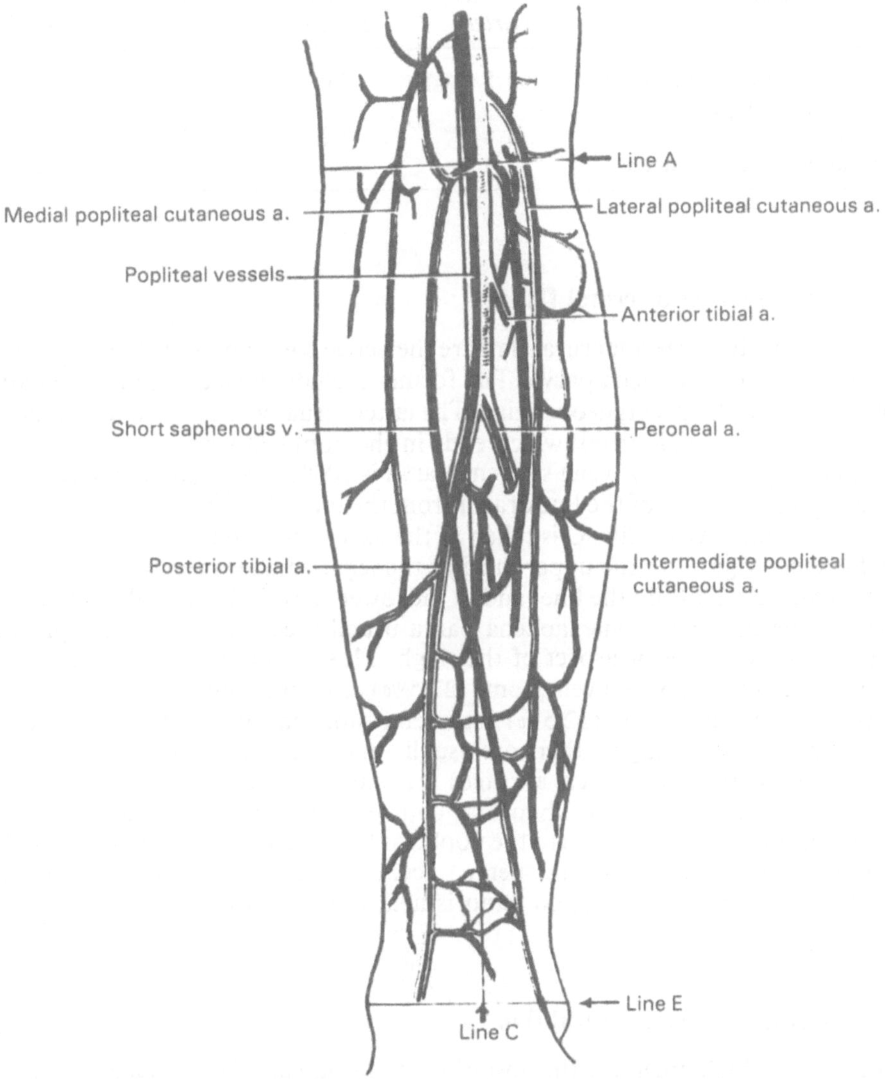

Figure 3.28 Schematic diagram of the arteries of the posterior crural flap

Most of them arise medial to line C, being 31 mm above line A. Its mean outer diameter is 1.4 mm. It pierces at the point 16 mm medial to line C and gives off all the way the ascending, lateral and descending branches. The descending branches may reach as far as 61 mm below line A. The three cutaneous arteries mentioned above anastomose freely to form a rich network.

Table 3.5 The outer diameter and vascular pedicle of popliteal cutaneous vessels (mm)

Name of vessel	*Diameter of artery*	*Diameter of vein*	*Arterial pedicle*	*Venous pedicle*
Lateral popliteal cutaneous	1.5	2.0	27	27
Intermediate popliteal cutaneous	1.5	2.2	24	24
Medial popliteal cutaneous	1.4	1.4	24	24

Veins of the posterior crural flap

The veins of the posterior crural flap are the venae comitantes of the cutaneous arteries and vena saphena parva. The former include the lateral, intermediate and medial popliteal cutaneous veins. The latter, usually one or two in number, unite to form a single trunk which ends in the popliteal vein.

The incidence rate of vena saphena parva is 100%. Its mean outer diameter measured at the level of the line drawn from the medial to the lateral malleolus is 2.9 (2–4) mm. When line C is taken as the axis, vena saphena parva presents an S-shaped figure. In the upper third of the leg it courses medial to line C; in the middle third it is on the line, and in the lower third it lies lateral to the line. Near its termination, vena saphena parva usually receives a femoropopliteal vein from the posterior aspect of the thigh. Most of the vena saphena parva (60%) end in the popliteal vein; some (27.5%) drain into the perforators of the femoral vein, and a few (12.5%) into vena saphena magna. Between venae saphena parva and magna, there are usually one or two communicating veins, the outer diameter of which averages 2.2 mm. In a few cases (2.5%) vena saphena parva assumes an abnormal course, ascending from the posterior aspect of the lateral malleolus to the popliteal fossa, and there it passes through the bifurcation of the sciatic nerve, accompanying the nerve upward to terminate in the vena profunda femoris near the fossa ovalis.

Nerves of the posterior crural flap

The nerves which innervate the posterior crural flap are the medial and lateral sural nerves and the sural communicating branch. The incidence rate of the lateral sural nerve is 100%. It arises from the trunk of the common peroneal nerve. Its breadth is 2.1 mm and the neural pedicle is 35 mm in length. The sural communicating branch is present in 90% of the cases, of which 85% share a common stem with the lateral sural nerve and 5% originate independently from the common peroneal nerve. Its breadth and length are 2.2 mm and 35 mm respectively. The communicating branch anastomoses with the medial sural nerve in 91% of cases. The site of anastomosis is 240 mm below line A. The medial sural nerve arises from the tibial nerve and measures 1.4 mm in breadth. It runs between the lateral and medial heads of the gastrocnemius and under cover of the deep fascia. After emerging from the deep fascia 224 mm below line A, most of them (77.5%) anastomose with the sural communicating branch and a few (22.5%) descend independently to the posterior aspect of the lateral malleolus. Its length available for isolation may attain 200 mm or more.

The taking of the posterior crural flap

In taking the posterior crural flap the lateral popliteal cutaneous artery should be first chosen as the pedicle because of its length and invariability as well as the large area it supplies. The X-ray film of the posterior crural flap, injected through the cutaneous arteries with red lead and latex, demonstrates that there are profuse anastomotic networks not only among the lateral, intermediate and medial popliteal cutaneous arteries but also between these arteries and those of the gastrocnemius and soleus (Figure 3.29). Moreover, the cutaneous branches, arising from the stem of the posterior tibial artery and supplying the posterior crural flap, also anastomose with these cutaneous arteries to form a network so as to enlarge the extent of supply of the lateral popliteal cutaneous artery. The injection of red ink into the lateral popliteal cutaneous artery of the lower

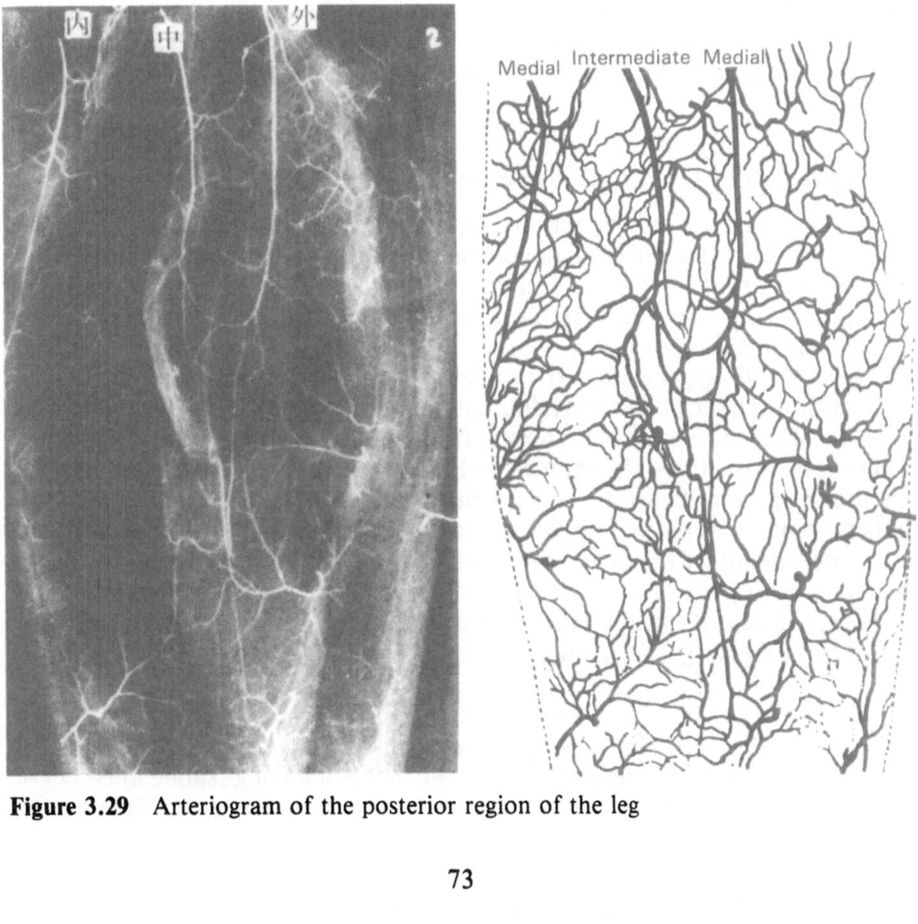

Figure 3.29 Arteriogram of the posterior region of the leg

limb of fresh cadaver indicates that the area supplied by this artery may be as large as 15 × 30 cm. Therefore the circulation in the flap will not be disturbed in the process of taking, provided the lateral popliteal cutaneous artery and its branches are kept intact. If flaps of small sizes are needed for grafting, various arterial pedicles can be selected in accordance with the requirement.

The maximal area of the flap to be taken should bear the following boundaries: line A as the upper limit, the line drawn from the lateral epicondyle of the femur to the lateral malleolus as the lateral limit, and another line joining the medial epicondyle of the femur and the medial malleolus as the medial limit. In order to avoid injury to the tibial nerve, the vascular pedicle can be divided against the lateral side of the nerve, where the outer diameter of the lateral popliteal cutaneous artery is 1.1 mm.

The medial sural nerve should be left in the donor site in the process of taking the posterior crural flap.

THE MEDIAL CRURAL FLAP

SUN BO AND CHANG JUNPING

The medial crural flap consists of the upper, and the middle and lower parts. The former belongs to those with the intermuscular septum vascular supply, and the latter to those with the intermuscular space vascular supply.

The upper part of the medial crural flap

In the medial intermuscular septum of the thigh the muscular and musculocutaneous branches given off from the femoral artery are of small calibre. Only the saphenous branch of the descending genicular artery (the highest genicular artery) from the lower end of the femoral artery is of great significance in clinical practice (Figure 3.30).

The descending genicular artery arises from the femoral artery just before it passes through the opening in adductor magnus, and immediately divides into the saphenous and articular branches. In the junction between the middle and lower parts of the thigh the saphenous branch pierces the aponeurotic roof of the adductor canal beneath the sartorius and descends in company with the saphenous nerve. It passes between the sartorius and gracilis for a long distance to the medial side of the knee joint, where it emerges from between the above muscles, piercing the deep fascia, to be distributed to the skin of the upper half of the medial side of the leg. The length of the saphenous branch from its origin to the site of emergence from the deep fascia averages 116 mm. The outer diameter at its commencement is 1.7 mm.

The saphenous branch of the descending genicular artery is easy to find by pulling laterally the lower segment of sartorius, and the sensation of the flap can be established by anastomosing the accompanying saphenous nerve (1.5–2.0 mm in breadth) with the nerve in the recipient area. Besides the

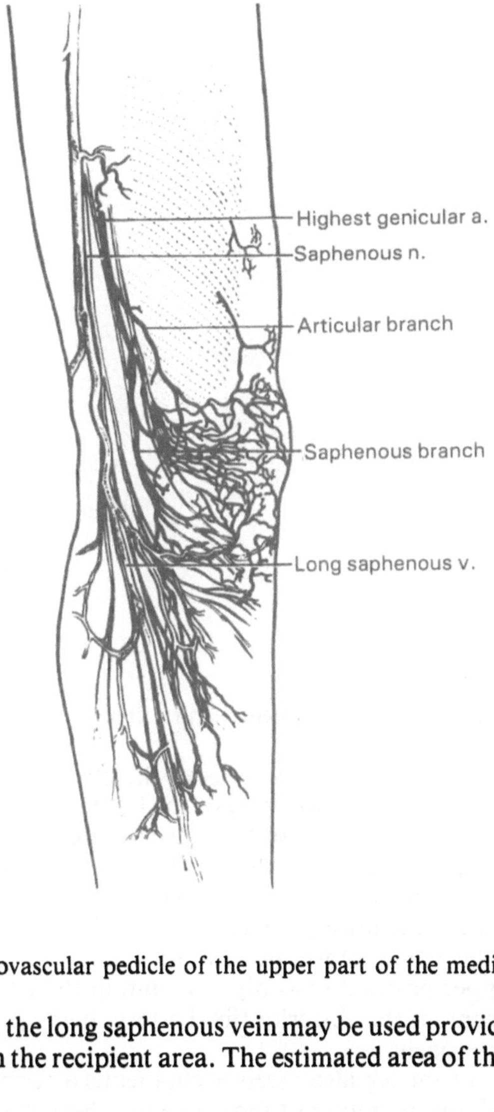

Figure 3.30 Neurovascular pedicle of the upper part of the medial crural flap

companion veins, the long saphenous vein may be used provided an appropriate vein is available in the recipient area. The estimated area of the flap is 7 × 13 cm.

Middle and lower part of the medial crural flap

The cutaneous arteries of the middle and lower part of the medial crural flap are derived from the posterior tibial artery. They pass between the soleus and the flexor digitorum longus, piercing the deep fascia on the medial side of the leg, to be distributed to the middle and lower part of the medial crural flap (Figure 3.31). The surface projection of the site of emergence of the cutaneous arteries from the deep fascia coincides with the line drawn from the junction of the upper middle thirds of the medial border of the tibia to the mid-point of a line drawn from the posterior border of medial malleolus to the tendo calcaneus.

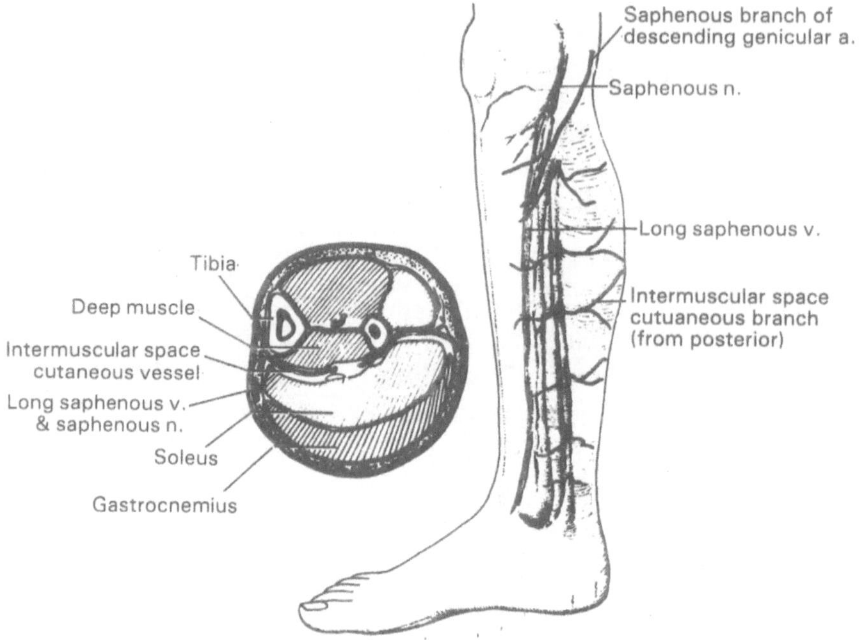

Figure 3.31 Vessels and nerves of the medial crural flap

The number of medial cutaneous arteries of the posterior tibial varies from two to seven, in the middle and lower part of the leg mostly two to four, which accounts for about 75%. The origin of these arteries lies mostly near the junction of the middle and lower thirds of the leg. Their outer diameter varies from 0.5 to 2.0 mm. Because the posterior tibial artery lies deep in the upper part of the leg and superficial in the lower, the length of the arterial pedicle of the flap diminishes gradually from above downward; viz., the pedicle measures 25–50 mm in the upper position but only 2–11 mm in the lower. At the lower end of the leg the trunk of the posterior tibial artery, being just under the deep fascia, is easy to approach.

The middle part of the leg also receives cutaneous arteries from the upper part of the leg. With the exception of the saphenous branch of the descending genicular artery coming from the subcutaneous tissue, all of the remaining arteries come from the posterior tibial artery at a higher level. They pierce the origin of the soleus obliquely to be distributed to the skin. A large periosteal branch is given off on the way. Moreover, there are a few cutaneous arteries passing between the flexor digitorum longus and the tibia to be distributed to the skin and periosteum. The above-mentioned cutaneous arteries from various origins form a rich arterial network in the subcutaneous tissue so as to increase the extent of the flap. The companion veins of the cutaneous arteries in the middle and lower part of the leg are mostly two in number, a superior and an inferior branch, which end in the posterior tibial vein. Their outer diameters are generally greater than those of the arteries but their pedicles are of the same length. There are many communicating branches between the cutaneous veins and the great saphenous vein near the junction of the middle and lower thirds of the leg.

Although the cutaneous arteries of the flap in the middle and lower part of the leg present an irregular segmental distribution, they are all linked to a longitudinal arterial trunk, the posterior tibial artery. Thus there are many choices for the flap to be taken. The cutaneous artery of a single segment can be taken as the pedicle for a small flap, and the trunk of the posterior tibial artery connected with several cutaneous arteries may be taken for a large one. According to the distribution of cutaneous vessels, the forward branches may reach the anterior midline of the leg, and the backward ones the posterior midline. The skin over the medial surface of tibia and in the vicinity of tendo calcaneus should not be used for grafting because of the scarcity of subcutaneous tissue, poor blood supply and liability to necrosis in these regions. Besides the companion veins of the arteries, the long saphenous vein and the saphenous nerve in the superficial layer may be chosen for anastomosis.

THE ANTERIOR CRURAL FLAP

LI JI

The anterior crural flap lies well concealed. The skin is of good quality and the arteries have large calibre. All these make the repair of skin defects of moderate degree suitable. However, the vascular pedicle lies deeply and is difficult to take. The arteries of the anterior crural flap belong to the intermuscular space vascular supply.

Arteries of the anterior crural flap

The blood supply of the anterior crural flap comes from the cutaneous branches of the anterior tibial artery, which arises from the popliteal artery, and passes through the interosseous membrane to the anterior region of the leg. It lies at first between the anterior tibialis and the extensor digitorum longus, which covers it, and then between the former and the extensor hallucis longus (Figure 3.32). Descending under cover of the extensor hallucis longus, the artery turns to lie between the extensor hallucis and digitorum longus above the intermalleolar line and continues on the dorsum of foot as the dorsalis pedis artery. In the anterior region of the leg the length of the anterior tibial artery averages 29 cm. The outer diameters measured at the upper, middle and lower portions of the leg are 3.6 mm, 2.9 mm and 1.4 mm respectively. It gives off one to five, usually three, cutaneous branches. The outer diameters of the cutaneous branches average 1.2 mm, mostly 1.0–1.6 mm. Most of the cutaneous branches arise from the anterior tibial artery in the upper and middle parts of the leg. They pass through the intermuscular space, emerging from the deep fascia, to be distributed to the skin and subdermis of a rather wide area of the upper and middle thirds of the leg (Figure 3.33).

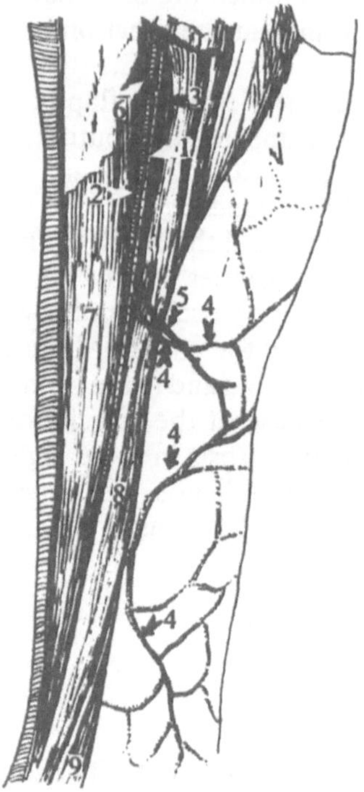

Figure 3.32 Cutaneous branches of the anterior tibial artery. **1**: Anterior tibial a.; **2**: anterior tibial v.; **3**: deep peroneal n.; **4**: cutaneous branches of anterior tibial a.; **5**: cutaneous tributaries of anterior tibial v.; **6**: anterior tibial recurrent a.; **7**: tibialis anterior; **8**: extensor digitorum longus; **9**: peroneus longus and brevis

Veins of the anterior crural flap

The anterior crural flap possesses only one set of veins in company with the stem of the anterior tibial artery and its cutaneous branches. There are no large subcutaneous veins. The anterior tibial veins, often two in number, have an outer diameter larger than that of the accompanying artery. Each of the cutaneous branches of the anterior tibial artery is accompanied by one or two cutaneous veins, the outer diameter of which averages 1.2 mm. It is sufficient for these cutaneous veins to drain the flap, thus assuring the establishment of circulation of the flap directly after grafting.

Nerves of the anterior crural flap

There is no cutaneous nerve trunk in the anterior crural flap, and the deep peroneal nerve, which accompanies the anterior tibial nerve, is mainly a muscular branch. The deep peroneal nerve is given off from the common

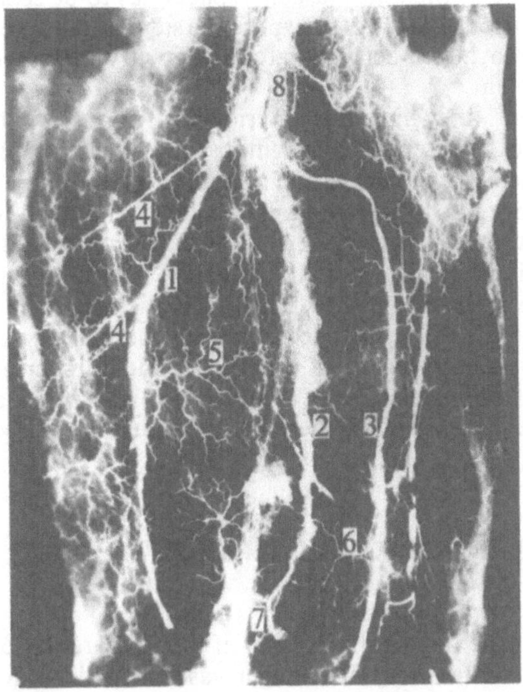

Figure 3.33 Arteriogram of the flap of the flap showing micro-vascular network. **1**: Anterior tibial a.; **2**: peroneal a.; **3**: posterior tibial a.; **4**: cutaneous branches of anterior tibial a.; **5**: musculocutaneous branches; **6**: cutaneous branches of posterior tibial a.; **7**: cutaneous branches of peroneal a.; **8**: popliteal a.

peroneal at the posteroinferior aspect of the head of the fibula. It courses among the muscles of the anterior compartment of the leg in company with the anterior tibial vessels, the topographical relation with which varies. It lies at first on the lateral side of the vessels, then in front of them, and again on its lateral side. This is the so-called lateral-anterior-lateral pattern. Another one is known as the lateral-anterior-medial pattern. Either of these two patterns accounts for half of the cases. Particular attention has to be paid to the nerve in dividing the anterior tibial artery during free flap grafting. The nerve should be carefully separated from the vessels along its course to avoid injury, which would lead to the paralysis of the muscles of the anterior region of the leg.

Applied anatomy regarding the anterior crural flap

According to the anatomical features of the origin of the cutaneous branches of the anterior tibial artery, the taking of the arterial pedicle is usually confined to the upper half of the artery. These cutaneous branches emerge from between the anterior tibialis and the extensor digitorum longus or between the extensor digitorum longus and the peroneus longus and brevis. Therefore, in taking the arterial pedicle, one of the intermuscular spaces has to be separated along the course of the cutaneous branches to expose the stem of the anterior tibial artery and keep these branches intact, so that a higher survival rate can be obtained after transplantation.

The experiment, in which the anterior and posterior tibial arteries are injected with black ink separately, demonstrates that though the cutaneous branches are gathered in the upper and middle parts of the leg, the ink injected may reach the knee above and the ankle below. Anteriorly it can reach the anterior crest of the tibia, and posteriorly it may exceed the line drawn from the head of the fibula to the internal malleolus. The area of the flap capable of being taken is estimated to be 25 × 7 cm. After the upper and middle portions of the anterior tibial artery have been excised, the blood supply to the deep structures of the anterior region of the leg and the dorsum of foot is mainly offered by the posterior tibial artery through the plantar arch and its branches ascending to these parts or via the perforating branches of the peroneal artery.

THE FLAP OF THE DORSUM OF THE FOOT

XU ENDUO

The advantages of the flap of the dorsum of the foot are: (a) better colour, (b) greater diameter of the artery and longer vascular pedicle, (c) the cutaneous nerve available for anastomosis to restore sensation after operation, and (d) the possibility of making a compound skin–tendon flap together with the extensor digitorum tendons. The disadvantages of the flap, however, are: (a) small area fitted only for the repair of small defects of the face, neck and hand and (b) little flexibility, so that the cut edges cannot be pulled together for suture, and the donor site has to receive a skin graft afterwards. Nevertheless, the flap of the dorsum of the foot can still be regarded as an excellent donor site.

The flap of the dorsum of the foot takes the arteria dorsalis pedis as its vascular pedicle, which gives off a lot of cutaneous branches to form a rich vascular network in the subcutaneous tissue and belongs to the flap with truncal and reticular arterial supply just as the forearm flap.

Arteries of the flap of the dorsum of the foot

The arteria dorsalis pedis is the continuation of the anterior tibial just below the mid-point of the intermalleolar line. It runs downward and forward between the extensor hallucis and digitorum longus over the dorsum of the talus, the navicular and the second cuneiform bone and then under the extensor digitorum brevis to the proximal end of the first intermetatarsal space, where it divides into a larger deep plantar branch and a smaller first dorsal metatarsal artery.

The stem of the arteria dorsalis pedis in adults is 6.5–8 cm in length and its outer diameter is 2–3.5 mm. If the artery is absent (0.5%) or belongs to the slender pattern (6.5%) with a diameter of less than 0.4 mm, it would not be advisable to use it as the free flap because it is too small to be anastomosed. The remaining patterns (straight pattern 59%; curved pattern 23% and medially or laterally deviated pattern 11%) may be used in grafting the vascularized flap.

Tiny cutaneous branches can be given off from any part of the arteria dorsalis pedis, but the major ones arise mostly from its proximal part, viz. within 20 mm from its origin and its distal part, i.e. within 20 mm from its termination. The former part usually gives rise to one or two major branches, the latter part usually to two or three major ones. The intermediate part of the arteria dorsalis pedis gives off a few major cutaneous branches only occasionally. In adults, the outer diameter of the major cutaneous branches from the proximal part of the arteria dorsalis pedis is 0.4–0.5 mm, that of the branches from the intermediate part is 0.3–0.5 mm, and that from the distal part has a diameter of 0.3–0.4 mm.

The chief branches of the arteria dorsalis pedis (the medial and lateral tarsal, the arcuate and the first dorsal metatarsal arteries) also give off many fine branches to the skin of the dorsum of the foot. These anastomose freely to form an arterial network (Figure 3.34), which extends horizontally to the medial and lateral margins of the dorsum of the foot, forward for 2–3 cm distal to the termination of arteria dorsalis pedis, and upward to the level of the ankle joint.

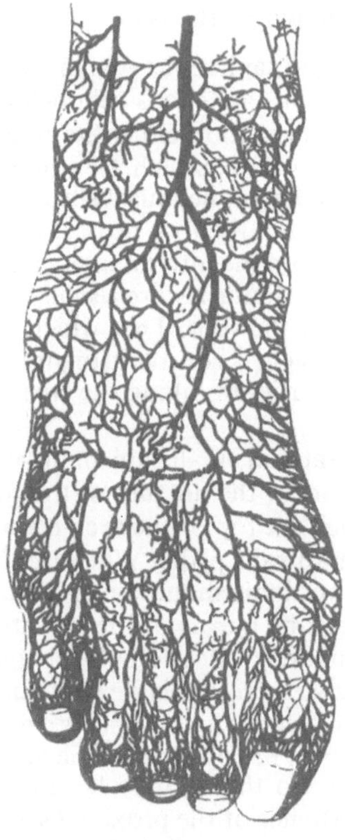

Figure 3.34 Cutaneous vascular network of the stem of the dorsalis pedis artery

Therefore, the arteria dorsalis pedis can be taken as an axis, about which the flap may extend for 4 cm both medially and laterally, downward to the proximal part of the web of toes, and upward to the level of the ankle joint, measuring about 8 × 10 cm.

Since the cutaneous branches arising from the lateral wall of the stem of arteria dorsalis pedis usually pierce the belly of the extensor hallucis brevis before being distributed to the skin, the latter should be preserved in the flap in order to ensure the blood circulation.

The angulation between the stem of the arteria dorsalis pedis and its cutaneous branches is usually 70–90 degrees. The cutaneous branches arising from the terminal part of the arteria dorsalis pedis may supply the skin overlying the dorsum of the first and second metatarsals, while those arising from the first dorsal metatarsal artery mainly supply the skin overlying the first and second phalanges. In taking the flap of the dorsum of the foot it is not necessary to include the first dorsal metatarsal artery, though the flap may extend to the base of the web of the toes. As the position of the first dorsal metatarsal artery varies greatly, the dissection of the deeply situated first dorsal metatarsal artery is very difficult. Therefore the omission of the procedure of dissecting this artery will save plenty of time.

Veins of the flap of the dorsum of the foot

The outer diameter of the great saphenous vein in front of the medial malleolus is 3–5 mm and that of the small saphenous vein behind the lateral malleolus is 2.2–3.0 mm. In the dorsum of the foot, either the great or small saphenous vein is provided with two or three valves, which are situated just about 1 mm distal to the large tributaries of the saphenous veins. Both the great and small saphenous veins in the dorsum of the foot possess one or two interosseous perforating tributaries, which drain the intermetatarsal spaces or the deep portion of the sole. The perforating tributaries are usually located in the middle and upper parts of the dorsum of the foot. That which ends near the termination of the first dorsal metatarsal vein is constant (Figure 3.35). However, attention has to be paid to these tributaries in taking the free flap of the dorsum of the foot.

In 90% of cases the great and small saphenous veins are united to form a venous arch in the distal part of the dorsum of the foot. This is known as the single-arch pattern, in which the top of the arch is not beyond the level 1.5 cm distal to the end of arteria dorsalis pedis. When the flap of the dorsum of the foot is to be taken, the lower limit should be at least 2 cm distal to the end of the arteria dorsalis pedis felt by means of the pulsation of the artery in order to avoid injury to the venous arch. Occasionally the top of the arch is far beyond the limit mentioned above so as to be liable to damage during operation.

In 9% of cases the dorsal venous arch presents a double-arch pattern (Figure 3.35), the lower limit of which nearly reaches the level of the second and third metatarsophalangeal joints, so that it may be injured in case of operation. However, thanks to the existence of the proximal series of arches, it is unlikely to cause circulatory disorders of the flap. In addition, as the dorsal venous

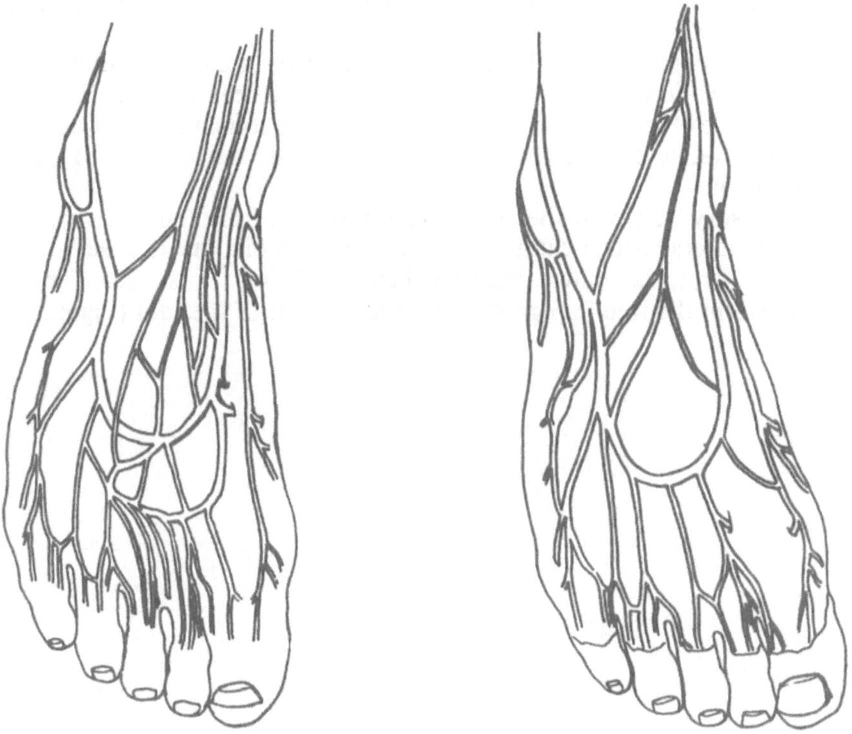

Figure 3.35 Patterns of the dorsal venous arch of the foot and the perforating tributaries

arch is absent in 1% of cases, the blood then returns through the venous network on the dorsum of the foot.

Since there is no valve within the dorsal venous arch, the blood can return in either direction. The outer diameters of the medial and the lateral ends of the venous arch are 2–3.3 mm and 1.2–2.2 mm respectively. The venous arch of the dorsum of the foot generally receives the first, second, third, and fourth dorsal metatarsal veins, each of which in turn receives in the proximal part of the web two or three neighbouring dorsal phalangeal veins including a small vein of the web. The dorsal phalangeal veins on the medial side of the great toe and the lateral side of the fifth toe return directly into the great and small saphenous veins respectively, or into either end of the dorsal venous arch. The medial dorsal phalangeal vein of the great toe is rather long. It is near the medial border of the dorsum of the foot. It would be best not to damage it while taking the flap of the dorsum of the foot together with the skin of the dorsum of the great toe.

In the middle of the dorsum of the foot there are still two or three smaller superficial veins, which communicate freely with one another and with the dorsal venous arch and the great and small saphenous veins. Owing to the absence of valves in these veins, the blood of the flap of the dorsum of the foot can also return to the great and small saphenous veins by way of them after transplantation.

The venae comitantes of the arteria dorsalis pedis are two in number. They accompany the deep plantar branches and drain the deep plantar tissues. Due to the existence of communications between the deep companion and superficial veins, these venae comitantes may be anastomosed accordingly to enhance venous return.

The sensory nerves of the flap of the dorsum of the foot are mainly the medial and lateral dorsal cutaneous nerves. The medial one is usually thicker than the lateral, its outer diameter being 1.9 mm. It is used for nerve anastomosis in the free flap grafting on the dorsum of the foot (Figure 3.36).

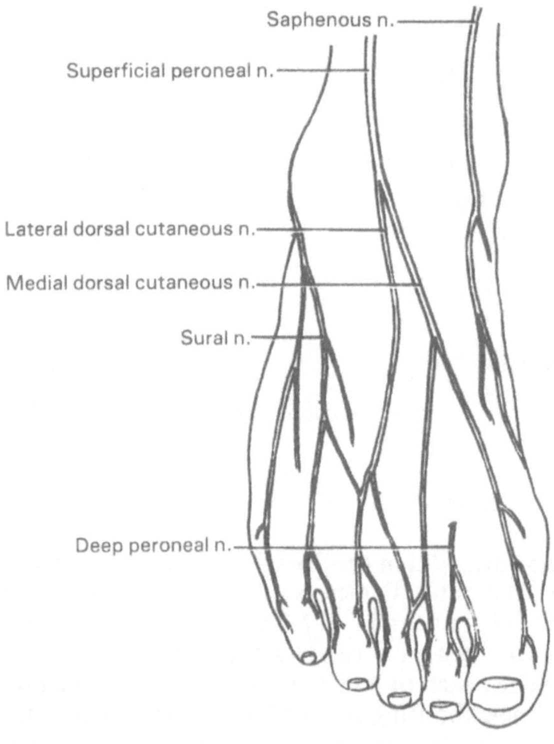

Figure 3.36 Cutaneous nerves of the dorsum of the foot

THE FIRST WEB FLAP OF THE FOOT

LUO LISHENG

The first web flap of the foot refers to the skin and subcutaneous tissue of the lateral part of the great toe and the medial part of the second together with the adjoining area. The flap lies concealed and no functional disorder will be left in the donor area after it has been excised. The skin is tender with rich subcutaneous fat, matching that of the hand in quality. The flap is provided with arteries, veins and sensory nerves suitable for anastomosis. It is thus often used for the repair of the skin defect of the finger pulp, the first web of the hand and the palm, with good results in external features, tenderness and sensation. It is generally an excellent donor of small flap.

Blood supply of the web flap

Arteries of the web flap

The first dorsal metatarsal artery has mainly been used as the vascular pedicle of the flap. It arises from the deep plantar branch of the arteria dorsalis pedis, running forward deeply or superficially through the first intermetatarsal space and accompanied by its venae comitantes. It gives off on the way several small branches to the interosseous muscles. Close to the metatarsophalangeal joint it divides into three phalangeal arteries, of which two medial ones are distributed separately to either border of the dorsal aspect of the great toe, a lateral one being distributed to the second toe. According to the deepness of the first dorsal metatarsal artery, it can be classified into three types, each of which will be described in detail in the section of Chapter 6 entitled 'Anatomy of Toe Transplantation for the Reconstruction of the Thumb'. Owing to the deep position of the first dorsal metatarsal artery in more than half of the cases, it is rather difficult to dissect the artery. However, since it always becomes superficial before reaching the first web, its terminal portion and the phalangeal arteries are easy to find by incising the skin over the transverse metatarsal ligament of the first and second metatarsal bones.

Though the outer diameter of the first dorsal metatarsal artery at its commencement measured from anatomical specimens is rather large (1.5–2.0 mm), its outer diameter measured at the point 1.0–1.5 cm distal to its origin is 0.8–1.0 mm. This is where the dissection in search for the artery stops in the taking of the first web flap of the foot. The first dorsal metararsal artery is 5–7 cm in length, which is enough for the operation, provided the length of a portion of the phalangeal artery and that of the web flap are included. If the length is not sufficient it has been suggested that the arteria dorsalis pedis could be used as the vascular pedicle. Nevertheless, we should be very cautious because this may add to the trauma of the dorsum of the foot, and the dissection of the deep branch of the arteria dorsalis pedis itself apears difficult.

Veins of the web flap

The veins of the web generally empty into the superficial venous system of the dorsum of the foot. On the lateral aspect of the great toe and the dorsomedial aspect of the second toe are observed thick dorsal phalangeal veins emptying into the dorsal metatarsal veins, which end in turn in the dorsal venous arch of the foot. In taking the web flap, either the dorsal metatarsal vein or the dorsal venous arch of the foot can be selected as the pedicle of the flap in accordance with the dimension of the recipient area. The outer diameter of the dorsal metatarsal vein at its termination is 1.5–2.0 mm. The deeply located venae comitantes of the first dorsal metatarsal artery are small in calibre, being unsuitable for vascular anastomosis.

Innervation of the web flap

The first web is innervated by the cutaneous branch of the deep peroneal nerve. In the dorsum of the foot the deep peroneal nerve accompanies the arteria dorsalis pedis, being lateral to the artery. At the posterior end of the intermetatarsal space the nerve crosses superficial to the artery to lie on the medial side of it. At the level of the transverse metatarsal ligament the deep peroneal nerve divides into the medial and lateral dorsal digital nerves which supply the adjacent borders of the great and second toes. The deep peroneal nerve is easy to find because of its superficial position. No matter whether the first dorsal metatarsal artery is superficially or deeply situated, the nerve is just beneath the skin.

The first web flap has a fine sensation. The acuity of the two-point discrimination of the first web flap is higher than that of the dorsum of the foot and averages 13 mm (11–16 mm) determined by various clinicians. That of the dorsum of the foot averages 30 mm (19–40 mm). Many authors held that the acuity of the two-point discrimination of the first web flap after being grafted to the hand may be markedly improved. This may be due to the acuity of sensation inherent to the skin of the hand and the increment in the receptor density around the regenerating nerve. We had a case in which the two-point discrimination of the first web before grafting was 11 mm, and it was improved to 6 mm 1 year after being transplanted to the finger pulp.

The extent of the flap to be taken

The size of the first web flap varies with individuals. In the adult the skin on the lateral side of the great toe that can be taken measures 3 × 5 cm to 4 × 6 cm, and that on the medial side of the second toe measures 2 × 4 cm to 3 × 5 cm. If a rather large flap is needed, the skin of the area between these two toes may be taken together. This may even include the skin on the dorsal and plantar aspects of the first web, the size of which may be from 5 × 10 cm to 7 × 12 cm. Buncke had reported a case of the first web flap in which the skin taken was up to 7.5 × 14 cm.

4

The applied anatomy of muscle and musculocutaneous flap transplantation

TAO YONGSONG AND ZHONG SHIZHEN

INTRODUCTION

A general survey of free muscular transplantation

The repairing of traumatic areas or the making up of tissue defects by means of muscle has roused the interest of surgeons for a long time. In 1889 Tubby took advantage of transferring the pronator teres for the replacement of the supinator. Later, the transfer of muscle with the neurovascular pedicle was used to replace disabled muscles or to repair defects of the soft tissue. However, this type of transferred muscle could not be used for remote parts because of the limitation in the length of the neurovascular pedicle, which led to the restriction of its practical application.

In 1970, Tamai first succeeded in carrying out free muscle transplantation by means of microneurovascular anastomosis. In 1971 Thompson performed the transplantation of free extensor digitorum brevis for the replacement of facial muscles. Again, in 1973, Harii carried out the gracilis graft with its overlying skin. In the same year the re-establishment of the flexion function of the hand by means of transplantation of the pectoralis major was successfully done in the Shanghai Sixth People's Hospital in China. The transplantation of the muscle or musculocutaneous flap by means of microneurovascular anastomosis is now extensively used.

Muscle flap

Principles for selecting the donor muscle

(1) The donor muscle must be free from any lesions.

(2) The donor muscle must not be indispensable functionally for fear that its resection should lead to definite functional disturbance.

(3) The muscle to be transplanted ought to be endowed with definite strength and size, and its position should be superficial so as to be easily dissected.

(4) The neurovascular pedicle of the donor muscle should be single or relatively concentrated. If the blood vessels are multiple, one of them should represent the large main vascular pedicle.

Characteristic features of the blood supply of muscles

(1) A muscle is an organ of active metabolism. It has profuse blood supply and is relatively sensitive and less tolerant to ischaemia. Intramuscular blood changes during ischaemia are most prominent, and these involve a decrease in blood pH and partial pressure of oxygen and an increase in partial pressure of carbon dioxide. As analysed by experiment, the pH value of the blood will decrease at room temperature from 7.40 to 7.19, the partial pressure of oxygen decreases from 45 to 20 mmHg, while that of carbon dioxide increases from 38 to 62 mmHg when the ischaemia of the limbs lasts 60 minutes. However the chemical composition of the blood recovers completely 5–10 minutes after the blood supply has been resumed. After the limb has been ischaemic for 90 minutes the blood pH will decrease to 7.04 and the partial pressure of oxygen to 10 mmHg, while that of carbon dioxide rises to 85 mmHg and it requires 10–15 minutes for these to recover to the normal state after the blood supply has been resumed. After 120 minutes of ischaemia of the limb the blood pH is reduced to 6.90, the partial pressure of oxygen reaches only 4 mmHg, and that of carbon dioxide rises to 104 mmHg, which leads to the lesion of the muscle fibres. If ischaemia continues degeneration and contracture of the muscle may ensue. Ischaemia for 6 hours will lead to muscular necroses. Therefore, when carrying out free transplantation of the muscle or musculocutaneous flap, we have to race against time, so that the period of ischaemia of muscle may not exceed 90 minutes lest the effect of transplantation should be altered. Temperature is closely connected with the rate of metabolism in muscle; lowering the temperature can retard the speed of changes within the muscles.

(2) The sources of blood supply of each muscle are usually multiple. They are from the neighbouring vascular stem or branches, and there are at least two sets of vessels for each muscle.

(3) Each muscle possesses one set of main vascular bundles for its blood supply, and there is rich anastomosis between it and other sources. Generally, the main vascular bundle enters the muscle in company with the nerves.

(4) The pattern of the vascular distribution of the muscle is related to its position and shape.

In case of broad muscles which originate from the trunk and insert to the limbs, e.g. the pectoralis major and the latissimus dorsi, there are generally two sets of vessels, of which one is the main set of longitudinal vessels, being relatively larger and distributed to the side of the muscle which is near the limb, while the other consists of segmental vessels, which are smaller and distributed separately to the medial portion of the muscle. The rectus abdominis includes an upper and a lower group of large vessels as well as many small segmental ones.

The muscles of deep layers of the trunks and most of the abdominal muscles usually have segmental blood supply but lack main vascular bundles.

The long muscles of the limb generally have a set of main vascular bundles, which gets into the muscle via the proximal end or the middle portion of the muscle, as do the gastrocnemius and the biceps brachii. In case of the lower extremity, some of the long muscles such as the sartorius and the gracilis have three or four vascular bundles of similar length and outer diameter. These vascular bundles are segmental in distribution. One or two sets of the bundles near the middle of the muscle are usually the main vascular bundles and appear slightly thicker.

The main vascular bundle of the muscles of the forearm and leg enters the muscle through its proximal end. As a rule, the muscle which is near the vessel often obtains some transverse branches from the vascular stem as the brachioradialis and the extensor carpi radialis.

(5) The site of entry of the vessel into the muscle takes the shape of a sulcus or a fissure, which can also be called the hilum of the muscle. The vessels and nerves often ramify into several small branches prior to their entrance into the muscle and are arranged linearly or in the form of a claw. Therefore, the site of entry of the vessels and nerves into the muscle frequently appears as a linear area.

The region through which the vessels get into the muscle is usually deep to the side near the vascular stem.

(6) From the standpoint of surgical manoeuvre, the methods of reaction of the vascular pedicle are quite flexible. One may directly resect the muscular branches as the pedicle, or may also cut the large branch or the arterial stem which gives off the muscular branches to make a composite pedicle, which includes one or several branches, e.g. the vascular pedicle of the musculocutaneous flap of the latissimus dorsi can be resected either from the dorsal thoracic vessels or much higher from the subscapular vessel; again, the vascular pedicle of the brachioradialis and the extensor carpi radialis longus can be resected either from the muscular branch of the radial artery or from the stem of the radial artery itself.

Characteristic features of the innervation of muscles

(1) Most of the muscles of the trunk, e.g. the intercostal and abdominal muscles and the deep muscles of the back, have multiple segmental nerve supplies, while others are of single innervation.

(2) The nerve of the muscle is more definite than its vessels in regard to the origin, course and site of entry into the muscle and has fewer variations.

(3) The nerve of the muscle often keeps company with the main vascular bundle and is consistent with the latter in the site of penetration into the muscle.

(4) The nerve distributed to the muscle is generally known as the muscular branch. It contains axons from the neurons in the anterior column of the spinal cord which maintain the tonus of the muscle and initiate muscular contraction. In addition, the muscular branch also contains the peripheral processes of the neurons in the spinal ganglia which are concerned with proprioceptive sensation as well as pain and temperature sensibilities. As a result, the muscular branch is pertaining to the mixed nerve. Some of the broad muscles of the trunk, e.g. the latissimus dorsi and the pectoralis major, have, in addition to the muscular branches of their own, cutaneous branches of segmental nerves emerging from the substance of the muscle. However, these cutaneous branches are not concerned with muscular movement and sensation.

Functions of the muscle

Strictly speaking, each muscle has generally more than two kinds of function, and any sort of joint movement is not accomplished by a single muscle, but is usually brought about by several muscles. It follows that the muscles involved in a joint movement may be classified as the prime movers, the synergists, the fixators and the antagonists. A muscle which is the prime mover of a type of movement of a joint can act as the synergist or even the antagonist for another movement. By reason of the synergic movement, after the resection of the prime mover, the functional movement of the joint can be compensated in part or largely by the synergist. Therefore, after the resection of a muscle of the body, except for some particular ones, it is not always necessary to have functional disturbances. This accounts for the possibilities of the muscles to be resected for muscular or musculocutaneous flap transplantation.

Musculocutaneous flap

The skin which covers the superficial surface of the muscle always receives nutrients from the musculocutaneous arteries. Therefore, as long as the vascular pedicle of the muscle is anastomosed, the muscle can be transplanted together with its overlying skin.

Musculocutaneous arteries are numerous minute branches which penetrate the substance of the muscle and enter the subcutaneous tissue separately and perpendicularly to be distributed to the skin. In addition there are some intermuscular cutaneous vessels entering the skin through the intermuscular connective tissue. The intermuscular cutaneous arteries arise frequently from the deep stem common to the adjacent musculocutaneous arteries and form again a network of anastomotic vessels in the subcutaneous tissue. Such an anatomical basis offers the possibility of widening the scope of supply of the musculocutaneous arteries. Clinical practice has proved that in the transplantation of musculocutaneous flaps by anastomosing the main vascular pedicle of the muscle, the area of the skin supplied by the arteries is always found much larger than the superficial area of the underlying muscle.

APPLIED ANATOMY OF THE THORACIC AND UPPER LIMB MUSCLES

TAO YONGSONG AND ZHONG SHIZHEN

Latissimus dorsi

Morphology

The latissimus dorsi, a triangular broad muscle, lies in the lumbodorsal as well as in the axillary region. The posterior layer of the lumbodorsal fascia serves as its origin and is attached to the spinous processes of the lower six thoracic, lumbar and sacral vertebrae, the supraspinous ligaments and the posterior portion of the iliac crest. The upper and anteroinferior parts of the muscular bundles are further attached to the inferior angle of the scapula and the lower three or four ribs.

The aponeurosis of the latissimus dorsi is narrow above and broad below with an average breadth of 50 mm and a thickness of 0.5 mm across its middle. The deep surface of the upper portion of the aponeurosis is fused to that of the serratus posterior inferior. The upper portion of the belly extends outward almost horizontally, covering up and encircling the teres major from behind. The middle and lower portions of the muscle direct upward and laterally and converge gradually to the insertion. The upper margin of the belly is 185 mm long, with a thickness of 4 mm at its mid-point. The inferior portion of the anterior margin is connected more or less closely with the external oblique muscle of the abdomen and the serratus anterior. Further upwards it is connected loosely with deep structures, from which it can be easily separated especially near the axilla. The upper portion of the anterior margin participates in the formation of the posterior axillary fold. The length of the anterior margin is 314 mm, with a thickness of 3 mm at its middle. The tendon of insertion is flat, covering up the tendon and part of the belly of the teres major anteroinferiorly and becoming inserted into the intertubercular sulcus. It is 41 mm long and 28 mm wide, fuses with that of the teres major for a length of 25 mm. The total length of the latissimus dorsi is about 300 mm.

Main neurovascular pedicle of the latissimus dorsi

The main neurovascular pedicle of the latissimus dorsi consists of the thoracodorsal vessels and nerve.

Thoracodorsal vessels

The thoracodorsal artery is the direct continuation of the subscapular artery and a few of them may come from the axillary artery or share a common stem with the lateral thoracic artery. The thoracodorsal artery passes downward across the teres major and then along the deep surface of the latissimus dorsi near its anterior border, and finally divides into a medial and a lateral branch to enter the muscle after giving off a constant branch to the serratus anterior and an inconstant one to the teres major. Accompanying the thoracodorsal artery are the thoracodorsal vein and nerve which are located respectively anteromedial and posterolateral to the artery. The artery is 81 mm long with an outer diameter of 2.4 mm. Mostly the vein is single, and if there are two companion veins they will combine into one near the subscapular vein. The point of termination of the vein is higher than the origin of the artery. The outer diameter of the vein is 4.0 mm. The point of entrance into the muscle of the lateral branch of the thoracodorsal artery is 72 mm from the end of the tendon, or 23 mm from the anterior border of the muscle. The part of the latissimus dorsi which is lateral to the scapular line and supplied by the thoracodorsal vessels represents two-thirds of the whole muscle (Figure 4.1).

The extramuscular length of the medial branch of the thoracodorsal artery is 21 mm, the outer diameter being 1.3 mm. The medial branch proceeds

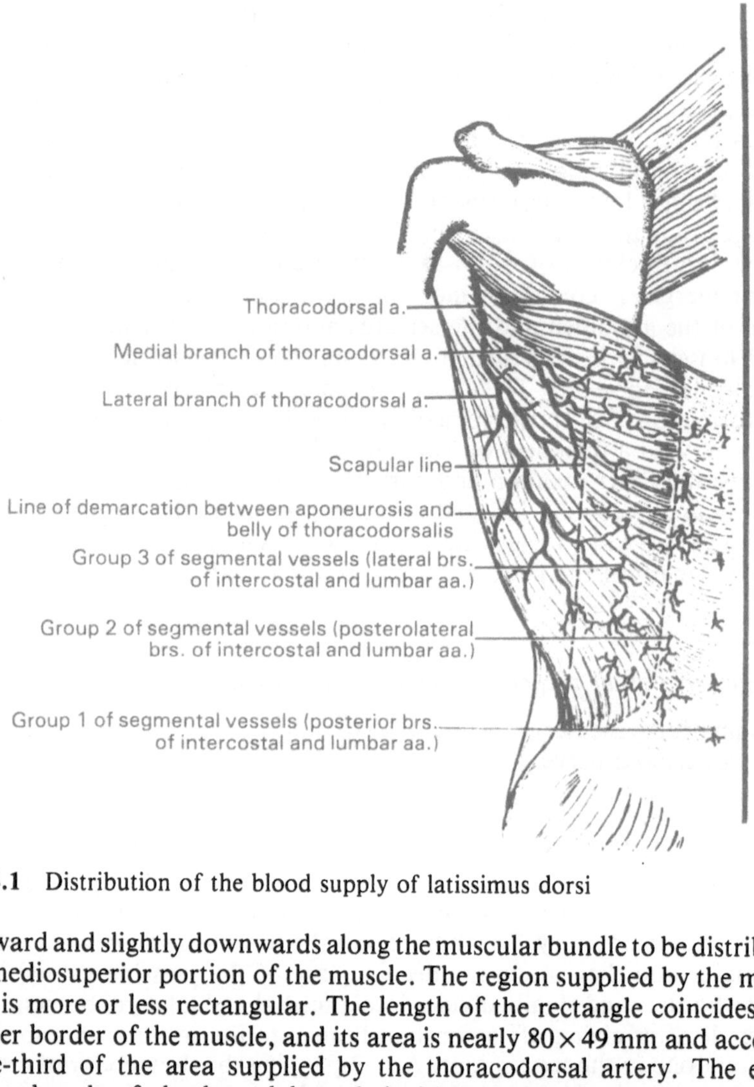

Figure 4.1 Distribution of the blood supply of latissimus dorsi

medialward and slightly downwards along the muscular bundle to be distributed to the mediosuperior portion of the muscle. The region supplied by the medial branch is more or less rectangular. The length of the rectangle coincides with the upper border of the muscle, and its area is nearly 80×49 mm and accounts for one-third of the area supplied by the thoracodorsal artery. The extramuscular length of the lateral branch is 24 mm, the outer diameter being 1.6 mm. The lateral branch proceeds downwards and slightly backward along the fascicles within the muscle and is distributed to a trapezoid area in the anteroinferior portion. The upper base of the trapezium is made by the insertion of the muscle, while the lower approaches the scapular line, the area of the trapezoid being $(33+96) \times 115 \div 2\,mm^2$. The medial and lateral branches usually give off some twigs to the insertion of the muscle prior to its entrance into the muscle. Sectioning these twigs may lengthen the extramuscular length of the medial and lateral branches. There are extensive anastomoses within the muscle among the twigs of the medial and lateral branches and between them and the segmental vessels, of which many can be observed with the naked eye. The outer diameter of these twigs at the site of anastomosis varies from 0.1 to 0.45 mm.

The thoracodorsal nerve

This nerve originates from the posterior cord of the brachial plexus and emerges from behind the axillary sheath. After descending for a certain distance, it accompanies the thoracodorsal vessel. Prior to its entrance to the muscle, the thoracodorsal nerve divides into the medial and lateral branches. The course and branching of these branches within the muscle keep pace with those of the medial and lateral branches of the thoracodorsal vessels. The resectable length of the nerve is 95 mm, the transverse diameter of the nerve being 2.1 mm.

The terminal end of the main neurovascular pedicle of the latissimus dorsi invariably divides into the medial and lateral branches, and their distribution within the muscle is quite definite. This affords a neurovascular pedicle for the resected muscle or musculocutaneous flap of the latissimus dorsi, thus increasing the number of chances to carry out various reconstruction operations, and, at the same time, maintaining functions of the donor area to some extent as well.

Other blood supplies of the latissimus dorsi

The latissimus dorsi is a muscle with multiple blood supplies. It has, in addition to the thoracodorsal artery and vein, three groups of segmental vessels and one descending branch of the transverse cervical artery for its blood supply, the latter being distributed to the upper portion of the muscle only.

The segmental vessels from the intercostal and lumbar vessels fall into three groups which are arranged longitudinally and are distributed to the aponeurosis and belly of the latissimus dorsi within the scapular line. The first group of segmental vessels, being near the posterior median line, comprises those posterior branches of the intercostal and lumbar arteries which are rather small and are distributed to the initial portion of the aponeurosis. The second group of vessels consists of posterolateral branches, which are slightly longer and more slender than those of the first group, emerging from between the spinalis and the longissimus thoracis 50–80 mm lateral to the posterior median line to be distributed to the initial portions of the aponeurosis and the muscular substance. The third group of vessels, being longer and thicker, comprises the lateral branches of the intercostal and lumbar arteries, which penetrate the intercostal space with the lateral cutaneous branches of the intercostal nerves 10 mm medial to the scapular line and incline downward and slightly laterally in the form of a claw to enter the muscular substance to be distributed along the muscular fascicles. Among the segmental vessels of these three groups are extensive anastomoses. Furthermore, there are thicker (0.1–0.45) anastomotic twigs between the vessels of the third group and the medial and lateral branches of the thoracodorsal artery.

Musculocutaneous vessels of the latissimus dorsi

Except for the skin near the axillary region which is supplied by the direct cutaneous arteries, the rest of the skin superficial to the latissimus dorsi is supplied by the musculocutaneous artery of the muscle. Both the medial and lateral branches of the thoracodorsal artery have many musculocutaneous arteries visible to the naked eye and distributed to the skin which overlies the muscle and is lateral to the scapular line. The musculocutaneous arteries, which are thicker near the insertion of the muscle, gradually become slender as they approach the scapular line. The three groups of segmental vessels, being the main blood supply of the skin of this region, penetrate the aponeurosis and muscular substance of the latissimus dorsi to be distributed to the skin within the scapular line. Moreover, the lateral cutaneous branches of the intercostal nerves are distributed to the skin in company with the segmental vessels of the third group.

The musculocutaneous vessels of the latissimus dorsi have profuse anastomoses and excellent collateral circulation in the muscular substance and the part superficial to it, but the anastomosis and collateral circulation are poor in the aponeurosis and the part overlying it. It follows that in the free transplantation of the musculocutaneous flap by means of the thoracodorsal vessels such as the pedicle, the skin overlying the muscle substance may survive quite well, while that on the superficial surface of the aponeurosis, especially near the median line and the lower part, is apt to undergo necroses.

Functions of the latissimus dorsi and the after-effects of its resection

The functions of the latissimus dorsi include the adduction, rotation and extension of the arm. When the arm is raised and fixed the latissimus dorsi, accompanied by the action of the pectoralis major, can draw the trunk upward. It can also draw the pelvis upward and forward. All of these functions are accomplished with the coöperation of other muscles, and resection of the latissimus dorsi will not lead to distinct functional disturbances.

Pectoralis major

Morphology

The pectoralis major is a fan-shaped, broad muscle situated in the anterior part of the chest. It can be divided into three parts according to its origins, viz., the clavicular, the sternocostal and the abdominal parts. The latter two may be grouped together to form the thoracoabdominal part.

Clavicular part of the pectoralis major

The muscular fibres of the pectoralis major take origin from the medial half of the clavicle. The belly inclines laterally and downward to be inserted into the anterior layer of its aponeurosis. The origin is 59 mm broad and 8 mm thick: the length of the belly is 123 mm; the insertion 48 mm in breadth and 7 mm in thickness. The superolateral border of the belly forms the deltopectoral sulcus with the anterior border of the deltoideus. Its lower border covers up the upper portion of the sternocostal part with traces of loose connective tissue and few blood vessels between them. Owing to a shallow sulcus visible superficially, these two parts are very easy to separate. However, the insertion fuses very tightly with the sternocostal part for a length of 34 mm. There is no natural boundary which can be used for the separation between the sternocostal and clavicular parts in about 5% of the specimens. The clavicular part is a strengthened mass with a definite length and thickness, suitable for functional reconstruction.

Thoracoabdominal part of the pectoralis major

Except for the origin, the sternocostal and abdominal parts have no natural boundary of separation. The thoracoabdominal part takes its origin from the lateral half of the sternum, the upper six costal cartilages and the anterior layer of the rectal sheath. The origin is 199 mm broad and 35 mm thick. The muscular fascicles of the upper part are situated almost horizontally and laterally to be inserted into the anterior layer of the tendon; those of the lower part incline gradually superolaterally to end in the posterior layer of the tendon. The upper margin, being covered up by the clavicular part, has a length of 152 mm, with a thickness of 5 mm at the mid-point; the lower border is 213 mm long and 6 mm thick at its middle. The belly gradually thickens as the insertion is approached. The muscular substance of the lower part, i.e. the abdominal part, is 20–40 mm broad and its medial three-quarters is parallel to the muscular fascicles of the sternocostal part, while the lateral one-quarter bends upward to reach the posterior aspect of the sternocostal part, shifting to the highest portion of the posterior layer of the tendon.

The tendon of insertion of the pectoralis major is flat and inserted onto the ridge of the greater tuberosity of the humerus and extends upward and downward to the greater tuberosity and the insertion of the deltoideus respectively. The length of the tendon of insertion (along the direction of the muscle fibres) is 36 mm, its breadth 55 mm and thickness 1.5 mm.

Main neurovascular pedicle of the pectoralis major (Figures 4.2–4.4)

The main neurovascular pedicle of the pectoralis major comes from the thoracoacromial artery and the pectoral branch of the axillary artery. The nerve to the pectoralis major comprises the lateral and medial thoracic nerves. The vessels and nerves of the pectoralis major are relatively complicated yet it is possible to discover a main neurovascular pedicle in each part, and the key is to give up those less important branches.

Main neurovascular pedicle of the clavicular part

The main vascular pedicle of the clavicular part is the deltoid branch of the thoracoacromial artery. The deltoid branch originates from the stem of the thoracoacromial artery, proceeds laterally into the deltopectoral sulcus and is distributed to the clavicular part by one or several branches which run into the deep surface of this part slightly lateral to its middle. The deltoid branch proceeds further laterally to be distributed to the muscle. The branch to the clavicular part often divides into a medial and a lateral branch prior to or after entry into the muscle. They proceed along the muscle fascicles and give off branches. The artery is 48 mm long measured from the origin of the deltoid branch to the site of its entrance into the muscle, and has an outer diameter of 1.9 mm. The veins are in company with the artery and a little thicker than it. The clavicular part also possesses veins emptying into the cephalic vein, which may be utilized as a vein for the vascular pedicle.

The nerve of the clavicular part is the clavicular branch of the lateral thoracic nerve, which arises as a short stem from the lateral cord of the brachial plexus. It usually consists of two, or rarely three, branches. One of the two branches is known as the clavicular branch of the lateral thoracic nerve and the other the upper pectoral branch of the lateral thoracic nerve. The clavicular branch makes its appearance above the terminal end of the cephalic vein, not in company with the deltoid branch of the thoracoacromial artery, and its entrance into the muscle is at the medial side of the vessel. The clavicular branch has a length of 43 mm and a transverse dimension of 1.6 mm.

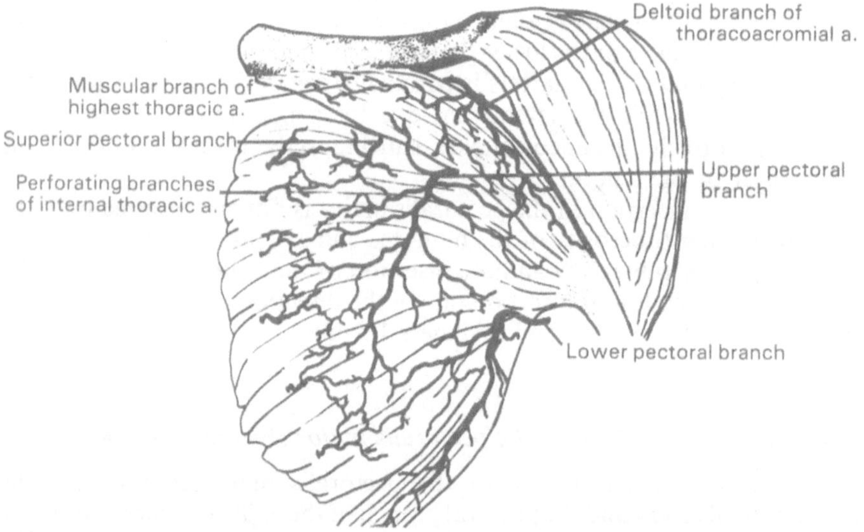

Figure 4.2 Distribution of the blood supply of the pectoralis major

Main neurovascular pedicle of the thoracocostal part

The main vascular pedicle of the thoracocostal part is the upper pectoral branch of the thoracoacromial artery. This branch passes over the upper border of the pectoralis minor after it arises from the stem of the thoracoacromial artery. It then goes medialward along the deep surface of the thoracocostal part and enters its middle part by means of two or three branches, which supply the lateral two-thirds of the muscle. The length of the upper pectoral branch is 80 mm, its outer diameter being 1.8 mm. The veins accompany the artery and are slightly thicker. Most of them empty into the axillary vein.

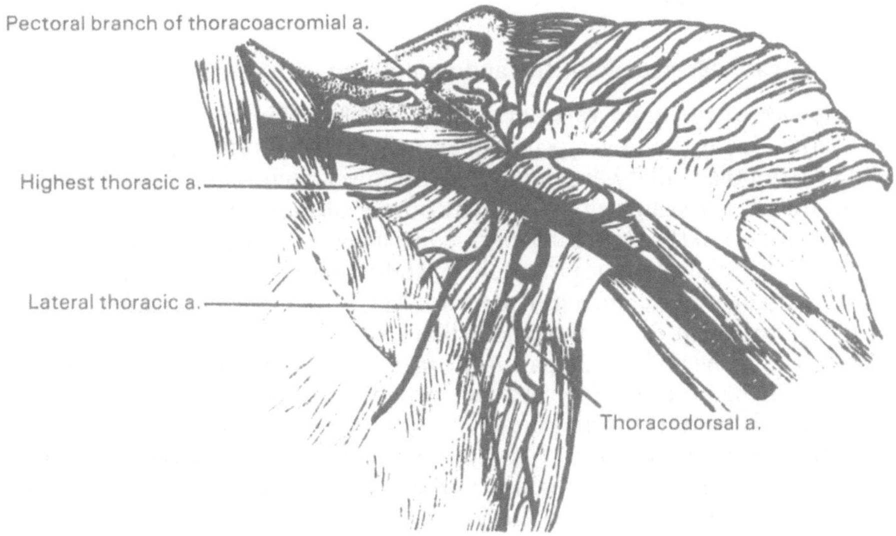

Figure 4.3 Main arteries of the latissimus dorsi and pectoralis major

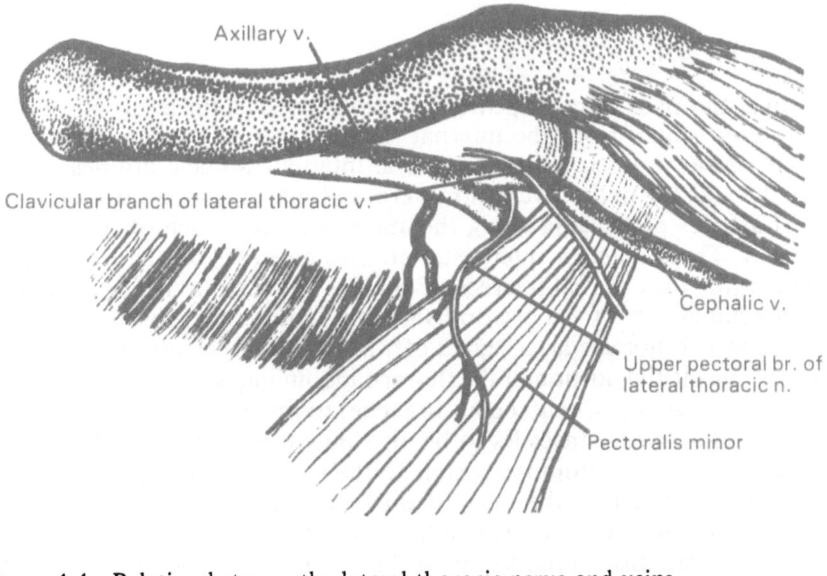

Figure 4.4 Relation between the lateral thoracic nerve and veins

The nerve of the thoracocostal part is the upper pectoral branch of the lateral thoracic nerve, which becomes visible between the cephalic and axillary veins. A few of them make their appearance above the terminal end of the cephalic vein together with the clavicular branch. The nerve is accompanied by the upper pectoral branch of the thoracoacromial artery and divides into two branches to get into the muscle. The nerve itself has a length of 78 mm and a transverse dimension of 1.4 mm.

Main neurovascular pedicle of the abdominal part

The incidence of the main vascular pedicle is 79%. The artery of the pedicle comes either from the lower pectoral branch of the thoracoacromial artery (36%) or from the axillary artery (43%). The lower pectoral branches proceed medialward after passing below the lower border of the pectoralis minor to get to the deep aspect of the abdominal part, while a few of them penetrate the lower portion of the pectoralis minor to reach the abdominal part. The artery is 77 mm in length with an outer diameter of 1.6 mm. The veins are in company with the artery; most of them empty into the axillary vein.

The nerve of the abdominal part is the medial pectoral nerve which emerges from between the axillary artery and vein, proceeding medially to be distributed to the pectoralis minor, the abdominal part of the pectoralis major and a portion of the thoracocostal part. Mostly, the medial pectoral nerve passes the lower border of the pectoralis minor and accompanies the vessels, but a few (35%) do not, but pass through the pectoralis minor to reach the abdominal part. The nerve is 73 mm long with a transverse diameter of 1.2 mm. The entrance of the vessels and nerve into the muscle is at the junction of the lateral and middle thirds of the abdominal part near the lower border.

Other blood supplies of the pectoralis major

In addition to the main vascular pedicle mentioned above, the pectoralis major gains its blood supply from the internal thoracic artery, the upper pectoral artery, the lateral thoracic artery, etc. The internal thoracic arteries, while travelling through the upper five or six intercostal spaces, give off two anterior intercostal arteries proceeding along the anterior part of each of these intercostal spaces. These anterior intercostal arteries give off, on the way, many twigs penetrating the external intercostal muscles and membranes to get to the thoracoabdominal part of the pectoralis major. In the upper five to six interspaces the internal thoracic artery gives off, in addition, perforating branches anteriorly to the medial portion of the thoracoabdominal part. The perforating branches, besides giving off cutaneous branches to the overlying skin, proceed laterally along the muscle fascicles to be distributed to the thoracoabdominal part. There are many anastomoses visible to the naked eye between their ends and the pectoral branches, the outer diameters of the vessels at the site of anastomosis being 0.1–0.4 mm. The anterior intercostal arteries and the perforating arteries are distributed to the medial third of the pectoralis major.

Musculocutaneous vessels of the pectoralis major

In addition to the blood supply from the perforating branches of the internal thoracic artery and the direct cutaneous arteries of the thoracoacromial artery, the skin overlying the pectoralis major is supplied by musculocutaneous branches from the pectoralis major. These branches penetrate the muscular substance of the pectoralis major and are distributed evenly to the skin. Many of them are visible to the naked eye.

Function of the pectoralis major

The main function of the pectoralis major consists of adduction and medial rotation of the arm. The clavicular part aids the anterior part of the deltoideus in the flexion of arm. After the arm has been raised the pectoralis major, joined by the latissimus dorsi, can draw the arm downward or raise the trunk. These actions of the pectoralis major are accomplished through the synergic actions of the deltoideus, the latissimus dorsi and muscle of the shoulder and arm. Resection of the pectoralis major, either a part or the whole of it, may not lead to obvious functional disturbances, provided that compensation by other muscles is available.

Biceps brachii

Reports on the clinical applications of the biceps brachii are not yet available. However, it is qualified to be a kind of muscular donor.

Morphology

The biceps brachii, being a long, spindle-shaped muscle, is situated in the anterior part of the arm and provided with two heads of origin.

The long head of the biceps brachii is lateral and a little posterior to the short head. It arises by a long narrow tendon from the supraglenoid tubercle of the scapula and passes in between two layers of shoulder joint, where it is wrapped by the synovial membrane and arches over the head of the humerus. Then it emerges from the interval between the greater and lesser tuberosities of the humerus, carrying with it a part of the synovial membrane to form a tubular sheath in the intertubercular sulcus. The length of the tendon, measured from the upper margin of the greater or lesser tuberosity, is 69 mm with a width of 9 mm and a thickness of 3 mm in the lower part. The muscular belly is 167 mm long with a breadth of 17 mm and a thickness of 13 mm in its middle part.

The short head of the biceps brachii is situated medially and slightly anteriorly and arises by muscular substance and flattened tendon from the apex of the coracoid process in common with the coracobrachialis, with which it fuses for a length of 64 mm. The tendon embraces the muscular substance from the lateral side, gradually gets thinner downwards and disappears from the anterior surface of the muscle. The belly measures, from the origin to the insertion, 225 mm in length with a width of 21 mm and a thickness of 10 mm at its middle.

The short and long heads unite to form a 51 mm long belly at the lower part of the muscle. There is only loose connective tissue and small vascular branches connecting the two heads above the union, so that they are easy to separate. The belly transfers downward to become the tendon and aponeurosis of biceps brachii. The tendon of the biceps brachii is shaped like a flattened cord and is inserted into the posterior part of the radial tuberosity inferolaterally. The tendon is 17 mm long, the width of its terminal part being 11 mm and its thickness 2.5 mm. The lacertus fibrosus is a thin layer of aponeurosis which diverges from the tendon downward and medially. It is about 35–40 mm in length, with a narrow beginning and a broad end which fuses with the deep fascia of the anterior aspect of the forearm.

Main neurovascular pedicle of the biceps brachii

The main neurovascular pedicle of the biceps brachii is the short stem given off by the brachial artery medially as the latter passes the middle of the muscle. This stem is 10–20 mm long and divides beneath the short head into two branches which enter the bellies of the long and short heads respectively, constituting their main vascular pedicles. The nerve to the biceps brachii is the musculocutaneous nerve, which proceeds deep to the biceps after penetrating the coracobrachialis and giving off branches to the bellies of the long and short heads (Figure 4.5).

Main neurovascular pedicle of the long head of the biceps brachii

The artery of the pedicle is given off by the short stem of the brachial artery. It passes deep to the short head and divides beneath the long head into an upper and a lower branch to get to the muscle. The artery is 28 mm long. Those with a length of more than 25 mm account for 70% of the cases. The outer diameter is 1.8 mm. The vein accompanies the artery and is mostly single and slightly larger than the artery. The point of entry of the vessels into the muscle is 140 mm away from the coracoid process. The nerve to the long head of the biceps brachii is situated deep to the belly and proceeds obliquely from above inferolaterally, not in company with the vessels. The nerve is 31 mm long with a transverse dimension of 1.4 mm and the entrance of the nerve into the muscle is near that of the vessels.

Main neurovascular pedicle of the short head of the biceps brachii

The artery of the pedicle arises mostly from a stem common to that of the long head. It is 33 mm long, and those with a length of more than 25 mm account for 88%, the outer diameter being 1.7 mm. The vein, mostly single, accompanies the artery and appears larger. The entrance of the artery into the muscle is at the middle of the muscle, being 134 mm from the coracoid process.

The nerve to the short head of the biceps brachii is deep to the belly, not in company with the vessels. The nerve is 24 mm long with a transverse dimension of 1.3 mm. The entrance of the nerve into the muscle is in the environ of that of the vessel.

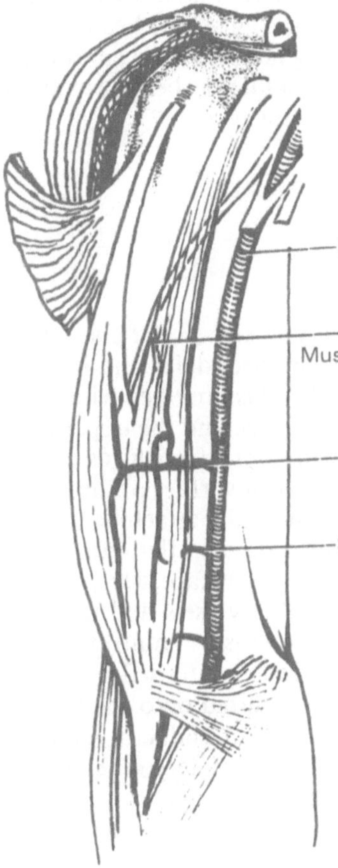

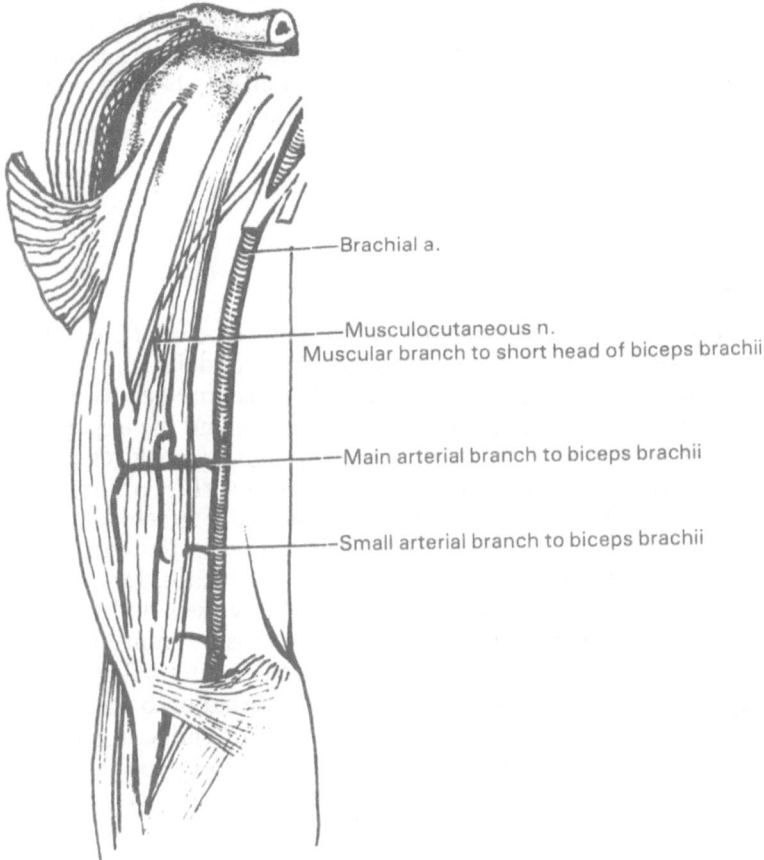

Figure 4.5 Arteries and nerves of the biceps brachii

Moreover, there are also some indefinite twigs to the muscle through both ends and the belly.

Function of the biceps brachii and the effect after its resection

The biceps brachii is chiefly a muscle for the flexion of the elbow and the supination of the forearm. Besides, the short head also takes part in the flexion and slight adduction of the arm, and the long head can draw the head of the humerus tightly to the glenoid cavity to prevent the head from upward dislocation and hence play an important role in increasing the stability of the shoulder joint. Resection of the biceps brachii as a whole must cause serious damage to the flexion of the elbow and supination of the forearm, and resection of the long head alone must in some ways disturb the stability of the shoulder joint. Excision, however, of the short head of the biceps brachii may not lead to definite disturbance in the flexion of the elbow and supination because of the compensation made by the branchialis, the supinator and muscles of the superficial layer of the anterior group of the forearm. The short head of the biceps brachii, which is more superficial than the long head and has an extensive area of contact with the subcutaneous tissue and the skin, may be used as an excellent donor of the muscle and musculocutaneous flaps.

Brachioradialis

Morphology

The brachioradialis is situated anterolaterally in the superficial layer of the forearm. The belly may be divided into the supracondylar and infracondylar parts. The former appears as pyramid-shaped and is provided with the medial, lateral and posterior surfaces. The posterior surface and the upper part of the lateral surface have their attachments on the proximal two-thirds of the lateral supracondylar ridge of the humerus and the anterior surface of the lateral intermuscular septum of the arm. The length of the muscular attachment on the bone is 50 mm. The infracondylar part of the belly appears flattened and can be divided into an anterolateral and a posteromedial surface. Deep to the infracondylar part are the vascular stem of the radial vessels and the superficial branch of the radial nerve. The belly as a whole is 219 mm long, 24 mm in breadth and 6 mm in thickness. The muscle transfers to a flat and cord-like tendon at the middle of the forearm, which is inserted onto the lateral aspect of the styloid process of the radius. The tendons of the abductor hallucis longus and the extensor hallucis brevis cross obliquely superficial to the tendon of the brachioradialis, while the radial vessels and the superficial branch of the radial nerve wind to its dorsal aspect. The tendon is 99 mm long, and the origin is 12 mm in breadth and 1 mm in thickness.

Main neurovascular pedicle of the brachioradialis

The brachioradialis has two sets of main vascular pedicles (Figure 4.6).

The first set of the main vascular pedicle

These are called the radial collateral vessels. They are the terminal branches of the direct continuation of the deep brachial artery, which pass to the lateral head of the triceps brachii and divide into anterior and posterior branches below the insertion of the deltoideus. The anterior branch penetrates the lateral intermuscular septum of the arm, in company with the radial nerve between the brachialis and the brachioradialis where it gives off a variable number of twigs, which are distributed to the brachialis and the brachioradialis and anastomose with the radial recurrent artery. The posterior branch descends along the posterior surface of the lateral intermuscular septum of the arm to the elbow. In addition to the branches distributed to the skin of the lower part of the arm and the upper part of the lateral aspect of the forearm, it also gives off larger

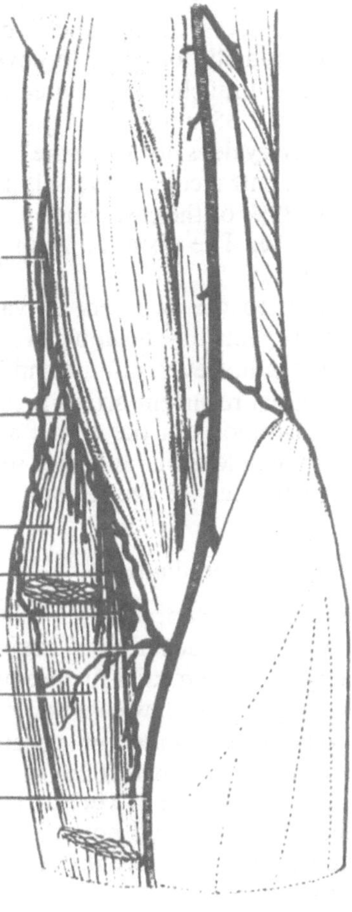

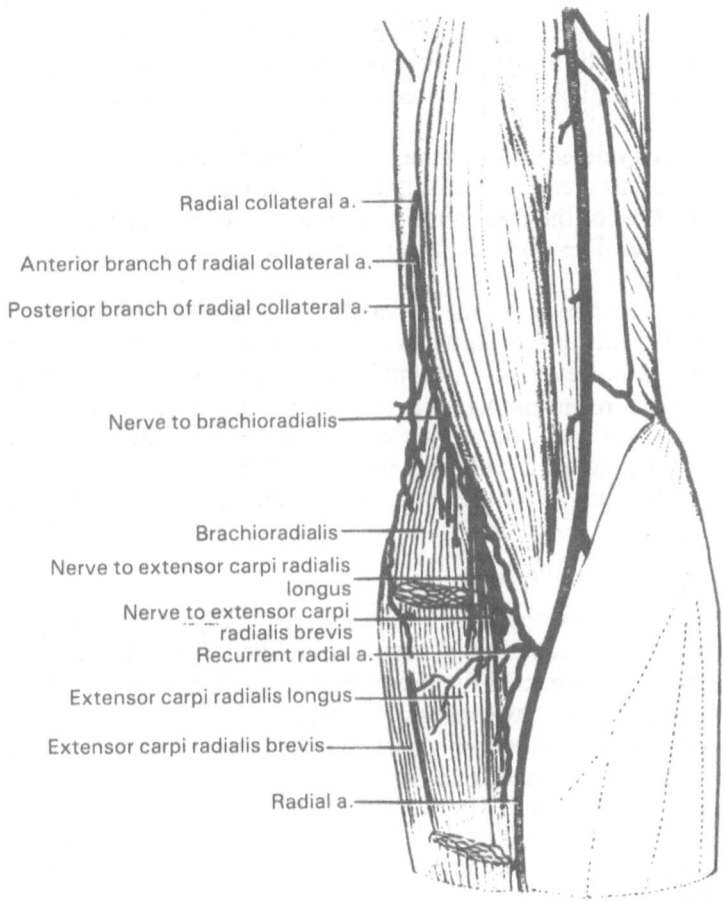

Figure 4.6 Vessels and nerves of the brachioradialis and the extensor carpi radialis

twigs which penetrate the lateral intermuscular septum of the arm to get to the brachioradialis and the extensor carpi radialis longus to constitute the first set of main vascular pedicle of these two muscles. The entrance of the artery into the muscle is 58 mm above the lateral epicondyle. From the entrance upward, the arterial trunk, which can be dissected free, is 48 mm long with an outer diameter of 1.3 mm. The vena comitans is mostly single and larger.

The second set of the main vascular pedicle

Most of the vessels are the branches of the radial recurrent artery and account for 75% of the cases. A few of them are the branches from the stem of the radial artery. The radial recurrent artery is a short stem with plexiform branching, which divides into the ascending, transverse and descending branches distributed to the muscles on the radial side of the forearm. The ascending and descending branches are the more definite. The former ascends along the radial nerve and, besides having anastomosis with the anterior branch of the radial collateral artery, gives rise to branches distributed to the brachioradialis and the extensor carpi radialis longus. Moreover, the radial recurrent artery also possesses transverse branches distributed to these two muscles. The length of the recurrent artery is 38 mm with an outer diameter of 1.8 mm. The vein accompanying the artery does not form the recurrent vein and empties into the radial vein alone. The entrance of the vessels into the muscle is 30 mm above the lateral epicondyle in 39% of the cases and just at the level of the lateral epicondyle or below it in 61%. The distance from the entrance to the lateral epicondyle averages 25 mm.

In addition to the two sets of vascular pedicles mentioned above, the brachioradialis gains blood supply from the transverse branches of the radial artery. They are, however, minute and indefinite. Considering the fact that the stem of the radial recurrent artery is too short to be resected and that there is sufficient anastomosis in the elbow and hand between the radial and ulnar arteries, it is possible to cut an upper segment of the radial artery including the radial recurrent artery as the second set of the main vascular pedicles.

Nerve to the brachioradialis

The nerve to the brachioradialis, which is given off by the radial nerve while passing between the brachialis and the brachioradialis, proceeds downward and slightly laterally to the medial surface or border of the muscle. In 85% of cases the nerve is single, and a few consist of a couple of nerves. The latter, however, turns out to be single, as the lower branch after being dissected upward will at length unite with the upper. The nerve is 25 mm in length with a transverse dimension of less than 1 mm. They do not accompany the artery and their points of entry into the muscle do not coincide. The entrance of the nerve into the muscle is mostly 15 mm above the lateral epicondyle, accounting for 75%, and a few are 16 mm below it.

Function of the brachioradialis and the effect after its resection

The function of the brachioradialis is to assist in the flexion of the elbow joint and to check the excess in pronation or supination of the forearm. This, however, is supplementary, as its resection will not affect the function of the forearm due to compensation made by the synergists.

Extensor carpi radialis longus

Morphology

The extensor carpi radialis longus is situated in the superficial layer on the lateral side of the posterior aspect of the forearm, and its belly is partially covered up by the brachioradialis. It takes its origin by muscular substance from the distal one-third of the lateral epicondylar ridge of the humerus, the anterior aspect of the lateral intermuscular septum of the arm, and the common extensor tendon of the forearm. The belly is flat, being 129 mm long, 24 mm wide at its middle and 11 mm thick. It becomes tendinous at the junction of the upper and middle thirds of the forearm and is inserted onto the dorsal surface of the base of the second metacarpus. The length of tendon is 162 mm, the width of the origin 12 mm, and the thickness 1.5 mm.

Main neurovascular pedicle of the extensor carpi radialis longus

The main vascular pedicle of the extensor carpi radialis longus is basically like that of the brachioradialis (Figure 4.6).

The first set of the main vascular pedicle

This is the posterior branch of the radial collateral artery of the deep brachial. This branch descends along the posterior surface of the lateral intermuscular septum of the arm, sending one or two branches to the lateral aspect of the supracondylar part of the muscle after giving off branches to the brachioradialis. The artery is 71 mm long, with an outer diameter of 1.3 mm. The entrance of the artery into the muscle is 36 mm above the lateral epicondyle. The vein is mostly single with an outer diameter slightly greater than that of the artery.

The second set of the main vascular pedicle

This comes from the ascending branch of the radial recurrent artery. The ascending branch sends a large branch to the medial border or aspect of the supracondylar part of the muscle before giving off branches to the brachioradialis and anastomosing with the anterior branches of the radial collateral artery. The artery of the second set is 38 mm long with an outer diameter of 2.0 mm. There are one or two venae comitantes, but mostly single with an outer diameter slightly greater than that of the artery. The entrance of the vessels into the muscle is 17 mm above the lateral epicondyle in 32%; and at the level of or 21 mm below the epicondyle in 68%.

The extensor carpi radialis longus gains, in addition, several small branches from the stem of the radial artery. It is not easy to make its resection because of the shortness of the radial recurrent artery. Nevertheless, owing to the presence of adequate anastomosis between the radial and ulnar arteries, it is also advisable to resect the upper segment of the radial artery, including the stem of the radial recurrent, as the main vascular pedicle.

The nerve of the extensor carpi radialis longus

This comes from the lower end of the stem of the radial nerve. The entrance of the nerve accounts for 19%. The nerve does not accompany the main vascular pedicle. It is 32 mm long with a transverse diameter of 1 mm. The entrance of the nerve into the medial aspect of the muscle is 12 mm above the lateral epicondyle in 21%, and the level of, or 14 mm below, the epicondyle in 79%.

In addition to extension of the wrist, the extensor carpi radialis longus can also act synergically with the flexor carpi radialis in the abduction of the hand.

Extensor carpi radialis brevis

Morphology

The extensor carpi radialis brevis is situated deep and a little lateral to the long extensor and covered medially by the extensors of the fingers. It follows that only a small spindle-shaped area of the muscle is in contact with the subcutaneous tissue and the skin. It takes its origin by muscular attachment from the lateral epicondyle of the humerus, the radial collateral ligament of the elbow joint and the intermuscular septum. The belly is 148 mm long, 25 mm wide and 12 mm thick. Its upper part fuses with the belly of the long extensor for a length of about 50 mm. The tendon measures 141 mm in length, 12 mm in width and 2 mm in thickness. It is overlapped by that of the long extensor and is connected with the latter by loose connective tissue. Both tendons pass deep to those of the abductor pollicis longus and the extensor pollicis brevis and the extensor retinaculum to be inserted onto the dorsal surface of the base of the third metacarpus.

Main neurovascular pedicle of the extensor carpi radialis brevis (Figure 4.6)

Main vascular pedicle of the extensor carpi radialis brevis

The artery of the vascular pedicle comes mainly from the descending branch of the radial recurrent artery (69%) and secondarily from the transverse branch of the radial artery. The descending branch is directed downward for some distance along the medial border of the muscle before entering it. The artery is 33 mm long with an outer diameter of 1.8 mm. The vein is mostly single and slightly larger than the artery. The entrance of the artery into the muscle is 58 mm below the lateral epicondyle. In addition to the main vascular pedicle, the extensor carpi radialis brevis gains some small branches from the stem of the radial artery and the dorsal interosseous artery. Owing to the fact that nearly 30% of the vascular pedicles originate from the stem of the radial artery, it is advisable to make the resection of the pedicle from the upper part of the stem.

Nerve to the extensor carpi radialis brevis

The nerve to the muscle is given off by the deep branch of the radial nerve prior to its penetration through the supinator. It passes through or deep to the branches of the radial recurrent artery and then accompanies the descending branch of the recurrent artery to the muscle. It is 48 mm long with a transverse dimension of 1 mm. The entrance of the nerve coincides with that of the vessels.

The extensors carpi radialis brevis and longus

These are identical in function. Owing to the close contact of these two muscles it is possible to make a conjoint muscle or musculocutaneous flap for transplantation. Similarly, the extensor carpi radialis longus may be made into a conjoint muscle or a musculocutaneous flap with the brachioradialis. The extensor carpi radialis brevis, however, is not suitable to be made into a musculocutaneous flap alone.

APPLIED ANATOMY OF THE LOWER LIMB MUSCLES

WANG QIHUA, LIN ZHENGYAN AND HUANG HONGJUN

Rectus femoris

Morphology

The rectus femoris, being a typical bipennate muscle and a part of the quadriceps femoris, is situated anteriorly along the midline of the thigh. It arises by a straight head and a reflected one from the anterior inferior iliac spine and the shallow groove above the brim of the acetabulum respectively. The two heads unite at an acute angle into a round tendon which is 38 mm in length and gradually becomes muscular fibres. Most of the muscles are provided with a prominent aponeurotic lamina on the deep surface which occupies the distal three-quarters of the muscle and narrows inferiorly into a tendinous fascicle of moderate thickness, uniting with the vastus medialis and lateralis to a considerable extent and subsequently inserting onto the base and either border of the patella. Some of the fibres pass over the patella to continue as the ligamentum patellae, which is inserted to the tubercle of the tibia.

The total length of the rectus femoris averages 377 mm, the belly being 287 mm and the tendon of insertion 69 mm. The widest portion of the belly, which resides 168 mm below the anterior superior iliac spine, is 38 mm in breadth and 11 mm in thickness. It is 17 mm wide and 9 mm thick at the site 60 mm below the anterior inferior iliac spine, and 17 mm wide and 7 mm thick at the site 100 mm above the upper border of the patella. The distance from the apex of the patella to the tubercle of the tibia, i.e. the length of ligamentum patellae, amounts to 42 mm, while at its mid-point the ligament is 20 mm in breadth.

Main neurovascular pedicle (Figure 4.7)

The neurovascular pedicle of the muscle flap comprises the rectus femoris branch of the descending branch of the lateral circumflex femoral artery and the branches of the femoral nerve.

The rectus femoris branch of the descending branch of the lateral circumflex femoral artery

This is the main nutrient artery of relatively constant incidence (66%). Its outer diameter is 2.5 mm and the extramuscular length is 38 mm. The main vessel constantly passes along the medial border of the rectus femoris where it enters the muscle 159 mm below the anterior superior iliac spine. After entering the muscle the main vessel descends in the direction of the longitudinal axis of the muscle fibres and gives off 7–18 branches from either side alternately, which are rarely symmetrical, the interval between the branches being 6–12 mm. The neurovascular pedicle is formed by the artery, vein and the branches of the femoral nerve. Owing to the fact that the fine branches have been given off prior to their entry into the muscle, and the artery and vein do not penetrate at the same point, the 'neurovascular door', through which the neurovascular bundle passes, does not appear as a point but is really a sort of linear area with a length of about 17 mm from above downwards.

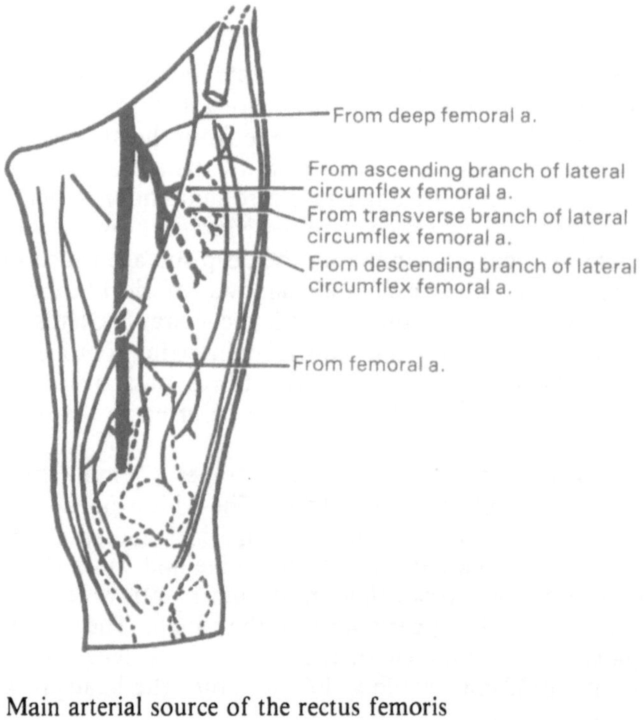

Figure 4.7 Main arterial source of the rectus femoris

The descending branch of the lateral circumflex femoral artery proceeds downwards and laterally deep to the rectus femoris and gives off regularly two or three tiny musculocutaneous branches to the rectus femoris and the overlying skin through the lateral border of the muscle. These vessels should be prevented from being injured during the taking of the musculocutaneous flap of the rectus femoris muscle. The accompanying vein is mostly single, its outer diameter being 3.4 mm and larger than the companion artery.

The rectus femoris branch of the femoral nerve

The nerve to the rectus femoris arises from the femoral nerve in the femoral triangle, 29 mm below the inguinal ligament. It is mostly a single stem (92%) and consists of two stems only in a few cases (8%). In the case of a single stem in 43% the nerve shares a common stem with other muscular branches, e.g. sartorius branch, vastus medialis branch, vastus lateralis branch or the anterior cutaneous nerve of the thigh. The numbers of rectus femoris nerves varies from two to five, and the two-branch pattern accounts for 58% of cases. The length of the nerve prior to branching is 41 mm with a calibre of 2 mm. They accompany the branchlets of the descending branch of the lateral circumflex femoral artery into the muscle constantly.

Other sources of blood supply

In addition to the descending branch of the lateral circumflex femoral artery, which is the main nutrient artery of the rectus femoris, there are four groups of vessels, viz. the femoral and deep femoral arteries and the ascending and transverse branches of the lateral circumflex femoral artery. Those from the ascending and transverse branches of the lateral circumflex femoral artery, the initial portion of the deep femoral artery and the rectus femoris branches of the lateral circumflex femoral artery are the more common of the neurovascular bundles in the upper fourth area of the rectus femoris muscle. Most of them get into the muscle through its deep surface, the site of entrance bing 80 mm from the anterior superior iliac spine. Those with an outer diameter of more than 2 mm represent 31%. The extramuscular length of the artery is 21 mm. The companion vein is of the same length as the artery and is mostly single. The outer diameter of the vein is usually smaller than that of the artery.

Essentials of applied anatomy

(1) The rectus femoris is the only head of the quadriceps femoris that is attached to the hip bone. Its function is concerned with the flexion of the hip and the extension of the leg. However, since the iliopsoas is the prime mover for the flexion of the hip and the other heads of the quadriceps take part in the extension of the leg, excision of the rectus femoris leaves no apparent functional defect. Moreover, the superficial position of the rectus femoris and the trace variations of its neurovascular bundle make it a choice for the muscle or musculocutaneous flap.

(2) The origin, course, outer diameter, length and companion veins and nerves of the main neurovascular bundle, constituted chiefly by the descending branch of the lateral circumflex femoral artery, remain rather constant. Hence, such a bundle is of the first choice for muscle transplantation.

(3) The nerve to the rectus femoris from the femoral nerve is often single and frequently shares a common stem with other muscular branches, which should not be injured during the management of the nerve to the rectus femoris.

Sartorius

Morphology

The sartorius, being the longest muscle in the body, arises from the anterior superior iliac spine by means of an inconspicuous short tendon. The muscle fibres pass obliquely from the upper lateral to the lower medial part of the thigh, reaching the back of the adductor tubercle of the femur to form a thin, flattened tendon 25 mm below the apex of the patella. The tendon is 59 mm long and is superficial to that of the gracilis muscle. It is inserted into the upper part of the medial surface of the shaft of the tibia after forming a goose pad with the semitendinosus tendon.

The whole muscle is narrow and ribbon-like from above downwards with an average length of 523 mm, the belly being 464 mm in length, 25 mm in width and 5 mm in thickness measured at the site 100 mm below the anterior superior iliac spine.

Main neurovascular pedicle (Figure 4.8)

The arterial supply of the sartorius displays a distinct segmentation from above downwards. The upper segment of the muscle, which resides in the femoral triangle, is supplied by the deep femoral artery, the lateral circumflex femoral artery or its descending branch and the branches from the proximal portion of

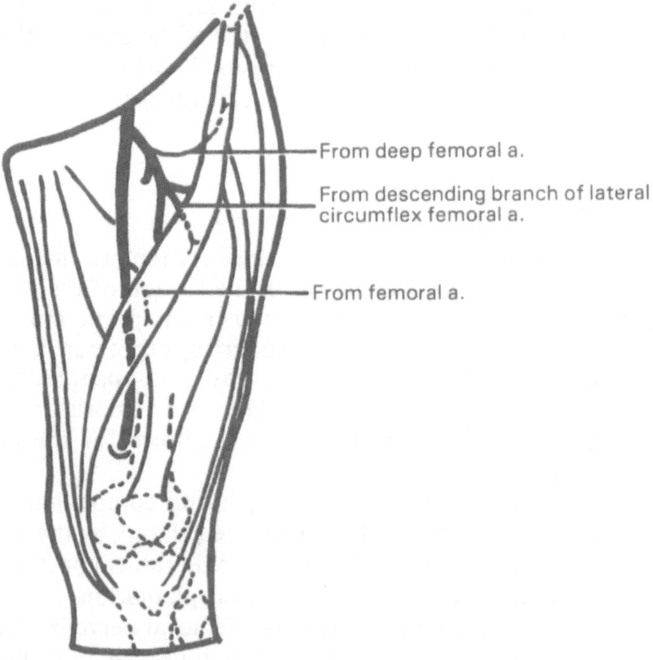

Figure 4.8 Main arterial supply of the sartorius

the femoral artery. The outer diameter of the arteries to the proximal portion of the sartorius is larger than that of the arteries to the distal portion, and the former have been thought to be the main vessels to the muscle and to form the neurovascular pedicle with the sartorius branches of the femoral nerve.

(1) The sartorius branches of the deep femoral artery arise from the deep femoral in the femoral triangle 98 mm below the anterior superior iliac spine. It ascends obliquely and laterally in front of or behind the branches of the femoral nerve or through them to enter the medial border of muscle. Its outer diameter is 1.3 mm and the extramuscular length 18 mm. In more than half of cases the artery has a couple of companion veins, the outer diameters of which are 1.7 and 1.4 mm respectively. Some have only one companion vein with an outer diameter of 1.9 mm. The vessels form a neurovascular pedicle to the muscle with the sartorius branches of the femoral nerve.

(2) The sartorius branch of the descending artery of the lateral circumflex femoral artery also arises in the femoral triangle 102 mm below the anterior superior iliac spine. It proceeds laterally or inferolaterally in front of or behind the femoral nerve to enter the muscle deep to its medial border. The outer diameter of the sartorius branch is 1.3 mm, the extramuscular length being 18 mm. There are mostly two companion veins for each artery. A neurovascular pedicle to the muscle is formed with the relatively constant sartorius branch of the femoral nerve.

(3) The sartorius branch arises directly from the lateral or anterolateral wall of the proximal segment of the femoral artery about 179 (25–275) mm below the anterior superior iliac spine. Its outer diameter is 1.3 mm, and the extramuscular length is 21 mm. There are mostly two veins accompanying the artery. They form the neurovascular pedicle with the sartorius branch of the femoral nerve.

(4) The sartorius branch of the femoral nerve usually arises as a single stem (82%) from the femoral nerve 0–2 mm below the inguinal ligament, and to a lesser extent shares a stem common to the anterior cutaneous nerve of the thigh. From the stem, two to six tiny branches are given off. Since the sartorius branch is the first one sent off by the femoral nerve, it may originate from the nerve at any level within the interval between the site 23 mm below the anterior superior iliac spine and the base of the patella. It forms the neurovascular pedicle with the companion vessels and enters the muscle within its upper third. The point of entrance varies considerably.

Other sources of blood supply

In addition to the main vessels in the femoral triangle, the sartorius owes its blood supply to the descending genicular artery of the femoral artery and the branches of the popliteal artery. These are mostly under cover of the sartorius and enter the muscle underneath its medial border. Their outer diameters are mostly smaller than those of the proximal sartorius branches. They usually own a couple of companion veins but the nerve is inconstant.

The sartorius branch from the superficial circumflex iliac artery is bound to the proximal part of the muscle 25 mm inferior to the anterior superior iliac spine. Its outer calibre is minute and only one companion vein is present.

Essentials of applied anatomy

(1) The long and ribbon-like sartorius is the muscular landmark in the anterior part of the thigh. It functions as the flexor of the hip and knee as well as the abductor and lateral rotator of the thigh. Its superficial position and the functional compensation offered by the hip muscles and the hamstrings after its excision all make it a muscular donor fit for clinical use. During the excision of its origin it is essential to note the lateral cutaneous nerve, which crosses the sartorius from medial lateralward 7 mm below the anterior superior iliac spine, and in operating on its insertion it is equally important to avoid injury to the saphenous nerve which proceeds between the sartorius and the gracilis at the level of the apex of the patella.

(2) The segmental arrangement of the blood supply of the sartorius is distinct, because the arteries to the muscle are given off at intervals of 70 mm on an average. The relatively constant major vascular pedicles are superficial in the femoral triangle and enter the muscle regularly along the medial border with clear markings. Therefore it will not be difficult to disclose the relevant vessels and nerves from that border of the muscle, which is an ideal site of approach. Moreover, since there is a moderately wide skin area in contact with the sartorius as well as a corresponding blood supply by the muscular and cutaneous arteries to the overlying skin, a relatively long and broad musculocutaneous flap may be accomplished.

Gracilis

Morphology

The gracilis is the most superficial muscle of the medial group of the thigh. It is thin, flattened and ribbon-like and is originated by a 14 mm long tendinous lamina from the inferior ramus of the pubis and the adjoining part of the ramus of the ischium. It gradually tapers downwards from the origin and, at the level of the upper border of patella, becomes a flattened round tendon in most cases (82%), which is inserted into the upper part of the medial surface of the shaft of the tibia below the condyle to form a part of the goose pad.

The total length of the gracilis averages 415 mm, that of the belly and the tendon of insertion being 289 mm and 125 mm respectively. The widest portion of the belly measured at the site 69 mm below the lower border of the pubis symphysis is 30 mm wide and 4.6 mm thick. It is 18 mm in width and 5.2 mm in thickness 100 mm above the upper border of the patella.

Main neurovascular pedicle (Figure 4.9)

The gracilis owns a neurovascular pedicle formed by the branches of the deep femoral vessels and the anterior branch of the obturator nerve.

(1) The gracilis branch of the deep femoral vessel is the most invariable and chief of the nutrient vessel. Its outer diameter averages 2.3 mm, and the

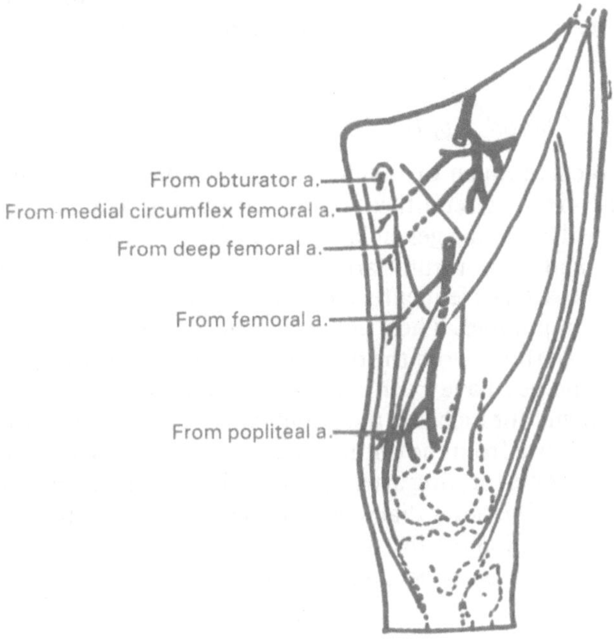

Figure 4.9 Main arterial source of the gracilis

extramuscular length 57 mm. The artery passes inferomedially in front of or behind the deep femoral vein and deep to the adductor longus, and penetrates through the lateral aspect of the muscle near its anterior border at the level of the junction between its upper and middle thirds. The main neurovascular pedicle of the gracilis is formed by the artery with one or two veins and the anterior branch of the obturator nerve. After entering the muscle, the main branches of the vessels travel downwards within the muscle parallel to the long axis of the muscular fibres. The outer diameter of the artery averages 1.2 mm. The artery gives off about 7–16 minute branches on either side alternatively, but rarely symmetrically. One may follow these branches up to the level of the upper border of the patella, i.e. the site of the junction of the belly and tendon. In case the gracilis branch from the femoral artery distributes its minute branches to the area 50–110 mm above the upper border of the patella, and its calibre is larger than 1 mm, the main vessels mostly end 50–100 mm above the upper border of the patella and anastomoses exist between the adjacent vessels. There are mostly two venae comitantes within the muscle with transverse communications between them.

(2) The gracilis branch of the obturator nerve exhibits excellent regularity. It comes from the anterior branch of the obturator nerve, shares a common stem with the adductor longus branch and divides 35–73 mm below the mid-inguinal point into two branches which innervate the adductor longus and the gracilis separately. The gracilis branch is 2.4 mm thick at its origin from the common

stem, the extramuscular length being 50 mm. It then divides into one to five twigs to enter the muscle. However, two or three twigs are the most common (71%).

Other sources of blood supply

Besides the gracilis branch of the deep femoral artery as the main vessel, the gracilis has the medial circumflex femoral artery, the femoral artery, the popliteal artery, the descending genicular branch of the femoral artery, the first perforating artery and the obturator artery as the other six sources. Of these, those from the femoral artery frequently enter the lower third of the muscle and may be one to three in number. Their outer diameters vary from 0.8 to 1.5 mm, all being smaller than those from the deep femoral artery. They have venae comitantes, but no nerves have been seen accompanying them. Those from the descending genicular branch and the popliteal artery enter the lower third of the muscle as well. Those from the obturator artery, the medial circumflex femoral artery and the first perforating artery get into the muscle within its upper third, i.e. near its origin. The outer diameters of these branches remain within 1 mm. There are venae comitantes in company with these branches. All except the obturator artery possess no accompanying nerve.

Essentials of applied anatomy

(1) The gracilis pertaining to the adductors of the thigh is endowed with the functions of the adduction of the thigh and the flexion of the leg. However, the gracilis is not the prime mover either. Its excision brings about no obvious functional disadvantages. Again, its position remains superficial and the neurovascular supply is invariable. All these make it a muscular donor suitable for clinical use.

(2) Though gracilis has multiple blood supplies, the gracilis branch from the deep femoral artery with the muscular branch of the obturator nerve is relatively constant. This neurovascular bundle can fulfil the requirements of muscle graft and therefore claims precedence over all others whenever gracilis flap is required.

(3) The nerve to the gracilis often has a stem common to that to the adductor longus and is given off 35–73 mm below the mid-point of the inguinal ligament. Hence, in isolating gracilis muscle, the gracilis branch has to be incised distal to the common stem to preserve the nerve to the adductor longus.

Semitendinosus

Morphology

The semitendinosus belongs to the posterior group of muscles of the thigh, taking its origin from the ischial tuberosity together with the semimembranosus and the long head of the biceps femoris. The muscle is fusiform and is provided with three surfaces: a posterior surface, narrow and in contact with the skin, a medial surface in apposition to the semimembranosus and a lateral surface adjacent to the long head of the biceps femoris. It is entirely separated from the long head of the biceps 84 mm on average below the ischial tuberosity, and then proceeds downwards and medialward, transforming completely into a round tendon at the level of the bend of the knee. It is finally inserted into the upper part of the shaft of the tibia medial to the tubercle of the tibia and the deep fascia of the leg. The tendon of insertion is 127 mm in length, which makes up 29% of the total length of the muscle. In fact, the aponeurosis beings 210 mm below the ischial tuberosity and measures 220 mm in length which corresponds to half of the length of the muscle. Hence, it has been called the semitendinous muscle.

The whole length of the semitendinosus averages 434 mm, the belly being 304 mm long. At the site 100 mm below the ischial tuberosity the greatest width of the belly is 19 mm and the thickness is 16 mm. As the belly proceeds downward, 150 mm below the ischial tuberosity, it is 13 mm wide and 17 mm thick.

Main neurovascular pedicle (Figure 4.10)

Semitendinosus branch of the first perforating artery

The first perforating artery pierces the adductor magnus to the back of the thigh 79 mm on the average below the ischial tuberosity where its average outer diameter is 2.6 mm. It passes downwards deep to the sciatic nerve and gives off two twigs to the semitendinosus. One of the branches arises from the first perforating artery 115 mm below the ischial tuberosity and enters the deep

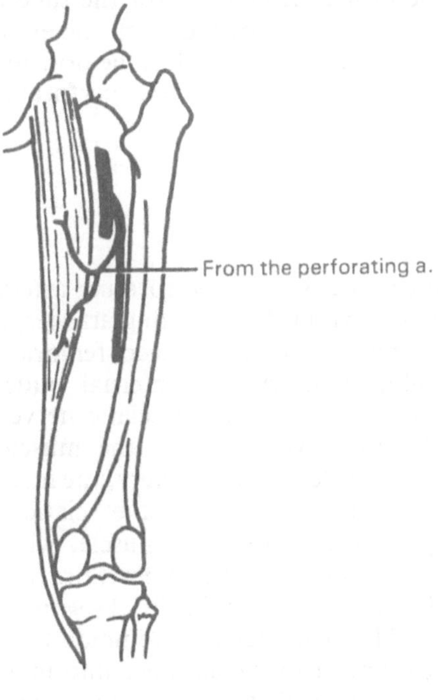

Figure 4.10 Main arterial source of the semitendinosus

surface of the muscle 126 mm below the tuberosity, its outer diameter being 1.5 mm and the extramuscular length 24 mm. Another branch is given off 150 mm below the ischial tuberosity. It enters the deep aspect of the muscle 177 mm below the tuberosity. Its outer diameter is 1.4 mm with an extramuscular length of 27 mm. The anastomoses between the perforating arteries, the branches of the perforating artery or the muscular branches of the perforating artery are plentiful whether they are within or outside the muscle. The semitendinosus branch usually has two companion veins, their outer diameters being 1.4 and 1.7 mm respectively.

Semitendinosus branch of the sciatic nerve

The nerve to the semitendinosus comes mostly from the sciatic nerve and is of two varieties. In about half of the cases (48%), it divides into an upper and a lower branch to innervate the semitendinosus. The upper branch is given off by the sciatic nerve 70 mm below the ischial tuberosity with a thickness of 2 mm and an extramuscular length of 40 mm and enters the muscle 130 mm below the ischial tuberosity. The lower branch is given off 139 mm below the ischial tuberosity, being 2–3 mm thick and with an extramuscular length of 52 mm. It enters the muscle 200 mm below the ischial tuberosity. Those with only one semitendinosus branch amount to 39%. Such branches divide into two or three twigs prior to entering the muscle and often arise 78 mm below the ischial tuberosity from the sciatic nerve with an extramuscular length of 52 mm. They enter the muscle 137 mm below the tuberosity. To judge from the rate of incidence, the thickness of the stem, the extramuscular length and the extent of innervation, the upper branch is the principal nerve, which forms the main neurovascular pedicle with the first perforating artery.

Other sources of blood supply

In adition to the branches of the first perforating artery, the semitendinosus is supplied by the second and third perforating arteries, the medial circumflex femoral artery, the femoral artery, the deep femoral artery, the popliteal artery, the inferior gluteal artery, the internal pudendal artery and the branches of the companion artery of the sciatic nerve. The semitendinosus branches given off by these vessels enter the muscle at different levels. Generally, the medial circumflex femoral artery, the inferior gluteal artery and the branches of the companion artery of the sciatic nerve of the internal pudendal artery supply the origin of the muscle, which is common to the biceps femoris and corresponds to the upper third of the thigh, while the popliteal artery and the branches from the distal segment of the femoral artery supply the distal third. The characteristics common to these branches are the interarterial anastomoses prior to the entrance into muscles and the presence of a couple of veins, the outer diameters of which are smaller than those of the corresponding arteries.

Essentials of applied anatomy

(1) Semitendinosus belongs to the hamstrings with the functions of flexion of the knee and extension of the hip. These functions may be compensated in its absence. Moreover, since it is superficial and easy to approach, it can be selected as a muscle donor for graft. However, due to its narrow posterior surface, limited contact with the skin and inadequate cutaneous vascularization, it is not an ideal musculocutaneous flap.

(2) The semitendinosus has a multiple blood supply as well as arterial anastomoses within and outside the muscle. The main vessels and nerves are present 130 mm below the ischial tuberosity. Hence it would be convenient to seek for its neurovascular pedicle in the environs of the junction of the upper and middle thirds of the posterior aspect of the thigh.

(3) As the nerve to the semitendinosus mainly springs from the sciatic nerve with considerable length and thickness, it may not be difficult to perform a neuroanastomosis. However, as it may share a common stem with that of the biceps or the semimembranosus, it is necessary to adopt blunt dissection to avoid injury to the latter.

Biceps femoris

Morphology

The biceps femoris belongs to the hamstring muscles and is situated on the posterolateral surface of the thigh. It has two heads of origin: one, the long head, arises from the ischial tuberosity in common with the semitendinosus and semimembranosus; the other, the short head, from the linea aspera of the femur and the lateral intermuscular septum by muscle fibres. The two heads unite in the lower portion of the thigh 133 mm above the capitulum of the fibula. The tendon is 82 mm in length with its upper end 16 mm in width and 2–6 mm in thickness and finally inserted into the head of the fibula.

The tendon of origin of the long head is 40 mm in length, 9 mm in width and 3 mm in thickness. The whole length of the muscle is 389 mm. The belly is fusiform in shape and descends to the level of the lateral condyle of the femur. The length of the belly is 267 mm, with a width of 31 mm and a thickness of 22 mm measured at the middle of its posterior surface. The upper end of the belly is completely separated from the semitendinosus 34 mm below the ischial tuberosity and descends inferolaterally. The medial surface of the biceps femoris adjoins the semitendinosus, the lateral surface is partly in apposition with the gluteus maximus, and the posterior surface is covered by the superficial fascia and skin.

The short head is 229 mm long, and prior to the union with the long head it measures 28 mm in width and 8 mm in thickness.

Main neurovascular pedicle (Figure 4.11)

The main neurovascular pedicle of the biceps femoris consists of the biceps branch of the first perforating artery and the branches of the sciatic nerve.

Long head branch from the first perforating artery

The first perforating artery is the main nutrient artery of the long head of the biceps. This amounts to 87% of the arterial branches which supply the long head. The first perforating artery approaches the posterior aspect of the thigh

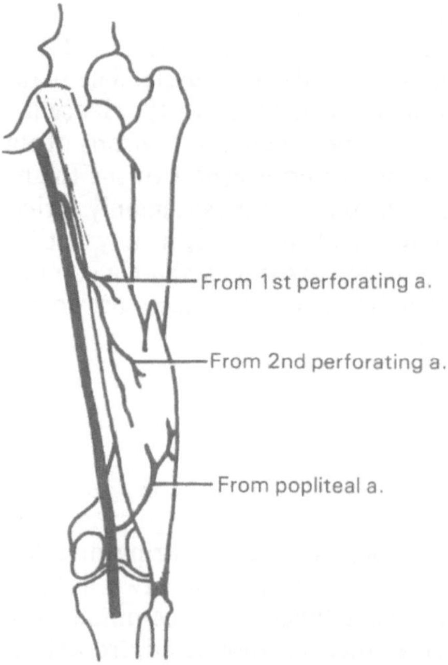

Figure 4.11 Main arterial source of the biceps femoris

79 mm below the ischial tuberosity where it resides between the lower border of the gluteus maximus and the long head of the biceps. It usually divides into an ascending and a descending branch. The ascending branch directs upwards and laterally, distributing principally to the lower part of the gluteus maximus and the part around the greater trochanter. The descending branch proceeds inferomedially deep to the sciatic nerve to its medial side. In addition to giving off branches anastomosing with the ascending branch of the second perforating artery, it invariably distributes to the long head of the biceps. The outer diameter of the artery is 1.7 mm, and the extramuscular length is 59 mm. It is accompanied by a couple of veins, the outer diameters of which are 2.3 and 1.7 mm respectively.

Branch of the sciatic nerve to the long head of the biceps femoris

The nerve to the long head arises from the upper end of the sciatic nerve and frequently has a common stem with the nerve to the semitendinosus, yet a single branch is the most frequent (98%). It divides into one to four twigs prior to the entrance into the muscle. The extramuscular part of the nerve is 44 mm long and

1.2 mm thick and mostly accompanies the muscular branch of the first perforating artery to form the neurovascular pedicle. The second branch, if present, would direct downwards and laterally after being given off from the sciatic nerve. It is 83 mm long and 1.3 mm thick. The nerve does not accompany the vessels, but passes by the side of them.

Vessels and nerves of the short head of the biceps femoris

The majority of the vessels of the short head of the biceps femoris come from the branches of the perforating arteries and the popliteal artery, those from the latter being shorter and thinner. The nerve to the short head springs from the common peroneal nerve, being 53 mm long and 1.2 mm thick, and enters the muscle via the posteromedial aspect of its upper part.

Other sources of blood supply

In addition to the branches of the first perforating artery, the long head of the biceps femoris draws its blood from the branches of the second and third perforating arteries and the medial circumflex femoral, inferior gluteal femoral and popliteal arteries. These branches are rather small and present a segmental distribution and profuse anastomosis outside the muscle.

Essentials of applied anatomy

(1) The long head of the biceps femoris has a superficial position and can be compensated, after its excision, by the gluteus maximus and other posterior femoral muscles without any functional disorders, thus fulfilling the requirements of a muscle donor. The long head can be used as a muscle or musculocutaneous flap, while the short head, owing to its superfluous attachment of origin and short vascular bundle, is not suitable for muscular translocation or free transplantation.

(2) The main vascular pedicle of the long head of the biceps femoris penetrates the deep surface of the muscle at about the middle of it; therefore it is possible to gain access to it through an incision along the posterior mid-line of the thigh at the level of the middle of the muscle. An inspection of the anterior border of the muscle will easily lead to the biceps branch of the first perforating artery which possesses sufficient length and outer diameter to meet the demand of a free muscle donor or a musculocutaneous flap.

(3) The nerve to the long head of the biceps femoris frequently occurs as a single twig. The site of entrance into the muscle is the same as the main vessels. They have adequate length but mostly share a common stem with the nerve to the semitendinosus. Hence, in making a free muscle flap one should be aware that the nerve to the semitendinosus should not be injured.

Tensor fasciae latae

Morphology

The tensor fasciae latae belong to the lateral group of the hip muscles and are located on the lateral side of the hip and thigh, residing between the sartorius and the gluteus medius. The belly, being 18 mm in width, arises by a conspicuous tendinous structure from the anterior part of the outer lip of the iliac crest and the anterior superior iliac spine. It is sandwiched between the two layers of fascia lata and gets thinner downwards to be inserted into the iliotibial tract of the fascia lata. The whole muscle is 159 mm long, the widest portion of the belly being 120 mm below the anterior superior iliac spine and measuring 33 mm in breadth and 8 mm in thickness. The lower border of the belly seldom appears to be horizontal, but often inclines anteriorly and exhibits a kind of faint serration gradually blending with the iliotibial tract, a thickened lateral portion of the fascia lata. The tract takes its origin from the outer lip of the iliac crest above and is attached below to the lateral condyle of the tibia. The tensor fasciae latae actually resides between the two layers of the upper third of the tract.

Main neurovascular pedicle (Figure 4.12)

The neurovascular pedicle of the muscle consists of the ascending branch of the lateral circumflex femoral artery and the branches of the superior gluteal nerve.

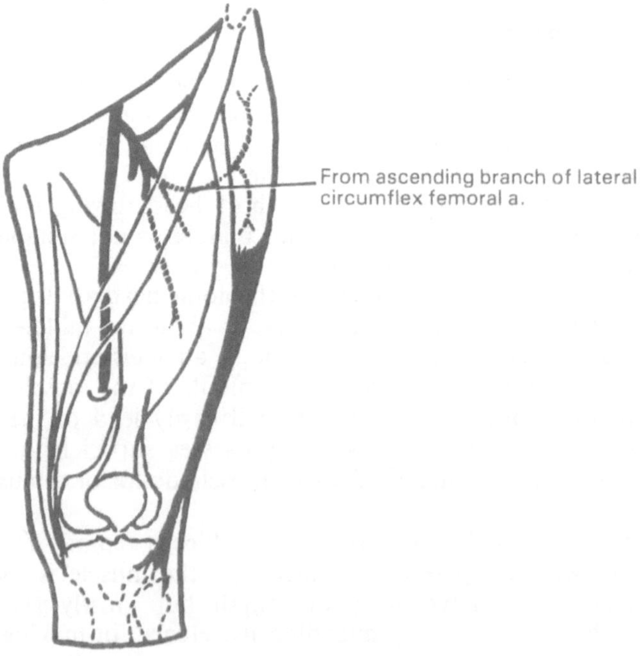

Figure 4.12 Main blood supply of the tensor fasciae latae

(1) The tensor fasciae latae branch of the ascending branch of the lateral circumflex femoral artery is the most constant of the main nutrient arteries to the tensor fasciae latae. The ascending branch given off by the lateral circumflex femoral artery, passes rather regularly deep to the branches of the femoral nerve and the rectus femoris and directs upward and laterally to divide into an upper and a lower branch to the muscle. The bifurcation is deep to the lateral border of the rectus femoris and the anterior border of the tensor fasciae latae, 80 mm from the anterior superior iliac spine. The outer diameter of the upper branch measures 1.6 mm, while that of the lower measures 1.4 mm. The entrances of the upper and lower branches into muscle are 54 mm and 86 mm below the anterior superior iliac crest respectively. The outer diameter of the initial part of the ascending branch is 2.5 mm, the extramuscular length 25 mm. The companion veins of the ascending branch are mostly double (68%), the outer diameters of which are 2.8 and 2.2 mm respectively. In case of a single companion vein, its outer diameter is greater than that of the artery, with a mean value of 3.6 mm.

After supplying the muscle, the upper and lower branches to the tensor fasciae latae given off by the ascending branch traverse the deep surface of the muscle to reach its posterior edge to be distributed to the neighbouring skin as the musculocutaneous branches 56 mm and 100 mm near the anterior superior iliac spine. Both the course and the direction of the ascending branch are rather invariable and the muscle–ascending branch angle exiting between the ascending branch and the tensor fasciae latae measures 66.5 degrees. During the skin flap transplantation, this angle should be preserved to facilitate the blood circulation and the survival of the flap.

(2) The tensor fasciae latae branch of the superior gluteal nerve is a slender branch, measuring 2.3 mm in width. Accompanied by the twigs of the superior division of the deep branch of the superior gluteal artery, it proceeds forward, deep to the gluteus medius. At the site 25 mm posteroinferior to the anterior superior iliac spine, the nerve gradually curves downwards under cover of the posterior border of the tensor fasciae latae to make entrance into the deep surface of the muscle 47 mm away from the anterior superior iliac spine.

Other sources of blood supply

The blood supply of the tensor fasciae latae, apart from that coming from the ascending branch of the lateral circumflex femoral artery which belongs to the femoral arterial system, has other sources, which consist of the branches of the deep division of the superior gluteal artery of the internal iliac system and the deep circumflex iliac artery of the external iliac system. Owing to the fact that these branches are rather slender and assume a deep position, it is not easy to take and anastomose; hence they are unsuitable for muscle transplantation.

Essentials of applied anatomy

(1) The tensor fasciae latae is superficial and easy to expose. Its function may be compensated by the gluteal muscles without appreciable defect after its excision. It gradually becomes flattened from above downwards, and is provided with

considerably constant musculocutaneous vessels and relatively profuse anastomoses existing among the vessels which make possible the preparation and utilization of a considerable-sized muscle donor.

(2) The vascular supply of the tensor fasciae latae is from multiple sources, but the main source is the ascending branch of the lateral circumflex femoral artery, which possesses adequate length as well as sufficient outer diameter. Furthermore, the management of the muscular pedicle is not troublesome. Ultimately, when a vessel of considerable calibre is needed for anastomosing, an extension toward the stem of the lateral circumflex femoral artery will provide considerable flexibility. The maintenance of the original position of the angle between the ascending branch and the tensor fasciae latae is significant in ensuring the patency of the circulation. The mean value of this angle is 66.5 degrees, which seems to be significant for reference, notwithstanding that the angle has to be determined during operations.

(3) The nerve to the tensor fasciae latae runs in an opposite direction to the main vascular pedicle to the deep surface of the muscle. When the muscle with its nerve is to be transplanted, this can be done by cutting the origin of the muscle and then gradually turning it downwards. Consequently, the nerve to the muscle may be sought for at its posterior border 47 mm below the anterior superior iliac spine. A small dissection on the deep surface of the gluteus medius will make a considerable length of the nerve available.

Gluteus maximus

Morphology

The gluteus maximus is situated in the buttock, belonging to the extracoxal muscles. It is an irregularly square muscle, rather flattened and thick. It takes its origin by a short tendon from the posterior gluteal line and the area behind it on the posterior surface of the ilium, from the posterior surfaces of the lower part of the sacrum and the coccyx, and from the sarcrotuberous ligament and the lumbodorsal fascia. The muscle fibres incline laterally and downwards and terminate as a thick aponeurosis. The upper fibres are connected with the iliotibial tract, while the lower fibres are inserted into the gluteal tuberosity of the femur. The gluteus maximus is the principal muscle for the extension of the hip. The upper border of the muscle is 147 mm wide, while its lower border is 150 mm with a thickness of 22 mm at its mid-point.

Main neurovascular pedicle (Figure 4.13)

The main neurovascular pedicle of the gluteus maximus comprises the inferior gluteal artery, the superficial branch of the superior gluteal artery and the inferior gluteal nerve.

(1) Gluteus maximus branches of the inferior gluteal artery and the superficial branch of the superior gluteal artery. The inferior gluteal artery is one of the terminal branches of the anterior division of the internal iliac artery. It gives off

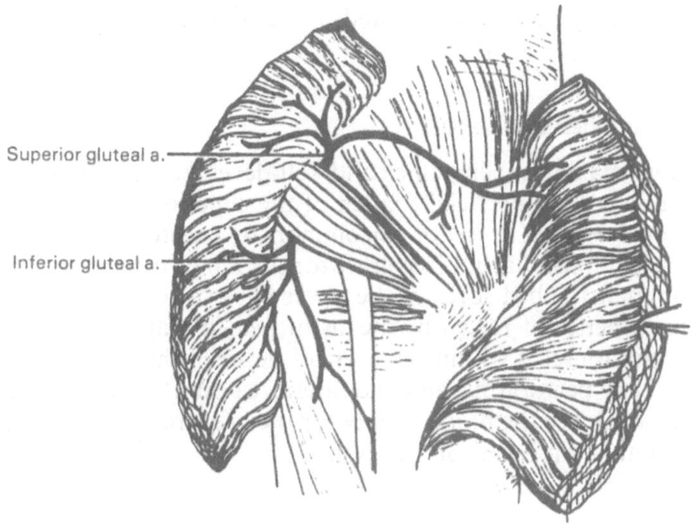

Figure 4.13 Main blood supply of the gluteus maximus

branches to the inferior portion of the gluteus maximus after emerging from the hiatus infra-piriformis where its outer diameter is 3.5 mm. The surface projection of the point of its exit coincides a bit medially with the junction of the middle and lower thirds of the line connecting the iliac crest and the ischial tuberosity, being 120 mm on the average from the iliac crest and 54 mm from the ischial tuberosity.

The superior gluteal artery divides into a superficial and a deep branch after leaving the suprapiriform hiatus. The deep branch is beneath the gluteus medius supplying the glutei medius and minimus, while the superficial branch, deep to the gluteus maximus, supplies the upper portion of the muscle and sends twigs to anastomose with the inferior gluteal artery. The outer diameter of the superior gluteal artery is 3 mm on leaving the suprapiriform hiatus, the surface projection of its exit being the mid-point of the line connecting the iliac crest and the ischial tuberosity, 87 mm on the average from either the iliac crest or the ischial tuberosity. Mostly, both the superior and inferior gluteal arteries own a couple of venae comitantes, the outer diameters of which are generally greater than those of the arteries.

(2) Gluteus maximus branch of the inferior gluteal nerve. The inferior gluteal nerve is a branch of the sacral plexus. It may comprise one to three, but mostly two, branches while leaving the infrapiriform hiatus. It is 1.7 mm thick, the extramuscular length being 63 mm. It generally enters the deep surface of the muscle accompanying the gluteus maximus branches of the inferior gluteal artery at the middle of the lower part of the muscle.

Other sources of blood supply

Besides the branches of the inferior and superior gluteal arteries, the ascending branch of the first perforating artery may be distributed to the insertion of the gluteus maximus, and the tensor fasciae latae branch of the lateral circumflex femoral artery may also be distributed to the muscle.

Essentials of applied anatomy

(1) The gluteus maximus, being thick and well-developed, has two large vascular pedicles, namely the superficial branch of the superior gluteal artery and the inferior gluteal artery. It is not uncommon to anastomose one of the two pedicles to accomplish partial free graft for the repair of breasts, and it is also possible to repair the bed sores of the lower back or to fix up the levator and to treat incontinence of faeces by means of pedicle flap transfer.

(2) The anastomoses within the muscles between the superior and inferior gluteal, the first perforating and the lateral circumflex femoral arteries are rather profuse. Hence the blood supply for the preparation of the vascularized gluteus maximus flap is out of question.

Gastrocnemius

Morphology

The gastrocnemius is situated superficially in the back of the leg. It has a medial and a lateral head, arising respectively from the medial and lateral condyles of the femur, the medial head being usually higher than the lateral. The two heads direct downwards and join each other 20–30 mm above or below the level of the head of the fibula whence the conjoint tendon proceeds downwards and unites with the tendon of the soleus to form the tendo calcaneus to be inserted into the posterior surface of the calcaneum. The full length of the gastrocnemius is 380 mm.

The medial head arises from the medial condyle of femur by means of a flattened tendon, which expands below as an aponeurosis that extends to the back of the belly. The major part of the aponeurosis invests the belly to a certain extent. The average width of the aponeurosis in the vicinity of the head of fibula measures 17 mm with an edge of 5 mm in thickness. The belly of the medial head is 214 mm long, the widest portion being 60 mm below the head of fibula where it is 58 mm wide and 11 mm thick. The terminal tendon, i.e. the part of the tendon from the lower end of the belly to the site of union with that of the soleus, is 111 mm long, being mostly shorter than the belly.

The origin of the lateral head is similar to that of the medial. The tendon of the origin spreads downwards into an aponeurosis, which is 14 mm wide and 3.3 mm thick and is attached to the posterior surface of the muscle at the level of the head of fibula. The belly, being 212 mm in length, has the widest portion 60 mm below the head of fibula where it is 46 mm wide and 9 mm thick. The tendon of insertion, being shorter than the belly, measures 95 mm in length.

Tendo calcaneus, which is the union of the tendons of the gastrocnemius and the soleus, is apparently stout with an average length of 72 mm. Its widest portion, which measures 21 mm, is situated 23 mm above the tuberosity of calcaneum. It is 14 mm wide and 6 mm thick along the line interconnecting the medial and lateral malleoli. The level of the union of the tendons is variable, so that the length of tendo calcaneus varies.

Main neurovascular pedicle (Figure 4.14)

Blood vessels of the medial and lateral heads of the gastrocnemius

The main vessel of the medial head of the gastrocnemius is the medial sural artery arising directly from the popliteal artery 37 mm above the head of the fibula. It is usually single, with an outer diameter of 2.3 mm and an extra-muscular length of 26 mm, and mostly enters the muscle through the thick portion of the belly with a range of 10 mm above or below the head of the fibula.

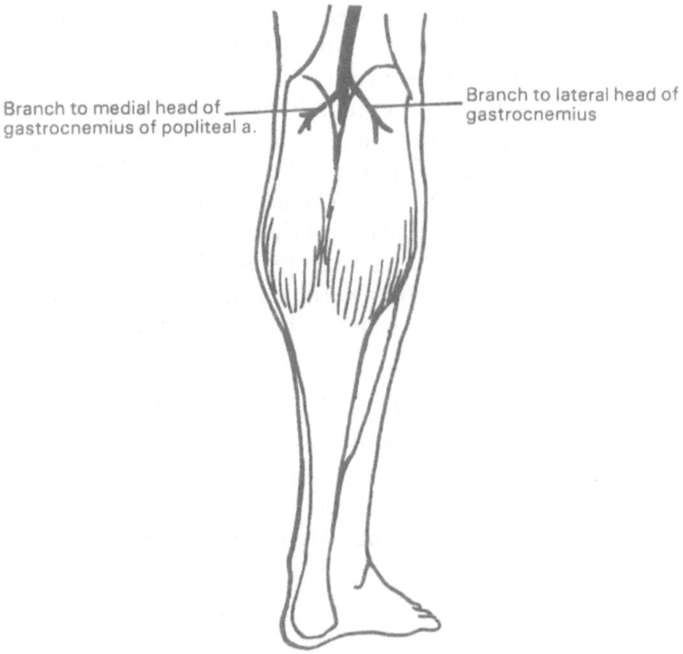

Figure 4.14 Main blood supply of the gastrocnemius

After entering the muscle the main arterial stem passes downwards along the long axis of the muscle fibres and gives off 4–29 tiny branches to either side alternatively, most frequently 8–15 branches. These branches send tiny twigs to the soleus, the fascia and skin overlying it and the medial head of gastrocnemius. The medial sural artery is usually accompanied by a couple of veins at the site of its entrance into the muscle. These veins in most cases unite into one companion vein with an average diameter of 3.7 mm, which ends into the popliteal vein above the origin of the corresponding artery or sometimes forms a common stem with the vein from the lateral head.

The main vessel of the lateral head of the gastrocnemius is the lateral sural artery which takes its origin from the popliteal artery 34 mm above the head of the fibula. This commencement is a bit lower than the medial one. The lateral sural artery is mostly single with an outer diameter of 2.2 mm and an extramuscular length of 22 mm. The arterial trunk descends parallel to the long axis of the fibres after entering the muscle and its mode of branching is generally similar to that of the medial sural artery. The artery is accompanied by a vein which is mostly single with an outer diameter of 3 mm and empties similarly into the popliteal vein.

Nerves to the medial and lateral heads of the gastrocnemius

The nerve to the medial head generally comes from the tibial nerve but a few may share a common stem with the nerve to the soleus or the lateral sural cutaneous nerve. The extramuscular length measures 29 mm with a thickness of 2.1 mm. It divides prior to its entrance to the muscle into one to three branches, of which one branch is the most frequent.

The nerve to the lateral head comes mostly from the tibial nerve. Some may have a common stem with that to the soleus. The origin of the nerve is somewhat below that of the nerve to the medial head. The extramuscular length is 25 mm and the thickness of the nerve is 2.2 mm. The mode of entrance into the muscle is similar to that of the medial sural nerve. If the epineurium is precisely incised it may be possible to dissect the nerves antidromically for a length of 58–185 mm without injury. This anatomical characteristic can be made use of in muscle translocation or transplantation in order to lengthen the nerve pedicle.

Characteristics of the mode of entry of the neurovascular pedicle

The vessels and nerves of the medial and lateral heads of the gastrocnemius are not enveloped in the fascia but are rather separated. They gather into bundles only when approaching the neurovascular door, the topographical relations being that the nerves remain superficial, while the arteries and veins are deep in the nerve.

Essentials of applied anatomy

(1) The gastrocnemius and the soleus form a muscular mass which is occasionally described as the triceps surae. It is superficial and possesses a constant neurovascular supply. Anatomical observations and clinical data all indicate that the removal of only one head of the gastrocnemius will have no apparent effect on striding or walking. Therefore, it is thought that the medial or lateral head of the gastrocnemius may be an ideal muscle donor. Owing to the presence of a considerable abundance of the musculocutaneous vessels and the wider area of contact with the overlying skin, considerably larger musculocutaneous flaps may be processed. The lateral head may sometimes be lacking; thus in operating

on this portion of the muscle the invariable position of the common peroneal nerve between the lateral head and the biceps femoris should be taken into account.

(2) Both the nerves to the medial and lateral heads of the gastrocnemius come from the tibial nerve. In case of the inadequate length of the nerve pedicle, antidromic dissection of the nerve for a certain distance to lengthen it may be considered. However, they may share a common stem with the nerve to the soleus, which must not be injured.

(3) The head of fibula, being prominent, may serve as a practical landmark. It corresponds to the site of union of the medial and lateral heads and also indicates the entrance of the vessels and nerves into the medial and lateral heads.

Extensor digitorum brevis

Morphology

The extensor digitorum brevis is a thin and flattened muscle often unnoticed beneath the skin of the dorsum of the foot. It is related to the tarsal sinus posteriorly and takes its origin from the upper and lateral surfaces of the calcaneum as well as the inferior extensor retinaculum. Its flattened thin belly directs enteromedially and transforms into four slender tendons at the level of the tubercle of the fifth metatarsal bone to be inserted into the proximal phalanx of the medial four toes. The muscle near its origin measures 35 mm in width and 3 mm in thickness, and 38 mm wide and 1.5 mm thick in the environ of the tubercle of the fifth metatarsal bone. The widest portion of the belly is 41 mm.

The data measured for the extensor digitorum brevis are listed in Table 4.1.

Table 4.1 The biometry of the extensor digitorum brevis (mm)

Distribution	*Length in whole*	*Length of the belly*	*Length of the tendon*	*Breadth of the tendon at the level of the heads of the metatarsus*
To first toe	137	55	82	2.3
To second toe	138	60	78	2.2
To third toe	130	68	63	2.3
To fourth toe	122	56	66	1.9

On the dorsum of the foot the extensor digitorum brevis is beneath the tendons of the extensor hallucis longus and the extensor digitorum longus, being crossed obliquely by the latter. At the level of the heads of the metatarsi the tendons of the long and short extensors become gradually approximated, forming acute angles pointing proximally. The measurements of these angles near the level of the heads are as follows: first toe, 10.5°; second toe, 7°; third toe, 11.8°; fourth, 14°, with an increment from the second to the fifth toe. Similarly, at the level of the head of the fifth metatarsus there is a great disparity in the width of the long and short extensor tendons, of which the former is wider than the latter.

Furthermore, some aspects of variations regarding the tendon of extensor digitorum brevis are of practical significance:

Increment in the number of tendons of the extensor digitorum brevis

The incidence of this variation is 13%, being more common in the tendon of the second toe. The tendon then divides into two branches, of which one maintains the usual position, while the superfluous one assumes a position medial to it and usually unites with the tendon of the long extensor at the level of the body of the metatarsus.

Decrement in the number of tendons of the extensor digitorum brevis

This incidence is 6.5%. Decrement in the fourth tendon of the short extensor is the commonest.

Conjunction of the short and long extensor tendons

The incidence is 6.5%. Such a conjunction is similar to the connexus intertendinous of the extensor digitorum on the back of the hand.

Main neurovascular pedicle (Figure 4.15)

The dorsalis pedis artery and its branch, the lateral tarsal artery, comprise the main vascular pedicle of the extensor digitorum brevis. The dorsalis pedis artery, being the direct continuation of the anterior tibial artery, is situated laterally to the extensor hallucis longus tendon on the dorsum of the foot. Its branches direct laterally and medially to supply the relevant structures. The outer diameter of the artery at the intermalleolar level is 3.3 mm. Two companion veins are invariably situated on either side of the artery, the outer diameter of the lateral vein being 2.2 mm, while that of the medial one 2.0 mm.

The extensor digitorum brevis branches of the lateral tarsal artery

The branches of the lateral tarsal artery, being the main and constant vessel of the short extensor, amount to one to five, of which two branches are the most common (78%). The lateral tarsal artery springs from the dorsalis pedis artery 3–52 mm distal to the intermalleolar line, and half of them within the range of 11–20 mm. The proximal one having an outer diameter of 1.8 mm is the thickest. In case there exist two branches the outer diameter of the proximal one must be greater than that of the distal; if there are three or four branches they generally become thinner from the proximal to the distal. These muscular branches proceed anterolaterally deep to the tendons of the extensor digitorum longus and brevis, and give off twigs to the deep surface of the muscle. A couple of veins accompany the artery. The proximal branch is generally accompanied by the extensor digitorum brevis branch of the deep peroneal nerve. Therefore

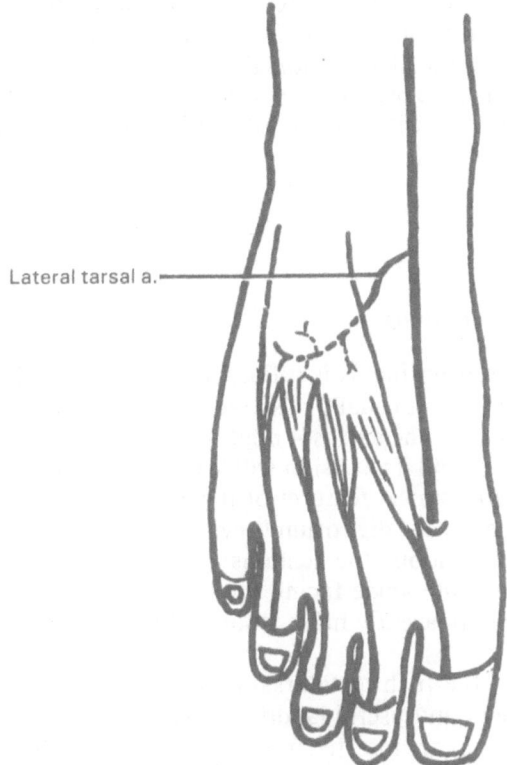

Figure 4.15 Main blood supply of the extensor digitorum brevis

the proximal lateral tarsal artery is thought to be the main neurovascular pedicle of the extensor digitorum brevis.

Extensor digitorum brevis branch of the deep peroneal nerve

At the intermalleolar line the deep peroneal nerve is situated superficial to the artery, sometimes medial or lateral to it. Those superficial to the artery are of the great majority (41%). The deep peroneal nerve divides into two terminal branches, at the intermalleolar line, i.e. the extensor digitorum brevis branch laterally and the terminal branch medially. The deep peroneal nerve measures 2.8 mm thick prior to its division.

The extensor digitorum brevis branch is generally given off from the deep peroneal nerve at the level of the intermalleolar line, passes deep to the extensor digitorum brevis accompanied by the proximal branch of the lateral tarsal artery and enters the deep surface of the muscle. The extramuscular length is 21 mm.

Other sources of blood supply

In addition to the branches of the lateral tarsal artery, the extensor digitorum brevis is supplied by the branches of the anterior lateral malleolar artery.

The substitution of the perforating artery of the peroneal artery for the dorsalis pedis artery occurs in 11% of cases. There are two possibilities: i.e. the perforating artery takes the place of dorsalis pedis artery and assumes the usual course; on the contrary, the perforating artery replaces the dorsalis pedis artery and forms an arterial ring with the anterior tibial arteries, and its courses and branchings are thus altered.

Essentials of applied anatomy

(1) The extensor digitorum brevis is a flattened thin muscle beneath the skin of the dorsum of the foot. It usually possesses four tendons inserted separately into the medial four toes. The extensor digitorum brevis plays no essential part in the extension of toes and its excision will leave no prominent defect. During transplantation the anatomical features of the muscles should be noticed; that is, the tendon of the extensor digitorum brevis always remains deep and lateral to the long extensor tendon, the tendons of the long and short extensors converge to form an acute angle facing proximally, and the tendon fibres of the long extensor are apparently more stout and prominent than those of the short extensor.

The tuberosity of the fifth metatarsal bone situated on the lateral side of the foot is a prominent and useful landmark. The peroneus tertius and brevis from different directions are inserted into it; therefore this tuberosity, together with the peroneus brevis tendon, can serve as the lateral border of the extensor digitorum brevis. The commencement of the short extensor is always approximated to the tendon of the peroneus brevis, yet they are easily separated.

(2) The vessels of the extensor digitorum brevis remain constant and have their origins from the dorsalis pedis artery. The dorsalis pedis artery has two sets of branches of different destinations: one set proceeds medialward and has nothing to do with the extensor digitorum brevis, and the other has a lateral course and consists of branches destined to the short extensor. Of the latter set the proximal branch of the lateral tarsal artery is the most constant one and needs protection.

Throughout its course on the dorsum of the foot the dorsalis pedis artery remains invariable on the lateral side of the tendon of the extensor hallucis longus. However, owing to the replacement of the dorsalis pedis artery by the peroneal that may occasionally take place, the course of the dorsalis pedis artery is thence varied, which needs attention.

(3) The extensor digitorum brevis branch of the deep peroneal nerve generally arises from the nerve at the intermalleolar line and proceeds anterolaterally to the deep surface of the muscle accompanied by the proximal branch of the lateral tarsal artery. In processing a muscle with its neurovascular pedicle one may dissect antidromically along the extensor digitorum brevis branch when a longer nerve for anastomosis is required.

APPLIED ANATOMY OF THE RECTUS ABDOMINIS

WU RENXIU

Morphology of the muscle

The rectus abdominis is situated bilaterally beside the mid-line of the anterior abdominal wall, separated by the linea alba and enveloped anteriorly and posteriorly by the vagina musculi recti abdominis (rectus sheath). It is attached above to the anterior aspect of the xyphoid process and the fifth, sixth and seventh costal cartilages, and below to the symphysis pubis and the anterior aspect of the body of pubis below the pubic crest. The average length of the rectus abdominis in the adult is 300 mm, the widths of its upper, middle and lower parts are 67, 56 and 21 mm respectively; the thicknesses of those parts are 5, 6 and 6 mm respectively. The muscle is fused in front with the anterior wall of the rectus sheath by the tendinous intersections. The intersections are usually three in number and are mostly found above the level of the umbilicus, though in some cases (39%), the third tendinous intersection may appear below that level. The pyramidalis is present in as many as 98% of the cases. The anterior wall of the rectus sheath in the adult is complete and may consist of, in addition to aponeurosis, a small number of muscle fibres. In the upper part of the posterior wall muscle fibres are found in most cases, but none in the lower part. There exists a distinct semicircular line at the lower end of the posterior wall of the rectus sheath in the adult, corresponding to the level 99 mm (74–114 mm) above the upper border of the symphysis pubis. Its surface projection falls within a range of 20 mm, that is, 10 mm above and below the junction of the upper and middle thirds of the line joining the umbilicus and the pubis. Below the semicircular line a parasemicircular line may sometimes be seen. The average length of the linea alba, which extends from the xyphoid process to the upper border of the symphysis pubis, is 320 mm (272–381 mm). The part of the linea alba above the navel is relatively wide and may be called the white band, whereas the part below the navel abruptly narrows to a mere line, and may be called the white string.

The main blood vessels and nerves of the muscle

The rectus abdominis is supplied mainly by the superior and the inferior epigastric arteries, and is innervated by the anterior branches of the seventh thoracic to the first lumbar nerves.

The superior epigastric artery and vein

The superior epigastric artery, which is the direct continuation of the internal thoracic artery, descends through the sternocostal triangle behind the rectus abdominis where it enters the muscle. Most of its branches anastomose with those of the inferior epigastric artery within the muscle near the navel. The origin of the superior epigastric artery is at the level of the sixth intercostal space in 57% of cases, and at the level of the seventh costal cartilage or its lower margin in the remaining 43% of cases. The average length of the vessel from its origin to the entrance into the muscle is 46 mm (22–73 mm), the outer diameter measured at its commencement is 2.1 mm (1.2–3.8 mm) and that at the site of the entrance 1.9 mm (1.2–2.6 mm), and the distance from the entrance to the anterior mid-line of the body is 37 mm (23–63 mm).

There are usually a couple of superior epigastric veins accompanying the artery. The outer diameter of its initial segment averages 2.8 mm (1.8–3.9 mm) and that at the site of the entrance into the muscle 1.3 mm (1.1–2.6 mm).

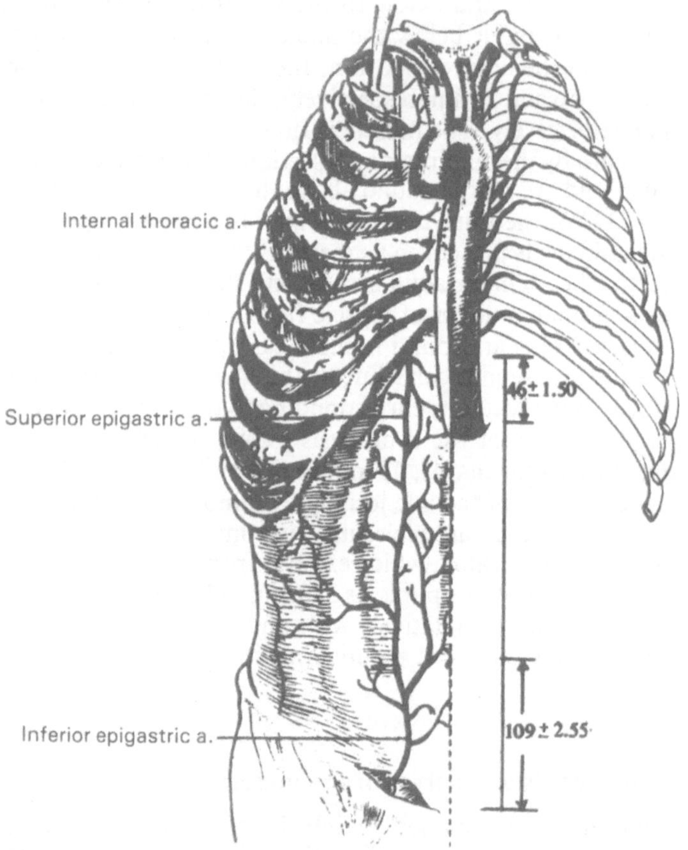

Figure 4.16 Blood supply of the rectus abdominis

The inferior epigastric artery and vein

The inferior epigastric artery arises from the anterior wall of the external iliac artery. The origin occurs above the inguinal ligament in 61% of cases, in which the average distance from the artery to the ligament is 6.6 mm (2–19.4 mm), just at the level of the ligament in 31% of cases, and below the ligament in 8% of cases, in which the average distance from the artery to the ligament is 12.9 mm

(2–21.3 mm). The inferior epigastric artery ascends upward and medialward to enter the rectus abdominis. The angle formed between the artery and the ligament averages 85° (70–120°). The length of the vessel from its origin to the entrance into the muscle is 109 mm (71–147 mm). The outer diameter measured at its commencement is 2.7 mm (1.6–3.5 mm), and that at the entrance 2 mm (1.5–2.6 mm). The distance from the origin of the artery to the pubic tubercle is 45 mm (32–58 mm), whereas the length of the inguinal ligament is 114 mm (100–136 mm), so that the inferior epigastric artery crosses the ligament at a point between the lateral three-fifths and the medial two-fifths of the ligament. The distance from the entrance to the anterior medial line is 34 mm (16–61 mm), and the level of the entrance of the vessel into the muscle is above the semicircular line.

There are two inferior epigastric veins accompanying the artery. The outer diameter at its origin is 3 mm (1.7–3.8 mm) and at the entrance 2.2 mm (1.7–3.8 mm).

The nerves of the rectus abdominis

The rectus abdominis is innervated segmentally by the anterior branches of the seventh thoracic to the first lumbar nerves. These branches are fine and enter the muscle from the posterolateral aspect of the muscle.

Other sources of the blood supply to the muscle

In addition to the superior and inferior epigastric arteries there are also other contributions from the anterior branches of the seventh intercostal to the first lumbar arteries, the fine vessels of which enter the rectus abdominis posterolaterally. Because of their small calibres these vessels are not important sources of blood supply to the muscle.

Owing to the fact that the rectus abdominis is a long, strap-like muscle, and that the superior and inferior epigastric arteries form an axial vascular pedicle, the rectus muscle or musculocutaneous flap can be used for pedicle flap transference or free transplantation. However, such cannot be used for function restoration, because the anterior branches of the segmental spinal nerves are too small to be anastomosed.

When the musculocutaneous flap from the lower abdomen is taken care must be exercised to protect the vulnerable abdominal wall behind the muscle where the posterior layer of the rectus sheath is lacking below the semicircular line.

An extensive rectus musculocutaneous flap may impair the strength and contractility of the anterior abdominal wall, and leave a rather long scar. Therefore, when young and middle-aged manual labourers are subject to such an operation the advantages and disadvantages should be carefully weighed beforehand.

5

The applied anatomy of bone transplantation

WU YONGMU

INTRODUCTION

The key to the success of bone graft lies in the blood supply of the donor bone. In the conventional non-vascularized bone transplantation the bone grafted is incapable of growth or union because of the interruption of blood supply. Only a few of the osteocytes beneath the periosteum are able to survive, and most of them are subject to necrosis and substitution. Therefore the transplantation can only play a role in a sort of bridging, which makes the periosteum at either end of the recipient bone creep on the donor bone in the course of intramembranous ossification, and is hence called substitution or creeping substitution. In bone transferring like this, the union needs a longer time; sometimes absorption or non-union of the bone may occur, which may even lead to a failure of operation.

In order to preserve the blood supply of the grafted bone, Hellstadin (1942), Davis and Taylor (1952), Kurada (1957, 1958) and others performed in succession bone transfer with muscular pedicle. The blood supply of such a graft is thus improved, but its clinical application has been restricted by the limited size of the bone to be grafted and the short distance in transplantation.

After Strauch, McCullough, Östrup (1971–74) and others had succeeded in transplanting vascularized ribs to the mandible in animal experiments, Taylor (1975) applied it clinically. Owing to the reservation of its blood supply, survival of the vascularized bone grafts makes the creeping substitution a simplified process as compared to that in bone healing after fracture, thus creating a new sort of therapy for the repair of massive defects of long bones, discovering a new approach to the treatment of pseudoarthrosis, opening up a hopeful prospect for the transplantation of the compound bone–muscle–skin flap, broadening the range of indication for surgical treatment and at length, leading bone transplantation to a new era.

Finley (1978) introduced the method of experimental graft with periosteum only, thus starting a new method of bone transplantation.

In 1977 the Shanghai Sixth People's Hospital of China achieved a stimulating success in vascularized fibular transplantation. In 1980 Huang Gongkang reported a case of transplantation of the iliac bone by anastomosis of the deep circumflex iliac vessels, and Fan Yieu reported satisfactory results in transplanting iliac bone by anastomosis of the superior gluteal vessels. In 1982 Yang Limin reported a case of free vascularized scapular transplantation.

FIBULA

WU YONGMU

The fibula belongs to a type of long bone. Its upper end is known as the caput fibulae while the lower end constitutes the malleolus lateralis. The constrictive part below the head is called the collum fibulae. On the anterior aspect of the body of fibula can be found the attachments of the extensor hallucis longus, the extensor digitorum longus and the peroneus tertius, and the medial surface affords the attachment for the tibialis posterior, while the posterior aspect is for the soleus and the flexor hallucis longus, and the lateral surface for the peroneus longus and brevis.

Length

According to the research data involving 6087 fibulae of adult Chinese, the length of the fibula averages 34 (24–47) cm. There is no obvious difference in respect to sides. Fibula in the male is about 3 cm longer than that of the female.

Nutrient foramen

Cases with one foramen are the commonest (88%); the next are those with two foramina (11%); those with more than three are uncommon (1%), while cases without nutrient foramen account for 2%. Most of them are located in the middle segment of the shaft (90%), some in the lower segment (8%) and only a few in the upper (2%).

Blood supply

There are three sources of blood supply of the long bone (Figure 5.1).

1. The nutrient artery, the principal arterial supply to the long bone, enters the narrow cavity via the nutrient foramen and divides into an ascending and a descending branch to supply the interior two-thirds of the compact bone of the shaft and bone marrow. It makes up 50–70% of the total blood supply of the long bone.
2. The metaphyseal and epiphyseal arteries come from the surrounding arteries. They enter the bone from its ends and anastomose with the nutrient artery, making up 20–40% of the total blood supply of the long bone.
3. The periosteal arteries are profuse and net-like, branching to supply the exterior one-third of the compact bone.

The fibula also gains its blood supply from the above-mentioned arteries: the middle portion receives its blood mainly from the nutrient artery, the arcuate artery and the muscular and perforating branches of the peroneal artery; the upper end is supplied by the branches of the anterior and posterior tibial arteries and the popliteal artery; the lower end by the branches of the arteries to the ankle joint.

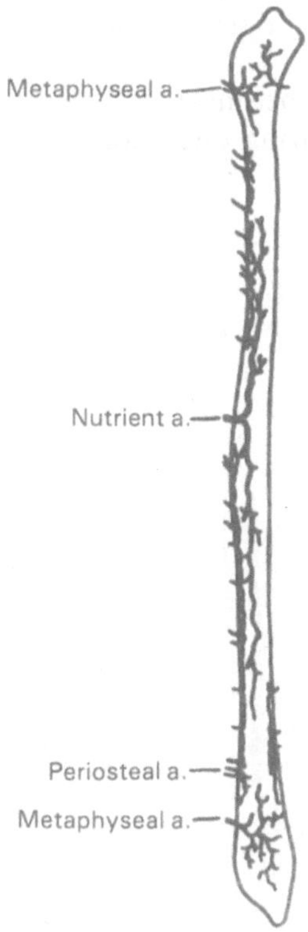

Figure 5.1 A schematic diagram of the blood supply of the fibula

Peroneal artery

The peroneal artery arises from the posterior tibial artery 30 (13–50) mm on average below the mid-point of the lower border of the popliteus muscle. Its average outer diameter is 4.0 (1.4–5.7) mm. It proceeds downwards and laterally, keeping at first some distance from the fibula, so that the upper end of the artery is about 10 mm from the latter. The further downward it proceeds, the nearer it approaches the bone. When an incision is made along the lateral border of the fibula through the posterolateral muscular septum of the leg between the peroneus longus and the soleus, the upper segment of the peroneal artery (about one-fourth of the length) may be exposed. The lower segment (about three-fourths of the length) is under cover of the flexor hallucis longus.

In case the muscle arises higher and happens to be well developed, it may cover the whole of the peroneal vessel. Therefore it is necessary to incise the muscle along its medial border so as to expose the vessel.

The peroneal artery, in the commencement of its course, is accompanied by the branch of the tibial nerve to the tibialis posterior. The nerve leaves the artery and enters the muscle at the junction of its upper and middle thirds. The nerve to the flexor hallucis longus is given off by the tibial nerve at the junction of the middle and lower thirds of the muscle. It is necessary to be aware of such topographical relations during operation in order to protect the nerve from injury.

The commencement of the peroneal artery varies considerably, so that careful attention is demanded during operation. The artery can be divided into

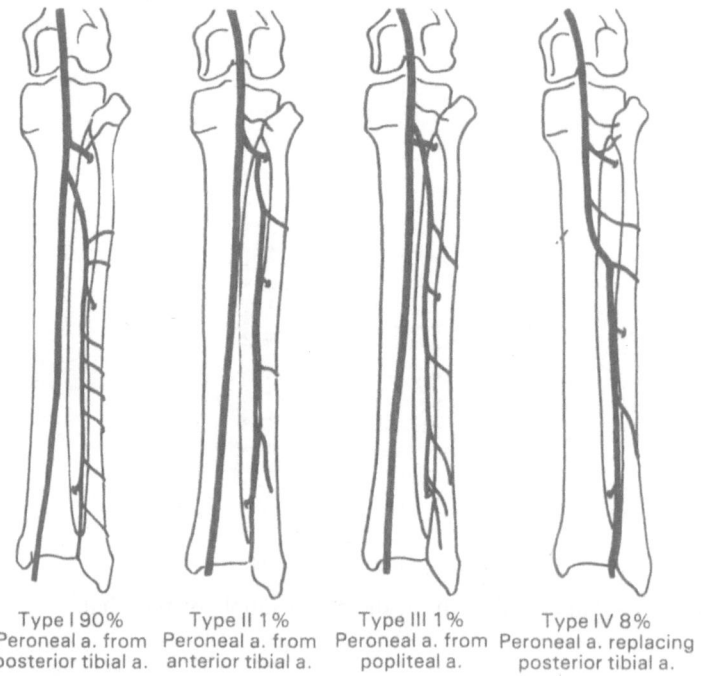

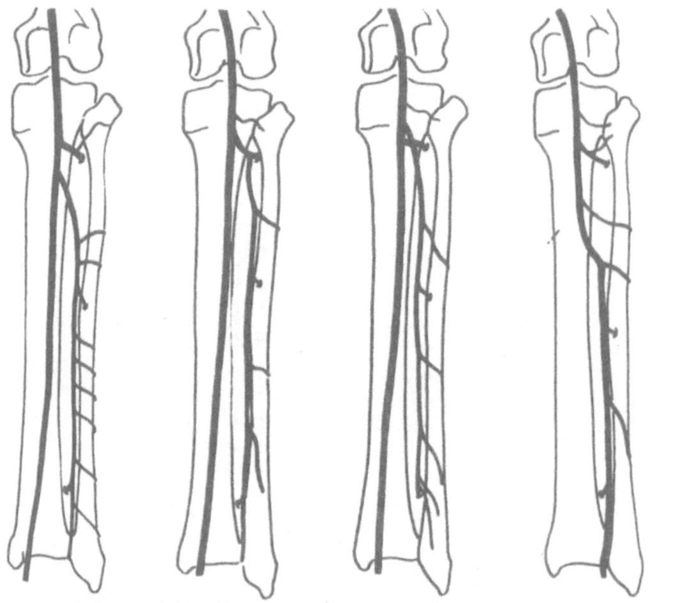

Figure 5.2 Types of origin of the peroneal artery

four types with regard to its origin, as shown in Figure 5.2. The branches of peroneal artery are:

(1) The nutrient artery of the fibula arises at the level 142 (103–234) mm on average below the head of fibula, viz. 68 (21–18) mm below the origin of the peroneal artery. Its length from the origin to the nutrient foramen averages 18 (3–69) mm and its outer diameter at its origin averages 1.2 (0.2–2.2) mm.

(2) The arcuate arteries, also known as the periosteal or musculoperiosteal branches, are about 9 (4–15) in number. They are arranged segmentally along the shaft of the fibula. Some of them are closely attached to the periosteal surface, while others reach the surface of the fibula after penetrating the muscle

fibres for a short distance and winds the fibula from behind forward and laterally to be distributed to the periosteum and muscles, viz. the peroneus longus and brevis and the flexor hallucis longus. The periosteal branches pass through Volkmann's canal, distributed to the outer one-third of the compact bone of the shaft. Between the arcuate arteries there are profuse anastomoses. In the absence of the peroneal nutrient artery most of the blood supply of the fibula comes from the arcuate artery.

The outer diameter of the initial part of the arcuate artery averages 1.4 (0.4–2.8) mm. Generally, they get thicker gradually from the upper part of the fibula downwards. They assume an almost horizontal course near the upper and middle segments of the fibula and gradually incline or take a spiral path downward and laterally near the lower segment.

Some individuals have stout arcuate artery, the branches of which incline laterally and downwards to the lateral portion of the fibula and become attached to the lateral aspect of the fibula with its terminal twigs as muscular branches, while some terminals of the arcuate artery go through the deep fascia of the lateral portion of the leg to become cutaneous arteries, some of which give off nutrient arteries to the fibula as well. These stout arcuate arteries, which give off the nutrient artery to the fibula, can also be called the second peroneal artery.

(3) Muscular branches: besides the muscular branches given off by the arcuate arteries, the peroneal artery sends those to the triceps surae, the flexor hallucis longus, the flexor digitorum longus and the tibialis posterior. The branch to the triceps surae is larger, while branches to the flexor hallucis longus and the flexor digitorum longus are smaller. The direction of their course is apt to be confused with that of the arcuate arteries, yet the latter are larger and do not penetrate into the periosteum of the fibula after having entered the muscle. The number of branches varies greatly; those to the flexor hallucis longus may amount to 16 at the most, while those to the tibialis posterior number as many as eight.

(4) The perforating branches vary between one and eight in number, of which one or two branches are the most frequent. Their outer diameters usually increase from above downwards. They pass through the interosseous membrane on the medial side of the fibula to get to the anterior aspect of the leg. Besides being distributed to the muscles of the anterior group of the leg, they send periosteal branches to the medial aspect of the fibula.

Peroneal veins

The peroneal veins are usually two in number. They course on either side of the artery and collect veins accompanying branches of the artery. They empty into the posterior tibial vein 52 mm on an average below the head of fibula, viz., 21 mm from the lower border of the popliteus, where they are slightly thicker than the companion artery with an average outer diameter of 4.5 (1.7–6.7) mm.

The blood supply of fibula in childhood

The minimum outer diameter of the peroneal artery of a child of 1 year approaches 1 mm. In children of 3 years, no matter whether it is an artery or a vein, the outer diameter of the vessels of the leg is above 1 mm on average and may reach 2 mm at most. As a result, the vessels in children are of sufficiently large calibre for anastomosis during transplantation.

Essentials in the applied anatomy of the fibula

As a donor for the vascularized free bone graft, the anatomical elements are as follows:

(1) Fibula, a long tubular bone, is the least important of the leg bones. It takes no part in the composition of the knee joint and hence is not responsible for bearing the body weight. Its upper three-quarters serve for the attachment of muscles and the weight-bearing function of the leg will not be affected much where the fibula is excised as a donor bone. Therefore, the upper three-quarters, including the head, can be chosen as the donor for transplantation. The lower quarter partakes of the composition of the ankle joint to which it affords stability. This part ought to be preserved in designing an operation. Excision of it will spoil the function of the ankle joint.

(2) The blood supply of the fibula is from multiple sources. In addition to the peroneal artery, both its upper and lower ends have their separate sources of blood supply. After a segment of the fibula with the peroneal artery as its vascular pedicle has been excised, the blood supply of the remaining parts of the fibula will not be affected.

(3) The nutrient artery of the fibula is the main blood supply of the body of the fibula and the protection of the artery during operation appears extremely significant. However, the nutrient artery is minute and short, the average length being only 18 mm and the external diameter 1.2 mm, which leads to considerable difficulty in surgical manipulations. As a result, it is not suitable for a vascular pedicle. It has appeared reasonable to use the peroneal artery and veins in clinical practice during recent years. Since the entrance of the nutrient artery into the bone is concentrated in the middle segment (90%) of the fibula, it is obvious that the blood supply of this segment is plentiful. Eventually, taking the middle segment of the bone will favour the survival of the grafted fibula.

(4) The arcuate arteries are the main source of blood supply of the periosteum. In case of obstruction of the nutrient artery, the arcuate arteries can penetrate into the marrow cavity from the outer one-third of the compact bone in place of the nutrient artery. In a minority of the cases (2%), in which the nutrient foramen is absent, the marrow cavity and the whole of the shaft are supplied entirely by periosteal vessels. Therefore, selecting the peroneal vessel as the vascularized pedicles will preserve the blood supply from the nutrient artery as well as a lot of arcuate arteries.

(5) The vascular network of the periosteum is composed, in addition to those from the arcuate arteries, of those through the muscular branches. Hence it is essential to preserve a layer of muscular sleeve around the fibula during its

resection to protect the relevant vessels. Through observation of the specimens, casts and roentgenography of the peroneal vessels, it is certain that the peroneal vessels are separated from the medial aspect of the upper segment of the fibula by about 1 cm before they gradually approach the posteromedial aspect of the lower segment. The muscular and periosteal branches of the arcuate arteries remain 0.3–0.5 cm from the lateral aspect of the fibula. Therefore in the preservation of the muscular sleeve, the thickness of the muscular layer to be left on the medial side of the upper segment of the fibula should not be less than 1 cm, and 0.5 cm is enough for its lower segment.

(6) The origin of the peroneal artery varies. In 8% of the specimens it may replace the stem of the posterior tibial artery. This should be taken into consideration in surgical operations. It is necessary, in case of suspicion, to try blocking this chief arterial stem in the posterior aspect of the leg, and ligation and excision are warranted only if no ischaemia is assured.

(7) The peroneal artery is distributed not only to the fibula and its periosteum and related muscles, but also to the skin in the neighbourhood of the posterolateral intermuscular septum of the leg. Therefore, vascularized fibula, together with the muscles and skin of the lateral part of the leg, can be used as a composite tissue graft.

RIB

WU YONGMU

Ribs are 12 in number on either side. Morphologically, the third to the ninth or the tenth ribs are known as the ordinary (standard) ribs, the rest being the special ribs.

As to the classification of the ribs, opinions differ as follows: some consider them as atypical long bones, yet owing to the lack of marrow cavity, they are sometimes grouped as atypical flat bones. A slender and bow-like rib has an anterior and a posterior end, a lateral and a medial surface and an upper and a lower border (in the case of the first rib, it is divided into an upper and a lower surface and a medial and a lateral border). Ribs are provided with the following structures: the costal tubercle, the costal angle, the body of rib and the costal sulcus, but the first rib is devoid of the costal angle and sulcus. The costal tubercle and sulcus are inconspicuous in the eleventh rib and no tubercle or angle is present in the twelfth rib.

For the sake of description of different parts of the rib, the costal angle (the tubercle of the first rib and the part of the twelfth rib corresponding to the costal angle of the eleventh rib) is adopted as a mark for demarcating a segment A facing backward and another segment B directing forward, which is again divided into three parts, namely, B_1, B_2 and B_3 from behind forward (Figure 5.3).

Nutrient foramen of the rib

These foramina are numerous and arranged all over the rib. Most of the foramina are distributed to its anterior and posterior ends, and the part near the costal sulcus, either scattered or in groups.

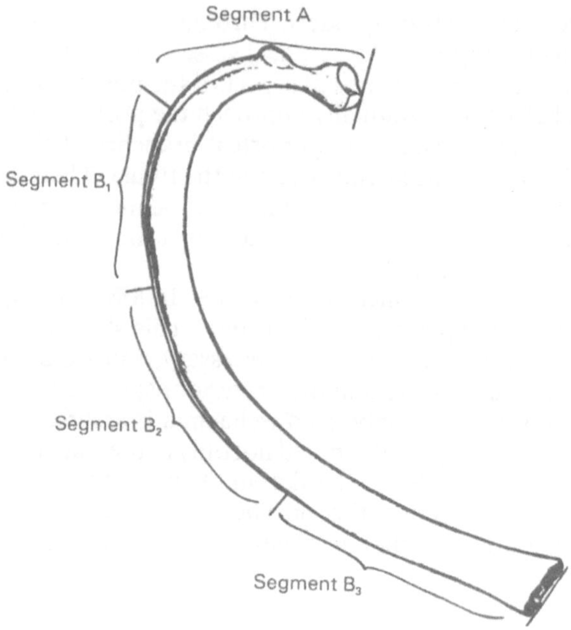

Figure 5.3 Segmentation of rib

Number of nutrient foramina

Dozens of nutrient foramina can be found in each rib. Those in the seventh rib are the most numerous, sixty-four on average.

The topographical distribution of the nutrient foramina

In the case of the third to the tenth ribs, most of the nutrient foramina are distributed over the medial surface of the rib (69%). Those distributed over the medial surface of each rib are concentrated on segment B (79%), especially on segment B_1, accounting for 46% of the total number of foramina on the medial surface of segment B, those in segments B_2 and B_3 being 27% for each. The nutrient foramina distributed over the external surface of each rib are comparatively less.

In view of the fact that the nutrient foramina are concentrated on a segment of a length of 6 cm anterior to the costal angle, this segment of the rib, being broad and straight, is often considered as a donor in transplantation.

Calibre of the nutrient foramina

The calibre of the nutrient foramina varies greatly: the minute ones are almost invisible to the naked eye, while the large ones may have a diameter of more than 1 mm. When the largest nutrient foramen on each of the 12 ribs is taken for measurement, the average value of the calibre has been estimated to be 0.6 mm.

Blood supply of the rib

Of the 11 intercostal spaces on either side the uppermost two are supplied by the highest intercostal artery (a. intercostalis suprema) of the costocervical trunk and the highest thoracic artery (a. thoracic suprema) of the axillary. The rest of the intercostal spaces are supplied by the intercostal arteries of the thoracic aorta. The artery below the twelfth rib is designated the subcostal artery. The anterior ends of the ribs are supplied by the anterior intercostal arteries of the internal thoracic artery. There are plentiful anastomoses between them.

The intercostal arteries (may be called the posterior intercostal arteries)

These arise from the thoracic aorta. They accompany the intercostal veins and nerves laterally and forward and divide into the upper and lower branches near the costal angle. The upper branch advances closely along the costal sulcus between the external and internal intercostal muscles. The lower branch proceeds along the upper border of the lower rib. The intercostal artery gives off, on the way, the muscular, periosteal and cutaneous branches to supply the ribs, intercostal muscles and the overlying skin.

(1) The outer diameters of the intercostal arteries at their commencement average 2.3 mm. Those of the left seventh and the right eighth intercostal arteries are the largest, with an average of 2.7 mm. The calibres of the arteries thence increase and decrease respectively up and down in the order of the ordinal numbers of the ribs.

(2) The outer diameters of the initial part of the upper branches of the intercostal arteries are generally greater than those of the lower. The outer diameter of the upper branch averages 1.4 mm and that of the lower 1.1 mm.

(3) Branches of the intercostal arteries. In addition to the upper and lower branches mentioned above, the chief branches of the intercostal artery are the nutrient arteries and the periosteal and muscular branches. The number of the nutrient arteries and that of the nutrient foramina are in perfect accord; however, their site of origin varies, and after emergence they may proceed upward, downward, forward or even backward as a recurrent branch to enter the foramen. Of these alternatives the last is the most common. The outer diameter of the nutrient artery of the rib varies between 0.01 and 0.06 mm, its length being about 10 mm. The periosteal branches are very profuse and interconnected to form a network, which is especially prominent on the head of the rib. Their outer diameters range from 0.01 to 0.07 mm. Muscular branches are more numerous and are generally given off from the lower branch of the intercostal arteries, their external calibres ranging from 0.1 to 0.12 mm. Both the periosteal and muscular branches supply the ribs.

The anterior intercostal branches (may also be known as the anterior intercostal arteries)

These arise from the internal thoracic artery. Each of the upper six intercostal spaces is provided with two anterior intercostal arteries of an outer diameter averaging 0.7 mm. Those of the seventh, eighth and ninth intercostal spaces are given off by the musculophrenic artery. The anterior intercostal arteries anastomose with the upper and lower branches of the posterior intercostals in the anterior one-third of the space.

The intercostal veins

These accompany the intercostal artery and nerve. The topographical relations of the initial portions of this triple are not constant, especially in the posterior part of the intercostal space. The outer diameter of the intercostal vein is generally greater than that of the artery and measures 3.5 mm at its posterior end.

Essentials in the applied anatomy of the rib

(1) Generally, with the exception of special ribs, most of the ribs can be used as donors. The donor area, after excision of the rib, shows little functional change.

(2) The rib has a flat and lengthened curvature. Its spongy bony character has the advantage of being a kind of skin-bearing bone graft. The part anterior to the costal angle also shows a certain degree of curvature and is suitable for curved bone graft such as that in the repair of mandibular defects.

(3) The body of the rib is the main portion of the bone, of which the segment anterior to the costal angle is the chief part, which usually appears flatter and thicker than other parts of the rib.

(4) The nutrient foramina of the rib are numerous. They are usually crowded anterior to the costal angle.

(5) The rib has a double source of blood supply. The posterior end is supplied by the posterior intercostal artery and the anterior end by the anterior intercostal arteries of the internal thoracic. The vessels are large and constant, easy to locate and dissect. Because of the dual source of supply at either end of the rib, there are few limitations to its excision.

(6) The body of the rib anterior to the costal angle, especially segment B_1 or the part with a length of 6 cm anterior to the angle, has so many advantages that it becomes the site of first choice as a bone donor. If the fourth to the sixth ribs are to be selected, the anterior intercostal arteries with or without the internal thoracic may be taken as the vascular pedicle. If the seventh to the ninth ribs are to be used, the posterior intercostal arteries can be adopted as the pedicle instead.

ILIUM

HUANG GONGKANG, MIAO HUA AND WU RENXIU

The ilium consists of a cancellous bone with a thin cortex on its surface. As a transplantation material the union rate of the cancellous bone is higher than that of the compact bone. Therefore, the iliac graft has a higher rate of success.

Transplantation of a vascularized free iliac bone was first successfully performed with its overlying skin. Taylor *et al.* (1978) and O'Brien (1970) reported the successful transplantation of the inguinal flap with a piece of iliac bone by means of anastomosis of the superficial circumflex iliac vessels. In 1979 Taylor *et al.* again used the deep circumflex iliac vessels as the blood supplier for the groin skin flap with iliac bone. Chinese microsurgeons Huang Gongkang *et al.* (1980) successfully carried out the transplantation of free iliac bone without overlying skin by anastomosis of the deep circumflex iliac vessels. Further investigation shows that there are still other nutrient vessels suitable for iliac bone grafting.

Morphology of the ilium

The ilium constitutes the upper part of the hip bone. It is somewhat irregularly fan-shaped and has a body and a wing, with an outer and an inner surface, and anterior, posterior and superior borders. The superior border (the iliac crest) presents a somewhat S-shaped curvature, its anterior and posterior parts being thick, and its middle part thin. Considering that the anterior part of the iliac crest is the most available donor in clinical practice the data of measurement relevant to the iliac crest are as shown in Table 5.1.

Table 5.1 Length and thickness of iliac crest (mm)

Specimen	*Whole length of iliac crest*	*Thickness of iliac crest*			
		Ant. sup. iliac spine	*Tubercle of crest*	*Middle of crest*	*Post. sup. iliac spine*
100 dry bones	233 (194–280)	13.8 (6.5–18.0)	16.8 (7.2–24.0)	7.6 (5.0–11.0)	21.0 (16.0–27.5)
100 wet bones	244 (201–288)	14.8 (7.4–24.0)	18.1 (9.1–30.2)	8.7 (6.2–15.4)	22.3 (23.8–34.0)

Blood supply of the ilium

The deep circumflex iliac artery

Origin of the deep circumflex iliac artery

Most of the deep circumflex iliac arteries originate from the femoral artery in male and from the external iliac artery in female.

The highest level of the origin is 13 mm above the inguinal ligament, while the lowest is 24 mm below it. The mean value is 1.4 mm below the ligament.

Table 5.2 Origins of the deep circumflex iliac artery in 200 specimens (%)

Sex	*External iliac artery*	*Femoral artery*
male	44.3	55.7
female	83.3	16.7
Total	59.5	40.5

Outer diameter of the deep circumflex iliac artery

The average diameter at the level of its origin is 2.8 (1–5) mm, in which sexual difference is not significant.

Course and branches of the deep circumflex iliac artery

The deep circumflex iliac artery runs laterally and upwards beneath the lateral half of the inguinal ligament to the anterior superior iliac spine. It then turns backwards along the inner lip of the anterior part of the iliac crest to the upper border of it. The artery thus has an inguinal and a suprailiac segment, as well as one medial to the iliac crest.

The inguinal segment of the deep circumflex iliac artery lies behind the inguinal ligament and is enclosed in a fibrous canal formed by the union of the fascia transversalis and the iliac fascia. The average length of this segment is 62 (41–81) mm. The accompanying vein is mostly single (88.4%) and lies antero-superior to the artery, its average diameter being 3.6 (2–6) mm. Most of them (72.9%) cross in front of the external iliac artery to end into the external iliac vein (Figure 5.4).

The origin of the deep circumflex iliac artery is hidden by the external iliac lymph nodes and is crossed by the femoral branch of the genitofemoral nerve. Near the anterior superior iliac spine and the lateral end of the inguinal segment, the deep circumflex iliac artery is crossed in front by the ilioinguinal nerve (36.5%) and from behind by the lateral femoral cutaneous nerve (84.6%). These nerves are closely related to the deep circumflex iliac artery, so that care must be taken to avoid injury to the nerves during the dissection of the deep circumflex iliac artery for iliac bone transplantation.

The inguinal segment of the deep circumflex iliac artery gives off on the way two to seven branches to the adjacent muscles. Most of them are three to five in number (69%) and their outer diameters range from 0.2 to 1.8 mm. A large branch arises from the artery 1 cm medial to the anterior superior iliac spine. It ascends on the anterolateral abdominal wall and is thus named the ascending branch. Führer called it the lateral epigastric artery. It almost solely supplies the muscles, and bears no relation to the supply of the iliac bone. As it has a diameter of more than 1 mm, care should be taken not to mistake it for the main trunk of the deep circumflex iliac artery.

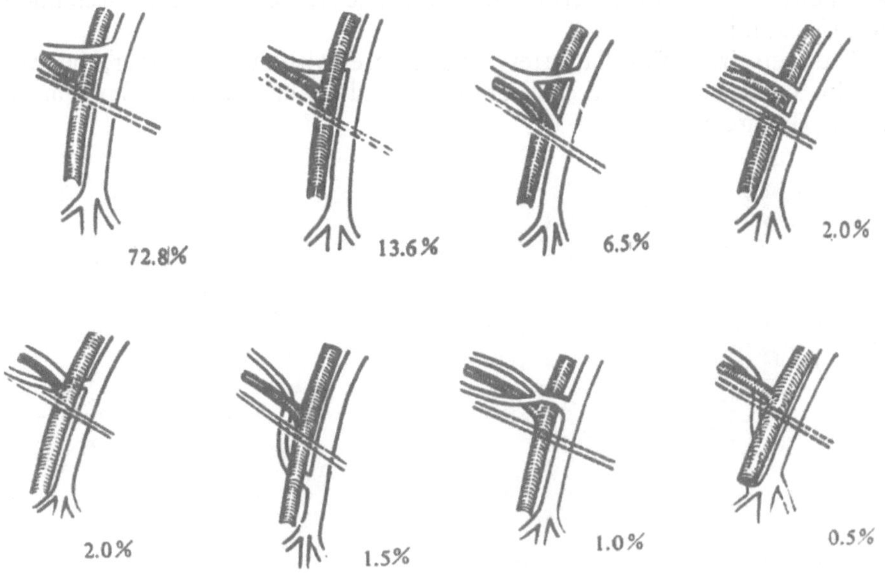

Figure 5.4 Patterns of the termination of the deep circumflex iliac vein

The segment medial to the iliac crest begins on the medial side of the anterior superior iliac spine and ends at a round hole formed by the union of the transversalis and iliac fasciae. This segment runs between two layers of the fascial sheath medial to the iliac crest, with an average length of 36 (11–58) mm and an average outer diameter of 1.5 (0.9–2.4) mm. Its vena comitans always lies above the artery, with an average outer diameter of 2 (1.2–4.1) mm. The distance between its commencement and the anterior iliac spine is 15.8 mm. It is crossed in front by the ilioinguinal nerve in 46.1% and from behind by the lateral femoral cutaneous nerve in 15.4%, and often gives off two to eight branches to directly enter the foramina in the inner lip of the iliac crest as the nutritive arteries of the anterior part of the ilium. Therefore, in performing iliac bone transplantation by vascular anastomosis with the deep circumflex iliac artery, care must be taken to preserve the attachment of the muscle to the inner lip of the iliac crest to avoid injury to the nutritive arteries of the iliac bone.

The suprailiac segment is the last segment of the deep circumflex iliac artery, which pierces the round hole formed by the union of the fasciae and runs upwards and backwards over the iliac crest. Its average length is 38 (14–65) mm and the average outer diameter is 1 (0.6–1.8) mm. In the course of this segment it is usually crossed by the iliohypogastric nerve, which runs therefrom forwards and downwards, accompanying the artery closely. The ilioinguinal nerve sometimes (17.3%) lies anterosuperior to this segment of the artery, but they are kept far apart.

The suprailiac segment of the deep circumflex iliac artery gives off two to nine branches to the iliac bone and the distance between two neighbouring branches varies from 2 to 22 mm. By the injection of black ink into the deep circumflex iliac artery in a fresh specimen, the ink within the vessels of the cancellous matrix of the anterior part of the iliac crest can be clearly seen under the surgical microscope.

The deep circumflex iliac artery anastomoses with the iliolumbar, the third and the fourth lumbar, the superior gluteal and the lateral circumflex femoral arteries (Figure 5.5).

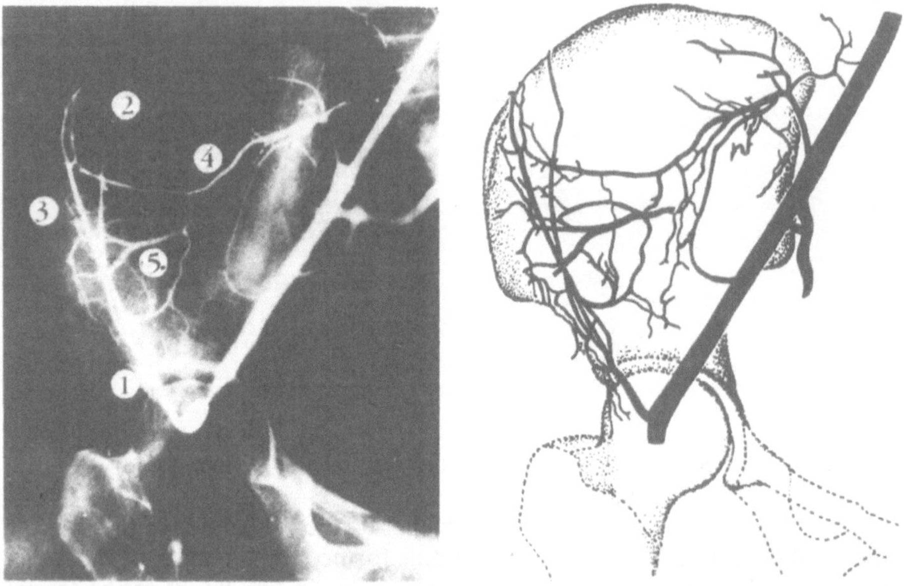

Figure 5.5 Anastomosis between the deep circumflex iliac artery and other arteries (X-ray film). **1**: Main trunk of deep circumflex iliac a.; **2**: ascending branch of deep circumflex iliac a.; **3**: terminal branch of deep circumflex iliac a.; **4**: iliolumbar a.; **5**: deep branch of superior gluteal a.

The superficial circumflex iliac artery

Origin of the superficial circumflex iliac artery

The origins of the superficial circumflex iliac artery are shown in Table 5.3. Most of them originate from the femoral artery. The distance from the origin to the inguinal ligament averages 14 mm.

Table 5.3 Origin of the superficial circumflex iliac artery (201 arteries)

Origin	*Percentage*
Femoral artery	75.1
Deep circumflex iliac artery	12.9
Lateral circumflex femoral artery	8.0
Profunda femoris artery	3.5
Medial circumflex femoral artery	0.5

The patterns of the branching of the superficial circumflex iliac artery can be classified into single-trunk type (79%), double-trunk type (3%) and the type with a trunk common to other arteries (18%).

Outer diameter of the superficial circumflex iliac artery

The average outer diameter of the superficial circumflex iliac artery is 1.5 mm and 1.3 mm in the single-trunk type and the type with a trunk common to other arteries respectively, and the common trunk itself is 2.1 mm in diameter.

Course, branches and distribution of the superficial circumflex iliac artery

In 69% of cases the superficial circumflex iliac artery as a single branch pierces the fascia lata lateral to the saphenous hiatus and runs upwards and laterally to enter the superficial fascia. It is distributed to the skin and subcutaneous tissue of the groin in the vicinity of the anterior superior iliac spine, and the superficial inguinal lymph nodes. In the remaining 31% the superficial circumflex iliac artery divides close to its origin into two terminal branches - a superficial and a deep branch. The course and distribution of the superficial branch is similar to that of the single-branch type, and most of the deep branches run beneath or between the two layers of the fascia lata to the anterior superior iliac spine and the neighbouring muscles. A number of the deep branches ascend or descend along the lateral aspect of the femoral artery to such deeper structures as the iliopsoas muscle. The superficial circumflex iliac artery is a subcutaneous artery. It supplies mainly the skin, and its muscular branches, which are distributed to the vicinity of the anterior superior iliac spine, may give some small branches to the anterior quarter of the iliac crest. If the superficial circumflex iliac artery is used as a nutrient artery in the transplantation of the iliac bone, the overlying skin must be grafted simultaneously to ensure the blood supply of the iliac bone.

In 79.49% of the cases the superficial circumflex iliac vein is single in number. It does not accompany the superficial circumflex iliac artery. Its average outer diameter is 2.5 (1–4) mm. It ends mainly into the greater saphenous vein.

Iliolumbar artery

The iliolumbar artery arises mostly from the trunk or posterior division of the internal iliac artery (79.6%) by a single stem or a double stem in 52.7% and 39.3% respectively. Its origin lies near the inlet of the pelvis. The average outer diameter of the iliolumbar artery is 2.5 (1–5.2) mm. The accompanying vein is single with an outer diameter of 3.5 (1.5–6) mm. The iliolumbar artery runs in front of the lumbosacral trunk and then passes laterally behind the obturator nerve, the external iliac vessels and the psoas muscle to be divided into an iliac (posterior) and a lumbar (anterior) branch. The iliolumbar artery rarely (8%) arises as three independent branches.

In general the iliolumbar artery is distributed mainly to the iliacus, the psoas major, the lower part of the abdominal muscles, the lumbosacral segment of the spinal cord and the superficial structures of the buttock. It gives off a large nutrient artery to the ilium and through the periosteum iliac and periosteal branches to the inner lip of the iliac crest. It also supplies a more extensive area of the iliac crest and wing indirectly via the rich anastomoses with other arteries. Because of its deep location it is difficult to operate over this region. That is why the iliolumbar artery is of no practical importance.

The fourth lumbar artery

The fourth lumbar artery lies below the third intervertebral disc or above the body of the fourth lumbar vertebra. It springs from the posterior wall of the abdominal aorta and passes backwards and laterally behind the psoas major, the lumbar sympathetic trunk and the roots of the first to third lumbar nerves. The average outer diameter of the fourth lumbar artery is 2.1 (1–4) mm. The accompanying vein is single and usually courses above the artery, its outer diameter being 2.6 (1–5) mm.

It is an indirect nutrient artery to the iliac bone through anastomosis with other arteries, so the fourth lumbar artery is of no practical value in the transplantation of iliac bone by means of microvascular anastomosis.

The lateral circumflex femoral artery

The lateral circumflex femoral artery generally springs from the profunda femoris artery. It runs laterally posterior to the rectus femoris and anterior to the iliopsoas muscles and ends by dividing into the ascending and descending branches. It rarely divides into three branches. The origin of the ascending branch lies 91.2 (60–118) mm below the anterior superior iliac spine. The length of the main trunk of the ascending branch before it enters the tensor fasciae latae is 41.6 (20–68) mm. The outer diameter is 2.6 (1.5–5) mm. There are two venae comitantes.

The ascending branch of the lateral circumflex femoral artery supplies only a small area of the iliac crest. Considering that a part of the main trunk of the ascending branch passes between the muscle fibres, it is difficult to isolate a sufficient length of the nutrient vessels from muscle fibres. Therefore, this artery is usually not selected as the nutrient vessel for iliac bone transplantation.

The superior gluteal artery

The superior gluteal artery is the continuation of the posterior division of the internal iliac artery. It leaves the pelvis through the suprapiriform foramen and enters the gluteal region, where it is divided into the superficial and deep branches. It enters the gluteal region 17.2 mm above the mid-point of the line joining the posterior superior iliac spine and the upper border of the greater trochanter of the femur, i.e. at the junction of the upper and middle thirds of the line.

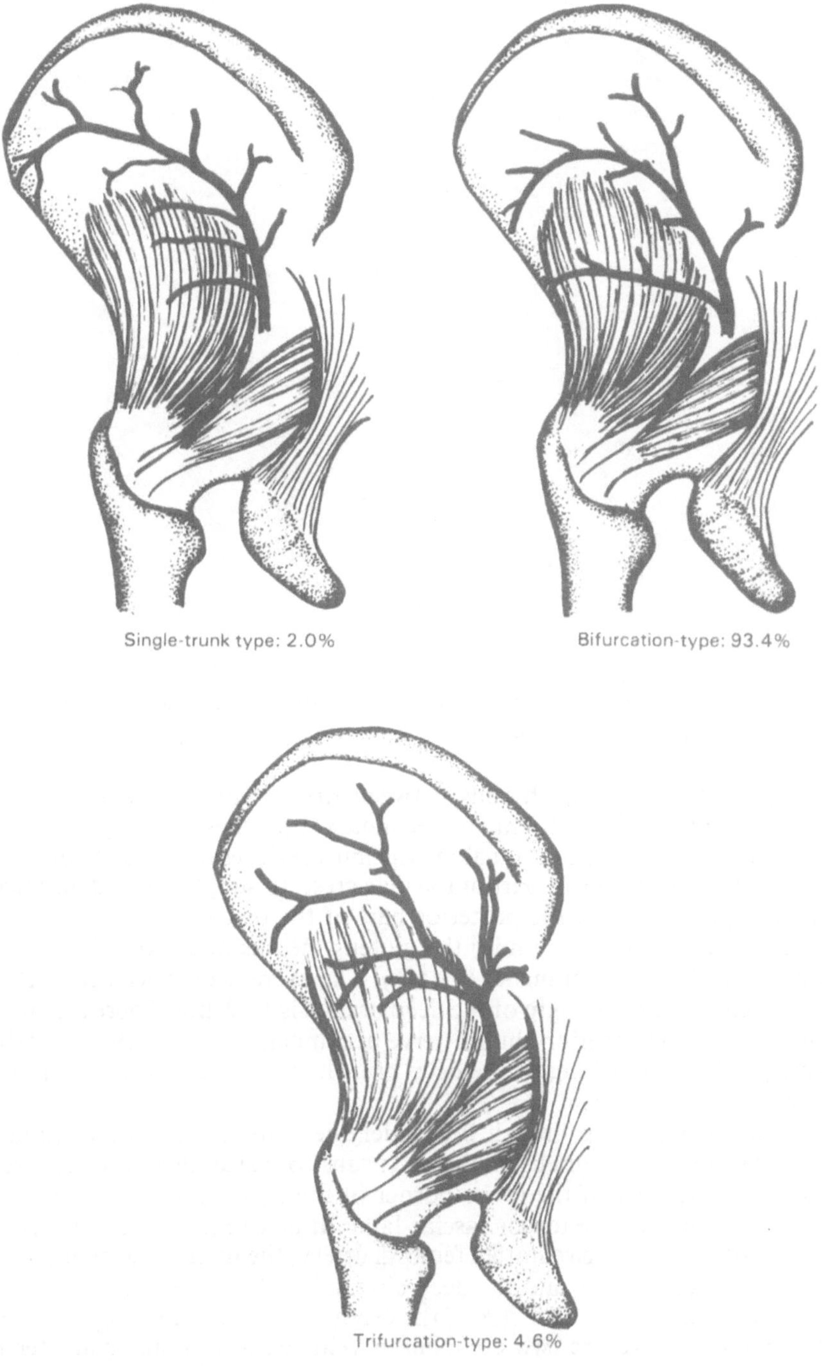

Figure 5.6 Pattern of the deep branch of the superior gluteal artery

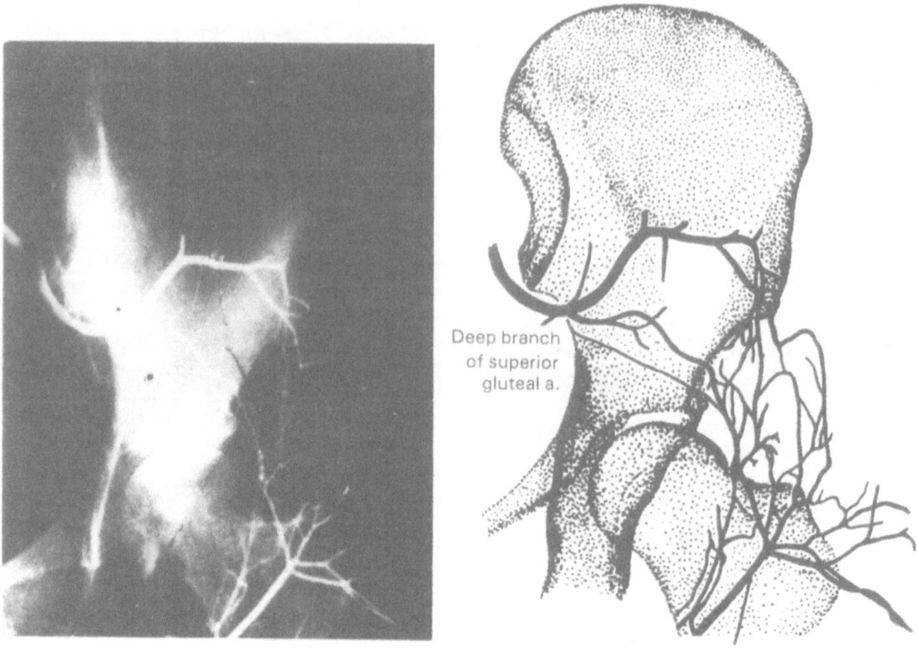

Figure 5.7 Arteriogram showing the anastomosis between the superior gluteal and lateral circumflex femoral arteries

The superficial branch runs between the piriformis and gluteus medius muscles and divides into many secondary branches to supply the gluteus maximus. These branches run along the muscle fibres towards the origin of the muscle, viz. the posterior part of the iliac crest, to supply the gluteus maximus, the overlying skin and the posterior part of the iliac crest.

The deep branch lies under the gluteus medius and soon divides into the superior and inferior branches (93.5%). The average distance between the site of branching and the origin of the deep branch is 13.2 mm. There are two venae comitantes. The superior gluteal nerve accompanies the artery inferiorly. The pattern of the branching of the deep branch can be classified into three types as shown in Figure 5.6.

The superior deep branch lies under the gluteus medius and follows the upper border of the gluteus minimus. It runs forwards along the iliac crest and ends in the vicinity of the lower border of the anterior superior iliac spine or under the cover of the tensor fasciae latae. It anastomoses with the ascending branch of the lateral circumflex femoral artery, the inferior deep branch of the superior gluteal artery and the deep circumflex iliac artery (Figure 5.7).

The average outer diameter of the origin of the superior deep branch is 2.9 (1.7–5) mm. There are two companion veins with an outer diameter of 3.7 (1–6.5) mm. An ascending branch of the superior gluteal nerve runs superficially. The superior deep branch of the superior gluteal artery gives off on the

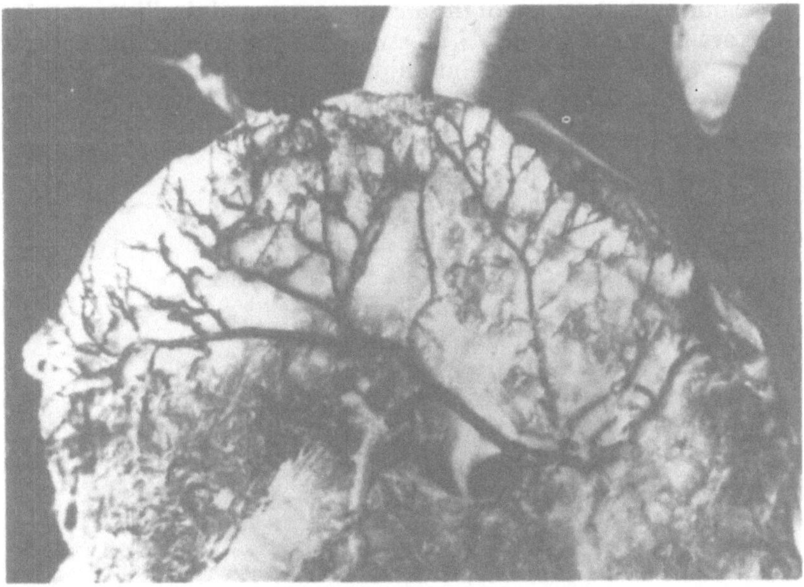

Figure 5.8 Iliac branches of the superior gluteal artery. A corrosion specimen of the superior gluteal artery filled with latex, showing numerous arterial twigs entering the cortex of the bone near the iliac crest

way 6–19 branches upwards to the iliac crest. After injecting black ink or red latex into the superior gluteal artery in fresh cadavers, followed by microanatomical dissection or corrosion (Figure 5.8), small branches of the superior deep branch of the superior gluteal artery have been proved to enter the iliac bone.

To map out the course and position of the superior and inferior deep branches of the superior gluteal artery and the superior gluteal nerve, we measured the distances between the upper border of the iliac crest and the respective points of the superior and inferior deep branches of the superior gluteal artery, and the superior gluteal nerve on the line drawn from the iliac crest to the apex of great trochanter of the femur. The data are shown in Table 5.4 and their surface projections are illustrated in Figure 5.9.

The superficial branch of the superior gluteal artery is distributed through its branches to the gluteus maximus to the posterior quarter of the iliac crest, while the superior deep branch of the superior gluteal artery is distributed by means of its branches to the gluteus medius to the outer aspect of the anterior three-quarters of the crest. Because of the easy identification of the location of the superior deep branch, its large calibre, numerous branches and greater extent of distribution to the bone, it is suitable for a massive iliac bone transplantation or for the condition when the deep circumflex iliac artery is injured.

Since the main trunk and the terminal segment of the superior deep branch run in the neighbourhood of the lower border of the iliac crest, it is convenient to take the anterior portion of iliac crest together with the terminal segment of the superior deep branch, which ascends in company with the muscular fibres of the gluteus medius to the iliac crest. A part of the muscle has to be preserved on the bone during the excision of the anterior portion of the iliac crest. Moreover, there are no important nerves crossing the operating field, so operation may be done without worrying about injuring any nerves.

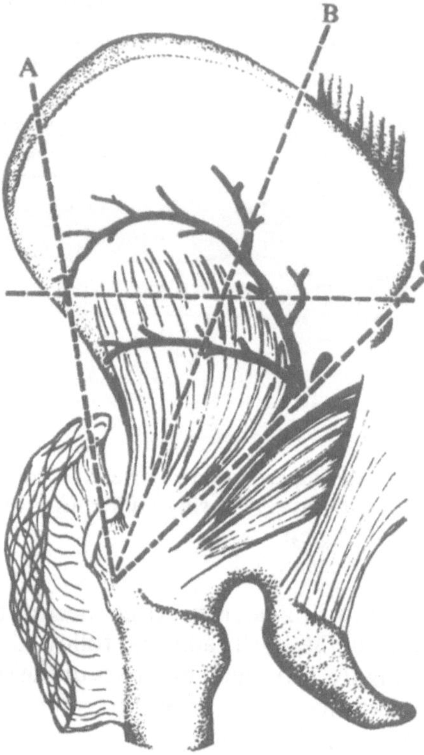

Figure 5.9 Surface projection of the deep branches of the superior gluteal artery. *Line A*: drawn from the posterior border of the tubercle of the iliac crest to the great trochanter; *line B*: drawn from the lateral border of the sacrospinalis to the greater trochanter; *line C*: drawn from the posterior superior iliac spine to the greater trochanter. Horizontal line drawn from the anterior to the posterior superior iliac spines

Table 5.4 The distances between the iliac crest and the superior gluteal artery and nerve on the line drawn from the iliac crest to the apex of the great trochanter (mm)

Intersection point on upper border of iliac crest	*Superior deep branch of superior gluteal artery*	*Inferior deep branch of superior gluteal artery*	*Trunk of superior gluteal nerve*
Outer border of sacrospinalis	63.9 (53–78)	85.0 (66–110)	88.7 (74–105)
Posterior border of tubercle of iliac crest	38.8 (28–52)	74.7 (51–98)	74.6 (52–97)

6

The applied anatomy for the functional reconstruction of the hands and fingers

WANG QIHUA AND ZENG YAOXIANG

INTRODUCTION TO THE FUNCTION OF THE HANDS

The highly developed intelligence of humanity has largely been manifested through the hands. The skilfulness reflected by the functions of the hands is most surprising. Our hands are not only organs for physical labour but also serve as tools for emotional expression and accessories for speech delivery.

Discrepancies in the working and living conditions exhibited by different individuals have cast definite effects on the structures of the hands. Those engaged in delicate and complicated yet not very laborious tasks have hands which reflect the characteristics of the refined and delicate skin with slight keratinization, of well-developed muscles and tendons though not thick and stout, of sensitive fingertips and free movement of the interphalangeal joints and fingers. On the contrary, those taking part in monotonous work and hard labour have muscles and tendons well developed but inclined to be thick and strong, their palms equipped with a thickened keratinized layer to meet heavy abrasions, poor movements of interphalangeal joints and the relative insensitiveness of the fingertips. Therefore, the effect of the working and living conditions on the hands has been so great that any post-traumatic management will accordingly be quite varied.

The basic postures of the hand consist of two types, i.e. those during motion and at rest. Though postures of the hand during motion vary, there is only one position at rest. The resting posture of the hand may be maintained for a relatively long time without fatigue. It comprises mainly overextension of the wrist for 10–15 degrees, with all fingers in the flexion state, the range of which increases from the radial to the ulnar side, i.e. the thumb assumes the least flexion and the little finger the greatest. The thumb flexes slightly beside the distal interphalangeal joint of the index finger. The tip of the index finger inclines to the ulnar side and that of the little finger to the radial side.

The resting posture of the hand varies with that of the wrist. When the extension of the wrist exceeds 15 degrees the range of flexion of the fingers increases accordingly. On the contrary, when the wrist flexes, the flexion of the fingers decreases as well. In complete wristdrop, the flexures of the fingers almost entirely disappear. All of these are the normal physiological state.

The functional position of the hand is different from its resting position. The functional position consists of the extension of wrist for 20–25 degrees, full abduction of the thumb, and slight flexion of the metacarpophalangeal and interphalangeal joints. The range of flexion of the interphalangeal joints is relatively uniform, the fingers being slightly separated. By means of such functional position the various functions of the hand can be fully performed, such as making a fist, grasping, extending the palm, etc. While managing a traumatic wound of the hand, especially in fixing a broken bone and bandaging, special attention should be paid to the maintenance of the functional position. If any joint is ankylosed in the non-functional position it will do some harm to the function of the hand as a whole.

STRUCTURES OF THE HAND

WANG QIHUA AND LIU QINGLIN

Skin and the superficial and deep fasciae

Skin

The skin of the palm and the dorsum of the hand have certain characteristics of their own and the structure varies accordingly. Owing to the direct contact of the palm with different objects during gripping, the skin of the palm is adorned with a thickened karatinized layer. Since it has no vigour, any incision made through it will be difficult to heal. If any loss of the palm skin is left to heal spontaneously, a great deal of cicatrices will result.

The hand is indeed a sensory organ, provided with a kind of special receptor made of a profuse collection of sensory nerve endings. Tactile sensation is dexterous, so is the stereognosis, through which the profile of objects and their weight and texture may be well recognized. It is known that blind people are able to be trained to appreciate braille through tactile sensibility by fingers.

There are three distinct dermatoglyphs on the skin of the palm. They are related to the movements of the thumb, the index and the rest of the fingers respectively. These are called the oblique stria of the thumb (the thenar stria or the proximal transverse stria), the middle palmar stria and the transverse palmodigital stria (the distal transverse stria). In making gypsum fixation for a broken hand or arm the length of the gypsum bandage must not exceed the limit of these striae, lest the movements of the thumb or the index finger should be restrained to impede the restoration of the function of the hand.

Furthermore, on the palmar surface of the finger there are three transverse striae, viz. the proximal, middle and distal striae. The proximal transverse stria in the middle of the proximal phalanx corresponds to the level of the finger webs and may sometimes be mistaken for the site of the metacarpophalangeal joints. As the range of flexion of the proximal interphalangeal joint is far greater than that of the distal joint during grasping, the middle transverse striae are more numerous than the distal. The skin of the finger is provided with many fine striae which are most distinct at the fingertip. Fine though they are, the striae are useful in nipping delicate objects. Fingerprints are characterized by individual differences, thus being significant in legal medicine.

As the skin of the palm is equipped with an abundance of sensory nerve endings and sweat glands, but without hairs, it is a type of highly differentiated structure in the body. Therefore it is difficult to satisfactorily substitute lost skin by using skin from other parts of the body.

The more prominent feature of the skin of the back of the hand in contrast to the palmar counterpart is that the skin of the dorsum remains thin, loose and soft and full of elasticity in order to meet the need of physical labour, e.g. the skin of the dorsum appears neither too tight in fisting nor superfluous in extension. Normally, the skin area of the dorsum of the hand is estimated to increase by some 25% more in fisting that it is in extension. Therefore, in skin graft, consideration should be taken of the relative lack of elasticity of the free flaps taken from other parts of the body, and the size of the flap should be increased accordingly in order to allow the hand to function normally after grafting.

There are many transverse striae and annular eminences in the skin around the back of interphalangeal joints. These are related to the movements of fingers. In a case where these striae are lost or replaced by cicatrices as a result of trauma or skin burn, the interphalangeal movements will be greatly restrained.

Subcutaneous tissue and deep fascia

The subcutaneous tissue of the palm abounds with fat, which is penetrated and divided into many small compartments by short dense connective tissue fibres firmly connecting the skin of the palm with the palmar aponeurosis. The subcutaneous tissue is almost lacking at the place of palmar striae, where the skin is in direct contact with the deep fascia. These structural characteristics prevent the skin of the palm from gliding, in order to obtain a steady grasp.

Since subcutaneous tissue of the dorsum of the hand is loose and devoid of fat, its skin has a great degree of mobility, which affords excellent conditions for free movements of the extensor tendons. However, the skin of the dorsum of the hand is vulnerable to trauma and laceration, which occur rather frequently in those who are engaged in mechanical work.

The deep fascia of the palm is dense, especially in its middle portion, where it becomes aponeurotic and is called the palmar aponeurosis. The palmar aponeurosis, being nearly triangular in shape, is a glistening fibrotic layer. The apex of the triangle is connected to the transverse carpal ligament and the palmaris longus tendon, while its base is divided into four slips on the line of metacarpophalangeal joints which are inserted separately into the flexor tendon sheaths, the deep transverse metacarpal ligament and both sides of the base of the proximal phalanx. The palmar aponeurosis sends off two prominent fibrous septa to reach the third and fifth metacarpal bones respectively, dividing the palmar space into three compartments: the thenar and middle palmar spaces and the hypothenar space.

The central part of the palmar aponeurosis is intimately bound to the skin to form a firm and thick structure, which stands as a good barrier for the deep structures and sets in a sense of protection for the deep vessels and nerves. However, during the infection of the palm, owing to the thickness of the aponeurosis, the redness and swelling of the palmar skin is far less prominent than it would be on the dorsum of the hand where the skin is thinner and softer, so that there is a certain possibility of misdiagnosis and false localization of the infection of palm.

Muscles of the hand

The muscles of the hand can be divided into the intrinsic and extrinsic ones.

The intrinsic muscles

These may be divided into the thenar, hypothenar and intermediate palmar muscles. The thenar muscles will be discussed in the section of this chapter entitled 'The functional anatomy of the thumb' (p. 168).

(1) The hypothenar muscles are four in number; viz. the palmaris brevis, the abductor digiti minimi, the flexor digiti minimi (brevis) and the opponens digiti minimi, of which the palmaris brevis assumes the most superficial position, being a kind of cutaneous muscle, situated on the ulnar part of the palmar aponeurosis and having transverse muscle fibres terminating in the skin on the ulnar border of the hand. Digital palpation and pressure on the ulnar nerve from the radial side of the pisiform bone will initiate contraction of the palmaris brevis, which is known as the palmaris brevis reflex, that vanishes in a case of injury of the ulnar nerve.

The flexor digiti minimi (brevis), the abductor digiti minimi and the opponens digiti minimi arise from the pisiform bone, the hamate and the flexor retinaculum. The two former muscles are inserted into the base of the proximal phalanx of the little finger. The opponens digiti minimi is inserted into the ulnar border of the fifth metacarpal. They are supplied by the ulnar nerve.

The intermediate palmar muscles include the lumbricals and the interossei.

There are four lumbricals in each hand, arranged in order from the radial to the ulnar side. The first and second lumbricals, being unipennate muscles, arise separately from the radial side of the tendon of the flexor digitorum profundus of the index and middle fingers; the third from the contiguous sides of the tendons of the middle and ring fingers, and the fourth from the contiguous sides of the tendons of the ring and little fingers. They are, however, bipennate muscles. Each of the lumbricals passes obliquely to the radial side of the corresponding finger, and is inserted into the base of the proximal phalanx, and also into the lateral margin of the dorsal digital expansion of the extensor digitorum, taking part in the formation of the galea aponeurotica of the extensors. The lumbricals are situated on the palmar surface of the transverse axis of the head of the metacarpals, so they can assist in the flexion of metacarpophalangeal joints. The tendons of the lumbricals join the dorsal digital expansions and can thus extend the interdigital joints.

There are seven interossei which reside in the intermetacarpal spaces. Abduction of fingers means that they move away from the longitudinal axis of the middle finger, the reverse being the adduction. The interossei palmares, three in number, arise separately from the ulnar side of the second metacarpal bone, and the radial sides of the fourth and fifth metacarpal bones. They are unipennate muscles and mainly adductors of the fingers. The interossei dorsales, four in number, are bipennate, each arising by two heads from the adjacent sides of the metacarpal bones. The first and the second are inserted into the radial side of the index and middle fingers respectively; the third and the fourth are inserted separately into the ulnar side of the middle and ring fingers. The dorsal interossei abduct the fingers; however, as they are inserted into the base of the proximal phalanges and the dorsal digital expansion of the extensor digitorum, they also join in the composition of galea aponeurotica of the extensors.

Though they are rather slender, the interossei and lumbricals remain extremely important in the coordination of delicate movements of the hand. They take part in the flexion of the metacarpophalangeal joints and the extension of the interdigital joints. Since the extension movement is requisite to the anticipation of the grasping movement, any loss of such a function will certainly lead to great difficulty in gripping. In case of paralysis of the interossei and lumbricals, the flexion of the metacarpophalangeal joints will then depend wholly upon the long flexors of the hand, so that the flexion movement of the metacarpophalangeal joints can be carried out only after full flexion of the interdigital joints, which affects the action of grasping and hinders the recovery of the delicate movements of the hand.

The first and second lumbricals are innervated by the median nerve; the third and the fourth and all of the interossei by the ulnar nerve.

Extrinsic muscles

The extrinsic muscles of the palm and dorsum of the hand all turn to be the tendons before they reach the hand. The movements of the thumb will be mentioned in the section of this chapter entitled 'The functional anatomy of the thumb' (p. 000). The tendons of the extrinsic muscles are fundamentally similar to the rest of the fingers in structure.

(1) The flexor tendons of fingers (Figure 6.1) comprise those of the flexor digitorum superficialis and profundus, each being four in number. The following is the biometry of the tendons of the flexor digitorum superficialis and profundus at the level of the styloid process of the radius. All of the tendons proceed by way of the carpal tunnel from the forearm to the distal stria of the palm, viz. the third area, in a divergent form, maintaining the topographical relation between the flexor digitorum superficially and the flexor digitorum profundus deeply. From the distal stria of the palm to the proximal interdigital joints the superficial and deep flexor tendons become surrounded by the tendon sheaths in the second area. The superficial and deep flexor tendons overlap each other at the level of the head of the metacarpal, and at the site of the proximal phalanges the tendons of the flexor digitorum superficialis become flattened

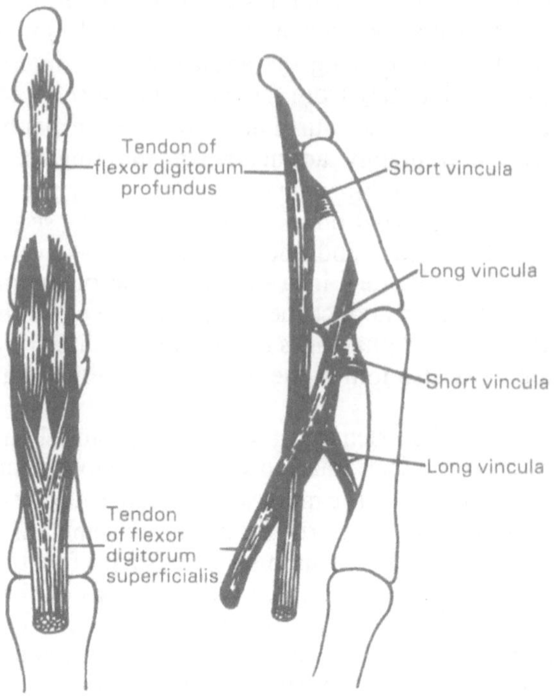

Figure 6.1 Flexor tendons of fingers

and folded, wrapping that of the deep flexor, and each divides to allow the passage of the tendon of the flexor digitorum profundus and then reunites. Finally the superficialis tendon divides again and is inserted into the base of the second phalanx. After passing through the superficialis tendon, the tendon of the flexor digitorum profundus enters the first area, which is located distal to the proximal interphalangeal joint. The deep tendon then widens and forms an extensive insertion at the base of the distal phalanx. Only the deep flexor tendon can be found in this area.

Each of the flexor tendons usually possesses two vincula longa and two vincula brevia. The short vincula are closer to the tendinous attachment than the long vincula. The blood reaches the flexor tendons within the tendon sheath by way of the vincula.

(2) The extensor tendons of fingers (Figure 6.2), six in number, belong to the dorsomedial group (the ulnar group). The following is the biometry of the extensor tendons at the level of the styloid process of the radius. The extensor tendons divert deep to the dorsal carpal ligament to the heads of the metacarpals of the dorsum of hand, viz. the third area. The extensor tendons become connected with one another by means of the juncturae tendinum (connexus intertendineus) within this area. Within the second area, i.e. from the level of the head of the metacarpal to that of the base of the middle digit, the extensor tendons send off transverse fibres extending bilaterally after passing through the heads of the metacarpals. These transverse fibres constitute what is called

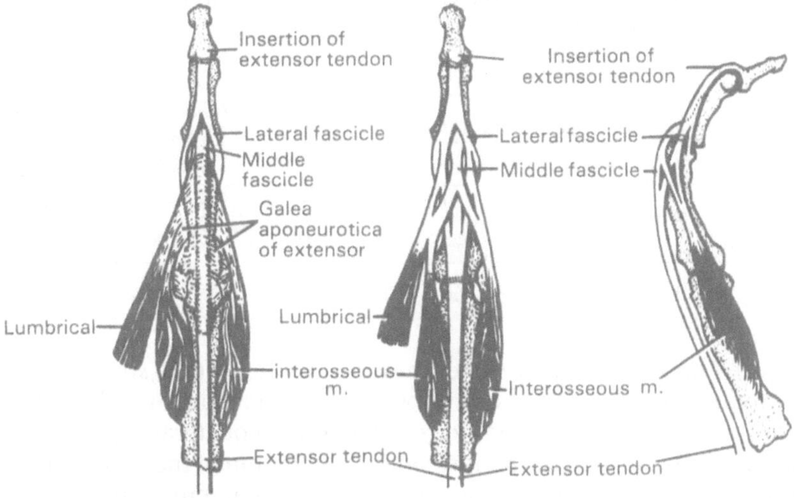

Figure 6.2 Extensor tendons of the fingers

Table 6.1 The biometry (mm) of the flexor tendons of fingers at the level of the styloid process of radius

	Index finger		*Middle finger*		*Ring finger*		*Little finger*	
	Width	*Thickness*	*Width*	*Thickness*	*Width*	*Thickness*	*Width*	*Thickness*
Tendon of FDS	4.2	2.0	4.7	2.4	3.9	2.2	1.7	1.3
Tendon of FDP	5.1	2.3	4.8	2.9	3.6	2.5	2.4	2.4

Abbreviations are explained in the text.

the dorsal digital expansion or the dorsal digital aponeurosis, which receives tendons of insertion of lumbricals at its radial side and those of the interossei at both sides to form the galea aponeurotica of the extensors. The dorsal digital expansion is connected proximally to the fibrous capsule of the metacarpophalangeal joint and the collateral ligaments. It divides distally into three small fascicles, i.e. the intermediate tendinous fascicles and the two lateral tendinous fascicles. The intermediate tendinous fascicle passes over the dorsal aspect of the proximal interphalangeal joint to be inserted into the base of the second digit, and as it passes over the proximal interphalangeal joint it fuses with the joint capsule. The lateral tendinous fascicles of either side proceed forward along the side of the dorsum of the digit to the proximal end of the middle digit and unite with each other into one band to end on the dorsum of the base of the distal phalanx and the capsule of the distal interphalangeal joint. In the lateral fascicles are decussating fibres, which connect with the intermediate tendinous fascicle to merge into the plate. These fibres are of great significance in preventing the lateral fascicles from slipping towards the palmar side during the flexion of fingers.

Table 6.2 The biometry (mm) of the extensor tendons of fingers at the level of the styloid process of the radius

Tendon of extensor digitorum								*Tendon of Extensor Indicis*		*Tendon of Extensor Digiti Minimi*	
Index finger		*Middle finger*		*Ring finger*		*Little finger*					
Width	*Thickness*	*Width*	*Thickness*	*Width*	*Thickness*	*Width*	*Thickness*	*Width*	*Thickness*	*Width*	*Thickness*
2.4	1.3	2.9	1.5	2.7	1.6	1.6	1.3	3.2	1.4	2.6	1.2

The galea aponeurotica of the extensors is an important structure of the extensor tendon on the dorsum of the finger. When passing over the first digit the extensor tendon is connected not only with the collateral ligament of the joint capsule, but also with the periosteum of the dorsum of the first digit. Thus, the hood plays an active part in the movement of the interdigital joint. When trauma occurs in the first digit the structure of the hood will be broken, causing its displacement and affecting the movement of the metacarpophalangeal joint. Therefore it is necessary to fix it up with care.

Blood vessels and nerves of the hand

Arteries

The arteries supplying the hand include the radial, ulnar and anterior and posterior interosseous arteries and the companion artery of the median nerve. There is a profuse anastomosis between them, constituting the volar and dorsal arterial retia and the superficial and deep palmar arches, of which the latter are the most important.

The superficial palmar arch (Figure 6.3)

This is situated deep to the palmar aponeurosis. It is formed by the anastomosis of the terminal part of the ulnar artery with the superficial palmar branch of the radial artery. The outer diameter of the ulnar artery superficial to the transverse carpal ligament averages 2.4 mm. On reaching the radial side of the pisiform bone the ulnar artery is situated on the radial side of the ulnar nerve and sends off a deep palmar branch. The terminal part of ulnar artery is 2–3 mm in outer diameter, curving superficial to the hypothenar muscles to form the superficial palmar arch with the superficial palmar branch of the radial artery deep to the palmar aponeurosis. The top of the superficial palmar arch corresponds to the distal transverse stria of the palm and gives off the following arteries in order from the ulnar to the radial side: the ulnar collateral artery of the little finger, to the ulnar side of the digit with an outer diameter of 1.2 mm; three common palmar digital arteries with an outer diameter of 1.5, 1.7 and

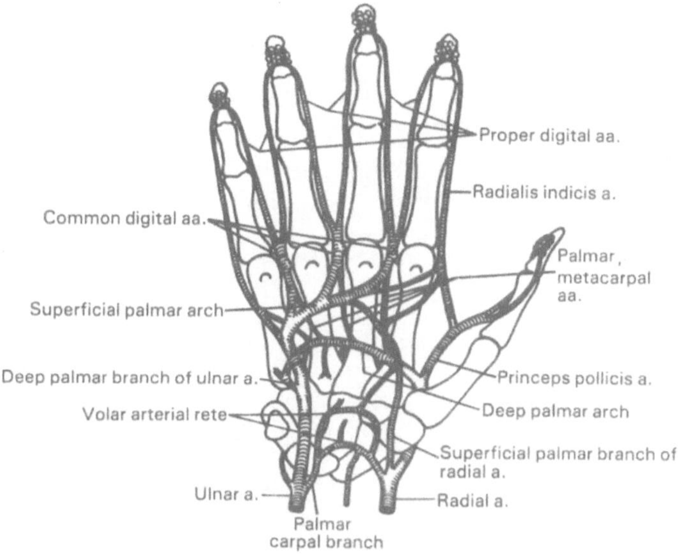

Figure 6.3 Superficial and deep palmar arches

1.5 mm respectively. The common palmar digital arteries proceed along the corresponding intermetacarpal space to the finger web where they divide separately into two proper palmar digit arteries, which are accompanied by small veins, situated on either side of the tendinous synovial sheath and destined to the ulnar side of the index finger, both sides of the middle and ring fingers and the radial side of the little finger separately. Two neighbouring proper palmar digital arteries anastomose with each other to form a rete to be distributed to the finger pulp.

The composition of the superficial palmar arch varies. There are four main patterns (Figure 6.4).

(a) Ulnar artery type This type of palmar arch is mainly formed by the ulnar artery, which gives off directly most of the common palmar digital arteries. The superficial palmar branch of the radial artery is minute, usually disappearing in the thenar muscles, or a few of them form a thready anastomosis with minute branches of the ulnar artery. In fact the superficial palmar branch of the radial artery does not give off directly any of the palmar digital arteries. This is the common type of the superficial palmar arch and amounts to 46–63%.

(b) Radial-ulnar artery type This is an arcuate anastomosis formed by the superficial palmar branches of the radial arteries with the terminal of the ulnar artery. It represents 41%.

(c) Median-ulnar artery type This type, representing 6%, is formed by the ulnar artery and the median artery accompanying the median nerve.

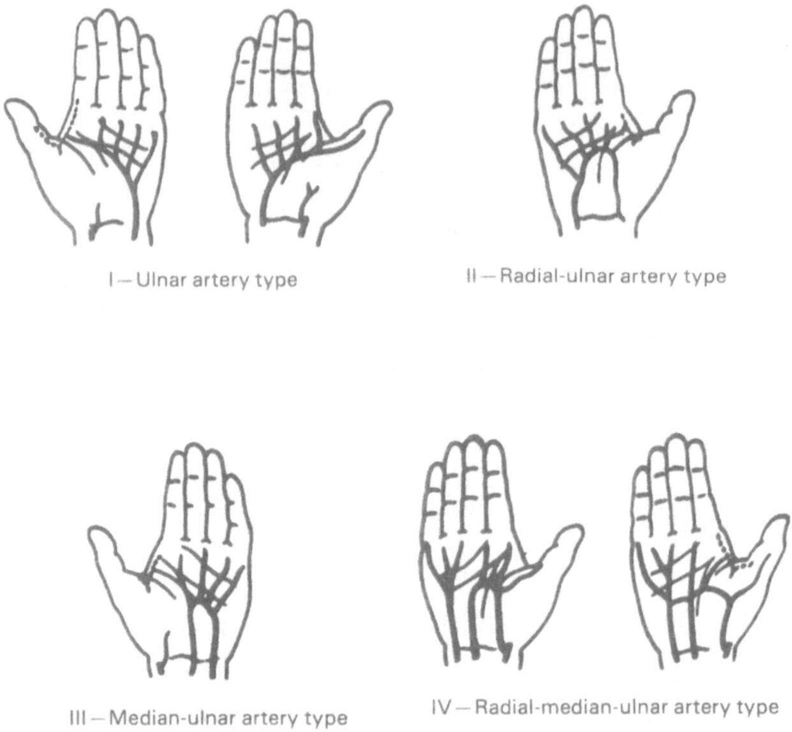

Figure 6.4 Four main categories of the superficial palmar arch

(d) Radial-median-ulnar artery type This type, being rare and representing only 0.5%, has two alternative conditions. One of them is that the superficial palmar branch of the radial artery, the median artery and the ulnar artery enter the palm as straight stems parallel to one another and connect by means of minute twigs to assume a railing form. The other condition involves the anastomosis formed at the radial side of the palm by the superficial palmar branch of the radial artery with the median artery to form an arterial arch which gives off branches supplying the opposite borders of the thumb and index finger as well as those of the index and middle fingers. The ulnar artery enters the palm alone and supplies the two and half fingers on the ulnar side.

Though the composition of the superficial palmar arch varies, the number and course of the common palmar digital arteries arising from the arch change a little, and the anastomosis with the arteria princeps pollicis is frequently present.

The deep palmar arch

This is formed by the terminal part of the radial artery and the deep palmar branch of the ulnar artery. The outer diameter of the radial artery measures 1.8 mm after it has given off the arteria princeps pollicis. The radial artery passes between the transverse and oblique hands of the adductor pollicis and anastomoses between the adductor pollicis and the flexor digitorum profundus with the deep palmar branch of the ulnar artery to form the deep palmar arch. The outer diameter of the deep palmar branch of the ulnar artery averages 1.4 mm. The composition of the deep palmar arch is relatively constant, so are the II, III and IV palmar metacarpal arteries arising from the arch with an outer diameter of 1.3, 1.1 and 1.0 mm respectively. The palmar metacarpal arteries anastomose with the common palmar digital arteries at the level of the metacarpophalangeal joints. The recurrent branch from the concave side of the deep palmar arch proceeds proximally, anastomosing with the anterior carpal arterial rete.

Veins (Figure 6.5)

The veins of the hand, like those of the other parts of the body, may be divided into superficial and deep ones. Of these, the superficial veins are particularly profuse and constitute the main channels for the return of the venous blood of the hand.

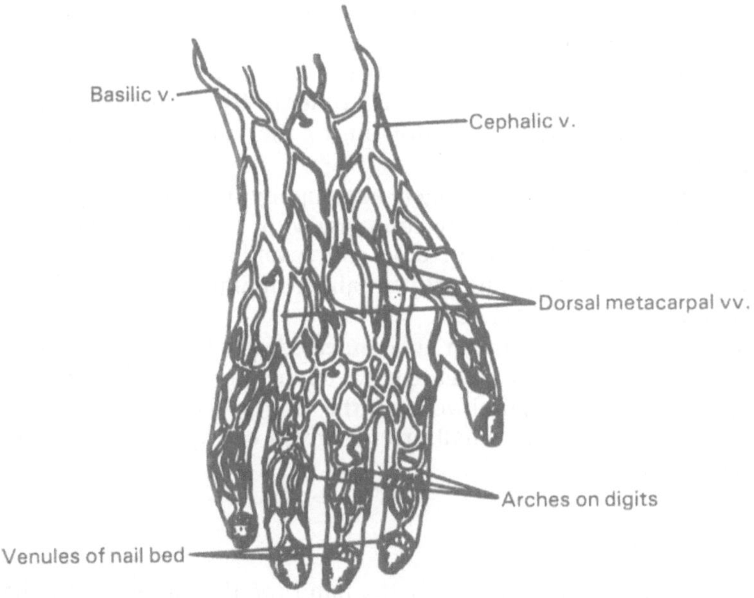

Figure 6.5 Superficial veins of the back of the hand

The veins of fingers

The superficial veins of the dorsum of finger have their origin from the small veins on either side of the nail bed which are about 1–2 mm away from the nail groove. The outer diameter of these small veins is about 0.3–0.4 mm. They move along the nail fold toward the median plane of the dorsum of the distal interphalangeal joint, where the outer diameter of the vein is 0.5–0.6 mm. The longitudinal superficial veins anastomose to form the venous network at the middle digit and separate from each other near the proximal interdigital joint. After passing over the joint, the superficial veins from four to six veins parallel to one another with outer diameters of 0.8–1.0 mm. Near the proximal digit the superficial veins anastomose again to form the venous network by one to three layers of venous arches, of which the single-layered arch is the more frequent with an outer diameter of about 1 mm, representing 74%. The veins of the thumb form no arch and their external diameters are slightly greater than those of the others, being about 1.8 mm. The arrangement of veins on the dorsum of the finger keeps the following rule. The vein on the dorsum of the middle finger is situated near the median plane, yet the veins on the dorsum of the index and thumb tend to shift to the radial side; those of the ring and little fingers to the ulnar side. At the metacarpophalangeal joint the veins on the dorsum of the second to the fifth finger usually appear at the sites, which correspond to the 10 o'clock 2 o'clock positions on a clock face. This rule has been followed in the search for veins when it is necessary to anastomose veins during the reconstruction of severed fingers.

The veins on the dorsum of fingers usually begin with venous arches, whence a kind of network is formed through anastomosis from the distal to the proximal phalanx, and end with another arch.

The superficial veins on the volar surface of the finger are more slender than those on the back and anastomose with each other to form a network. Most of them are connected to those on the dorsum of the hand by means of communicating branches.

The deep veins on the back of fingers accompany the dorsal digital artery. The proper palmar digital veins are in company with, but are smaller than, the accompanying artery which has a tortuous course and is usually single. Rarely a couple of veins may be seen. The proper palmar digital vein eventually flows into the common palmar digital vein.

The superficial veins of the finger are connected with the deep ones by communicating branches, most of which are between the proper palmar digital vein and the superficial dorsal digital vein of the finger. These communicating branches often accompany the small arteries given off by the proper palmar digital artery.

The veins of the hand

The superficial veins on the dorsum of the hand are the largest of the hand, being the main channels of venous drainage of the hand. The veins on the dorsum of the hand originate from the dorsal digital veins, which anastomose with those of the neighbouring fingers to form the dorsal metacarpal veins. The four dorsal metacarpal veins become confluent at the level of the head of the metacarpus into the dorsal network or arch which receives veins of the palm and finally empties into the cephalic vein on the radial side and into the basilic vein on the ulnar side respectively.

The superficial veins of the palm, being smaller than those on the palmar surface of the finger, anastomose with each other to form a network, which is relevant to the dermal striae of the hand in its arrangement and draws the blood of palmar veins into those on the dorsum of the hand.

All of the deep veins of the palm, as well as those on the back of the hand, are in company with the arteries. Thus there are the superficial and deep palmar venous arches, the common palmar digital vein, the palmar metacarpal vein, etc., yet the outer diameters of the veins are much smaller than those of the accompanying arteries. There are many communicating branches between the deep and superficial veins of the palm and back of the hand. The anastomosis between the superficial and deep veins of the palm resides in the venous plexus in the middle of the palm, especially between the superficial and deep palmar venous arches. Most of the communicating branches between the deep and superficial veins on the back of the hand can be found near the heads of metacarpi or adjacent to the wrist. Owing to the relative abundance of the communicating branches, the venous return will not be affected in the various functional positions assumed.

The veins of the hand possess numerous valves, especially in the case of communicating branches which connect the superficial and deep veins. Most of the valves are bicuspid, univalves are fewer. Seventy-three per cent of the valves of the superficial veins of the finger can be found in the middle part of the proximal phalanx, less in the middle phalanx and least in the distal. There are more valves on the dorsal than on the volar surface of the digit.

In view of the structures of the veins of the hand as a whole, the direction of blood flow is from the deep to the superficial veins, and from the palm to the back of the hand. Thus, the superficial veins of the back of hand are the most important. In replantation of severed fingers it is necessary to reserve the superficial veins on the dorsum of the finger. This is the key to the success of the operation.

Nerves

The nerve supply of the hand consists of the median and ulnar nerves on the palmar aspect and the superficial branches of the radial and ulnar nerves on the back, all of which are sensory. Of these, the median nerve will be described in connection with the functional anatomy of the thumb.

Ulnar nerve

The ulnar nerve trunk proceeds on the superficial aspect of the flexor retinaculum and divides into a superficial and a deep ramus at the site where the bifurcation is radial to the pisiform bone and 5 mm below the styloid process of the ulna. The transverse dimension of the ulnar nerve at the site of bifurcation is 4.3 mm; the anteroposterior dimension, 2.9 mm; the cross-sectional area, 9.8 mm^2, the number of fascicles, 19. The deep ramus is proportionally smaller than the superficial ramus, the ratio of the deep to the superficial ramus being 4:6. The deep ramus, being a motor branch, has a transverse diameter of 1.4 mm on average and a number of fascicles of 4.2 mm. The length of the nerve capable of being dissected proximally is 46 mm. At first the deep ramus passes from between the abductor digit minimi and the flexor digiti minimi brevis medial to the pisohamate ligament and then becomes deep to the tendon of the flexor digitorum profundus but superficial to the interossei palmares. It gives off branches to the interossei, the hypothenar muscles, the third and fourth lumbricals and the abductor pollicis. The superficial ramus consists of sensory fibres aside from those to the palmaris brevis. The sensory fibres are represented by three branches: the ulnar collateral branch of the little finger, the ulnar collateral branch of the palm and the fourth proper palmar digital nerve supplying the relevant area of the skin.

Radial nerve

The deep ramus of the radial nerve may also be called the posterior interosseous nerve, being the main motor nerve to the extensors of the forearm. The superficial ramus is mainly sensory, accompanying the radial artery to the site 60–70 mm above the styloid process of the radius whence it parts from the radial artery and passes deep to the brachio-radialis, crossing the bottom of the 'anatomical snuffbox' to get into the back of the hand, supplying sensory fibres to the skin of the 3½ fingers on the radial side.

THE FUNCTIONAL ANATOMY OF THE THUMB

WANG QIHUA, LIU QINGLIN AND ZENG YAOXIANG

The thumb possesses only two phalanges, being the shortest of the fingers and occupying one-fifth of the volume of the hand, but functionally it represents 50% of the hand as a whole. The functional significance of the thumb can be recognized only when disturbances occur with loss of functions. The perfect functions of the thumb are closely connected with the structural features of the bone and joint, as well as numerous muscles, the profuse blood supply and innervation.

Bones and joints of the thumb

Skeleton (Figure 6.6)

The skeleton of the thumb comprises the phalanges, metacarpals and the trapezium bone.

The thumb possesses only two phalanges, of which the proximal one is shorter than that of the other fingers, yet is longer than their middle phalanges. Each of the phalanges can be divided into three parts: the head, shaft and base. The head, equipped with a larger articular facet, is broader than the shaft. Owing to the unequal size of the two condyles of the facet, the flexion of the interdigital joint of the thumb is always accompanied by anterior rotation to facilitate the opposition of fingers. The nutrient vessels generally enter through the volar surface of the base. There is a ridge on the dorsum of the base.

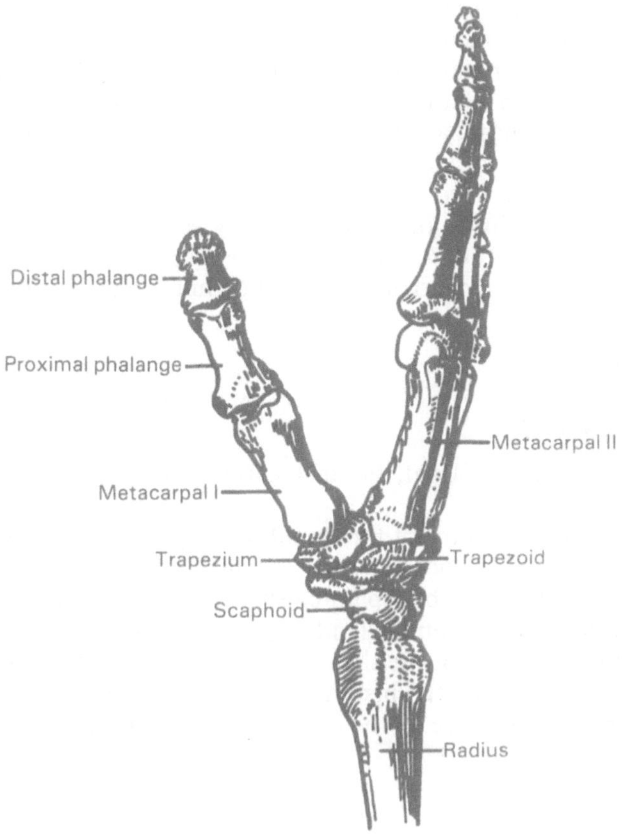

Figure 6.6 Skeleton of the thumb

The central prominence is for the attachment of the tendon of the extensor pollicis brevis. It separates the facet from the shaft and has a thickness of about 5–6 mm, which corresponds to that of the first digit of the index finger.

The distal phalanx of the thumb is similar to those of other fingers. It is longer by 2–4 mm and is also broader and thicker. On the volar aspect of the base are depressions and rough surfaces which represent the insertion of the flexors of the thumb. The distal end of the dorsal articular facet is equipped with a ridge, the central prominence of which affords attachment to the extensor pollicis longus and divides the articular surface into two depressions to conform the head of the first digit in making up the interphalangeal joint.

The first metacarpus is the shortest of the metacarpal bones, with a broad shaft, the midst of which is about 6–11 mm thick. This offers some idea of reference for the choice of thickness of the intramedullary needle for internal fixation of broken metacarpus. The morphological features of the extremities of the first metacarpus are as follows: the head is different from that of other metacarpals in that the articular facet appears to be quadrangular, with a larger volar surface to be articulated to the base of the proximal phalanx to form a kind of hinge joint. So is the base of the first metacarpus which also shows some peculiarities that make it different from that of other metacarpals: it presents a concave surface from the palmar to the dorsal aspect and a convex surface from the radial to the ulnar side. The trapezium bone is just the opposite: it presents a convex surface from the palmar to the dorsal aspect and a concave surface from the radial to the ulnar side. The first metacarpus and the trapezium bone fit together and form a saddle-shaped joint which offers an anatomical basis of significance for the functional flexibility and stability of the thumb. Therefore, in traumatic injuries of the thumb, any stump of the first metacarpal, even as short as 10–15 mm, should never be discarded, as this is of the utmost importance in the reconstruction of the thumb and its functional recovery afterwards.

Articulations (Figure 6.7)

These include the carpometacarpal, the metacarpophalangeal and the interphalangeal joints.

(1) The carpometacarpal joint of the thumb belongs to the type of saddle joint. As the capsule is rather loose and the articular surfaces are not closely attached to each other, they can be separated slightly in some localities. If the thumb is pulled in its abducted and extended state, the ulnar and volar parts of the carpometacarpal joints may be slightly separated. The radial and dorsal parts of the joint may come apart when the thumb is pulled in adduction and flexion. The extensor tendons are on the dorsal aspect of the carpometacarpal

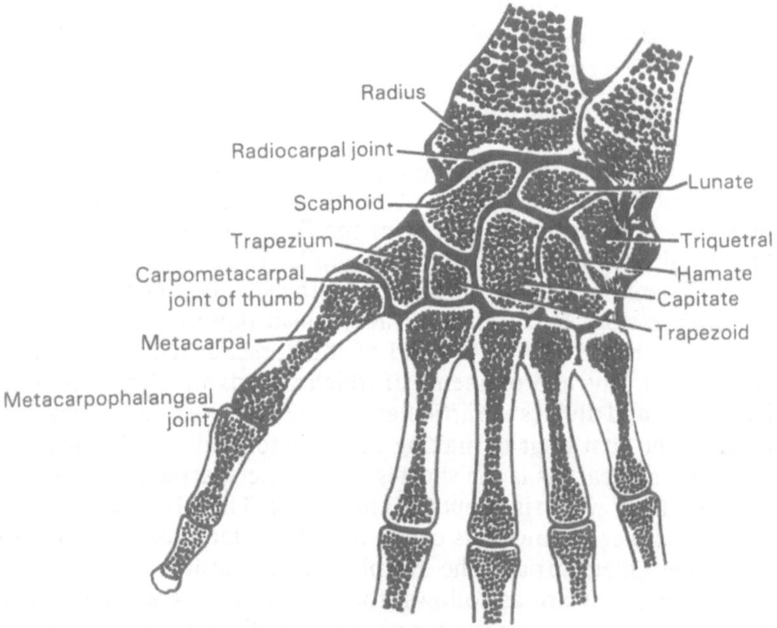

Figure 6.7 Articulations of the thumb

joint of the thumb, and the palmar surface of the capsule is strengthened by the insertions of the thenar muscles. The radiocarpal and ulnocarpal ligaments adhere to the respective side of the joint capsule.

The structural features of the carpometacarpal joint of the thumb afford it the movements of flexion, extension, adduction, abduction and opposition. The first metacarpal can rotate anteriorly, i.e. towards the palm, for 15–20 degrees in full flexion of the metacarpophalangeal joint.

(2) The metacarpophalangeal joint of the thumb belongs to the type of hinge joint. There are two sesamoid bones on either side of the volar aspect of the joint. The sesamoid bone on the radial side is larger than that on the ulnar side. The dorsal part of the capsule is thinner than its volar part, and the radial and ulnal collateral ligaments help to strengthen both sides of the joint capsule. Two parts of the collateral ligament may be distinguished in accordance with its attachment. The thicker part arises from the head of the metacarpus and directs obliquely from the dorsal to the ventral side to be inserted into the base of the phalanx. This part represents the collateral ligament generally referred to. The other part is slightly broader and thinner and is situated proximal to the former, being inserted into the sesamoid bone and the volar plate (Figure 6.8). The volar plate is a kind of fibrocartilaginous plate, the distal end of which is strong and connected to the base of the proximal phalanx, while its proximal end appears to be thin at the site of its connection with the head of the metacarpus. The tendinous sheath of the flexor pollicis longus is intimately connected with it; therefore the tendinous sheath also links with the sesamoid bones and the collateral ligaments. The tendon of the flexor pollicis longus passes from between the two sesamoid bones.

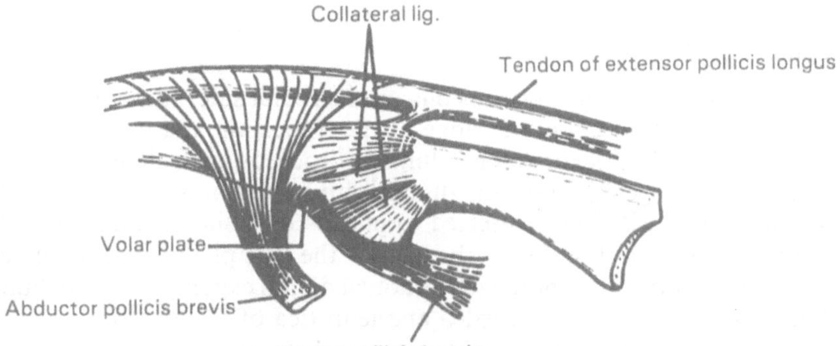

Figure 6.8 Metacarpophalangeal joint of the thumb

The metacarpophalangeal joint of the thumb carries out chiefly a flexion-extension movement. The extent of flexion is smaller than that of other metacarpophalangeal joints, while that of extension may reach 180 degrees but individual differences exist. Flexion leads to the tension of the collateral ligaments which allows no movement; extension loosens ligaments, leading to a slight degree of collateral movement. The collateral movement is under the influence of the abductor pollicis brevis, the adductor pollicis and the extensor pollicis longus, resulting in slight adduction and abduction.

(3) The interphalangeal joints of the thumb have collateral ligaments on either side for strengthening. The collateral ligaments also link with the volar fibrocartilaginous plate. The tendon of the flexor pollicis longus penetrates the fibrocartilaginous plate to end on the base of the distal phalanx. On the back of the digit, as the tendon of the extensor pollicis longus crosses the interphalangeal joint, it is connected with the joint capsule by fibres.

Because of the unequal size of the two condyles on the distal end of the proximal phalanx, the finger pulp will undergo slight anterior rotation when the thumb is flexed. This is in favour of the action of opposition and can be proved by the fact that the plane of the nail of the thumb inclines obviously to the radial side during the action of flexion. This should be observed in carrying out anthrodesis of the interphalangeal joint of the thumb by fixation of the joint in a slight flexion and anterior rotation to facilitate opposition of the thumb.

Muscles of the thumb

Intrinsic muscles

The intrinsic muscles of the thumb are known as the thenar muscles. All of them are on the radial side of the palm and can be distinguished into two layers: the superficial and the deep layers, each of which consists of two individual muscles. They are, from the radial to the ulnar side, the abductor pollicis brevis and the flexor pollicis brevis of the superficial layer, and the opponens and adductor pollicis of the deep layer.

The abductor pollicis brevis

This is a thin muscle, being subcutaneous on the radial side. It arises from the tubercle of the scaphoid bone, the ridge of the trapezium and the lateral half of the distal end of the flexor retinaculum. It proceeds anterolaterally across the metacarpophalangeal joint of the thumb with some fibres connected to the articular capsule and is finally inserted by means of a short tendon into the sesamoid bone on the radial side of the base of the first phalanx. A small part of the fibres direct dorsally, ending in the dorsal digital expansion of the thumb to add into the formation of the galea aponeurotica of the extensor.

The abductor pollicis brevis passes over two joints and it is thus known as a two-joint muscle. It can carry out flexion, abduction and anterior rotation of the carpometacarpal joint of the thumb, and abduct the metacarpophalangeal joint as well. Because of the connections made by its fibres with the dorsal digital expansion, thus strengthening the interphalangeal joint of the thumb, the great finger remains powerful in grasping. Normally, this function, being not apparent, is apt to be neglected. However, judging from cases of paralysis of the median nerve, the reduction of extension strength of the thumb appears unequivocal. During the transplantation of the tendon for the restoration of the ability of abduction of the thumb, the transplanted tendon should be ultimately sutured on the ulnar side of the tendon of the extensor pollicis longus in order to rotate the thumb anteriorly with the possibility of strengthening the act of extension.

The flexor pollicis brevis

This is situated on the ulnar side of the muscle mentioned above. It is equipped with a superficial and a deep head. The superficial head arises from the flexor retinaculum, the tendinous sheath of the flexor carpi radialis and the ridge of the trapezium bone; the deep head is weaker and arises from the volar aspect of the trapezoid bone and the bases of the second and third metacarpals. The two heads converge anterolaterally with the tendon of the flexor pollicis longus passing underneath them. In exploring the tendon of the flexor pollicis longus, an incision should be made along the ulnar border of the flexor pollicis brevis and the tendon is to be found amidst the two heads of the short flexor. The flexor pollicis brevis transforms into a slender tendon near the metacarpophalangeal joint with which it is linked by a small amount of fibres. Eventually the tendon is inserted into the radial side of the base of the first digit and the sesamoid bone of that side, part of the tendinous fibre extending to the dorsal digital expansion. The main function of the flexor pollicis brevis is to flex the thumb and assist it in adduction and opposition.

The opponens pollicis

This is a broad and flat muscle deep to the flexor pollicis brevis. It originates from the tubercle of the trapezium and the flexor retinaculum. The muscle fibres direct anterolaterally to end on the lateral border of the first metacarpal, almost reaching its head. It is the chief muscle of opposition of the thumb.

The adductor pollicis

This, the deepest of the thenar muscles, is under the cover of the tendons of flexor pollicis brevis and longus. It has two heads: the transverse head arising from the capitate and the volar aspect of the third metacarpal; the oblique head from the capitate, the part of the flexor retinaculum near the trapezoid and the tendinous sheath of the flexor carpi radialis. The fascicles of the two heads give some fibres to the joint capsule and the dorsal digital expansion and converge toward the radial side to form a short tendon to end in the ulnar side of the base of the first phalanx and the sesamoid bone of that side. It adducts and flexes the thumb.

Except for the adductor pollicis and the deep head of the flexor pollicis brevis which are supplied by the deep branch of the ulnar nerve, the rest of the thenar muscles are innervated by the median nerve.

The extrinsic muscles

All of these muscles except the flexor pollicis longus are on the back of the hand. They are extensor tendons originating from the dorsolateral side of the forearm:

the abductor pollicis longus and the extensor pollicis brevis and longus. The biometry of these tendons at the level of the styloid process of the radius is as follows.

All of these long tendons, except that of the abductor pollicis longus, end in the base of the first metacarpus. The tendon of the extensor pollicis longus passes superficial to those of the long and short extensors on the radial side, but deep to the dorsal carpal ligament. After passing medial to the dorsal tubercle of the lower end of the radius, the tendon directs obliquely to the radial side, forming the ulnar border of the anatomical snuff box and remaining on the ulnar side near the first metacarpus and the metacarpophalangeal joint. It forms the dorsal digital expansion or the galea aponeurotica of the extensor, just as the other extensor tendons do. The tendon of the extensor pollicis brevis remains on the radial side, dividing into a superficial and a deep fascicle on passing over the metacarpophalangeal joint. The deep fibres end in the middle of the base of the proximal phalanx; the superficial fibres continue forward to form the radial portion of the dorsal digital expansion and, together with that of the flexor pollicis longus, are inserted into the distal digit. Owing to such anatomical facts the interdigital joint of the thumb may reserve its function of extension even in case of paralysis or injury of the extensor pollicis longus.

Table 6.3 The biometry of the extrinsic muscle tendons on the back of the thumb in mm (at the level of the styloid process of radius)

Tendon of FPL		*Tendon of EPB*		*Tendon of EPL*		*Tendon of RCRL*		*Tendon of RCRB*	
Width	*Thickness*	*Width*	*Thickness*	*Width*	*Thickness*	*Width*	*Thickness*	*Width*	*Thickness*
4.7	2.3	2.3	1.5	3.7	1.2	5.0	2.1	5.0	2.1

Abbreviations are explained in the text.

The dorsal digital expansion of the thumb, like those of the other fingers, forms the galea aponeurotica on the dorsum of the metacarpophalangeal joint (Figure 6.9). It is formed mainly by the tendons of the extensor pollicis longus and brevis, with the tendons of the abductor pollicis brevis and the flexor

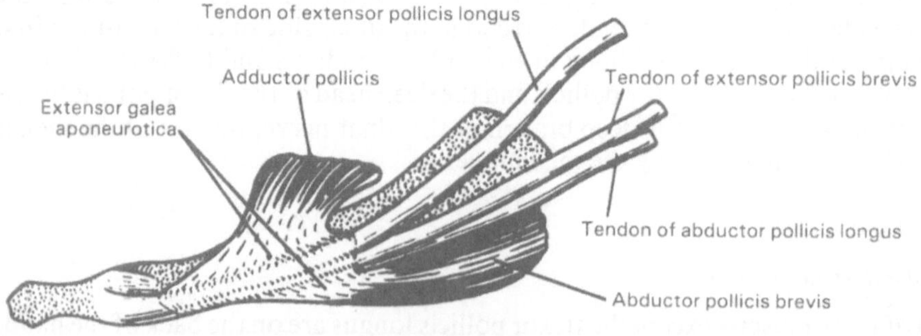

Figure 6.9 Extensor galea aponeurotica of the thumb

pollicis brevis ending on its radial side and the tendinous fascicles of the adductor pollicis on the ulnar side. These tendinous fascicles from the thenar muscle pass directly over the two extensor tendons of the thumb on the proximal end of the dorsal digital expansion and then obliquely to its distal end. The galea aponeurotica of the thumb is structurally similar to those of the other fingers, but since all of the extensors of the thumb are supplied by the radial nerve, the interdigital joints of the thumb may still carry out the action of extension in paralysis of the radial nerve or injury of the extensor pollicis longus due to the action of the thenar muscle. Attention should be paid to this in examining traumatic lesions of the hand.

Vessels and nerves of the thumb

Vessels (Figure 6.10)

The blood supply of the thumb comes chiefly from the principal artery of the thumb (a. princeps pollicis) given off by the radial artery.

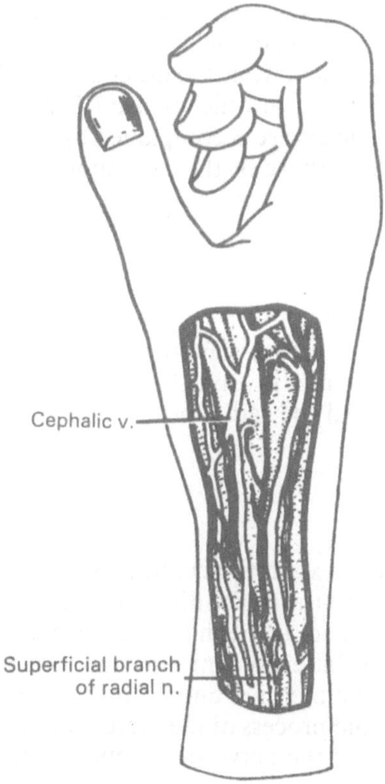

Figure 6.10A Vessels and nerves of the thumb (superficial layer in anatomical snuff box)

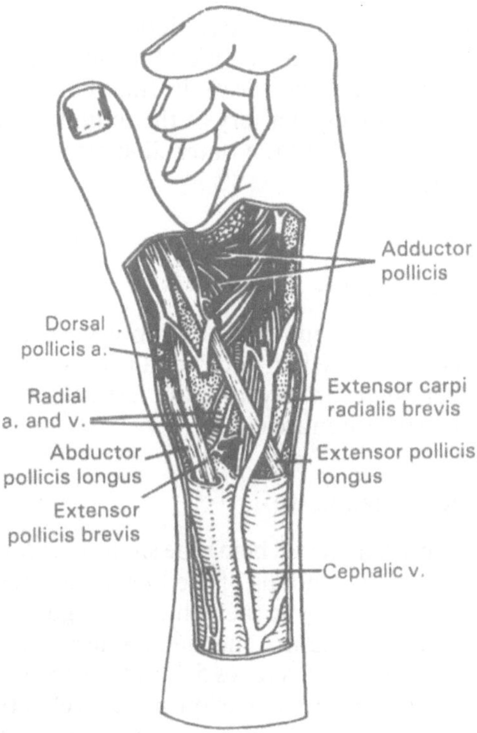

Figure 6.10B Vessels and nerves of the thumb (deep layer in anatomical snuff box)

The radial artery remains lateral to the tendon of the flexor carpi radialis in front of the wrist. Here it assumes a very superficial position. It then passes deep to the tendons of the extensor pollicis longus and brevis and the abductor pollicis longus at the distal end of the styloid process of the radius to the back of the hand, where it lies at the bottom of the anatomical snuff box. The outer diameter of the radial artery averages 2.7 mm near the styloid process of the radius. It is accompanied by a couple of veins with outer diameters of 1.8 and 1.5 mm respectively.

The radial artery gives off the principal artery of the thumb and the deep palmar branch as it passes between the anatomical snuff box and the first dorsal interosseus, where it corresponds to the base of the first metacarpus. The deep palmar branch anastomoses with the deep branch of the ulnar artery to form the deep palmar arch.

The principal artery of the thumb is one of the chief terminal branches of the radial artery and has an outer diameter averaging 1.9 mm at its origin. It proceeds distally through the first dorsal interosseus for 21 mm, where it divides into a radial and an ulnar branch at the level of the head of the first metacarpus. The radial branch with an external diameter of 1.1 mm is distributed to the radial aspect of the thumb; the ulnar branch proceeds a little forward as a short stem and divides into two small branches near *hukou*, i.e. part of the hand between the thumb and the index finger. One of the small branches with an outer diameter of 1.2 mm ends on the radial side of the index, while the other is distributed to the ulnar side of the thumb, the outer diameter of which is also 1.2 mm.

The principal artery of the thumb and its branches are accompanied by two small veins, with the outer diameters smaller than those of the corresponding arteries.

Nerves (Figure 6.11)

The innervation of the thumb is complicated and varied. The sensory nerves include the median and radial nerves; the motor nerves involve the median and ulnar nerves innervating the intrinsic muscles, and the radial nerve supplying the extrinsic muscles.

The median nerve

The median nerve, being the shallowest above the flexor retinaculum, is situated between the tendons of the flexor carpi radialis and the flexor digitorum superficialis and deep to the palmaris longus. It then passes through the carpal canal to get to the palm. The median nerve presents a flattened configuration in the wrist area and averages 5.5 mm for its transverse dimension and 2.2 mm for its anteroposterior dimension at the level of the styloid process of the radius, where the cross-sectional area amounts to 10.4 mm^2 and the nerve stem contains 22 fascicles.

The median nerve lies deep to the superficial palmar arch after getting to the palm and gives off the thenar branch. This branch has a transverse diameter of 1.0 mm and contains 1.3 fascicles on the average. Its site of emergence from

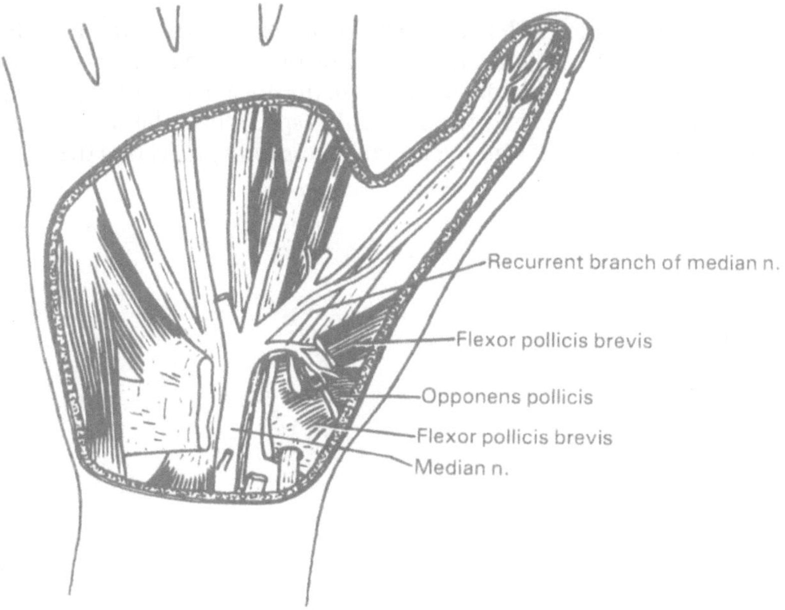

Figure 6.11 Nerves of the thumb

the median nerve is known as the 'forbidden area'. Any incision in this area is apt to injure the thenar branch. The topography of the 'forbidden area' corresponds to the proximal half of the thenar area.

Ulnar and radial nerves (see above)

Anatomical snuff box (Figure 6.12)

The anatomical snuff box is a clear landmark with the following boundaries: the ulnar limit is the tendon of the extensor pollicis longus; the radial, the tendons of the abductor pollicis longus and the extensor pollicis brevis; the base of the first metacarpus is the distal limit, and the proximal limit is the styloid process of the radius; the floor is composed of the tendons of the extensor carpi radialis longus and brevis and the scaphoid bone. The main structures in the box are the terminal segment of the radial artery, the superficial branch of the radial nerve and the initial end of the cephalic vein. It appears to be most prominent when the radiocarpal joint assumes the neutral position with the extension of the thumb. The width of the snuff box is 10–12 mm and its length 16–20 mm. During the fracture of the scaphoid bone the snuff box disappears owing to the local swelling, and distinct tenderness is exhibited within the box, which is the important site for examining the fracture of the scaphoid bone.

Essentials of applied anatomy

(1) Under normal conditions the index, middle, ring and little fingers are parallel to one another when they are stretched. As they are flexed the axis of each points

towards the scaphoid bone. Hence, when it is necessary to do traction during fracture of the phalanx or metacarpal, the direction of traction should always point to the scaphoid bone in order to maintain the normal anatomical position, lest abnormal positions of fingers should result, especially in the case of fracture of the little finger, which will lead to permanent disability affecting the function of the hand as a whole.

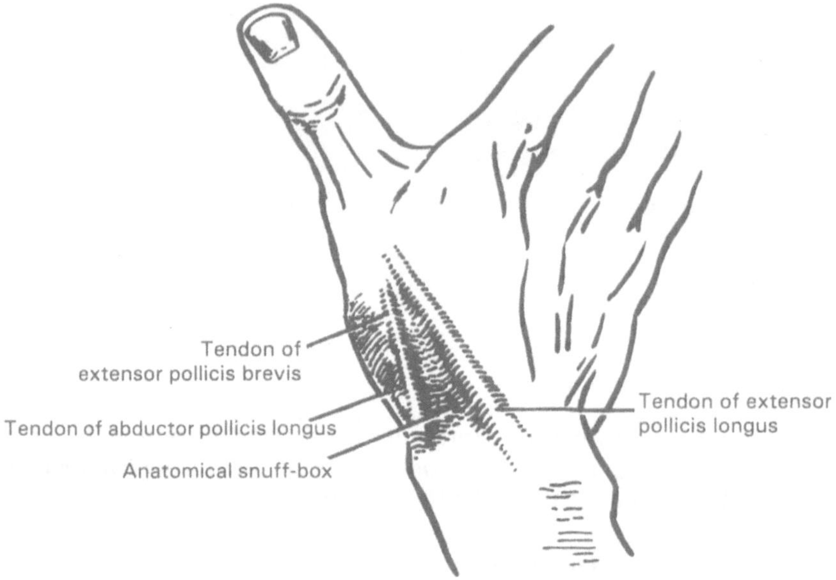

Figure 6.12 Anatomical snuff box

(2) Though the hand is only a part of the upper limb, all of the important activities are manifested through it. Therefore as the functions of the hand face disruption, those of the upper limb will be so greatly affected as to bring inconvenience to life and work. Sometimes, traumatic lesions are not found on the hand, as in the case of paralysis owing to nerve injury and Volkmann's ischaemic contracture, but all symptoms are referred to the hand. Hence, a thorough knowledge of the regional structures of the hand is essential for the understanding of the activities of its muscles, nerves and vessels which are intimately connected with one another. As to the management of trauma of the hand, only by comprehensive consideration will a genuine and satisfactory therapeutic effect be achieved.

(3) During the full opposition of the pulps of the thumb and little fingers the thenar and hypothenar muscles contract apparently. Viewing from the palmar aspect, one can observe a hollow rhomboid, the distal boundaries of which are the thumb and little finger; the proximal boundaries are the edges of the thenar and hypothenar eminences. The maintenance of this anatomical gesture requires the integrity of the functions of the median and ulnar nerves that supply the thenar and hypothenar muscles. Injury to either nerve will

certainly lead to difficulty in restoring this movement and the rhomboid profile in spite of any repair whatsoever.

(4) The dexterity and variability of movements of the hand can be fully expressed only under a normal state of the thumb. The principal features of the function of the thumb are the massive and powerful movement and the part it plays in accurate clench; all these need a sound background of stability. As long as the reconstructed thumb is provided with sufficient stability, and is able to contact the other four fingers freely, the perfect action of nipping can be recovered regardless of its ugly profile. The thumb has sometimes been compared to the immovable mandible of an alligator, which can still take part in the action of powerful biting provided that the maxillae are in action. Nevertheless, since the thumb is the shortest of the fingers and its normal length makes its distal end come to somewhere near the proximal interphalangeal joint of the index, a reconstructed thumb of excessive length will do no good and, on the contrary, will cause trouble.

(5) The depth of the *hukou* is one of the anatomical attributes necessary for the variability and dexterity of the thumb movements. By *hukou* is meant the first finger web, situated between the thumb and the index. The maintenance of its definite depth and width is essential for repairing any case of trauma or defect of the thumb. Too shallow a *hukou*, as well as an exceedingly narrow one, will certainly hinder the thumb from executing the normal functions of the hand.

(6) The act of opposition carried out by the thumb bears much significance to working and living conditions. This is due to the anatomical characteristics exhibited by the carpometacarpal joint of the thumb which is not arranged in the same plane as other joints of the same kind. Thus a reconstructed thumb should not be arranged with other fingers in the same plane but has to be kept at 10–15 degrees in the state of opposition (flexion plus anterior rotation). A thumb reconstructed in the position of opposition, less mobile though it may be, can still play a better part in the act of nipping provided a certain degree of stability can be maintained and at the same time other fingers remain capable of motion.

(7) The carpometacarpal joint of the thumb affords an anatomical basis for the great mobility of the thumb. Thus, there is much difference between the methods of functional rehabilitation in accordance with whether the defect of the thumb is proximal or distal to the first carpometacarpal joint.

(8) In reconstruction of the thumb using a toe, the anatomical snuff box is of the first choice as the recipient area, because the vessels and nerves here have definite courses and clear marks. Besides, the vessels have adequate outer diameters and sufficient length available for dissection.

(9) In the replantation of severed fingers one should look for the flexor tendons first and then the following structures on either side of the tendinous sheath in order from the volar to the dorsal aspect: the proper palmar digital nerves, and then the proper palmar digital artery, usually accompanied by a small vein. Either end of the transverse dermal stria of the finger may serve as markings denoting the limit of the digital vessels and nerve. In case of difficulties in seeking for the superficial veins of the finger, the head of the metacarpus can be regarded as a clock face, on which the superficial veins of

the thumb usually appear at the sites of 1 o'clock, 2 o'clock, 10 o'clock or 12 o'clock; those of the index, middle and ring fingers at the sites of 2 o'clock or 10 o'clock and that of the little finger at the sites of 2 o'clock, 9 o'clock or 10 o'clock.

ANATOMY OF TOE TRANSPLANTATION FOR THE RECONSTRUCTION OF THE THUMB

CHEN YAOLIANG AND CHEN ZHIYI

In 1966 Yang Dongyue first succeeded in transplanting the vascularized second toe for the reconstruction of the thumb. This procedure has the advantage of substituting the thumb with restoration of the function of the hand but not at the expense of the function of the foot. Though it has recently been widely adopted all over the world, failures still occur. One of the reasons is that research on the anatomy of the toe, a composite entity for the transplantation, cannot satisfy surgical demands. This is especially true in the variations of the dorsalis pedis artery and the varying origin and course of the first dorsal metatarsal artery. All these problems concern orthopaedic surgeons greatly.

Recently, Gilbert (1975) and O'Brien (1975) reported the regional anatomy of the dorsalis pedis artery, the first dorsal metatarsal artery and the deep plantar artery. In 1980 Wu Jinbao *et al.* described the variations of the dorsal pedis and deep plantar arteries in 100 cases. In 1981 Ling Tong *et al.* reported the course, branches and diameters of the same vessels in 120 cases with special reference to their clinical significance. All these papers are of great value to orthopaedists.

Topographical structures on the dorsum of the foot

Skin and subcutaneous tissue

The skin is thin and tender, and the subcutaneous tissue loose and rich in vessels. Therefore, they can be used as vascularized free island flaps.

Cutaneous veins

The cutaneous veins in the superficial fascia drain into the long saphenous vein medially and the short saphenous vein laterally. They form a dorsal venous arch at the distal part of the dorsum of the foot, which collects the dorsal metatarsal and digital veins of the foot (Figure 6.13).

Cutaneous nerves

The cutaneous nerves on the dorsum of the foot are (Figure 6.14):

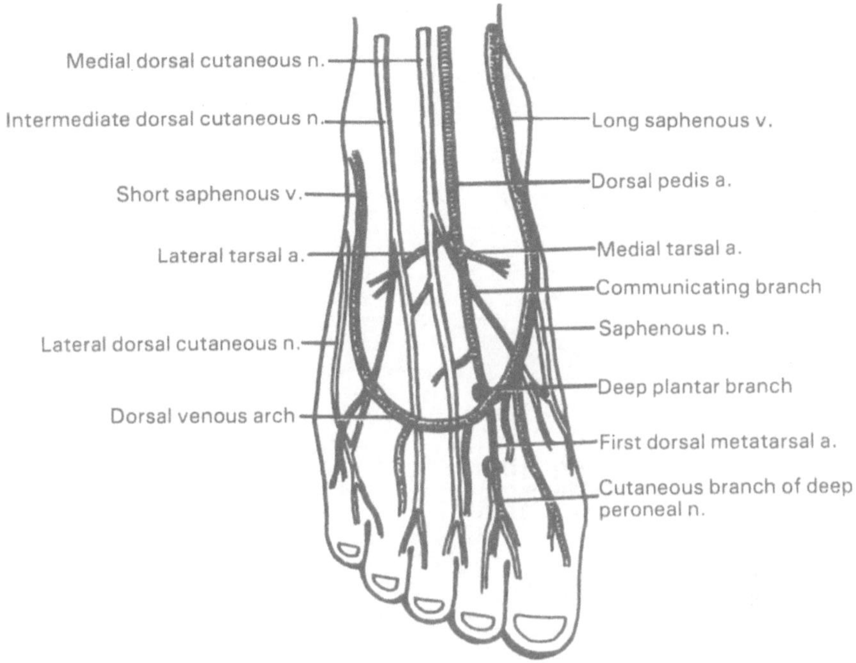

Figure 6.13 Arteries, veins and cutaneous nerves on the dorsum of the foot

1. The saphenous nerve supplies the medial border and the adjacent dorsal part of the foot.
2. Cutaneous branches of the deep peroneal nerve emerge from the deep fascia at the first web of the toes and supply the adjacent borders of the great and second toes.
3. The medial and intermediate dorsal cutaneous nerve of the foot take origin from the superficial peroneal nerve and supply the skin of the medial side of the great toe, and the adjacent sides of the second, third, fourth and fifth toes.
4. The lateral dorsal cutaneous nerve is the terminal branch of the sural nerve. It passes below the lateral malleolus and divides into two branches, of which one supplies the lateral side of the fifth toe and the other anastomoses with the intermedial dorsal cutaneous nerve to supply the adjacent side of the fourth and fifth toes.

Muscles of the dorsum of the foot

These can be divided into two layers. The superficial layer consists of the tendons of the long extensors, i.e. the tendons of the tibialis anterior, the extensor hallucis longus, the extensor digitorum longus and the peroneus tertius from the medial to the lateral side. In the deep layer there are the extensor hallucis brevis and extensor digitorum brevis (Figure 6.14).

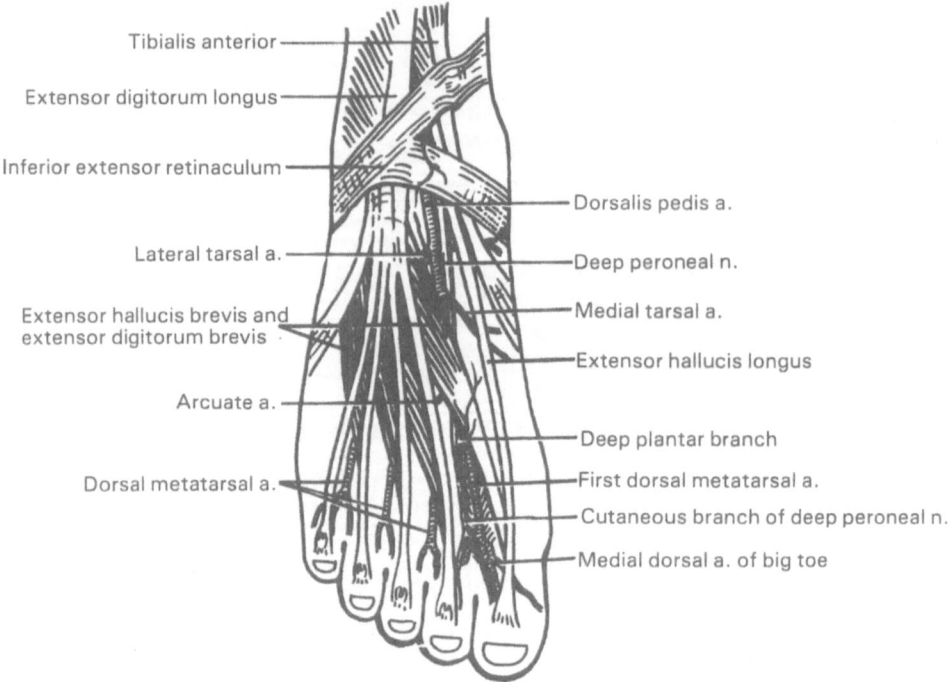

Figure 6.14 Dorsalis pedis artery and muscles of the dorsum of the foot

Dorsalis pedis artery and deep peroneal nerve

The dorsalis pedis artery crosses the ankle joint midway between the two malleoli, and runs deep to the inferior extensor retinaculum. It continues forward, crossing in turn the talus, the talonavicular joint, the navicular, the naviculocuneiform joint, the middle cuneiform and the fascia covering the first dorsal interosseous. At the middle of the foot the artery runs deep to the tendon of extensor hallucis brevis. The artery is rather superficial and distal to the inferior retinaculum. Its pulsation can be palpated lateral to the tendon of the extensor hallucis longus. The terminal branch of the deep peroneal nerve passes along the medial side of the dorsalis pedis artery.

Arteries on the dorsum of the foot

The blood supply of the dorsum of the foot originates from the dorsalis pedis artery, which is the direct continuation of the anterior tibial artery. The dorsalis pedis artery commences proximally midway between the two malleoli, and ends at the base of the first intermetatarsal space. It divides into the first dorsal metatarsal artery and deep planter artery (83.3%). It also gives off the medial, lateral tarsal arteries and the arcuate artery. In 4.2% of cases it is displaced medially from its usual position; in 5.8% it deviates laterally. The latter often arises from the peroneal artery, while the stem of the artery often runs deep to the tendons of the extensor digitorum longus and brevis. In 6.7% the dorsalis pedis artery is slender or absent. It is often accompanied by two veins.

(1) The first dorsal metatarsal artery lies between the skin and the first interossei muscle, accompanied by the first dorsal metatarsal vein. The cutaneous branch of the deep peroneal nerve lies medial to it. At its commencement the outer diameter of this artery is 2–2.9 mm (84.4%). Approaching the metatarsophalangeal joints it divides into three branches, which are given off to both sides of the dorsum of the big toe and the medial border of the second metatarsus. According to the classification by Gilbert, the course of the first dorsal metatarsal artery in the first intermetatarsal space appears to be of three types:

Type I: the first dorsal metatarsal artery runs over or through the first dorsal interossei muscle. On reaching the distal end of the first interosseous space (Figure 6.15 a,b), it is dorsal to the deep transverse metatarsal ligament and becomes the dorsal digital artery.

Type II: the first dorsal metatarsal artery is deeper than that of Type 1. It originates from the distal part of the deep plantar artery or from the plantar arch by a stem common to the first plantar metatarsal artery and runs through the dorsal interosseous muscle. In the distal third of the interosseous space it often traverses the interosseous muscle, or it is covered by a thin layer of interosseous muscle. Sometimes a slender artery springs from the proximal part of the deep plantar artery and runs over the surface of the dorsal interosseous muscles (Figure 6.15c,d).

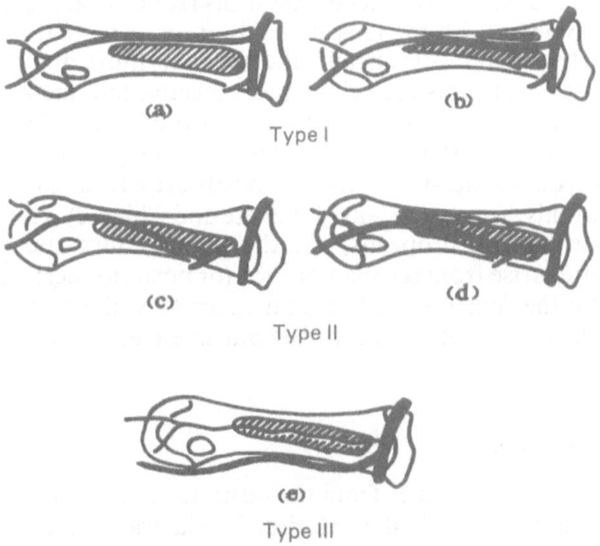

Figure 6.15 Types of the first dorsal metatarsal artery

Type III: The artery is very slender or sometimes missing. Its outer diameter is less than 1 mm. The slender first dorsal metatarsal artery often originates from the deep plantar artery (or plantar arch). In this pattern the blood supply of the first and second metatarsals comes mainly from the plantar metatarsal artery (Figure 6.15e). It will add difficulty to the operation and utmost patience is required to dissect into the depth in order to find out the first plantar metatarsal artery.

Table 6.4 Number of cases of different types of the first dorsal metatarsal artery (%)

Type	*Wu Jinbao* (100)	*Ling Tong* (120)	*Gilbert* (50)
Type 1	45 (45.0)	58 (48.3)	33 (66.0)
Type 2	46 (46.0)	52 (43.3)	11 (22.0)
Type 3	9 (9.0)	10 (8.4)	6 (12.0)

(2) The deep plantar artery springs from the dorsalis pedis artery and passes from between the two heads of the first dorsal interosseous muscle at the proximal end of the intermetatarsal space to join the lateral plantar artery to form the plantar arch. In free graft of the second toe, if the first dorsal metatarsal artery belongs to type 3 the operation must be carried out with extreme care. Because of the deep position of the terminal of the deep plantar artery, which is difficult to tie, it will soon shrink back, and bleeding can be stopped only with difficulty. The outer diameter of the deep plantar artery, measured at the point where the deep plantar artery penetrates the interosseous, is 1.8–3.0 mm (89.5%).

(3) The arcuate artery is one of the branches of the dorsalis pedis artery. It commences near the base of the metatarsal, runs laterally on the dorsum of the foot, and anastomoses with the lateral tarsal artery to form the arterial arch. The arcuate artery gives off distally the second, third and fourth dorsal metatarsal arteries, which proceed along the respective intermetatarsal space to the web of the toe. Each of them divides into two dorsal digital arteries. The incidence of the arcuate artery in Europeans is higher (54%) and the second, third, and fourth dorsal metatarsal arteries mostly arise from the arcuate artery. The incidence of this artery in Asians (Japanese and Chinese) is lower (35–47%) in contrast with that in Europeans, and the second, third and fourth dorsal metatarsal arteries arise from the plantar arch (or posterior perforating artery). Of the second to the fourth dorsal metatarsal arteries, the more lateral one is found to arise less frequently from the dorsal side (see below).

III. Arteries of the sole

The plantar blood supply comes from the posterior tibial artery which divides into the medial and lateral plantar arteries. The lateral plantar artery anastomoses with the deep plantar artery to form the plantar arch. The plantar arch is situated near the base of the metatarsal. From the convex side of the arch spring the first, second, third and fourth plantar metatarsal arteries, each of which divides into two plantar digital arteries supplying the opposite borders of two neighbouring toes from the first to the fifth. Each plantar metatarsal

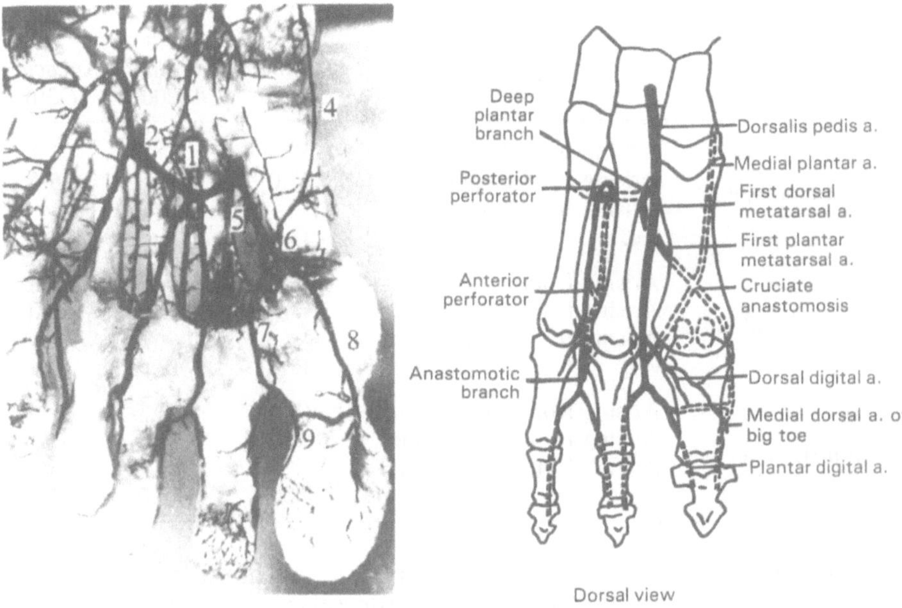

A

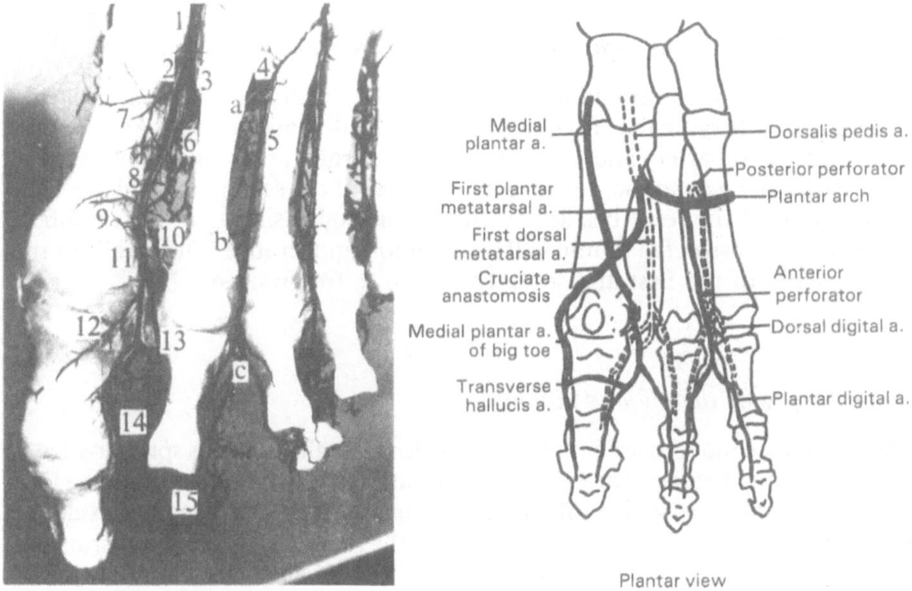

B

Figure 6.16 Blood supply of the great and second toes

Table 6.5 The origins of the second, third and fourth dorsal metatarsal arteries (cases) (%)

	Origins	*Wu Jinbao* (100)	*Huber* (200)	*Acachi* (230)
Second metatarsal a.	Arising from dorsal side	30.0	55.0	36.1
	Arising from plantar side	37.0	33.5	56.5
	Arising from both sides, etc.	33.0	11.5	7.4
Third metatarsal a.	Arising from dorsal side	18.0	59.0	35.6
	Arising from plantar side	43.0	23.0	57.0
	Arising from both sides, etc.	39.0	18.0	7.4
Fourth metatarsal a.	Arising from dorsal side	17.0	40.5	33.9
	Arising from plantar side	55.0	37.5	63.5
	Arising from both sides, etc.	28.0	22.0	2.6

artery gives off one perforating artery in the proximal and distal end of the inter-metatarsal space to connect with the respective dorsal metatarsal artery in order to establish an extensive arterial linkage between the sole and the dorsum of the foot. The plantar and dorsal digital artery are also connected by anastomotic branches on the anterior margin of the deep transverse metatarsal ligament.

Blood supply of the big and second toes (Figure 6.16)

In vascularized toe transplantation for the reconstruction of the thumb, the big or second toe carrying the vascular pedicle of the dorsalis pedis artery, the first dorsal metatarsal artery and digital artery is generally used. Nowadays it is the trend to use the second toe, because the removal of the second toe will not alter the function of the foot; besides, as the second toe is similar to the thumb in shape, the reconstructed thumb will have a good appearance. The details of the blood supply of the first and second toes are as follows:

Blood supply of the big and second toes

The big and second toes are supplied by the dorsal digital arteries springing from the first dorsal metatarsal artery. When the latter artery passes through the first intermetatarsal space it gives off three to four branches supplying both sides of each toe. These include the nutrient artery of the first metatarsal bone, branches to the interossei, the periosteal branches and the articular branches. Owing to the presence of a large number of branches, bleeding usually occurs during the dissection of the first dorsal metatarsal artery. When the big toe is to be freed it should be dissected along the lateral side of the first dorsal metatarsal artery.

When the second toe is to be transplanted the dissection should be carried out along the medial border of the vessel. In this way, not only can the main stem be well taken care of, but the branches that must be retained will also be preserved in good condition without being damaged.

The first dorsal metatarsal artery passes over the deep transverse metatarsal ligament to become the first dorsal digital artery. It divides into three branches. One of them passes deep to the tendon of the extensor hallucis longus to the medial border of the big toe and is named the medial dorsal artery of the big toe. The other two branches run forward to the opposite borders of the first and second toes.

The blood supply of the plantar side of the first and second toes

This comes mainly from the first plantar metatarsal artery, which arises from the deep plantar artery (or plantar arch) and runs medially to the plantar side of the first metatarsal, anastomosing with the medial plantar artery behind the sesamoid. After having passed the sesamoid it runs forward and divides into two branches, one of which runs to the medial border of the big toe to form the medial plantar artery of the big toe, while the other divides into two plantar digital arteries, which supply the opposite borders of the first and second toes.

The middle part of the plantar side of the first phalanx of the big toe has a large, constant and transverse anastomotic branch named the transverse hallucis artery. It connects the plantar digital artery on either border of the big toe. The vascular anastomoses at the distal end of the toe are rich and often form a network.

The blood supply of the second toe

This comes from the first dorsal and plantar metatarsal arteries as well as from the second dorsal and plantar metatarsal arteries. The second dorsal metatarsal artery often arises from the branches of the posterior perforating artery, while the second plantar metatarsal artery often arises from the plantar arch. These two arteries send off some branches bilaterally. There are anterior and posterior perforating arteries connecting the dorsal and plantar metatarsal arteries.

Applied anatomy regarding the transplantation of the third type of the first dorsal metatarsal artery

Since the third type of the first dorsal metatarsal artery is very slender or sometimes missing, and the position of the plantar metatarsal artery is very deep, the relevant operations were once abandoned. According to the anatomical characteristics, the following measure can be taken into consideration.

(1) If the second dorsal metatarsal artery originates directly from the arcuate artery of the dorsalis pedis artery and its diameter is larger than that of the first

dorsal metatarsal artery, the second dorsal metatarsal, the arcuate, and the dorsalis pedis arteries can be preferably chosen as the vascular pedicle.

(2) If the second dorsal metatarsal artery originates from the plantar arterial arch with a diameter of over 1 mm, and meanwhile the first dorsal metatarsal artery is missing, the second dorsal metatarsal artery can be cut and connected directly with the dorsalis pedis artery. This re-formed artery may substitute the first dorsal metatarsal artery to give the second toe an adequate blood supply. This has been proved effective in clinical practice at the Huashan Hospital in Shanghai.

(3) As the first intermetatarsal space is quite narrow it is impossible to manage a very deeply seated plantar metatarsal artery. Therefore, by incising the lateral half of the first metatarsophalangeal joint and forcing the big toe and the first metatarsus medially, the first intermetatarsal space can be widened for operation.

(4) According to anatomical statistics, the patterns of branching of the left and right dorsalis pedis arteries are mostly asymmetrical. If the artery of one foot is not suitable for operation, the other one can be the alternative.

Dorsal superficial veins of the foot

The success of a vascularized toe transplantation depends not only upon the anastomosis of the arteries, but also on the venous return.

The great saphenous vein

This is the main vascular channel for the venous return of the dorsum and digits of the foot, especially the first and second digits. Its outer diameter measured in front of the medial malleolus is 3–5 mm (93.3%).

Small saphenous vein

The outer diameter of the small saphenous vein behind the lateral malleolus is 2.2–3 mm (80.7%).

Dorsal venous arch

The distal border of the dorsal venous arch is 20–40 mm away from the second metatarsophalangeal joint (88.6%).

Of all the dorsal venous arches, 92.5% are typical, 3.3% are missing and 4.2% are incomplete. At the medial end of the dorsal venous arch (near the deep plantar artery in the first intermetatarsal space), there is usually a valve which indicates that the blood of the first dorsal metatarsal vein ends mainly into the great saphenous vein. The lateral end of the dorsal venous arch usually possesses no valve.

7

The applied anatomy of intestinal transplantation

ZHONG SHIZHEN AND TAO YONGSONG

GENERAL CONSIDERATIONS

The intestine is the longest part of the alimentary tract. Resection of a considerable part of it does not necessarily interfere with its normal function. The greater part of the intestine is provided with mesentery which allows a great range of mobility, so that intestinal segment with its vascular pedicle can be transferred to repair an oesophageal defect or to replace the urinary bladder or stomach which is out of order. These operations had been put into practice long before the development of microsurgical technique. However, owing to the limitation of the distance of transference of a segment of the intestine, such as the transthoracic replacement of the upper part of the oesophagus by jejunum or colon, the distal end of the intestinal loop often becomes necrotic due to deficient blood supply. In 1950 Androsov, a Russian surgeon, succeeded in avoiding necrosis of the distal end of jejunum by anastomosing vessels of the upper part of the jejunum with the internal thoracic vessels while the abdominal vascular pedicle of the jejunum was preserved. With the microvascular anastomosis technique, in 1957 Seidenberg was the first to succeed in reconstructing the cervical part of oesophagus by free vascularized jejunum (Seidenberg 1959).

As the calibre of the blood vessels of intestine is rather large it was not necessary to use the operating microscope for the free grafting of intestinal segment in former days. However, since microsurgical technique became available the rate of success of vascular anastomosis has increased. Recently, due to further progress in microsurgical technique, operations using microvascular anastomosis such as the reconstruction of urethra by vermiform appendix grafting has been successfully developed. It is anticipated that vaginoplasty by free intestine graft will be realized in due time.

The anastomosis of blood vessels to guarantee the blood supply is the key to the success of intestinal transplantation and it is therefore important to learn some data on the anatomy of the blood supply of intestine.

Blood supply of the intestinum tenue mesenteriale

The intestinum tenue mesenteriale consists of the jejunum and ileum which adhere to the posterior abdominal wall by the mesentery. They are movable and convenient for operation and are the first choice for free intestinal transplantation. The average length of the jejunum and ileum in an adult is 531 cm. The blood supply comes from the intestinal arteries given off by the superior mesenteric artery. These intestinal arteries pass to the gut between two layers of the mesentery, ramifying and anastomosing repeatedly to form several layers of arterial arches. From the last series of arches arise many small straight arteries which pass toward the mesenteric border of the intestine where they divide into two branches to enter the intestinal wall. Though anastomoses exist beneath the serous membrane and in the muscular and submucosal layers, collateral circulation still seems insufficient, especially on the free antimesenteric border of the intestine. Therefore, there are two major points about the blood supply of the intestine that are worthy of mention.

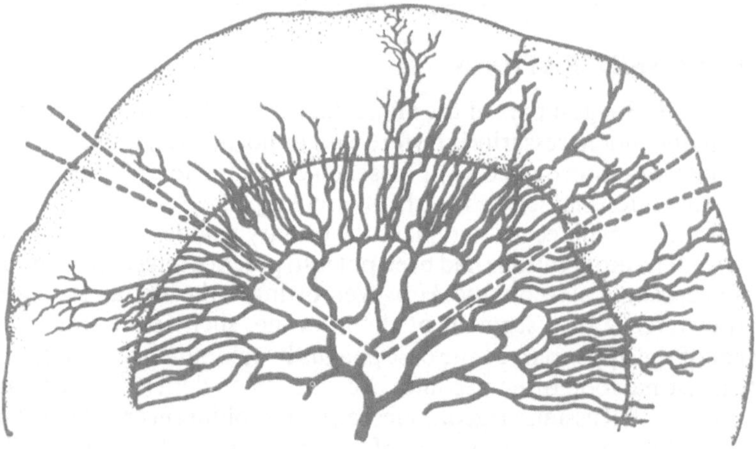

Figure 7.1 The blood supply and incision of small intestine

1. Intestinal arteries have rich anastomoses of arterial arches and a very good circulatory potentiality. When the intestinal loops are straightened in operation, these arches have to be preserved to ensure blood circulation.
2. Although there are intramural anastomoses of straight arteries, the collateral circulation is still insufficient for compensation. Hence, during intestinal resection and anastomosis, it is necessary, in addition to the fan-shaped resection of the mesentery, to increase the fanning on the intestinal wall by 20–30 degrees, the angle of which faces the antimesenteric border (Figure 7.1).

Blood supply of the colon

The large intestine includes the caecum, the vermiform appendix, the ascending colon, the transverse colon, the descending colon, the sigmoid colon and the rectum. Of these only the vermiform appendix, the transverse colon and the sigmoid colon have mesentery and are also of choice for intestinal graft. The average length of the colon in adults is 150 cm.

The blood supply of the colon comes from the ileocolic, the right colic and the middle colic arteries, which are the branches of the superior mesenteric artery, and also from the left colic and sigmoid arteries of the inferior mesenteric. Near the mesenteric border of the colon, neighbouring colic arteries anastomose with each other to form a continuous arterial arch, which is called the marginal artery, along the ascending colon to the distal end of the sigmoid colon. From the marginal artery arise many straight arteries perpendicular to the long axis of the colon. Each straight artery gives off a long and a short branch. The short branches are more numerous. They pierce the taenia mesocolica to enter the wall of the colon, supplying one-third of the wall near the mesenteric border. The long branches are fewer and run beneath the serous membrane on either side of the wall. When they reach the other two taeniae they get into the wall and are distributed to the remaining two-thirds of the wall, giving off a few twigs to the appendices epiploicae. According to the pattern of blood supply of colon, the following two aspects should be noticed.

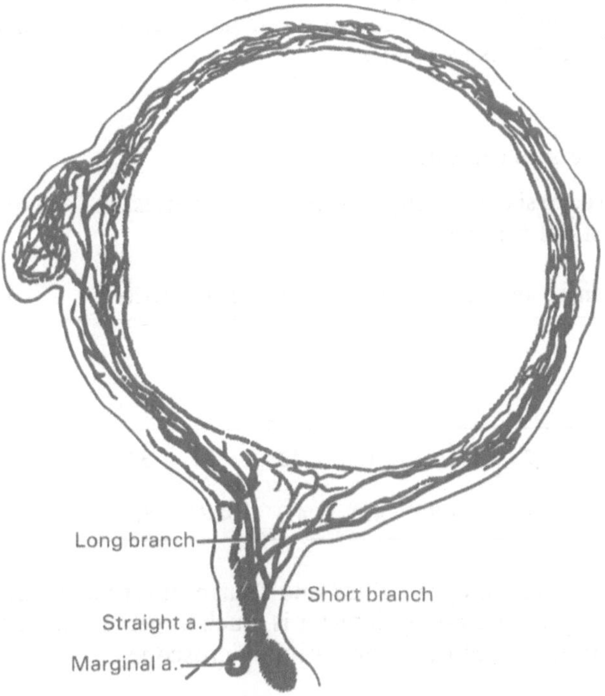

Figure 7.2 Blood supply of the colon

1. The marginal artery is formed by the anastomosis of the colic arteries. Some of the anastomotic vessels may, however, be slender. In the replacement of oesophagus by colon, the sites of ligation of colic arteries have to be selected carefully. Prior to the ligation the marginal artery should always be clamped temporarily on either side to see if there is an efficient collateral circulation.

2. Though the intramural branches of the straight arteries anastomose freely, the anastomosis is insufficient, so that effective collateral circulation cannot be set up easily. Therefore, all of the straight vessels should be adequately protected during operation, and the appendices epiploicae should not be pulled excessively, thus avoiding injury to the long branches of the straight arteries which would lead to necrosis of the wall due to ischaemia.

APPLIED ANATOMY IN RELATION TO THE REPLACEMENT OF OESOPHAGUS BY SMALL INTESTINE

The repair of total or partial defects of oesophagus by intestinal transplantation can be effected in two ways: one is completely free vascularized intestine grafting and the other is partially free grafting by anastomosing the vessels of the upper part of intestine with the thyroid or the internal thoracic vessels and preserving simultaneously the abdominal vascular pedicle. The anatomy concerning these operations is as follows.

Arteries of the small intestine

There are three to six averaging 5.4, intestinal arteries. In 44% of the cases there are five intestinal arteries.

Table 7.1 Length and outer diameter of intestinal arteries

Ordinal no. of intestinal arteries	*1*	*2*	*3*	*4*	*5*	*6*	*7*	*8*	*Ileocolic artery*
Length (mm)	25	36	45	42	32	32	15	11	64
Outer diameter (mm)	3.5	3.8	4.0	4.3	4.8	5.0	5.5	5.5	4.1

The average length of the third and fourth intestinal arteries is comparatively greater, and their outer diameter is much larger, so that anastomosis can be done without the aid of an operating microscope.

Table 7.2 Number of layers of arterial arches of the small intestine

Ordinal no. of intestinal arteries	*1*	*2*	*3*	*4*	*5*	*6*	*7*	*8*	*Ileocolic artery*
Average no. of layers of arches	1.5	2.4	2.7	3.2	3.4	3.5	3.5	4.5	3.0

The arterial arches formed by the anastomosis of intestinal arteries are the important regulation mechanism for the blood supply of small intestine. The number of layers of arches increases from above downwards but decreases in the territory of the ileocolic artery.

Table 7.3 Mean value of the diameter of arterial arches of the small intestine

Ordinal no. of intestinal arteries	*1*	*2*	*3*	*4*	*5*	*6*	*7*	*8*	*Ileocolic artery*
First layer of arches	1.9	2.6	2.7	2.9	2.9	3.0	3.1	3.8	2.7
Second layer of arches	1.1	1.4	1.6	1.9	1.8	2.1	1.9	2.3	1.6
Third layer of arches	0.8	1.2	1.0	1.3	1.3	1.3	1.4	1.3	1.2
Fourth layer of arches	0	0.8	0.9	0.9	0.9	1.0	0.8	0.9	0.7

The outer diameter of the arterial arches of the small intestine gradually diminishes with the ascent of layers. Up to those of the last layer the outer diameter is always less than 1 mm.

Table 7.4 Length of intestinal segment supplied by each of the intestinal arteries (mm)

Ordinal no. of intestinal arteries	*1*	*2*	*3*	*4*	*5*	*6*	*7*	*8*	*Ileocolic artery*
Length of intestinal segment	37	53	60	100	133	153	228	253	49

The extent of the intestinal segment supplied by the intestinal artery is often increased from above downwards. However, the ileocolic artery supplies a relatively small segment.

Ratio of the length of the straightened mesentery to that of the straightened upper part of the jejunum

In order to preserve the necessary arterial arches during operation, the gut should be straightened as far as possible. We made a trial in the upper part of jejunum. To preserve arterial arches of a diameter of more than 1.0 mm we need to straighten the mesentery to 25 cm and the free border of jejunum is measured at 64 cm, i.e. 2.6 times the length of mesentery. It follows that in order to raise the mesentery to 1 cm an intestinal segment of 2.6 cm should be resected.

Veins of the small intestine

Veins of the small intestine are short venous trunks with large calibre, which are less numerous than the intestinal arteries. The first-grade tributaries always accompany the intestinal arteries.

Table 7.5 Length and diameter of intestinal veins (mm)

Ordinal no. of intestinal veins	*1*	*2*	*3*	*4*	*5*	*Ileocolic veins*
Length	32	34	33	49	28	58
Diameter	7.0	8.2	7.5	7.5	10.0	5.0

Vessels of the recipient area

The superior thyroid artery is the artery of first choice in the recipient area in the replacement of oesophagus by intestine. Its location is comparatively constant and its diameter relatively large. The diameter of the right superior thyroid artery averages 2.8 mm and that of the left, 3.1 mm.

The internal thoracic artery is also an important vessel in the recipient area. The diameters of it measured in the second and third intercostal spaces are as follows.

Table 7.6 Outer diameter of internal thoracic arteries (mm)

	Intercostal space					
	Second			*Third*		
Vessels	*Artery*	*$Vein_1$*	*$Vein_2$*	*Artery*	*$Vein_1$*	*$Vein_2$*
Outer diameter	2.8	3.1	2.6	2.7	2.6	2.3

In the second intercostal space the distance from the internal thoracic artery to the margin of sternum averages 13 mm. The internal thoracic vein is usually single (85%) and medial to the artery. In the third intercostal space nearly half of the internal thoracic veins are in pairs (51%), guarding the artery on both sides.

Applied anatomy

The vessels of jejunum and ileum have comparatively large calibre and sufficient length to meet the need of vascular anastomosis in completely free intestinal transplantation. Owing to the preservation of the abdominal vascular pedicle the vascular anastomosis in the partially free transplantation of the small intestine involves many anatomical details to be discussed below.

First intestinal artery

The first intestinal artery is generally not fit for vascular anastomosis because of the following facts.

1. Frequent variation: the first intestinal artery often arises by a common stem with the inferior pancreatico-duodenal artery (12–17%).
2. High origin: the origin of the first intestinal artery is above the duodenojejunal flexure in about half of cases. This deep position of the commencement of the artery adds to the difficulty of operation.
3. Insufficient length: the first intestinal artery is mostly short, averaging only 25 mm.
4. Small area of supply: most of the first intestinal arteries give off branches to the terminal part of the duodenum and the duodenojejunal flexure. However, the extent of jejunum supplied by this artery is rather small, averaging 37 mm in length.
5. Incompleteness of arterial arch: the first intestinal artery is devoid of arterial arches in 19%. Its branches then do not have macroscopic anastomoses with those of the second intestinal artery.

Second, third and fourth intestinal arteries

With respect to their position, length and diameter, these three intestinal arteries are more suitable for anastomosis. The third intestinal artery is especially ideal for such purpose or for the preservation of the vascular pedicle.

Short trunk of the intestinal artery

In many cases the small intestinal artery is a short trunk, giving off two, three or even four branches immediately. Though the length and diameter of the trunk are not uniform, there must be one or more branches which have a longer span and a wider diameter. Thus branches of the short trunk can be used for vascular anastomosis just as the intestinal artery itself.

Preservation of the arterial arches

Within the intestinal wall the collateral circulation formed by the intramural twigs of the straight arteries arising from the last layer of arterial arches is poor. Thus it is necessary to preserve the arches when the intestinal loop is straightened. If the diameter of arterial arches of the last layer is less than 0.8 mm and it is predicted that the circulation is inadequate, two layers of arches should be preserved during operation.

Veins of the small intestine

The number of tributaries of a small intestinal vein is far less than that of the branches of a small intestinal artery, and veins and arteries do not always accompany each other during their course. However, since the tributaries of the first grade basically correspond with the intestinal artery, they are directly selected for venous anastomosis. Owing to the especially large calibre of intestinal veins, being more than 5.0 mm in the majority of cases, the calibre of the veins in the recipient area selected for anastomosis should be as large as those of the donor area.

Vessels in the recipient area

The superficial vessels easily approachable in the neck and chest can generally be chosen for anastomosis. These are the superior and inferior thyroid, the facial, transverse cervical, internal thoracic and external carotid or the common carotid arteries as well as the external jugular, thyroid, anterior jugular or internal thoracic veins. Of these the thyroid artery is ideal because of its superficial position and ease of exposure. Its calibre, being about 3 mm, appoximates to that of the second to fourth small intestinal arteries. The internal thoracic artery is also an ideal one for its constant position near the transposed small intestine. As to the veins in the recipient area, the external or the anterior jugular vein may be chosen to match the intestinal vein because of its large calibre.

APPLIED ANATOMY IN RELATION TO THE RECONSTRUCTION OF URETHRA BY THE TRANSPLANTATION OF VERMIFORM APPENDIX

The vermiform appendix is a degenerated organ, the resection of which has no ill-effects on health. It has a mucous membrane and a muscular layer consisting of inner circular and outer longitudinal fibres, and the repair of urethral defect with vermiform appendix seldom leads to constriction. In 1979 Zhang Zhaowu and others succeeded in repairing defects of the posterior urethra by autologous free vermiform appendix transplantation.

Topography and morphology of vermiform appendix

The vermiform appendix may assume one of the several positions: (1) retrocaecal, 28%; (2) pelvic, 26%; (3) subcaecal, 22%; (4) retroileal, 22%; and (5) preileal, 2%. The position of vermiform appendix is directly influenced by that of caecum, which may reach as high as the inferior surface of liver in childhood, though this seldom occurs in adults. The high caecum of children may account for 21%. Real absence of vermiform appendix is very rare. Nevertheless, when it is extraperitoneal and retrocaecal in position, being entirely covered by the parietal peritoneum, it cannot be approached unless the peritoneum is incised.

The length of vermiform appendix averages 7.8 cm. Its outer diameter averages 7.2 mm measured at its middle portion. The length of the free border of mesoappendix, being only 4.1 cm in average, is smaller than that of vermiform appendix, so that the appendix presents some tortuosity and is hooked, spiral, arched or sigmoid in form.

Blood vessels of vermiform appendix

The appendicular artery may arise from one of the branches of the ileocaecal artery: the ileal branch (45%), the posterior caecal branch (24%) or the trunk of ileocaecal artery (12%). Those arising from the trunk of ileocolic artery reach 18%. The single appendicular artery amounts to 92%, and double arteries 8%. When the appendicular artery is duplicated, that which is distributed to the proximal part of the vermiform appendix also supplies the neighbouring part of the caecum and the maximal range of supply will not exceed the proximal one-third of appendix, so that the distal branch is the main one. The average length of appendicular artery measured from its origin to the tip of appendix is 56 mm and that of the accompanying vein 52 mm. The outer diameters of the artery and vein are 1.5 mm and 1.7 mm respectively.

Applied anatomy of the vessels of perineum

Perineal vessels

The perineal artery arises from the internal pudendal artery in the anterior part of the anal triangle. It pierces the superficial transverse perineal muscle (66%), or passes superficial to the muscle (34%), to enter the urogenital triangle and divide into two terminals, the posterior scrotal artery and the transverse perineal artery. In the course from behind forwards, the perineal artery proceeds from a deep to a superficial position and moves medially. After it has given off the transverse perineal artery, the outer diameter of the perineal artery gets wider, averaging 1.7 mm.

The perineal vein may be single (78%) or double (22%). Its outer diameter averages 2.0 mm.

Posterior scrotal vessels

The posterior scrotal artery, a branch of the perineal artery, is a single trunk on either side of the central perineal point. It runs forward to the base of scrotum, dividing into two branches (Figure 7.3). At the level of central perineal point the distance from the perineal artery to the midline is 14.6 mm. In the urogenital triangle the posterior scrotal artery lies deep to the superficial perineal fascia (Colles' fascia), between the bulbospongiosus and ischiocavernosus. The depth from the surface of the posterior scrotal artery on either side of the central perineal point averages 12.7 (8–17) mm. The outer diameters of the arteries on both sides are mostly approximate, averaging 1.3 mm.

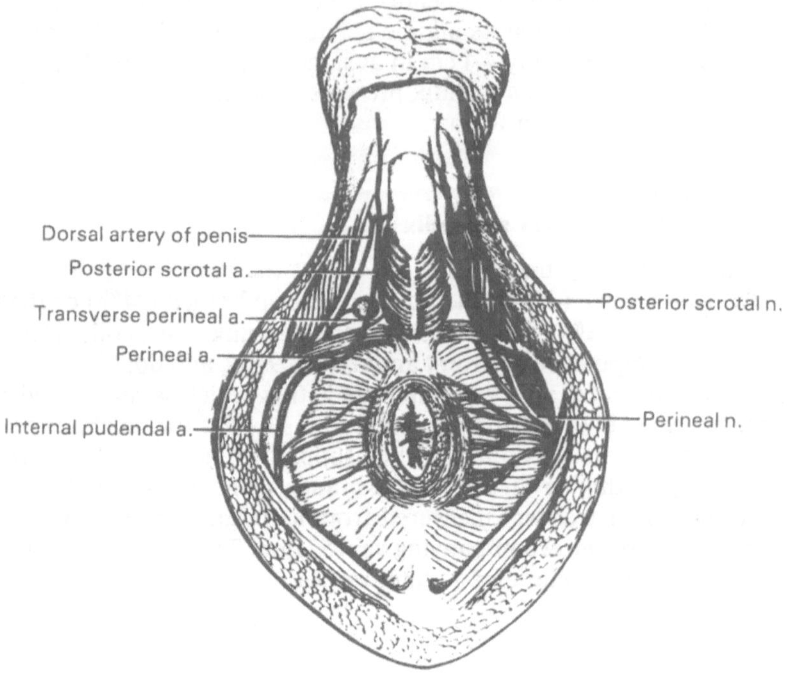

Figure 7.3 Arteries and nerves of the male perineal region

Most of the posterior scrotal veins are single (82%) and a few are double (18%). Its outer diameter averages 1.7 mm.

Applied anatomy of the donor area

The tailoring of vermiform appendix

The length of appendix in adults is mostly long enough for repairing the posterior urethral defect, except for those of less than 4 cm in length (6%), which are too short to be operated on. The circular muscle at the base of appendix being comparatively thick has a similar function to sphincter muscle. This makes the basal part look a little bulky, while its lumen is rather narrow. Moreover, the distal branch of double appendicular arteries is easier to dissect in contrast with the proximal one. Therefore, when the superfluous part of appendix is to be excised, the basal segment of appendix has to be cut off first, so as to prevent the site of anastomosis from ischaemic necrosis.

Lengthening of appendicular artery

The appendicular artery of some people is short, and it tends to retract after excision. This leads to a shortening of the artery, which is then not fit for anastomosis. Therefore, isolating a segment of the trunk of ileocaecal artery or its continuance to increase the available length of appendicular artery may be taken into consideration. Due to the complication of the arterial pattern in the ileocaecal part of the gut, in order to prevent inadequacy of the blood supply of caecum following ligation of the trunk of ileocaecal artery, it has been suggested that the artery which is to be cut, be clamped temporarily to see if there is any aura of ischaemia and the site of ligation of the artery is eventually decided.

Applied anatomy of the recipient area

Based on the analysis of topographical relations, the posterior scrotal artery in the recipient area is of the first choice for vascular anastomosis in the repair of the posterior urethral defect. The external superficial pudendal artery comes next. Other neighbouring arteries such as the superficial epigastric and the deep external pudendal are not suitable, because their location and course will undergo greater rearrangement during operation, which may lead to the compression and traction of the arteries and add much inconvenience to surgical manoeuvre. In the repair of hypospadias of urethra the dorsal artery of the penis is one appropriate to vascular anastomosis in the recipient area.

The posterior scrotal artery has a superficial position, constant course and few variations. The posterior scrotal artery and vein can easily be approached on either side of the central perineal point, 1.5 cm lateral to the midline, after the skin is incised and retracted. Here the posterior scrotal nerve accompanying the corresponding vessels has divided into two branches. Since the nerve is superficial and lateral to the vessels it can be used as an accessory mark in searching for the vessels. The posterior scrotal artery moves from lateral medialward as it courses from behind forwards. Therefore it can be approached laterally in its anterior portion and medially in its posterior portion. Moreover, the posterior scrotal artery is situated just between the bulbospongiosus and ischiocavernosus on either side of the central perineal point, the depression between these muscles can be felt by palpation and be used as a reliable guide to the vessels.

As the posterior scrotal artery runs forward, it tapers off gradually and is no longer suitable for anastomosis. If it is traced backward its calibre becomes larger, especially prior to the commencement of the transverse perineal artery where its outer diameter averages 1.7 mm. Therefore, when the posterior scrotal artery is found to be too narrow to anastomose, it would be advisable to trace it backward. However, the topographical relationship should be kept in mind that the more backward it courses, the more deeply and laterally it lies.

The calibre of the posterior scrotal arteries of both sides varies greatly (4%). When the calibre of the artery of one side is found to be too small to operate, its fellow of the opposite side can be approached in the corresponding position.

The dorsal vessels of the penis, being superficial, are easy to find. The superficial and deep dorsal veins of the penis are situated above and beneath the Buck's fascia respectively. On either side of the deep vein lie the dorsal arteries of the penis: they are of unequal size. The calibres of the dorsal vessels measured at the root of the penis are as follows: 2 mm for the superficial dorsal vein;

2.5 mm for the deep dorsal vein and 1.5–2.0 mm for the dorsal artery. These vessels can be selected for anastomosis in the recipient area when repairing hypospadias.

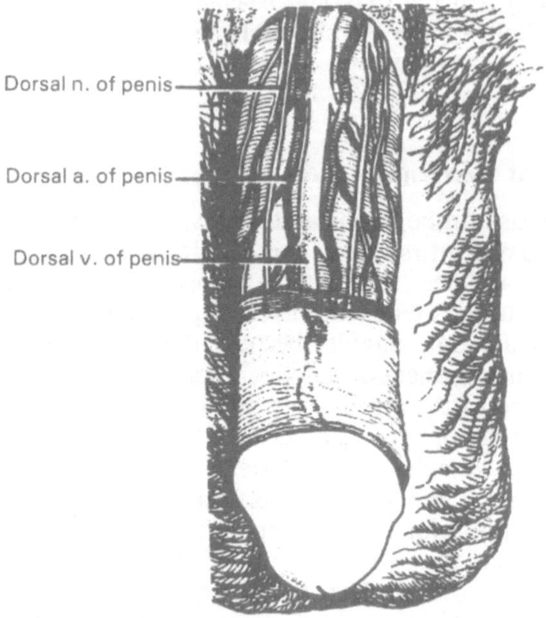

Figure 7.4 Vessels and nerves on the dorsum of penis

APPLIED ANATOMY OF INTESTINAL GRAFTING FOR VAGINOPLASTY

Vaginoplasty consists of creating a cavity between the rectum and urinary bladder and transplanting the appropriate tissue to form its wall. The materials used for reconstructing the vaginal wall have been skin flaps, amnion and intestinal loops. Of these the intestinal loops are of better quality, because of the presence of mucous membrane with circular or semicircular plicae and intestinal glands, which help lubricate the organ and make it pliable.

The key to successful vaginoplasty lies in the total survival of the transplanted wall of the cavity. It was impossible to perform vaginoplasty without vascularized free intestinal grafts before the development of microsurgical technique. Free non-vascularized transplants of small intestinal segment, sigmoid colon or rectum often lead to ischaemic necrosis, infection and very few survivals with a high rate of mortality. The transplantation of sigmoid colon or rectum with vascular pedicle for vaginoplasty is very difficult because of limitation of the length of pedicle. The development of microvascular anastomosis, however, makes the vascularized free graft of intestinal segment possible for vaginoplasty.

Applied anatomy of the donor area

The intestinal segments of choice should be those which are convenient for operation. Jejunum, ileum, transverse or sigmoid colon are ideal donors because they possess mesentery and have a great mobility. Moreover, these intestinal segments have a longer vascular pedicle with large calibre, which adds convenience to operation. Jejunum and ileum have layers of arterial arches. The calibre of those of the last layer is often small and probably unsuitable for vascular anastomosis. However, that of the arches of the layer next to the last is large and suitable for anastomosis. The data of calibre of the blood vessels of different intestinal segments are listed below. They provide a reference for the design of operation. The calibres of arterial and venous arches of the last layer of jejunum and ileum are 0.9 and 1.1 mm respectively; those of the layer next to the last, 1.2 mm and 1.4 mm; those of the middle colonic artery and vein, 1.7 mm and 2.0 mm; and those of the sigmoid artery and vein, 1.8 mm and 2.1 mm.

Applied anatomy of the recipient area

The posterior labial artery is the most ideal for vascular anastomosis in the recipient area. The posterior labial artery, homologous to the posterior scrotal artery in male (Figure 7.5), is the continuation of the perineal artery and lies 22 mm lateral to the midline at the level of the central perineal point. In the urogenital triangle the posterior labial arteries are under the superficial perineal fascia and are 14 mm (9–18 mm) deep on either side of the central perineal point.

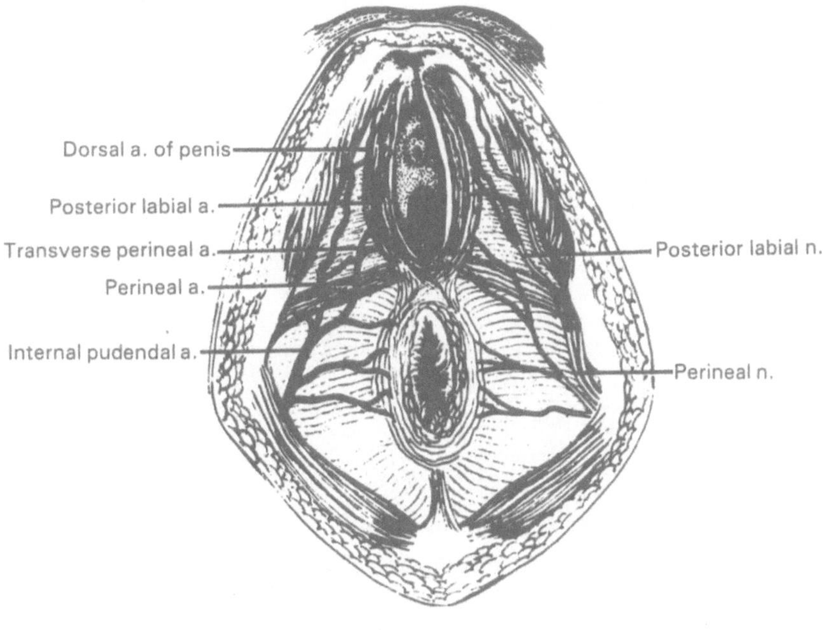

Figure 7.5 Arteries and nerves of the female perineal region

The outer diameter of the artery at its posterior end averages 0.8 mm and that of the accompanying vein 1.3 mm.

The distribution of blood vessels and nerves in the female perineum is similar to that in the male, and the details of applied anatomy are identical with those described on page 199 of this chapter. However, the calibre of the blood vessels of female perineum is smaller than that of the male. This will certainly add difficulty to the operation.

8

The applied anatomy of the omental transplantation

ZHU JIAKAI AND YU GUOZHONG

INTRODUCTION

The greater omentum is a part of the visceral peritoneum. It comprises four layers, passing downwards to the pelvis like an apron in front of the small intestine. The two anterior layers commence at the greater curvature of stomach and the first part of the duodenum, descend as low as the pelvic brim and then turn upward, becoming the two posterior layers to be attached to the transverse colon. The omental bursa is thus formed between the anterior and posterior layers, which are, however, inseparable. Within the layers there is a profusion of arteries, veins, lymphatics and adipose tissue. The omentum thus has the ability of absorption, adhesion, repair and localization of inflammation.

The greater omentum is endowed with great activity, so that it can reach any part of the abdominal cavity to localize any inflammation that occurs. Therefore, Morison (1906) called it 'the policeman in the abdomen'. Meanwhile, it was known to receive a split-skin graft on its surface and was greatly valued by anatomists and clinicians in former days.

In 1888 Senn discovered, in his experiment with dogs, that the pedicled or free omentum could protect the anastomosis of the gastrointestinal tract. He was the first to use the omentum to fill perforations of the stomach and to protect the stump of duodenum and the gastrointestinal anastomosis. Complications of fistula or rupture from anastomosis were thus greatly reduced. Thereafter, clinical reports successively appeared concerning the usage of omentum to repair defects in respiratory and urinary tracts and to shunt portal hypertension as well as lymphoedema of the lower limb. The greater omentum can also provide blood for ischaemic organs in coronary heart disease and for the limb in arteriosclerosis. It can be used to reconstruct the breast and to protect the great vessels exposed in irradiated or infected wounds so as to prevent secondary bleeding.

In 1972 McLean and Buncke, using microvascular technique, first succeeded in the repair of scalp by omental transplantation followed by split-skin graft. In recent years there have been many successful reports regarding vascularized omental transplantation, such as the repair of large skin defects resulting from the excision of tumour or scar, filling of the cavity left by sequestrectomy in osteomyelitis, orthopaedic reconstruction for hemifacial atrophy and improvement in circulation in the limbs with thrombophlebitis.

In China, Zhang Disheng *et al.* began vascularized omental transplantation in 1977. Sheng Zuyao *et al.* (1979) adopted the operation and initiated the omental axial skin graft. In the past few years omental transplantation has been widely available in China. Yu Guozhong *et al.* (1980) made some observations with regard to the anatomy of greater omentum during operation, and some measurements in the diameter and thickness of the wall of its vessels.

As to the applied anatomy of the greater omentum, Alday (1972) and Das (1976) and others made a survey of the distribution of its vessels as well as its area. Colleagues in Ningxia Medical College (1977) analysed the patterns of the vessels of greater omentum, and Mo Jingguo *et al.* (1980) made the same observation.

APPLIED ANATOMY OF THE GREATER OMENTUM

Blood supply of the greater omentum

The blood supply of the greater omentum comes chiefly from the left and right gastroepiploic arteries. The veins accompany the arteries. The vessels of the greater omentum are thin-walled and should be carefully handled in the course of surgical manoeuvre.

Left gastroepiploic artery (LGEA)

The LGEA is a branch from the splenic artery which arises from the coeliac artery. The splenic artery passes horizontally to the left along the upper border of the pancreas deep to the omental bursa. Near the tail of the pancreas it divides into two to four short gastric arteries to the fundus of stomach and then gives off the LGEA which proceeds in the gastrosplenic ligament and skirts the greater curvature of stomach, or 1–2 cm below it, to the right to form the gastroepiploic arterial arch by anastomosing with the right gastroepiploic artery.

Sometimes the LGEA does not arise from the trunk of the splenic artery but from its branches. Occasionally the LGEA gives off a branch to the lower pole of spleen as well as several twigs to its tail and the posterior layers of the greater omentum. It then runs to the right along the greater curvature in the anterior layers of the greater omentum, giving off many gastric branches to the anterior and posterior walls of stomach adjacent to the greater curvature. Therefore, much attention should be paid to the ligation of these small branches in dividing the omentum, to prevent them from bleeding.

The mean outer diameter of LGEA is 1.84 (1.0–3.0) mm, and that of the accompanying LGEA, 2.4 (1.0–4.5) mm. Clinically, the LGEA is seldom used as a pedicle for the omental graft, because it is fragile and apt to be torn near the hilum of spleen, and bleeding ensues once the gastrosplenic ligament is tightly stretched. Besides, the calibre of LGEA is smaller than that of the right artery.

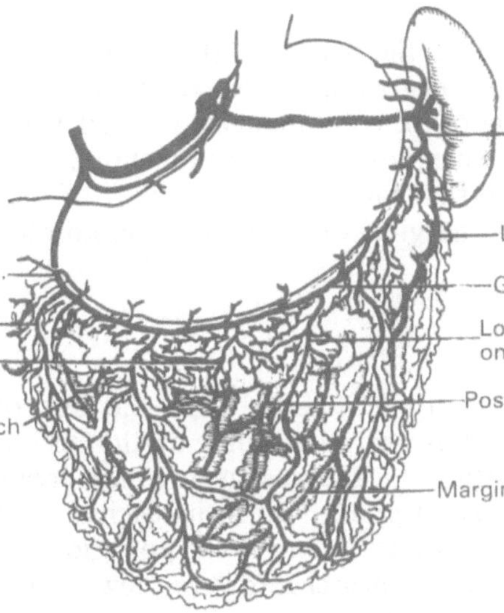

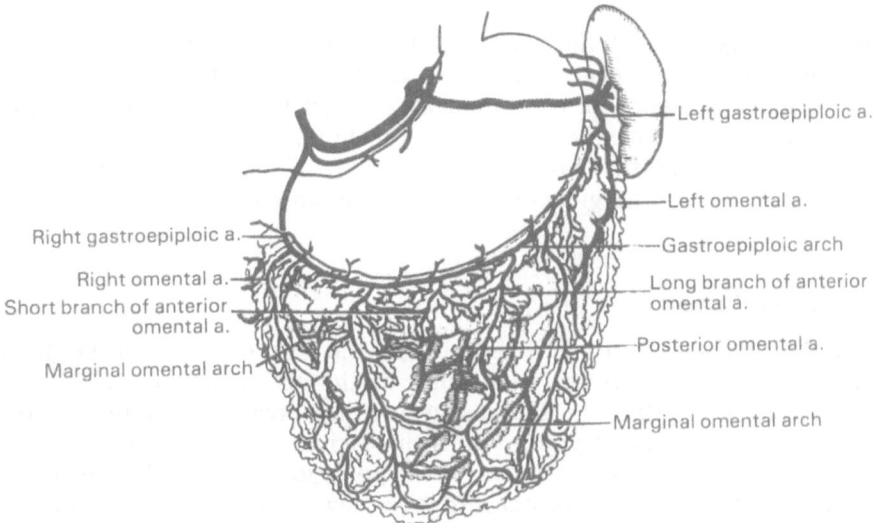

Figure 8.1 Vascular distribution of the greater omentum

Right gastroepiploic artery (RGEA)

The RGEA is one of the terminal branches of the gastroduodenal artery, which arises from the common hepatic artery. It commences from the lower margin of the bulbous portion of the duodenum and then turns left, skirting the greater curvature of the stomach, or 1–2 cm below it. It gives off several gastric branches to the anterior and posterior walls of the stomach and finally anastomoses with the left gastroepiploic artery to form the gastroepiploic arterial arch.

The mean outer diameter of the RGEA is 2.8 (1.5–4.5) mm. The thickness of its wall averages 0.3 (0.2–0.5) mm. The diameter of the right gastroepiploic vein is 3.2 (1.5–4.5) mm and the thickness of the wall, 0.1 (0.1–0.2) mm. As the RGEA is larger than LGEA, most of the anterior omental arteries come directly from it in the absence of the gastroepiploic arterial arch. It is preferable to choose RGEA in either pedicled omental transplantation or vascularized omental graft.

Gastroepiploic arterial arch

The gastroepiploic arterial arch gives off many branches to the greater omentum in addition to the gastric branches. Of these, there are two large branches given off from the commencement of the right and left gastroepiploic arteries, known as the right and left omental arteries. The rest of the branches vary in length and they are named collectively as long and short branches of the anterior omental arteries.

Left omental artery

The left omental artery is the thicker of the anterior omental arteries. It may be as large as the left gastroepiploic artery. Its mean outer diameter is 1.6 (0.5–3.0) mm and that of the accompanying vein is 1.9 (0.8–4.0) mm. They run within the posterior layers of the greater omentum. The left omental artery anastomoses with the right one in the lower part of the omentum to form a constant and distinct marginal omental arch (Barkow's arch).

Right omental artery

The right omental artery is smaller than the left one. Its mean outer diameter is 1.2 (0.5–2.0) mm, while that of the accompanying vein is 1.5 (0.8–3.0) mm. It is within the anterior layers of the greater omentum near the right edge of the omental apron. When it reaches the lower margin of the omentum it turns upward, ascending in the posterior layers of the omentum, and joins the marginal omental arch. However, few of the right omental arteries may originate from the pancreatic branch of the splenic artery.

Anterior omental arteries

Anterior omental arteries are numerous, being 7–13 in number. The longer and larger ones may reach the lower free margin of the greater omentum, then turn upward in its posterior layers and anastomose with the marginal omental arch. The shorter and smaller ones do not reach the marginal omental arch, but divide repeatedly within the anterior layers of the omentum and anastomose with the neighbouring omental arteries. Arterior omental arteries of variable location and length were called by some authors (Alday, Ningxia Medical College, etc.) the short, long or accessory omental artery. Of these, the largest was also termed the middle omental artery and the arteries of the greater omentum were further classified into five patterns according to the level of branching of the middle omental artery. However, we have found that two or three branches with almost the same calibre are often given off from the gastroepiploic arch, and it is difficult to distinguish the so-called middle omental artery from other branches. Moreover, the crucial vessels in tailoring the omentum during operation are the gastroepiploic arch, the marginal omental arch, and the right and left omental arteries. It seems likely that these have nothing to do with the pattern of the anterior omental arteries. We agree to the suggestion by Mo Jingguo and Li Zhikun (1980) that the so-called middle omental arteries be named the anterior omental arteries.

Marginal omental arch

Most of the marginal omental arches (Bardow's arch) are located in the posterior layers of the greater omentum, except for a few cases where they are in the anterior layers. It is formed mainly by the left omental artery which anastomoses with the right. It is further joined by the long branches of the anterior omental arteries. The arch is constantly present though it varies in its position. The most highly situated arch is, however, 4 cm from the transverse colon. Its presence is significant in the communication of vessels between the right and the left sides of the omentum. It also serves as an important guide during omental tailoring and lengthening so far as the origin of blood supply is concerned.

Posterior omental arteries

Several posterior omental arteries arise from the marginal omental arch. They ascend in the posterior layers of the greater omentum to be distributed to the transverse colon, either superficially or deep into the wall. In addition to the middle colic artery which anastomoses with the right and left colic arteries to form the marginal artery of the colon, the transverse colon gains its blood supply partly from the posterior omental artery, which is, however, small in calibre and cannot completely compensate the middle colic artery during its injury.

The dimensions of the greater omentum

The length of the omentum refers to the distance between the greater curvature of the stomach and the free margin of the greater omentum, and its width is the widest transverse dimension. The length and width of the omentum measured from cadavers do not correspond to those obtained from patients during operation. The omentum is about 25 cm long and 30 cm wide. It is shorter in children, yet the width of the omentum shows less distinct age differences.

Dissection and lengthening of the greater omentum

In the free or pedicled transplantation of the greater omentum it is necessary to choose the omental vessels or vascular pedicle as the course of blood supply. Judging from the distribution of omental vessels, the right and left gastroepiploic arteries are the source of blood supply. These, together with the gastroepiploic arch, the right and left omental arteries and the marginal omental arterial arch, form a complete vascular circle of the greater omentum to provide a rich collateral circulation. Therefore, in omental transplantation the gastroepiploic arteries are of first choice. Of these, the right gastroepiploic artery is more often used in clinical practice because of its greater calibre.

The lengthening of the greater omentum may be done according to the method shown in Figure 8.2. On the premise of preserving the right or left gastroepiploic artery as the major source of blood supply, the omentum can be tailored in accordance with the arrangement of the omental vascular circle. If it is used to wrap the finger, set one anterior omental artery in the omental stuff of each finger. Since the long branches of the anterior omental artery join

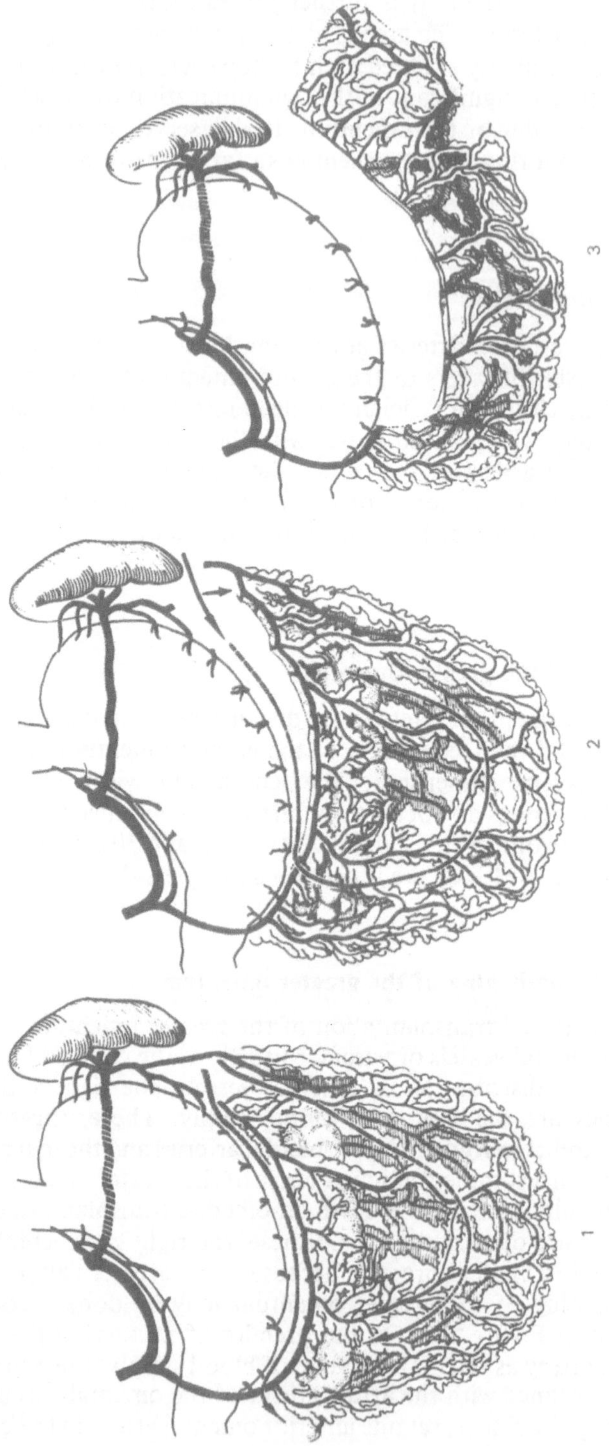

Figure 8.2 The lengthening of the greater omentum in accordance with its vascular distribution

directly the anastomosis between the gastroepiploic arch and the marginal omental artery, it can be chosen in the process of further tailoring. Nevertheless, as long as the continuity of the omental vascular arch is well kept, the anterior omental arteries can be divided without any ill effect. The omental vascular pattern has to be examined first before the method for lengthening the omentum can be decided. The omental vessels to be cut may be clamped to see whether the omentum can get its blood supply as expected. If not, the design should be modified.

The greater omentum is adhesive to the head of pancreas but is separable from the body and tail, so that its separation from the greater curvature of the stomach and transverse colon is easy to carry out from left to right. The gastroepiploic arterial arch is near the greater curvature and gives off many large gastric branches which should be well ligated in the course of separation. The marginal omental arch is more remote from the transverse colon, and the posterior omental arteries are few and small and difficult to dissect.

The greater omentum can be wrinkled up to reduce its area but can never be folded, especially in compression bandaging so as to avoid circulatory disturbance. It should be noticed that in lengthening the greater omentum, tension from over-pulling has to be avoided. When the recipient area is far from the abdomen it is better to perform free omental transplantation.

THE OMENTAL AXIAL SKIN FLAP

This is a newly designed method for the enlargement of donor flap and was successfully carried out in 1979 by Shen Zuyac *et al.* in Jishuitan Hospital, Beijing. The operation is based on the characteristics of the greater omentum, i.e. the abundance of blood vessels and the ease of establishment of collateral circulation with other tissues. The omentum with the right gastroepiploic artery as its pedicle is transplanted into the abdominal subcutaneous tissue. After the union between the greater omentum and the subcutaneous tissue has been completed and the blood circulation between them established, the abdominal subcutaneous tissue and the overlying skin with the omental pedicle can be taken en bloc and grafted as the omental axial skin graft to the recipient area.

9

The microsurgical anatomy of the central nervous system

ZHANG WEILONG AND ZHENG ZHILIANG

INTRODUCTION

It is not long since microsurgical technique was applied to the central nervous system. The history may be traced to as early as 1957, when Kurze in the United States used the operating microscope in neurosurgery and designed the subtemporal transmental approach for the removal of acoustic neurinoma. The first report on microsurgical operation for brain tumours was given by House in 1961 and then by Kurze and Doyle in 1962. In the field of microvascular brain surgery, Jacobson and Donaghy were the first to employ microsutures in intracranial vascular anastomosis. In 1960 they carried out an endarterectomy on the middle cerebral artery in Burlington, but the first successful surgical case was reported by Shelley Chou in 1963. Thenceforth successful cases in which the microscope was used in the management of intracranial aneurysm were published successively by Adam and Witt (1964), Pool and Colton (1966), and Rang and Zanetta (1967). On 30 October, 1967 Yasargil in Zurich performed for the first time the anastomosis of the superficial temporal artery with the middle cerebral artery using microsurgical technique. The same operation was done the next day by Donaghy in Burlington to establish an artificial collateral circulation for a patient who suffered from cerebral occlusion. Such operations have now been improved to some extent, and much progress has been made in respect of basic theory, operative technique, indications and choice of cases. In the People's Republic of China the application of extra- and intracranial vascular anastomosis for the relief of ischaemic cerebral vascular disease was first reported by the Xinjiang Medical College in 1976. Anastomosis of the occipital artery with the posterior inferior cerebellar artery was performed in Beijing in 1978. Recently, extra- and intracranial arterial bypass has been reported in many provincial and municipal hospitals in China, and the microsurgical ligation of the neck of the intracranial aneurysm, microsurgical operations for intracranial tumours and those on the vertebral column and spinal cord have also been carried out in some local hospitals.

The structures and functions of the brain and spinal cord are quite different from those of the other organs of the body. For example, nerve cells possess high metabolic rate and demand a rich supply of oxygen so that the brain and spinal cord are provided with an abundance of vessels. The processes of the neuroglia enclose the body and processes of the neuron and adhere to the walls of the capillaries. In consequence, the intercellular spaces are so narrow that a minute injury may often involve a number of neurons.

Notwithstanding the enveloping meninges, the absence of connective tissue framework within the brain and spinal cord makes the brain tissue very soft and fragile. Since part of the brain is deeply seated in the skull, exposure becomes very difficult. Neurons, being capable of conductivity, take part in the most important regulatory functions of the body. However, they are incapable of mitosis after birth, and nerve fibres in the brain and spinal cord seldom regenerate. Eventually, a minute lesion in the central nervous system could cause widespread functional disturbance or even irreversible damage. These characteristics demand a high standard of neurosurgical technique, i.e. they require accuracy and gentleness, elaborate haemostasis and the least traction and injury to the brain tissue so as to promote recovery of nervous function. Microsurgical technique is destined to show its superiority in this field.

The main applications of microsurgery to the central nervous system at present are in the aspect of tumour of the brain and spinal cord, aneurysm, arteriovenous malformation, and precise resection of cranial nerve roots. These also involve such operations as endarterectomy, repair of blood vessels and artificial bypass, and bridging for cerebrovascular occlusive diseases.

In recent years, along with the development of microsurgery of the central nervous system, relevant literature has appeared widely. Some of the important reports by Chinese colleagues are: *The Surgical Anatomy of the Vessels for Extra- and Intracranial Bypass* (Zhong Shizhen, 1979), *The Microanatomy of the Anterior Portion of the Circles of Willis* (Zhang Weilong, 1980), *The Distribution and Measurement of the Superficial Temporal and Occipital Arteries in the Scalp* (Li Shufen, 1980), *A Preliminary Survey of Fifty Cases of Cavernous Sinus in Chinese* (Lin Kai, 1980), 'Microsurgical anatomy of cortical branches of middle cerebral artery' (Zhang Weilong, 1982) and *A Study of the Venous System of the Brain in Chinese* (Zeng Silu, 1981).

VESSELS OF THE BRAIN

ZHAO MINXUE, QIN DENGYOU, ZHANG SHIXING,
ZHANG WEILONG AND ZHENG ZHILIANG

Arteries of the brain

The arterial blood supply of the brain is derived from two systems: internal carotid and vertebrobasilar systems. Branches of the cerebral arteries fall into two types: central and cortical branches. The central branches arise from the internal carotid artery and the proximal segments of the anterior, middle and posterior cerebral arteries. They penetrate into the parenchyma of the brain to supply such structures as the diencephalon, corpus striatum, and internal capsule. The cortical branches arise from the anterior, middle and posterior cerebral arteries and pass along the cerebral sulci and gyri to form rich anastomoses within the leptomeninges. Arising from the network formed by these anastomoses, the short arteries supply the adjacent cortex while the long ones pass through the cortex to the medullary substance. Cerebral arteries are generally more crowded in the sulci than on the surface of the gyri. Consequently the cerebral cortex should not be incised along the sulci in order to avoid bleeding.

Internal carotid arterial system

Internal carotid artery

At the commencement of the internal carotid artery (71%) or at the point of bifurcation of the common carotid (9%), the artery shows a slight fusiform dilatation termed the carotid sinus. In the tunica adventitia of the sinus there is the pressor-receptor, which is able to react to changes in blood pressure. Atherosclerosis and stricture are apt to occur at the carotid sinus and the carotid bifurcation. The calibre of the internal carotid artery at the carotid sinus averages 6 (3–10) mm, and that of the intracranial segment, 3.3 (2–5) mm. The calibre of the artery may be somewhat larger in a living body. Normally, the internal carotid arteries are mostly equal in size on both sides, but the left one may sometimes be wider than the right.

The internal carotid artery can be divided into extra- and intracranial portions. The intracranial portion may be further divided into five segments: the petrous, cavernous, siphonic, supraclinoid and terminal segments. They are designated as C_5, C_4, C_3, C_2 and C_1 respectively in carotid angiogram (Figure 9.1).

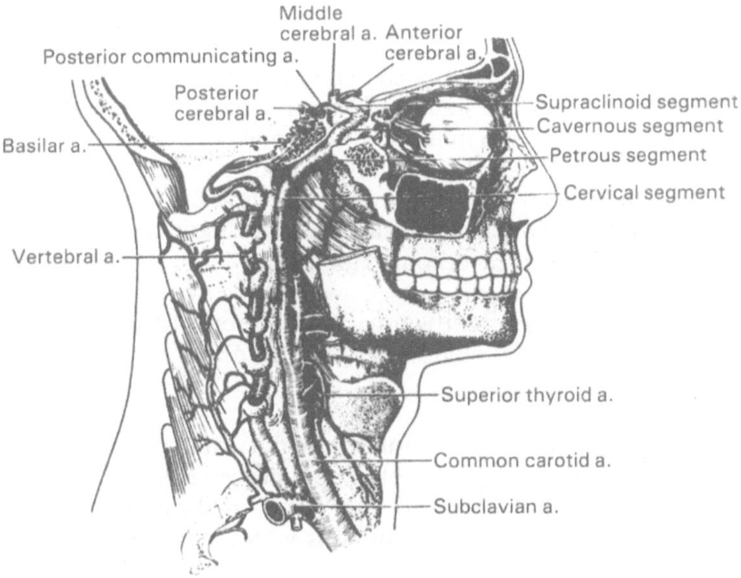

Figure 9.1 Segmentation of the internal carotid and vertebral arteries

The petrous segment This is situated in the carotid canal of the petrous portion of the temporal bone. It can be divided into a vertical and a horizontal segment. The part connecting these segments is called the genu and measures 5 cm in its outer diameter. The vertical segment is the part of the internal carotid artery which ascends vertically after entering the canal. The length of this segment is 10.5 (6.0–15.0) mm. It is related to the pharyngotympanic tube anteriorly, the jugular fossa posteriorly and the tympanic portion of the temporal bone laterally. The horizontal segment proceeds from the genu anteromedially and horizontally to the apex of the petrous temporal bone. It is about 20 (15–20) mm in length, and is separated from the cochlea by a thin osseous plate. The medial part of the roof of the horizontal segment is formed by the dura mater or a thin bony plate that separates the carotid artery from the Gasserian ganglion. The horizontal segment emerges from the foramen lacerum to enter the cavernous sinus immediately. After entering the carotid canal the carotid nerve, a branch of the superior cervical ganglion of the sympathetic trunk, accompanies the artery and divides into a larger anterosuperior and a smaller posteroinferior trunk. The two trunks give off the deep petrosal nerve and send some branches to join the trochlear, trigeminal and abducent nerves. The vessels given off by this segment are the caroticotympanic artery and the pterygoid branch.

The petrous segment of the internal carotid artery is closely related to the facial canal, internal acoustic meatus, cochlea, geniculate ganglion, facial nerve, greater and lesser petrosal nerves, trigeminal nerve, tympanic cavity, auditory tube, middle meningeal artery and the tensor tympani. When it is to be exposed from the lateral side of the trigeminal nerve and the floor of the middle cranial fossa for a common carotid–petrous segment bypass with a venous graft, all of the above-mentioned structures must be protected carefully from injury.

The cavernous segment This is situated in the cavernous sinus. It first ascends for a short distance within the sinus and then proceeds horizontally forward along the carotid sulcus at the junction of the body and greater wing of the sphenoid bone to the under-surface of the anterior clinoid process. It finally curves upwards and backwards to become the siphonic segment, and then traverses the dura mater to be continued as the supraclinoid segment (for details see the section entitled 'The cavernous region').

The siphonic segment This signifies the turning point where the cavernous segment becomes the supraclinoid segment. The ophthalmic artery usually arises from this segment.

The supraclinoid segment This is situated slightly above an imaginary line drawn from the anterior to the posterior clinoid processes and runs backwards in the opposite direction to the cavernous segment. On the under-surface of the anterior perforated substance it is continuous with the terminal segment.

The terminal (or cerebral) segment This is very short and divides into the anterior and middle cerebral arteries immediately.

The course of the intracranial portion of the internal carotid artery is tortuous. It possesses four bends. The first bend is located in the carotid canal where the vessel turns from the ascending to the horizontal position. The second is located where the petrous segment turns to the cavernous segment. The third sits at the siphon and the fourth bend lies above the trigeminal ganglion before the terminal segment divides into the anterior and middle cerebral arteries. These bends can be seen clearly on a normal lateral arteriogram of the internal carotid artery. Their physiological significance may be concerned with the buffering of blood pressure within the arteries.

The cavernous (C_4), siphonic (C_3) and supraclinoid (C_2) segments are together called the carotid siphon. According to Chinese data there are four types regarding the configuration of the carotid siphon (Figure 9.2): 'U' type in 40%; 'V' type in 48%; 'C' type in 10%; and 'S' type in only 2%. Each of these types may be subdivided into several subtypes. The configuration of the carotid siphon is related to the age: the more advanced in age the more tortuous the siphon.

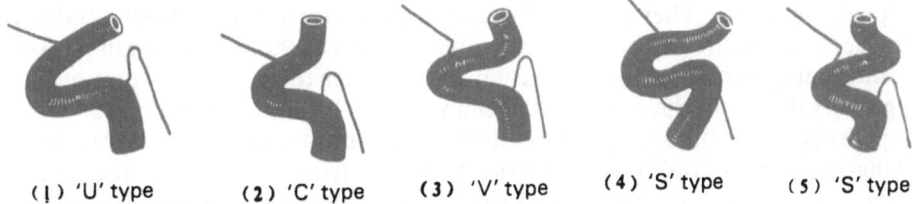

Figure 9.2 Configurations of the carotid siphon

Variations in the internal carotid artery

The internal carotid artery varies in its origin, position, configuration and branches. These may influence the blood circulation of the brain to a certain degree and have practical significance in the diagnosis and treatment of cerebral vascular disease.

(1) Absence of the unilateral internal carotid artery and absence of aplasia of a segment of it. The former occurs very rarely. It was first reported by Tode in 1787, and up to 1973 a total of only 25 cases has been reported abroad. In the presence of these variations the blood supply of the affected side may come from the basilar artery and the contralateral internal carotid artery, or from the branches of the internal maxillary artery, which enter the cranium through the foramen rotundum and foramen ovale to form a common trunk, from which the ophthalmic artery, the anterior and middle cerebral arteries arise. The blood may even come from the enlarged posterior communicating artery, from which the ophthalmic artery springs.

(2) In the absence of the common carotid artery the internal and external carotid arteries arise directly from the aortic arch.

(3) The common carotid artery does not bifurcate but extends directly into the internal carotid artery, whence the branches of the external carotid artery arise.

(4) The level of origin of the internal carotid artery may be as high as the first cervical vertebra and as low as the second thoracic vertebra.

(5) In rare cases (3.8%), the internal carotid artery seems to be the direct continuation of the common carotid, the internal carotid artery being medial to the external carotid artery. Therefore in ligation of the external carotid artery it may be distinguished on the basis of its branches and not simply on its position, in order to evade errors in ligation.

(6) Tortuosity, coiling and kinking. The cervical portion of the internal carotid artery may exhibit angular, S-shaped, C-shaped or even coiling tortuosity. Metz reported that the incidence of carotid tortuosity in angiograms was 16%, while that found in autopsy in the Chinese was 11%. These variations usually cause no symptoms. However, in severe cases they may affect the blood supply of the brain and be a cause of cerebral ischaemia.

(7) In rare cases the ascending pharyngeal artery may arise from the cervical portion of the internal carotid artery.

(8) Caroticobasilar anastomoses. There are three anastomotic channels in the 3–4 mm embryo. These are the primitive trigeminal artery, otic artery and hypoglossal artery. They connect the internal carotid artery with the longitudinal arteries of the neural tube. The longitudinal arteries of the neural tube in the 3–4 month embryo are fused into the basilar artery. When the posterior communicating artery develops, the primitive trigeminal artery begins to degenerate and disappears at the 14 mm stage of the embryo. The primitive otic artery is transient, being the first to disappear, while the primitive hypoglossal artery disappears right after it, when the embryo gets to the 5 mm stage. These primitive arteries, when persistent, are known as the caroticobasilar anastomoses in adult.

(a) The primitive trigeminal artery is the most common of the caroticobasilar anastomoses and was first recorded by Quain in 1844. The incidence of it found at autopsy was 0.3–1.5%, and in angiography 0.1–0.6%, averaging around 0.23%. It arises from the proximal end of the cavernous segment of the internal carotid artery, runs backwards in the sinus medial to the trigeminal nerve and penetrates either the diaphragma sellae or the dura mater near the clivus to anastomose with the basilar artery between the commencements of the superior and anterior inferior cerebellar arteries. It varies in calibre. The clinical significance of this anastomosis is that it may be the site of aneurysm or be the point of weakness on the wall of the internal carotid or basilar artery. It is believed that it may compress the trigeminal and abducent nerves, resulting in trigeminal neuralgia and esotropia respectively.

(b) The primitive otic artery is rare, its incidence being about 0.1%. It arises from the petrous segment of the internal carotid artery, emerges from the internal auditory meatus with the statoacoustic nerve, and turns medially to join the basilar artery between the anterior and posterior inferior cerebellar arteries. The larger the otic artery, the smaller the vertebral artery.

(c) The primitive hypoglossal artery is also of rare occurrence, with an incidence of 0.1%. This artery arises from the internal carotid artery at the level of C_1–C_3. After a tortuous course it passes through the hypoglossal canal to enter the posterior cranial fossa and connect with the commencement of the basilar artery.

Branches of the internal carotid artery

The ophthalmic artery This artery arises from the siphonic segment at an obtuse angle, but may sometimes originate from the cavernous or the terminal segment. It passes anterolaterally below the optic nerve and enters the orbit through the optic canal. In the orbital cavity it gives off the central artery of retina, ciliary arteries, lacrimal artery, frontal artery and dorsal nasal artery to supply the eyeball, ocular muscles, lacrimal gland and the skin and muscles over the forehead and the dorsum of the nose. It also anastomoses with the superficial temporal, the facial and the maxillary arteries of the external carotid artery by its branches, i.e. the frontal, the dorsal nasal and the lacrimal arteries. In the occlusion of the internal carotid artery the blood in the external carotid artery may shunt through the ophthalmic artery into the brain via these anastomoses. As the ophthalmic artery is a branch of the internal carotid artery, the blood pressure within the carotid can be shown by measuring that of the ophthalmic artery.

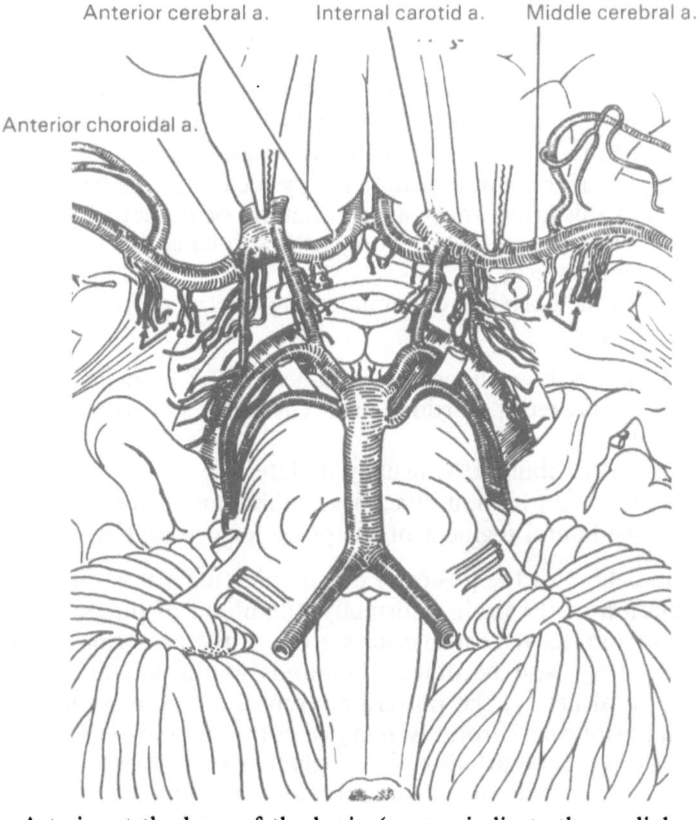

Figure 9.3 Arteries at the base of the brain (arrows indicate the medial and lateral perforating arteries of the middle cerebral artery)

The posterior communicating artery (PCOA) This artery arises from the dorsal convex border of the terminal segment of the internal carotid artery and proceeds posteromedially below the optic tract and above the oculomotor nerve to anastomose with the posterior cerebral artery. Its outer diameter averages 1.3 (0.3–3.1) mm. In 50% of cases it is equal size on both sides. Its length averages 14 (9–34) mm, the right one being relatively longer in 50% of the cases. The number of perforating branches arising from the posterior communicating artery averages 7 (4–12). Their diameters average 0.3 (0.1–1.1) mm. They pass through the tuber cinereum, optic tract and chiasma, corpus mammilare, cerebral peduncle and the posterior perforated substance to get into the brain. Four of the perforating branches arising from the anterior half of the posterior communicating artery usually supply the hypothalamus, the ventral thalamus, the anterior one-third of the optic tract and the posterior limb of the internal capsule. The other three arising from the posterior half of the artery are distributed to the posterior perforated substance and the subthalamic mucleus. In 80% of cases the largest of these perforating branches is called the 'thalamotuberal artery' or 'premamillary artery' with an average outer diameter of 0.6 (0.3–1.0) mm. It enters the brain between the mamillary body and the optic tract to supply the lateral and anterior portions of the thalamus and the hypothalamus. This artery originates from the middle third of the posterior communicating artery in 67% of cases, from the anterior third in 20%, and from the posterior third in 13%. It is of significance in the angiographic diagnosis of tumours of the third ventricle, the thalamus, and the hypothalamus. The thalamotuberal artery may be absent (20%) and replaced by two or three branches of unequal size to enter the premamillary area.

Since the posterior communicating artery is close to the oculomotor nerve, the aneurysm of this artery may cause ipsilateral oculomotor palsy. Occlusion of the perforating branches which supply the subthalamic nucleus will lead to contralateral hemiballism.

Variations in the posterior communicating artery are frequent. They are as follows (Figure 9.4).

(a) Configuration: bow-shaped or S-shaped, 48%; loop-shaped, 5%; plexiform in its posterior portion, 2%. The latter two types are frequently unilateral.
(b) Total absence: about 1%, usually unilateral.
(c) Calibre: less than 1.0 mm, 9%; large calibre and extending posteriorly to become the lateral segment of the posterior cerebral artery, 11%.

Variations in calibre of the posterior communicating artery directly affect the blood circulation of the brain. Normally, the blood of the posterior cerebral artery comes from the vertebrobasilar system. If the posterior communicating artery is very large and becomes continuous as the lateral segment of the posterior cerebral artery, the posterior cerebral artery may obtain its blood chiefly from the internal carotid system just as the embryo. The medial segment of the posterior cerebral artery is thus slender, so that ligation of the internal or common carotid artery may cause severe visual damage due to lack of compensation. Berry investigated some patients suffering from cerebral malacia and found that tiny posterior communicating arteries occurred in 49%.

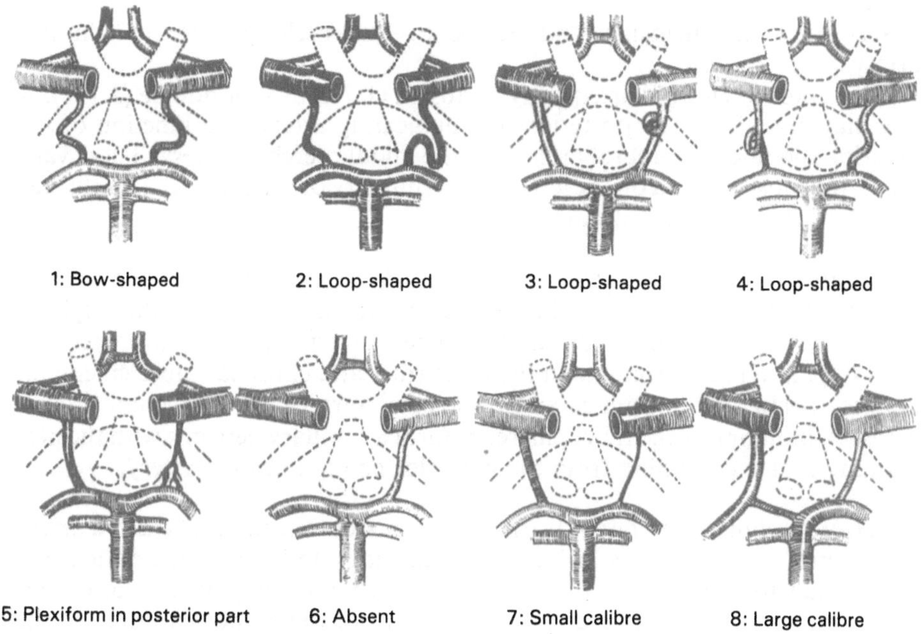

Figure 9.4 Variations of the posterior communicating artery

The anterior choroidal artery This artery is mostly the first branch of the internal carotid artery distal to the origin of the posterior communicating artery (67%). A few of them may be the second branch (15%), the third branch (11%) or the fourth branch (7%). The distance between its origin and the posterior communicating artery averages 2.7 (1–5) mm. It runs backwards, and crosses the optic tract from the lateral to the medial side. At the anterior margin of the cerebral peduncle it inclines posterolaterally, crossing the optic tract from its medial to the lateral side. It enters the lower and anterior part of the choroid fissure between the lateral geniculate body and the uncus to terminate in the choroid plexus of the inferior horn of the lateral ventricle. The outer diameter at its origin averages 1.1 (0.6–1.6) mm. The length from its origin to the entrance into the choroid plexus averages 26 (15–35) mm. It gives off branches on the way to the uncus in the temporal lobe, optic tract, part of the lateral geniculate body and optic radiation, the genu and posterior limb of the internal capsule, tail of the caudate nucleus and the medial part of the globus pallidus, part of the lateral thalamic nucleus and the subthalamus, and the middle third of the cerebral peduncle and the substantia nigra. From the PCOA also arise some branches which supply the optic tract, cerebral peduncle, lateral geniculate body and the choroid plexus of the lateral ventricle, and they anastomose with the perforating branches of the PCOA and the branches of the posterior choroid artery (Figure 9.3).

The typical symptoms of the occlusion of the anterior choroid artery are contralateral hemiplegia, hemianopia and hamianaesthesia. Owing to the wide distribution of, and variations in, this artery, symptoms may not always manifest themselves. In some cases of parkinsonism, ligation of this artery may give a noteworthy improvement. According to pathological observations the incidence and degree of atherosclerosis are low in this artery.

The anterior choroid artery may be absent (1.7–2.0%) or double (2.7%). A few may arise from the posterior communicating artery, the junction of the anterior and middle cerebral arteries or the middle cerebral artery. These variations are mostly found on the left side. Asymmetry of calibre is frequently seen (37.8%). The left one is usually larger.

The perforating branches of the internal carotid artery These are two or three in number and originate from the internal carotid artery distal to the origin of the posterior communicating artery. Their outer diameter averages 0.3 (0.1–1.0) mm. They terminate in the optic tract and chiasma, tuber cinereum, anterior perforated substance and the medial surface of the temporal lobe. Those terminating at the tuber cinereum form a capillary network with the perforating branches coming from the posterior communicating artery.

Anterior cerebral artery (ACA) After arising from the internal carotid artery the anterior cerebral artery inclines anteromedially and crosses the optic nerve or chiasma to the Sylvian fissure. It curves round the genu of the corpus callosum, and runs backwards along the sulcus of the corpus callosum to the splenius, where it anastomoses with a branch of the posterior cerebral artery. The anterior cerebral arteries of the two sides join above or in front of the optic chiasma by the anterior communicating artery. The part of the ACA between the internal carotid and anterior communicating arteries is usually called the proximal segment (A_1), and the part distal to the anterior communicating artery the distal segment (A_2).

Proximal segment of the anterior cerebral artery The average length of the proximal segment is 14 mm on the left and 15 mm on the right. The outer diameter averages 2.5 mm on the left and 2.4 mm on the right. This segment often exhibits various bends (Figure 9.5). The most common of these consists of the proximal half which curves inferomedially and the distal half which curves superolaterally.

Hypoplasia of A_1 is the most frequent variation in the anterior cerebral artery. Its incidence is about 10% and it usually occurs on the right side. The hypoplastic A_1 is rather thin, its outer diameter being 0.5–1.5 mm, while the contralateral A_1 is thicker and divides into right and left A_2 to supply two hemispheres. Kirgis called this variation 'the anterior trifurcation of the internal carotid artery'. It is generally believed that the hypoplasia of A_1 is correlated with the occurrence of the aneurysm of the anterior communicating artery. This may be due to the asymmetry of the vessels of the two sides which produces a local alteration in the intravascular hydrokinetics and provides a mechanical factor for the development of aneurysm. Other variations are rare; these include mainly the absence of A_1, double trunk, partial double trunk and the island-shaped anterior end of A_1 (Figure 9.6). The bends and variations of A_1 can be referred to in cerebral angiograph.

The central branches arising from A_1 are also called perforating arteries. According to the course and distribution these can be divided into three groups: the recurrent artery, the anterior perforating and the hypothalamic branches.

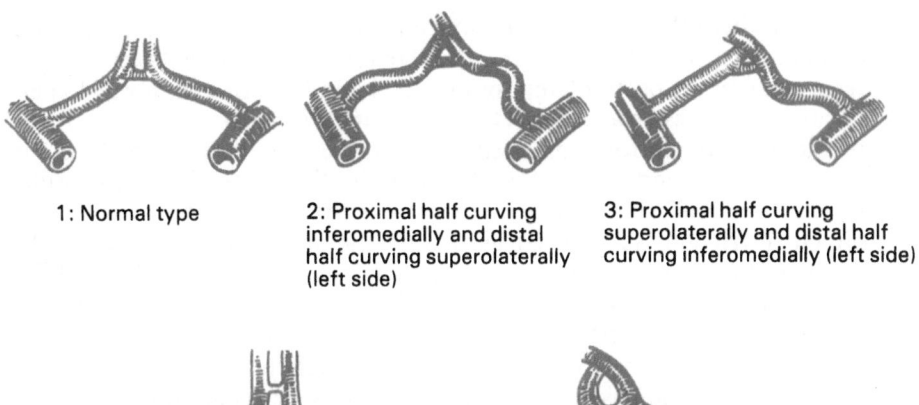

1: Normal type

2: Proximal half curving inferomedially and distal half curving superolaterally (left side)

3: Proximal half curving superolaterally and distal half curving inferomedially (left side)

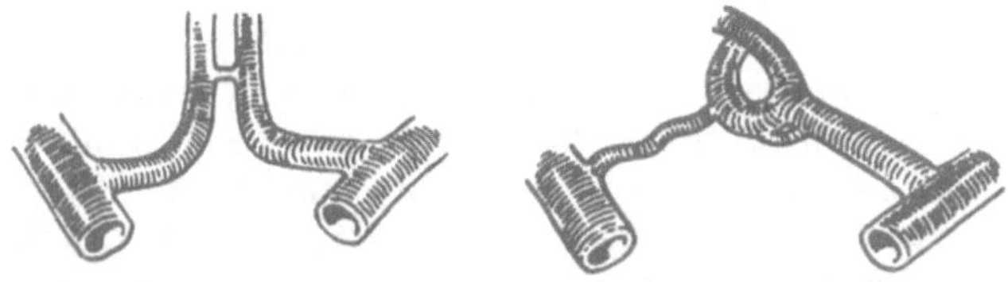

4: A_1 dividing into horizontal and ascending segments

5: Hypoplasia of A_1 with more bends (right side)

Figure 9.5 Bends of the proximal segment of the anterior cerebral artery

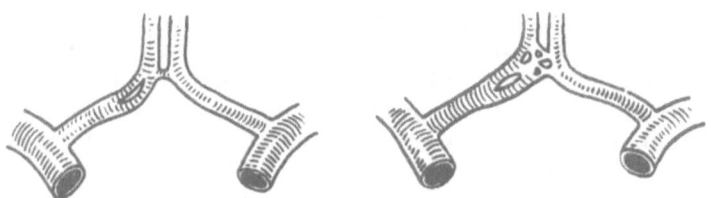

1 and 2: Island-shaped anterior end

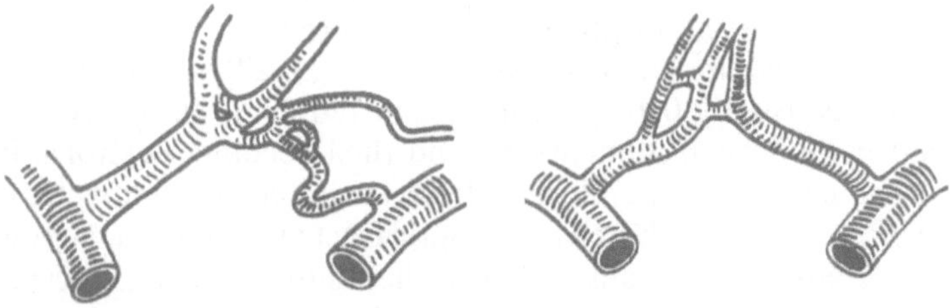

3: Hypoplasia of left A_1 with marked bends

4: Partial double trunk of A_1

Figure 9.6 Variations of the proximal segment of the anterior cerebral artery

1. *The recurrent artery*. Since it was first recorded by Heubner in 1874 it has also been named the Heubner's artery. It may be single (65%) or double (30%), but there may be as many as four. The outer diameter averages 0.8 (0.2–2.0) mm. Heubner's artery is larger in cases of hypoplasia of A_1. It usually arises from the lateral wall of the anterior cerebral artery as the level

of the origin of the anterior communicating artery (more than 50%). A few of them may arise from A_1 or A_2. Heubner's artery assumes various recurrent courses posterolaterally and divides into 4.5 or as many as 13 perforating branches on average. The latter branches penetrate the lateral area of the anterior perforated substance to supply the anterior part of the caudate nucleus and putamen, and the anterior limb of the internal capsule. It also gives off some small branches on the way to the orbital gyri, olfactory trigone, subcallosal gyrus and the suprachiasmatic area. The course of the recurrent artery may be divided into four groups (Figure 9.7): (a) parallel to and in front of A_1; (b) parallel and deep to A_1; (c) looped; and (d) arising proximal to A_1, running for a distance, and then coming back in front of or deep to A_1. It must be indicated that the recurrent artery arising from the anterior communicating artery or A_2 is often connected closely to A_1 by fibrous tissue when it is parallel to A_1. Inadvertent observation will mistake its origin for being proximal to A_1. Those advancing with a looped course or arising proximal to A_1, running distally, and then coming back, usually cannot easily be seen on the surface, and their origin is often apt to be mistaken for being distal to A_1. Attention should be paid to these conditions during operation so as not to injure the recurrent artery while clamping A_1. Injury to the recurrent artery will not only cause softening of the anterior limb of the internal capsule to produce corresponding symptoms, but will also lead to frontal lobe ataxia and intellectual disturbances.

2. *The anterior perforating artery* is mostly single (43%) or double (35%), but there may be as many as 10. The outer diameter averages 0.45 mm. It is larger when single and smaller when multiple. A total of 65% of the arteries arise from the posterosuperior wall of the lateral third of A_1, the rest being from the middle third (32%) and the medial third (3%). It perforates the anterior perforated substance singly or in the form of several branches (usually two to four in number, or up to 11) to supply the head and the medial aspect of the anterior part of the body of the caudate nucleus. A few of them may be traced to the olfactory tract and trigone, gyrus rectus, subcallosal gyrus and optic chiasma (Figure 9.8).
3. *The hypothalamic branches* average 8.6 (3–20) in number. The outer diameter is usually 0.1–0.2 mm, and infrequently 0.5–0.6 mm. The large ones usually branch immediately and then become plexiform in distribution. These branches mainly arise from the anteroinferior wall of the lateral third of A_1 to be distributed to the optic tract and chiasma, suprachiasmatic area and lamina terminalis. A few of them supply the optic nerve, olfactory tract, subcallosal gyrus and the genu of the corpus callosum. As most of the hypothalamic branches and the anterior perforating arteries arise from the lateral third of A_1, good care must be taken in the management of aneurysm to avoid injury to these branches when the lateral portion of the A_1 is to be clamped (Figure 9.8).

Distal segment of the anterior cerebral artery The distal segment of the anterior cerebral artery may be single or double. The single-trunk type which is more frequent (78%), gives off the orbital, frontopolar, anterior frontal,

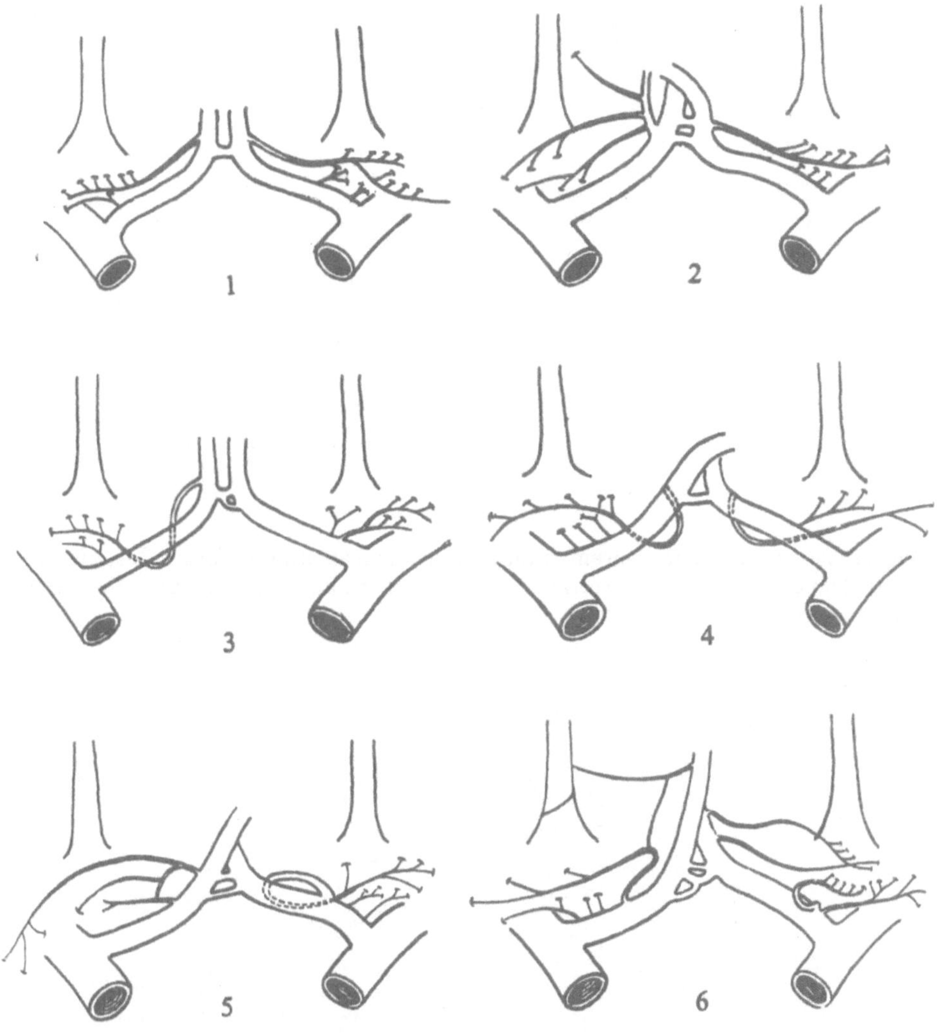

Figure 9.7 Course of the recurrent artery. **1** and **2**: normal course, parallel with A_1 anterolaterally; **3–6**: various looped courses

middle frontal, posterior frontal, paracentral, precuneal and callosal arteries to the cerebral cortex. The double-trunk type is less frequent (22%), its inferior trunk being called the pericallosal artery which courses similarly to the single-trunk type. Its superior trunk is named the callosomarginal artery and runs along the cingulate sulcus and gives off the anterior, middle and posterior frontal arteries. These cortical branches are more frequently single; few may be double. It may arise independently or join its neighbours (Figure 9.9).

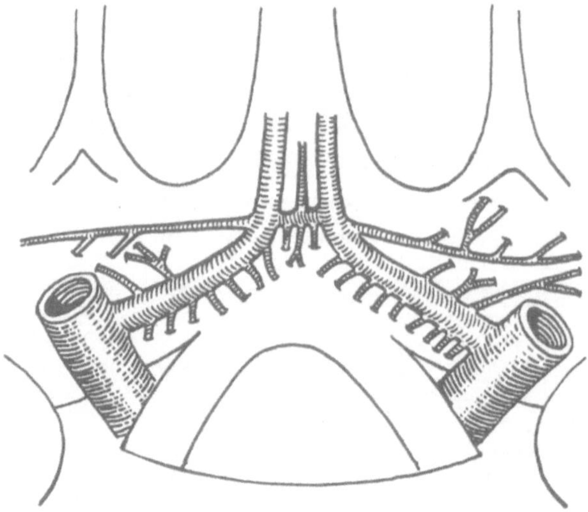

Figure 9.8 A schematic diagram of the recurrent and anterior perforating arteries, the subthalamic branches, the perforating branches of the anterior communicating artery and the median callosal artery

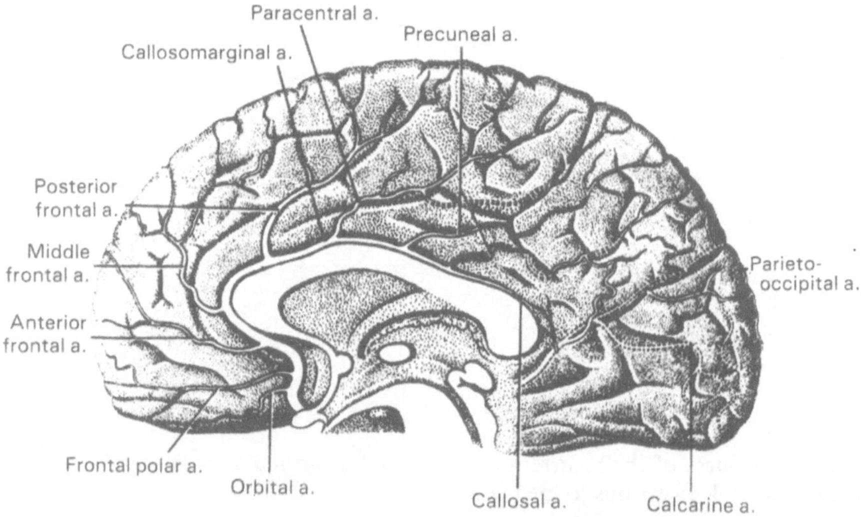

Figure 9.9 Cortical branches of the anterior cerebral artery

1. The orbital artery most commonly arises from A_2 several mm distal to the origin of the anterior communicating artery. After crossing over the gyrus rectus it divides into two branches to be distributed to the medial portion of the orbital part of the frontal lobe. The orbital artery sometimes possesses two trunks, known as the anterior and posterior orbital artery respectively.

2. The frontopolar artery commences under the genu of the corpus callosum and arborizes to supply the medial and lateral aspects of the frontal pole.
3. The anterior frontal artery arises near the genu and courses forwards and upwards on the medial aspect of the frontal lobe. It divides into two or three branches which cross the dorsomedial margin of the hemisphere to its dorsolateral surface to supply the cingulate gyrus and the upper portion of the superior and middle frontal gyrus.
4. The middle frontal artery arises from the ACA above the trunk of the corpus callosum, extends backwards and upwards, and crosses the cingulate gyrus to divide into two or three branches. These branches run round the dorsomedial margin of the hemisphere to its dorsolateral surface and divide into several branches to the cingulate gyrus and the upper portion of the superior and middle frontal gyri.
5. The posterior frontal artery arises from the ACA above the trunk of the corpus callosum, runs backwards and upwards and crosses the cingulate gyrus obliquely to divide into two or three branches. At the posterior portion of the superior frontal gyrus these branches wind round the dorsomedial margin of the hemisphere to its dorsolateral surface to supply the cingulate gyrus, the superior frontal gyrus, the upper part of the middle frontal gyrus, and the upper fourth of the precentral gyrus.
6. The paracentral artery arises from the ACA at the posterior or middle portion of the trunk of the corpus callosum. It extends backwards and upwards, crossing the cingulate gyrus obliquely to the paracentral lobule, where it divides into two or three branches, which wind round the dorsomedial margin of the hemisphere to the upper portion of the pre- and postcentral gyri to supply the cingulate gyrus, paracentral lobule and the upper fourth of the pre- and postcentral gyri.
7. The precuneal artery is usually the continuation of the anterior cerebral artery as it turns upwards just in front of the splenium. It is divided into two or three branches, which wind round the dorsomedial margin of the hemisphere to the superior parietal lobule to be distributed to the cingulate gyrus, the anterior part of the precuneus and the superior portion of the superior parietal lobule.
8. The callosal artery is small, and usually arises from the trunk of the anterior cerebral artery in front of the splenium. It passes backwards along the sulcus of the corpus callosum to be distributed to the corpus callosum and the adjacent cortex. Sometimes it may reach the parieto-occipital sulcus.

In brief, parts of the brain supplied by the distal segment of the anterior cerebral artery comprise the medial surface of the hemisphere in front of the precuneus, the upper half of the dorsolateral surface of the middle frontal gyrus, the superior frontal gyrus, the upper fourth of the pre- and postcentral gyri, the upper portion of the superior parietal lobule and the medial half of the orbital portion of the frontal lobe. Occlusion of this segment may cause central paralysis of the opposite limbs (sometimes monoplegia of the contralateral lower limb), dysaesthesia of the opposite lower limb, mental dullness and confusion, incontinence of urine, and apraxia.

Most of the initial portions of the right and left A_2 are overlapping (77%). They usually cannot be distinguished very well on the posteroanterior and lateral carotid angiograms, except in the oblique position.

The anterior communicating artery (ACOA) This artery connects the right and left anterior cerebral arteries and is extremely variable in number and pattern. It can usually be divided into two types: the simple type, including those with a single trunk running transversely or obliquely, and the complex type, involving those with more than one trunk as well as such patterns as V-shaped, Y-shaped or reticular. These two types are of equal incidence. However, it may be completely absent in rare cases (Figure 9.10). Those of the simple type are 3.0 (0.5–5.0) mm in length and 1.8 (0.5–3.5) mm in outer diameter. When the communicating artery appears as two trunks, the anterior one is shorter and wider and may be regarded as the main channel, whereas the longer and thinner posterior one may be regarded as an accessory branch which may become obviously tortuous or even coiled. From the dorsal surface of the anterior communicating artery are given off about five (from one to eight) perforating branches, most of which are relatively small. Their outer diameter is 0.1–0.2 mm (a few of them may be 0.5–0.6 mm and a few may be 1.0 mm). The perforating branches are further divided into twigs to supply the optic chiasma, suprachiasmatic area, lamina terminalis, subcallosal gyrus, area parolfactoria, genu of the corpus callosum and the anterior part of the cingulate gyrus (Figure 9.11). The permanent mental disturbance caused by impairment of the anterior communicating artery may be ascribed to the insufficient blood supply of these areas. For this reason in managing aneurysms of the anterior communicating artery these perforating branches must be carefully protected. A median callosal artery may sometimes arise from the anterior aspect of the dorsal surface of the anterior communicating artery. This vessel, also known as the median anterior cerebral artery or the third anterior cerebral artery, was first reported by Windle in 1888. Its incidence is about 16%, and the outer diameter averages 0.8 (0.5–1.0) mm. Accompanied by the anterior cerebral artery this vessel ascends to the genu of the corpus callosum. A few of them may reach the trunk of the corpus callosum as far as the parieto-occipital sulcus, and supply the adjacent cortex and the corpus callosum along its course.

The anterior communicating artery is closely related to the optic chiasma. In 56.0% of cases it is located in front of the chiasma within a range of 5 mm. In 44.0% of cases it is located above the chiasma. Some reported that it was situated on the lateral side of the chiasma (Figure 9.12); therefore, aneurysm of the anterior communicating artery may compress the chiasma to cause bitemporal hemianopia. Care must be taken to avoid accidental injury of the chiasma during operation on the aneurysm.

The middle cerebral artery (MCA) This is the largest terminal branch of the internal carotid artery and may be regarded as its continuation. It crosses the anterior perforated substance horizontally to enter the lateral cerebral fissure. It then passes backwards and laterally and gives off branches near the island of Reil. The segment proximal to its bifurcation is called the main stem of middle cerebral artery or M_1. This segment may be S-shaped, bow-shaped or

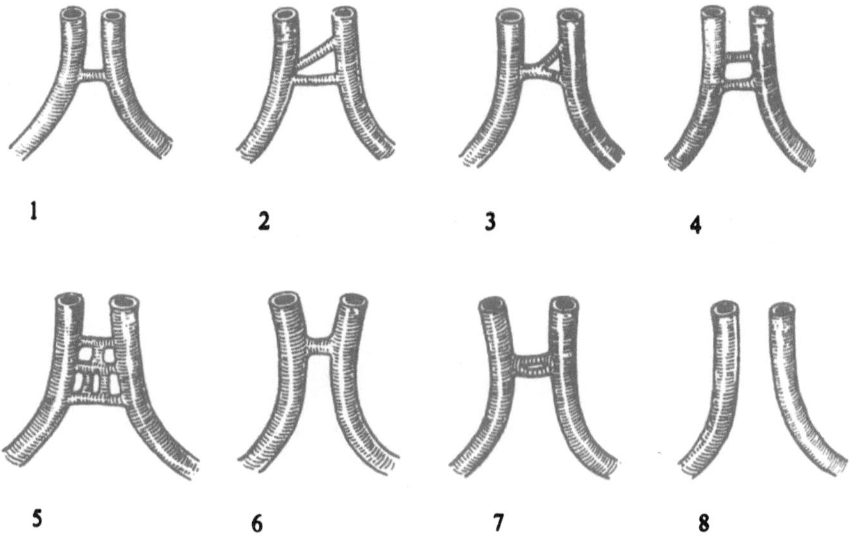

Figure 9.10 Anomalies of the anterior communicating artery. **1**: Normal type; **2–8**: abnormal type

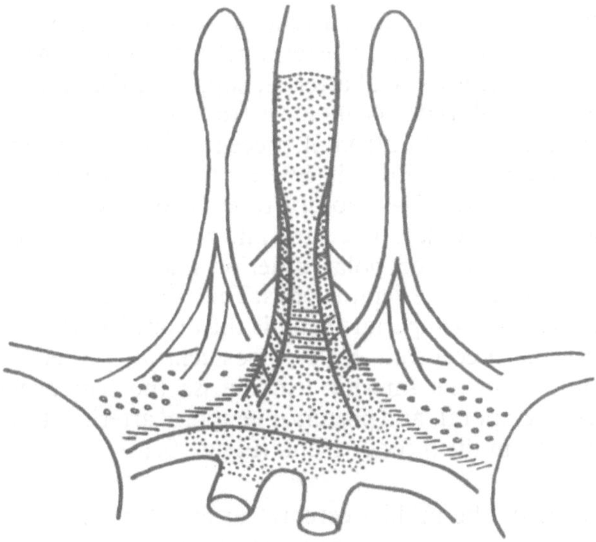

Figure 9.11 Distribution of the anterior communicating artery

straight, being 15 (3–28) mm long and 3 (2–4) mm in its outer diameter. It gives off central branches supplying the deep part of the brain. Near the island of Reil it sends of cortical branches, which assume single-, double- or triple-trunk types, supplying the cerebral cortex. The single-trunk type occurs in about 13%. The temporopolar and anterior middle and posterior temporal arteries arise from its inferior wall, supplying the temporal lobe. The orbitofrontal,

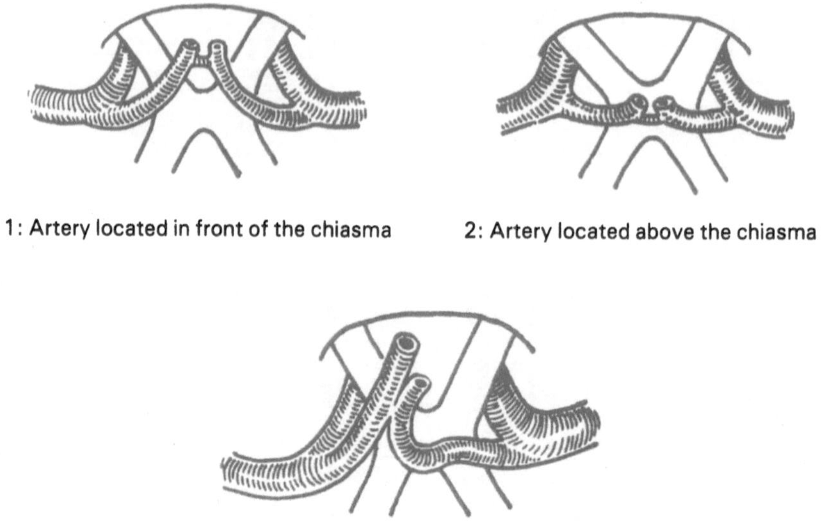

1: Artery located in front of the chiasma

2: Artery located above the chiasma

3: Artery located on the lateral side of the chiasma

Figure 9.12 Relationship between the anterior communicating artery and the optic chiasma

precentral, central, and postcentral arteries arise from its superior wall, supplying the frontal and parietal lobes. The terminal end of the main stem divides into the angular and posterior parietal arteries, supplying the occipital and parietal lobes. The double-trunk type occurs most frequently in about 76%. Its upper trunk usually gives off the orbitofrontal, precentral, central, postcentral, inferior parietal and angular arteries. From its inferior trunk arise the temporopolar and anterior, middle and posterior temporal arteries. In other cases the superior trunk may give off the temporopolar, precentral and postcentral arteries, and from the inferior trunk arise the temporopolar, anterior, middle and posterior temporal, the angular and the inferior parietal arteries. The triple-trunk type occurs in about 11% of cases. Usually its superior trunk is the orbitofrontal artery; its middle trunk gives off the precentral, central, postcentral, posterior parietal, and angular arteries. From its inferior trunk arise the temporopolar, anterior temporal, middle temporal, and posterior temporal arteries. The angular artery sometimes arises from the inferior trunk (Figure 9.13).

Cortical branches of the middle cerebral artery (Figure 9.14) The cortical branches are one or two in number and they arise alone or with a neighbour by a common trunk.

1. The orbitofrontal artery, one to three in number, runs upwards and forwards, and then divides into three to five branches. The anterior one or two branches supply the lateral portion of the orbital surface of the frontal lobe and anastomose with the branches from the anterior cerebral artery. The posterior two or three branches supply the pars triangularis and pars opercularis of the inferior frontal gyrus, and the inferior part of the middle frontal gyrus.

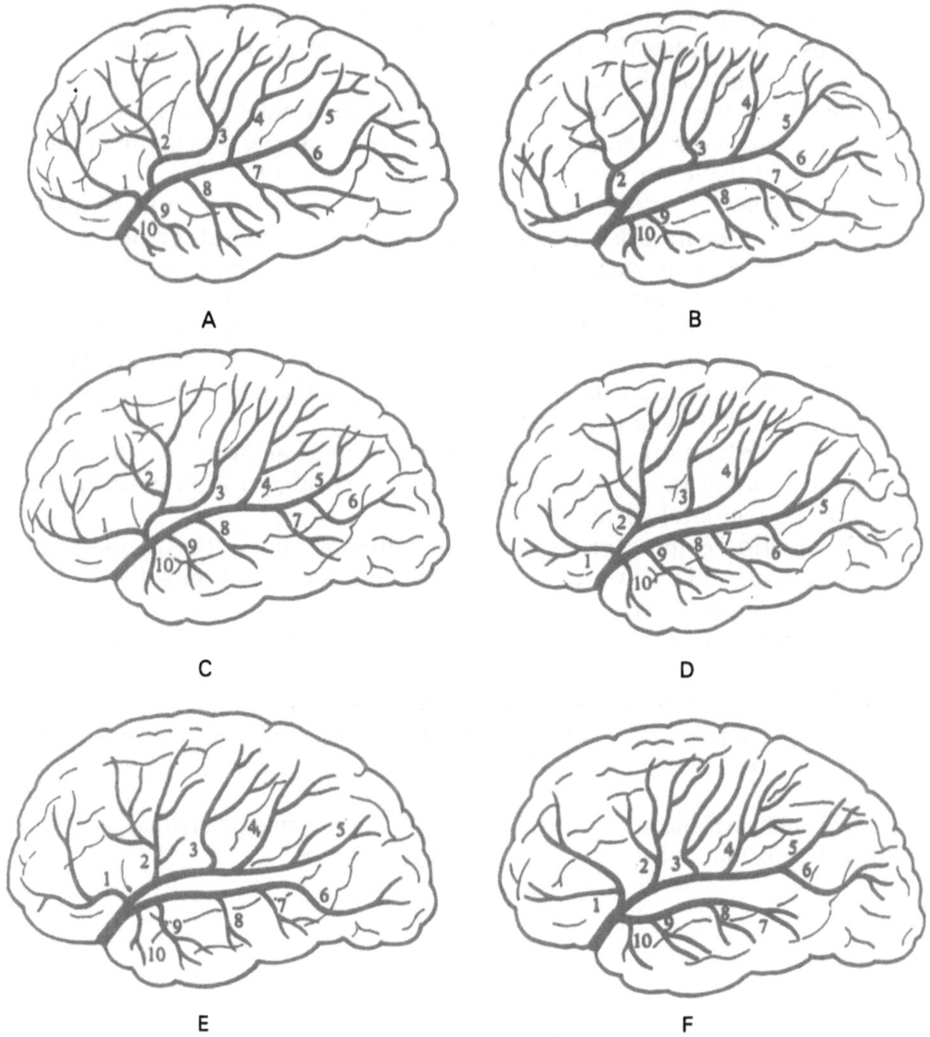

Figure 9.13 Patterns of the bifurcation of the middle cerebral artery. **A**: Single-trunk type; **B–E**: double-trunk type; **F**: triple-trunk type: **1**: orbitofrontal a.; **2**: precentral a.; **3**: central a.; **4**: postcentral a.; **5**: posterior parietal a.; **6**: angular a.; **7**: posterior temporal a.; **8**: middle temporal a.; **9**: anterior temporal a.; **10**: temporopolar a.

2. The precentral artery runs obliquely upwards and backwards and usually divides into two branches ascending along, or in front of, the precentral sulcus to supply the posterior part of the pars opercularis of the inferior frontal gyrus, the posterior part of the middle frontal gyrus as well as the anterior part of the precentral gyrus.
3. The central artery usually runs upwards and forwards round the gyrus, which encloses the central sulcus inferiorly to the central sulcus or along its shores. It sends off small branches supplying the lower three-quarters of the pre- and postcentral gyri.

4. The postcentral artery runs upwards and backwards in the postcentral sulcus and supplies the greater part of the inferior portion of the postcentral gyrus and the supramarginal gyrus.
5. The posterior parietal artery crosses the supramarginal gyrus to the interparietal sulcus or its adjacent area. Its branches supply the supramarginal gyrus and the lower part of the superior parietal lobule.
6. The angular artery is always single. It describes at first a curve with the convexity downwards, crossing the superior temporal gyrus to the superior temporal sulcus, and then divides into branches supplying the angular gyrus and the greater part of the occipital gyri.
7. The posterior temporal artery usually lies within the lateral cerebral sulcus. When emerging from this sulcus it crosses the superior temporal gyrus obliquely and runs backwards to supply the posterior part of the superior and middle temporal gyri.
8. The middle temporal artery runs downwards and backwards to supply the middle part of the superior and middle temporal gyri after crossing the superior temporal gyrus.
9. The anterior temporal artery crosses the superior temporal gyrus obliquely downwards and backwards to supply the anterior part of the superior and middle temporal gyri.
10. The temporopolar artery usually varies in origin. It may sometimes arise from the main stem or the inferior trunk of the middle cerebral artery, the anterior choroidal artery, or a common trunk which it shares with the anterior temporal artery. It is small and supplies two or three branches to the temporal pole.

Central branches of the middle cerebral artery These may be divided into two groups: the medial and the lateral perforating arteries.

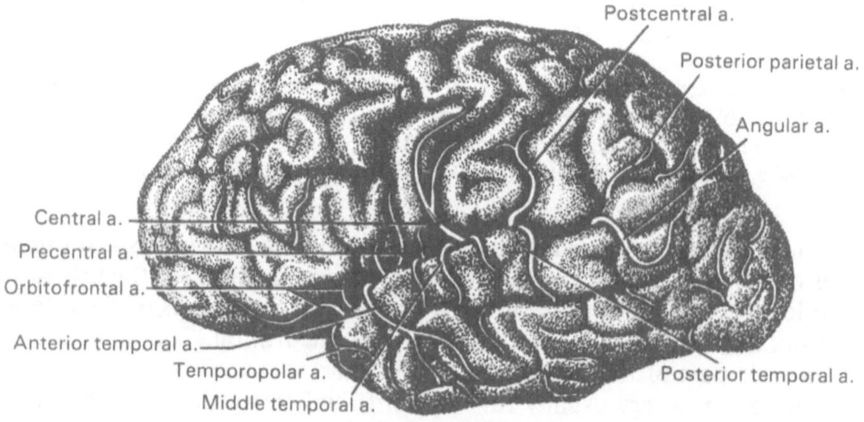

Figure 9.14 Cortical branches of the middle cerebral artery

1. The *medial perforating arteries* are one to nine in number, mostly two or three (48%), being very small, with an outer diameter of 0.4 (0.2–1.2) mm. They arise mostly from the stem of the middle cerebral artery at right angles (97%), but a few of them may arise from the bifurcation of the stem, the superior trunk or the cortical branches. They pass for a distance in the subarachnoid space and then enter the brain through the anterior perforated substance to supply the putamen of the lentiform nucleus, caudate nucleus and the frontal part of the internal capsule (Figures 9.15 and 9.16).

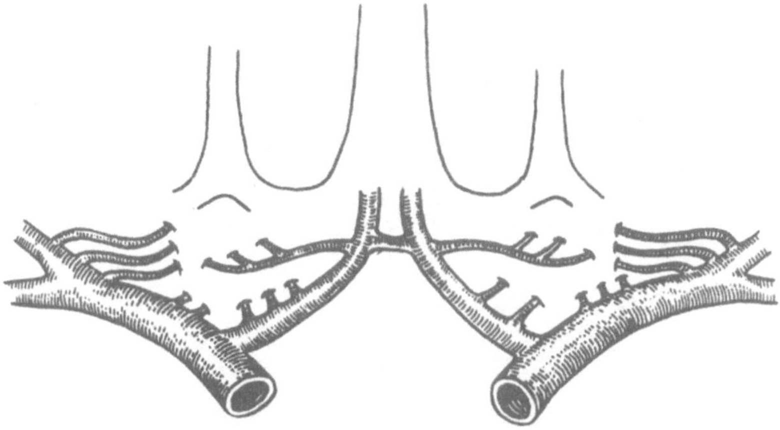

Figure 9.15 Medial and lateral perforating arteries of the middle cerebral artery

2. The *lateral perforating arteries* are one to nine in number, mostly two or three (51%). Their outer diameter measures 0.55 (0.2–1.5) mm. In about 55% of cases these arise from the stem or the bifurcation of the middle cerebral artery; the rest may arise from its superior trunk, inferior trunk or cortical branches. The middle cerebral artery, especially its site of bifurcation, is frequently subject to cerebral aneurysm (38.9%) and therefore, in surgical treatment of aneurysm, care must be taken to avoid injury to these perforating arteries. The lateral perforating arteries usually arise at an acute angle from MCA and then course in an opposite direction to the main stem just as the recurrent artery does; that is, they run first inwards and upwards, then curve outwards and upwards to get into the brain through the anterior perforated substance, and fan out to traverse the putamen to supply the putamen, the body of the caudate nucleus and the occipital part of the internal capsule (Figures 9.15 and 9.16). That the perforating arteries proceed in an opposite direction to MCA is of certain clinical significance. Ohone considered that according to Hagen-Poiseuille's law, the peculiar reversed siphonic course extends the length of the vessel. Under normal conditions it possesses the function of regulating blood pressure, but in patients suffering from high blood pressure the regulating mechanism would be impaired. Furthermore, due to the

presence of four curvatures in its course, which are almost at right angles, the vascular wall of these curvatures is subject to the powerful haemodynamic load, which may rupture the vessel to cause intracerebral haemorrhage in a case of hypertension.

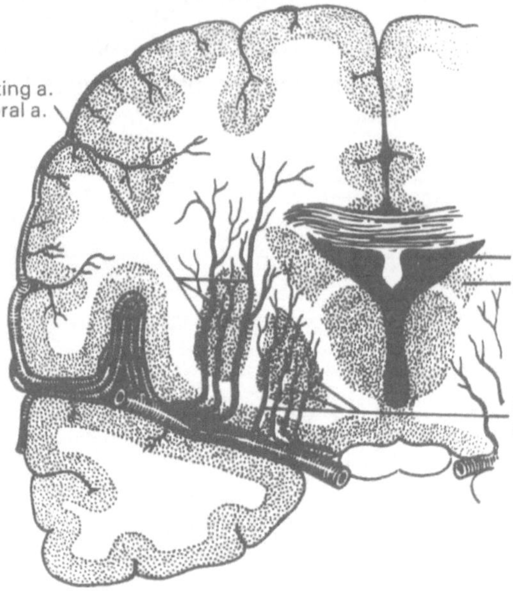

Figure 9.16 Distribution of the central branches of the middle cerebral artery

As mentioned above, the middle cerebral artery supplies a much larger area than either the anterior or the posterior cerebral artery. Its cortical branches mainly supply the middle and inferior frontal gyri, lower three-quarters of the precentral gyrus, lower part of the superior parietal lobule, inferior parietal lobule, superior and middle temporal gyri, the upper half of the inferior temporal gyrus, the greater part of each of the occipital gyri, the medial and lateral surfaces of the temporal pole, the lateral half of the orbital surface of the frontal lobe and the insula. Its central branches supply the body of the caudate nucleus, the lentiform nucleus and the anterior three-fiftns of the internal capsule. Occlusion of the middle cerebral artery and its branches is more often seen than that of any other intracranial arteries. Obstruction of the proximal part of its stem leads to massive necrosis of the area supplied by the central and cortical branches. Its main clinical symptoms are: contralateral hemiplegia, hemianaesthesia, hemianopia, and functional disturbance of the parietal lobe. If it occurs in the dominant hemisphere it is often accompanied by aphasia. If the central branches are occluded, hemiplegia usually ensues with or without slight hemianaesthesia and ipsilateral hemianopia. If the obstruction occurs distal to the origin of the central branches it may cause symptoms similar to those due to obstruction of its main trunk; that is, the hemiplegia of the arm will be more severe than that of the leg. This is because the centre which controls the movements of the lower limbs is represented in the paracentral lobule, which is supplied by the anterior cerebral artery. Occlusion of certain cortical branches produces corresponding symptoms due to encephalomalacia of the area which it supplies. For example, the occlusion of the central artery (the rolandic branch) may produce contralateral monoplegia of the upper limb or incomplete hemiplegia (more severe in the arm) by slight paraesthesia; the occlusion of the orbitofrontal artery at the dominant hemisphere may result in motor aphasia, and that of the posterior temporal gyrus may cause sensory aphasia. The occlusion of the angular artery may produce visual aphasia, etc.

Variations in the middle cerebral artery are less frequent than those in other intracranial great vessels and mainly comprise double-trunk, early bifurcation, accessory middle cerebral artery, fenestration and absence.

Vertebrolbasilar arterial system

The vertebrobasilar arterial system consists of the intracranial portion of the vertebral artery, the stem of the basilar artery, the cerebellar arteries, the posterior cerebral artery, and their branches.

Intracranial portion of the vertebral artery (VA)

After emerging from the foramen transversarium of the first cervical vertebra, the vertebral artery winds round the lateral mass of atlas, pierces the atlanto-occipital membrane and enters the skull through the foramen magnum. Most of its course is tortuous. Its position in the lower segment of the cranium is constant, being lateral to and then in front of the medulla oblongata. In the adult the union of the vertebral arteries takes place at the level of the bulbopontine groove in 41.0%, at the level of the pons in 39.6% and at the level of the medulla in 19.4%. It lies on the mid-line in 54% of cases and slants to the left in 40% and to the right in 6%. The deviation of the point of union from the mid-line may be as much as 10 mm to the left and 8 mm to the right.

The left vertebral artery has a calibre larger than that of the right in 47.9%, but smaller than the right only in 18.2%. They are equal in 33.9%. The outer diameter of the left one averages 3.13 (1–5) mm and that of the right 2.91 (0.74–6.5) mm. Hypoplasia or fenestration of this artery is rare. The length of the intracranial portion of the vertebral artery averages 31.4 (24.5–47.0) mm on the left, and 31.0 (24.5–45.0) mm on the right.

The main branches of the intracranial portion of the vertebral artery are as follows:

The anterior spinal artery (ASA) This artery arises from the medial aspect of the upper one-third of the intracranial portion of the vertebral artery by a right and a left root. The origin of the left artery averages 5.4 (0–11.5) mm apart from the junction of the vertebral arteries and that of the right artery 5.9 (0–11.5) mm. From their origin the two roots units mostly on the mid-line to form the anterior spinal artery. The distance between the union of these two roots and the junction of the vertebral arteries varies greatly. The maximal distance may be 32 mm; that is, the roots of ASA may unite at the level of the lower end of the medulla oblongata.

There is an anastomotic branch between the two roots of the anterior spinal artery in 74% of the cases, and it is absent in 26%. In some cases it may arise from either vertebral artery. The anterior spinal artery mainly supplies the anterior part of the medulla oblongata and gives off branches to join the anterior group of arteries on the medulla. The anterior group of arteries may be divided into the anteromedial and anterolateral arteries. All of them have many branches anastomosing with those of the neighbouring arteries to supply the anteromedial and anterolateral parts of the medulla respectively. The main stem of the anterior spinal artery is a single trunk running in the anterior median fissure of the spinal cord.

The ventral part of the medulla oblongata is mainly supplied by the branches of the anterior spinal artery, and may be supplemented by the terminal segment of the vertebral artery and a branch of foramen caecum of the basilar artery. Obstruction of the anterior spinal artery may produce medial medullary syndrome, which manifests itself as the cross paralysis with the injury of the unilateral or bilateral hypoglossal nerves and the pyramidal tract.

The bulbar branches (Figure 9.17) These originate from the upper and middle segments of the intracranial vertebral artery. Usually, one or two of them join the anterior group of arteries of the medulla oblongata.

The short circumferential arteries of the vertebral artery are frequently one to three in number, winding round the pyramid and olive to the lateral recess of the medulla oblongata. They give off fine branches to the IX, X, XI cranial nerves, and anastomose with the branches of the basilar artery and the anterior and posterior inferior cerebellar arteries. They chiefly supply the lateral part of the medulla oblongata.

The posterior spinal artery (PSA) The PSA, one on each side, most frequently arise from the lower end of the intracranial vertebral artery in 60.5%, and from the posterior inferior cerebellar artery in 39.5% of cases. The artery gives off one to three bulbar branches which, together with the branches of the posterior inferior cerebellar artery, join the posterior group of medullary arteries to supply the posterior part of the medulla oblongata (Figure 9.18). The posterior spinal artery may extend directly to the termination of the spinal cord.

The posterior inferior cerebellar artery (PICA) This springs mostly from the middle third of the intracranial portion of the vertebral artery (the origin corresponds to the level of the lower end of the olive). It may also come from the lower third, but rarely from the upper third of the intracranial vertebral artery. All of the PICA arising from the VA account for 94% of the cases (Figure 9.19); a few of them also arise from the basilar artery. We found a case in which the PICA arose bilaterally from the occipital artery of the external carotid artery; no similar cases have been reported in China. It is likely that the collateral branch between the external carotid artery and the vertebrobasilar system existed in the embryonic stage. It is the remnant of this collateral branch which becomes the 'extracranial segment' of the posterior inferior cerebral artery.

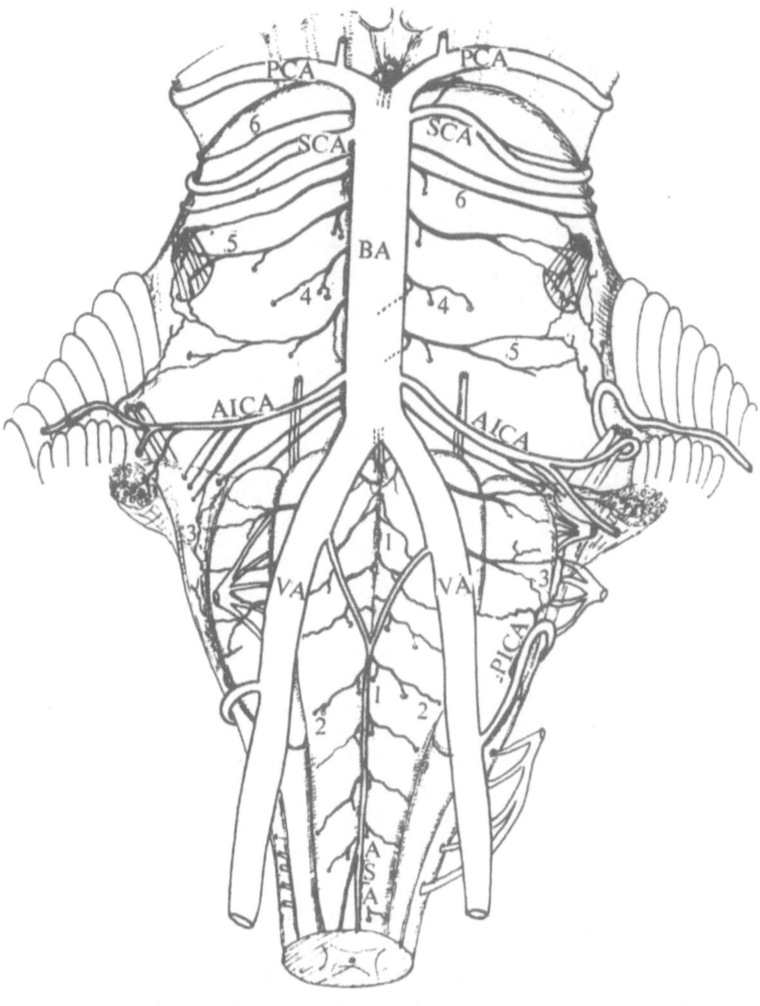

Figure 9.17 Arterial branches on the ventral side of the brain stem. **1**: Anteromedial a.; **2**: anterolateral a.; **3**: lateral group of arteries of medulla; **4**: paramedian a.; **5**: short circumferential a.; **6**: long circumferential a.

The course of the posterior inferior cerebellar artery is tortuous (Figure 9.20). After arising from the vertebral artery it courses backward and downward around the ventral surface of the medulla oblongata. This initial segment is referred to as the anterior medullary segment. The artery continues encircling the lateral aspect of the medulla, where it is known as the lateral medullary segment. It descends on the posterolateral surface of the medulla, describing a U-shaped caudal loop. It then ascends on the posterior surface of the medulla as the posterior medullary segment. Most of them reach the space between the upper border of the cerebellar tonsil and the inferior vermis and curve again posteriorly over the superior pole of the tonsil to form the cranial

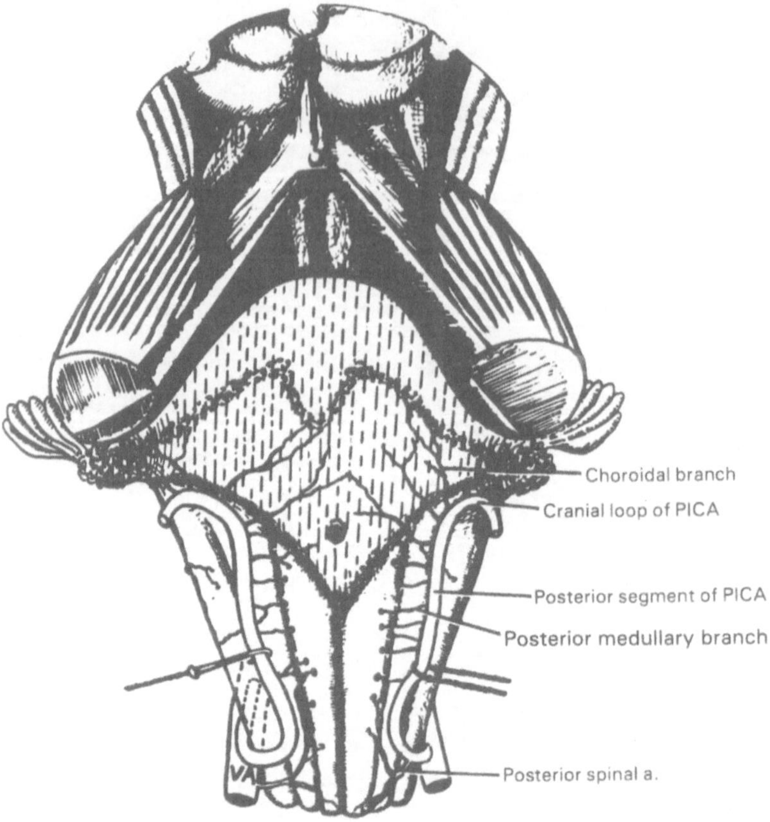

Figure 9.18 Posterior group of the arteries of the medulla oblongata

loop. The artery finally divides into medial and lateral branches. The medial one supplies the inferior vermis, while the lateral one supplies the hemisphere and tonsil of the cerebellum.

In about 50% of cases the lateral segment forms the lateral loop, which is convex upward and makes the PICA closely related to the IX–XI cranial nerves. This loop may extend as far as the level of the lower part of the pons in touch with the VII and VIII cranial nerves (Figure 9.21). The PICA may sometimes be connected to the anterior inferior cerebellar or the basilar artery by an anastomotic branch. The caudal loop is mostly at the level of the middle part or the lower pole of the cerebellar tonsil, whereas the cranial loop adheres to its ventromedial surface and more frequently to its upper pole.

Branches of the posterior inferior cerebellar artery

1. The bulbar branches arise from the anterior and lateral segments of the PICA and supply the olive with small twigs. The lateral bulbar branch anastomoses freely with those from the vertebral, basilar and anterior inferior cerebellar arteries, and sends some small branches to the XI–XII

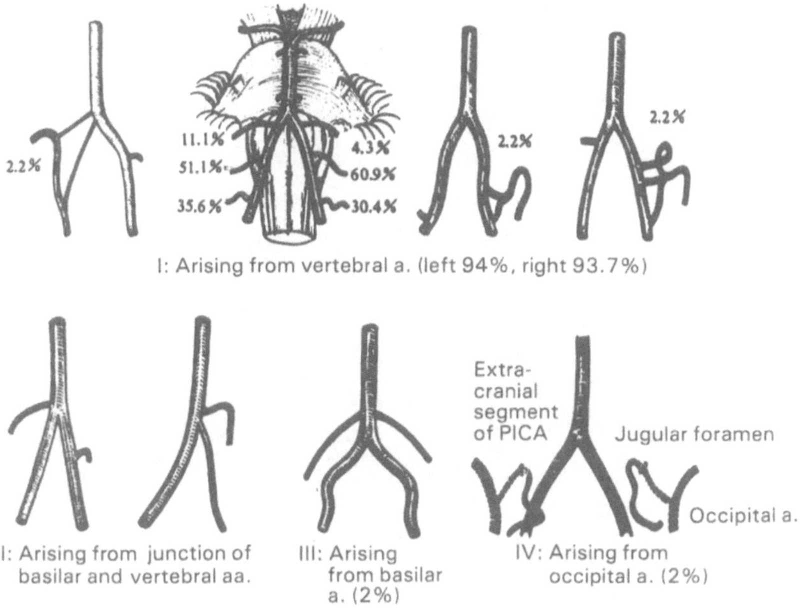

Figure 9.19 Origin and variations of the posterior inferior cerebellar artery

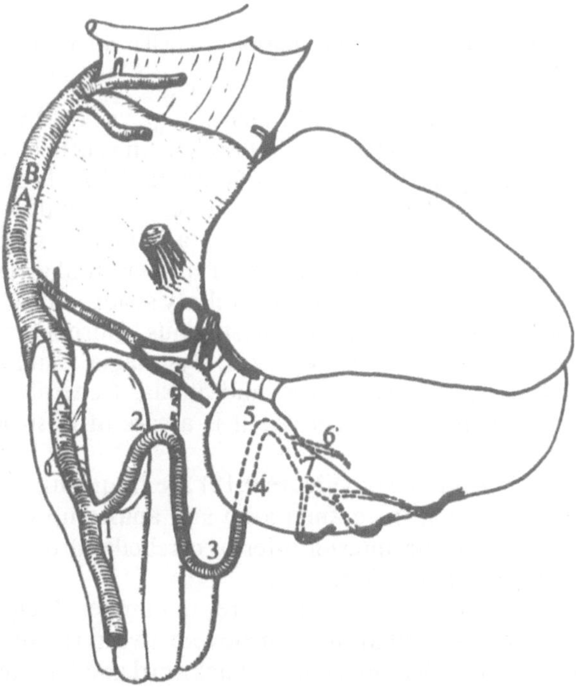

Figure 9.20 Course of the posterior inferior cerebellar artery. **1**: Anterior segment; **2**: lateral segment; **3**: caudal loop; **4**: posterior segment; **5**: cranial loop; **6**: medial branch; **7**: lateral branch

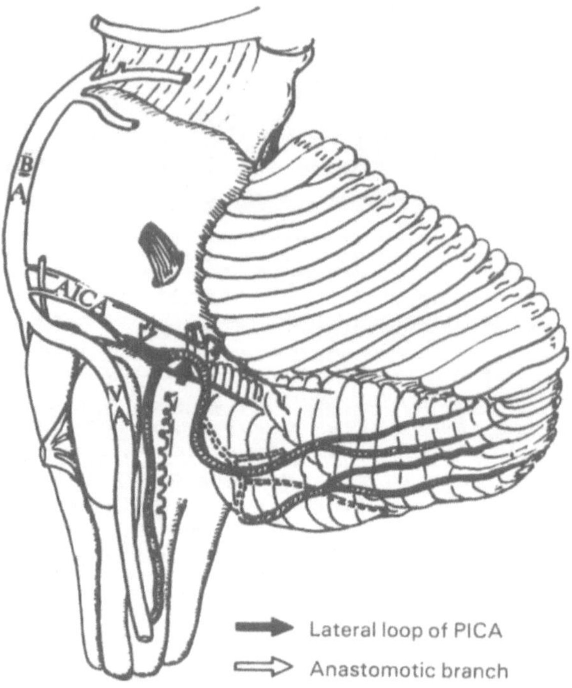

Figure 9.21 Lateral loop of the posterior inferior cerebellar artery in touch with the VII and VIII cranial nerves

cranial nerves. The posterior bulbar branches are given off by the posterior segment, running along the lateral wall of the fourth ventricle, and dividing into some twigs to supply the medulla oblongata. Their lower twigs may anastomose with the bulbar branches of the posterior spinal artery.

The lateral part of the medulla oblongata is mainly supplied by the PICA and short circumferential branches of the vertebral artery. Vascular occlusion of PICA may lead to lateral medullary syndrome, which consists of sudden onset of vertigo, vomiting, nystagmus, Horner's syndrome on the ipsilateral side, crossed hypoaesthesia, dysphagia resulting from the paralysis of IX and X cranial nerves, and ataxia. Generally, it does not present any pyramidal signs; otherwise it is a case of obstruction of the vertebral artery.

2. Branches of the choroid plexus (Figure 9.18) are frequently three to six in number. They arise from the cranial loop and anastomose with the corresponding branches of the anterior inferior cerebellar artery at the lateral foramina of the fourth ventricle.
3. Branches to the hemisphere are usually three in number (Figure 9.22). The inferomedial branch is located in the groove between the inferior vermis and the tonsil of the cerebellum, running backward and lateralward medial to the inferior margin of the tonsil to the horizontal fissure of the cerebellum. The intermediate branch runs backward and lateralward on the ventral surface of the lower part of the tonsil. The inferolateral branch crosses the middle part of the tonsil, and runs posterolaterally.

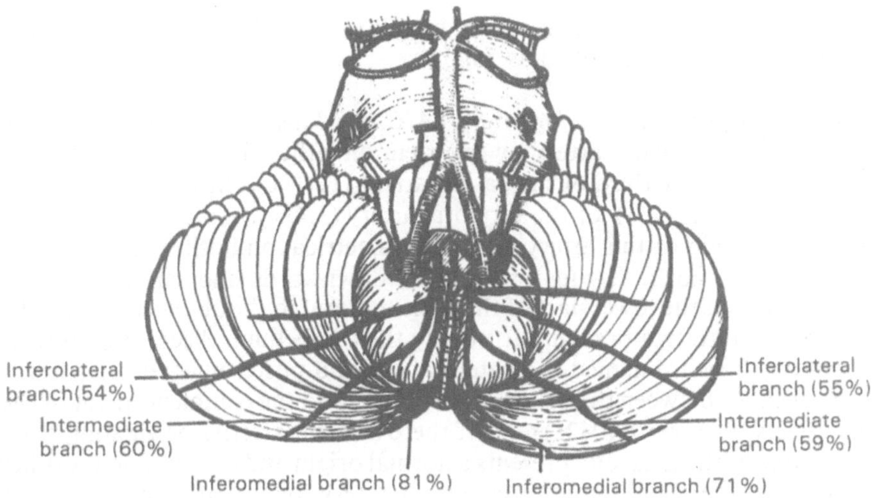

Figure 9.22 Incidence of hemispheric branches of the posterior inferior cerebellar artery

4. Branches to the vermis supply the inferior vermis. They are not always present on both sides. If they are absent on either side the blood supply may then be compensated by those of the opposite side or by the branches from the superior vermis. Most of them run longitudinally, vary greatly in number and anastomose with one another.

The PICA supplies the greater part of the inferior surface of the hemisphere in 47%, the smaller part in 36%, and the posterior half of the inferior surface in 17%. Thus, it is clear that the blood supply from the posterior and anterior inferior cerebellar arteries to the inferior surface of the cerebellar hemisphere is not equalized. The area supplied by the PICA is generally larger than that by the anterior inferior cerebellar artery. More than half of the area of the inferior surface is supplied by the PICA.

Basilar artery (BA)

The stem of the basilar artery arises from the junction of two vertebral arteries. Bending, fenestration and some other variations may exist in its course. Only 45% of the stems run straightly along the mid-line on the ventral surface of the brain stem, the rest showing some bending, of which the simple bending represents 37%, double bending 15%, and triple bending 3%. Fenestration in its lower segment represents 2%. In about 50% of cases there is a stricture at its upper end. It is situated mostly between the origins of the posterior cerebral and superior cerebellar arteries or below the origin of the latter. The termination of the basilar artery lies above the groove between the pons and mesencephalon in 54% of cases, and may be as high as 5 mm above this groove to touch the mamillary bodies. It may be parallel to this groove (36%) or below it (10%). The diameter of the middle part of this artery averages 3.6 (2.54–4.7) mm and its length averages 28.6 (21.5–37.5) mm.

The branches of the basilar artery mainly supply the brain stem and the cerebellum. They are described as follows.

The anterior inferior cerebellar artery (AICA) This arises mostly from the lower third of the basilar artery by one stem on either side (66.5%). The rest arise from the middle third of the basilar artery (12.1%), the posterior inferior cerebellar artery (11.2%), or the vertebral artery (3.4%). It may also be absent (6.3%). The origin of this artery may be symmetrical on both sides (34%), or asymmetrical in 66%. It runs backwards, downwards and laterally on the ventral surface of the lower part of the pons. Lateral to the abducent nerve, the artery divides into two branches to supply the cerebellum. According to their distribution, they are named the anterolateral and posteromedial branches.

The distance between the origin of the AICA and the commencement of the basilar artery averages 8 (0–21) mm. If there are two arteries originating from one side, one of them usually presents a normal origin and course, and the other may be called the middle inferior cerebellar artery, or the superior or inferior accessory anterior inferior cerebellar artery according to the level of their origins (Naidich, 1976).

The branches of the anterior inferior cerebellar artery are as follows.

(1) The hemispheric branches are divided into the anteromedial and the anterolateral branches. The incidence of the latter accounts for 96% of cases. It runs upwards and laterally, forming with the main stem a caudal loop at or above the pontomedullary groove, and then bends upwards and laterally to form another two loops below the VII and VIII cranial nerves and on the brachium pontis, i.e. the loop of the internal auditory meatus and the loop of brachium pontis (Figure 9.23). The loop of the internal auditory meatus protrudes into or close to the internal auditory meatus, and then passes from between the facial and auditory nerve (or between the auditory nerve and the flocculus) to the brachium pontis to form the loop of the brachium pontis bent upward.

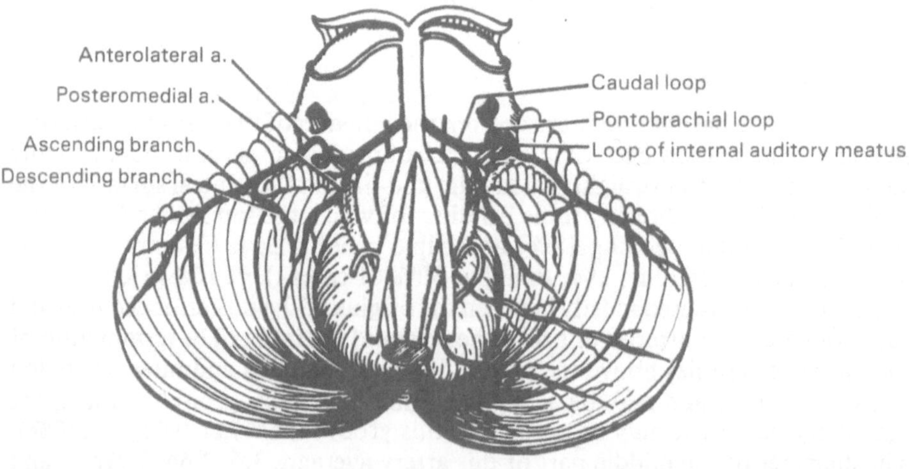

Figure 9.23 Course and branches of the typical anterior inferior cerebellar artery

The summit of the latter loop may be in contact with the posteroinferior aspect of the sensory root of the trigeminal nerve. Finally, the anterolateral branch enters the horizontal fissure of the cerebellum and divides into an ascending and a descending branch above or lateral to the flocculus.

The incidence of the posteromedial branch is 62%. It may terminate in the pontomedullary groove or the upper part of the lateral recess of the medulla oblongata. Generally, it arises from the stem lateral to the abducent nerve, passes backward and downward over the pontomedullary groove and the lateral recess of the medulla oblongata to the cerebellar hemisphere. It supplies the flocculus or the biventer lobule, and sends some twigs to the choroid plexus of the fourth ventricle. In about 40% of cases the posteromedial branch is enlarged to replace the posterior inferior cerebellar artery (Figure 9.24). In the absence of the posteromedial branch it will be compensated mostly by the inferior accessory AICA (38%) (Figure 9.24).

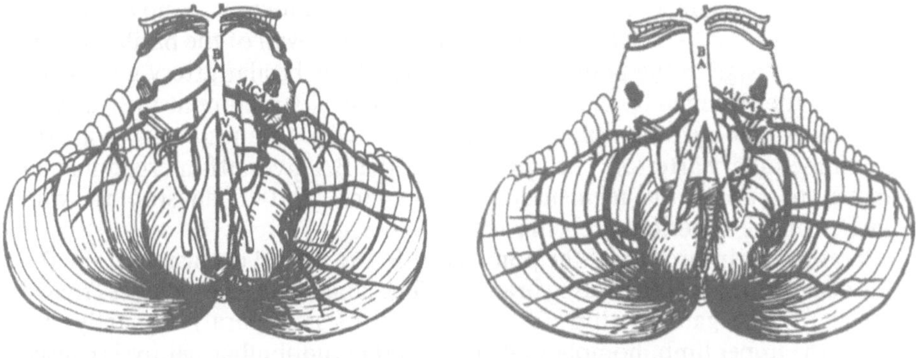

Enlarged posteromedial branch compensating posterior inferior cerebellar artery

Posteromedial branch compensated by enlarged inferior accessory artery

Figure 9.24 Posterior inferior cerebellar artery compensated by the anterior inferior cerebellar artery

(2) The labyrinthine artery arises from the anterior inferior cerebellar artery (72–90%). A few of them arise from the basilar artery. Its diameter averages 0.20 mm. The difference in respect to sides or age is very small.

(3) The choroidal branches are either the descending branches from the posteromedial and anterolateral branches, or the twigs from the inferior accessory artery supplying the choroid plexus of the fourth ventricle. At times a single slender recurrent choroid artery may arise independently from the anterolateral or posteromedial branch, running downwards and backwards over the flocculus to the choroid plexus.

(4) The medullary branches average three in number. They pass downward and laterally across the pontomedullary sulcus to supply the superolateral portion of the medulla oblongata. They accompany the corresponding branches from the vertebral and posterior inferior cerebellar arteries to form the lateral medullary arteries (Figure 9.17).

(5) The pontine branches average four in number. They usually spring from the loop of the brachium pontis from the anterolateral branch to supply an area under the root of the trigeminal nerve on the lateral side of the pons, and send

some twigs to the brachium pontis. The pontine branches accompany the short circumferential artery of the basilar artery and the branches of the superior cerebellar artery to form the lateral pontine arteries (Figures 9.17 and 9.18).

In the surgical management of the pontocerebellar angle tumour the anterior inferior cerebellar artery must be carefully protected. Most of the postoperative infarction of the pons is due to adverse ligation of the anterior inferior cerebellar artery. The inferolateral pontine syndrome (of Marie-Foix) reflects its clinical picture which includes the ipsilateral cerebellar dysfunction, facial palsy, deafness, impairment of sensations to light touch, pain, and temperature of the face and contralateral loss of pain and temperature sensibility over the trunk and extremities.

Pontine branch of the basilar artery The basilar artery gives off five to seven pontine branches of unequal length from either side. These branches may be distinguished as follows.

(1) The paramedian arteries (Figure 9.17) are the anterior group of arteries supplying the pons, which arise from the dorsolateral wall of the basilar artery, and give off twigs to the pons. The lower end of the basilar artery gives off a branch to the foramen caecum supplying the central structure at the junction of the pons and medulla oblongata as well as twigs to anastomose with the anterior medullary arteries. The upper end of the BA gives off interpeduncular branches to supply the tegmentum of the pons, and to anastomose with branches of the superior cerebellar artery.

Paramedian infarction of the pons is due to the partial occlusion of the BA or the occlusion of its penetrating branches. The clinical picture includes crossed paralysis of conjugate gaze towards the side of the lesion, paralysis usually confined to the upper limb, homolateral ataxia and pseudobulbar paralysis caused by bilateral lesions.

(2) The short circumferential arteries (Figure 9.17) arise directly or by a common trunk with the paramedian artery from either wall of the basilar artery. They turn up to the ventrolateral surface of the pons to supply the ventromedial portion of the trigeminal root, and anastomose with the pontine branches of the anterior inferior and superior cerebellar arteries to form the lateral group of arteries.

Infarction of the lateral portion of the pons is caused by partial occlusion of the basilar artery and the occlusion of the short circumferential arteries. There may be crossed sensory disturbance and paralysis, and ataxia on the side involved.

(3) The long circumferential artery (Figure 9.17) arises directly from the lateral wall of the upper segment of the basilar artery. It winds round the upper part of the ventral surface of the pons to the posterolateral area to enter the pons. These arteries also anastomose with branches of the superior cerebellar artery.

The superior cerebellar artery (SCA) This is a larger branch of the basilar artery. It arises from its upper end proximal to the origin of the posterior cerebral artery and winds to the posterolateral aspect of the pons ventral to the oculomotor nerve. Its trunk bends in varying degrees near the trigeminal nerve, with which it may sometimes make contact (44.4%). When the superior cerebellar artery arrives at the lateral side of the midbrain it divides into the medial and lateral branches.

There is one superior cerebellar artery on either side in about two-thirds of cases. It arises from the basilar artery in 96.8%, and from the posterior cerebral artery in 3.2%. The latter type can only be seen in cases of unilateral multiple origination of the superior cerebellar artery. Based on the number of branches, origin and ramification, the superior cerebellar artery may be classified into three types (Figure 9.25). The single-branch type (76%) arises alone from the basilar artery and then divides into a hemispheric and a vermian branch. The double-branch type (22%) arises from the BA by two separate origins or, in addition to the origin from BA, the superior branch arises from the posterior

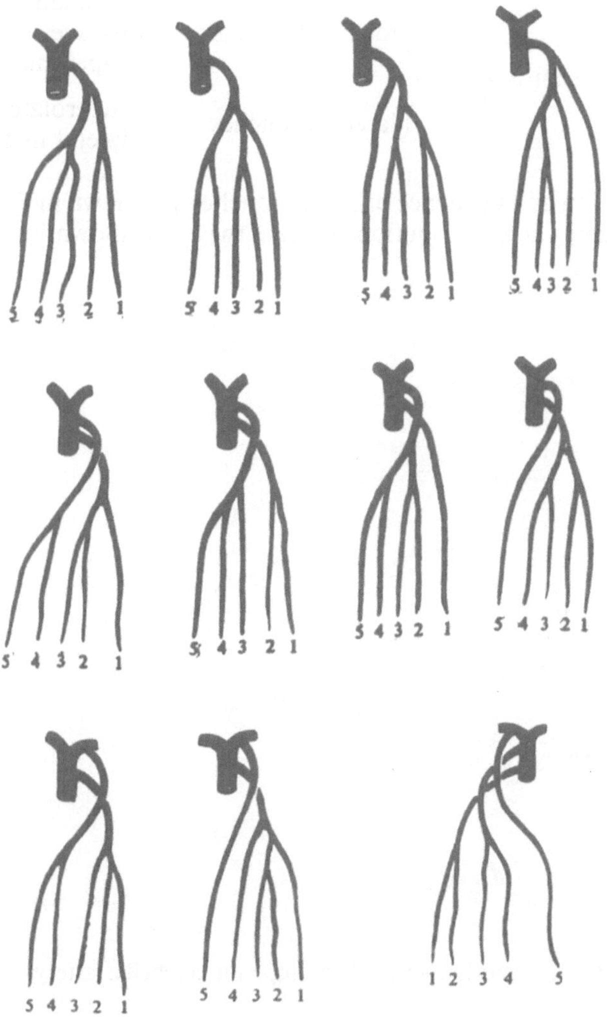

Figure 9.25 Types of the superior cerebellar artery. **1**: Lateral marginal branch; **2**: superolateral branch; **3**: superomedial branch; **4**: paravermian branch; **5**: vermian branch

cerebral artery. The triple-branch type (2%) has three origins: the upper one arises from the posterior cerebral artery, the lower two from the BA.

In the Chinese, the calibre of the superior cerebellar artery averages 1.43 mm on the left and 1.45 mm on the right. It is of equal size on both sides in 52.7%, whereas the left one is larger than the right in 25.4%, and on the contrary, the right one is larger than the left in 21.9%.

Branches of the superior cerebellar artery supplying the cerebellum are as follows.

The superior cerebellar artery gives off twigs along its course to supply the parenchyma of the midbrain and the pons.

superior cerebellar a.
- medial branches
  - vermian branch
  - paravermian branch
  - superomedial branch
- lateral branches
  - superolateral branch
  - lateral marginal branch

The distribution and incidence of these branches are shown in Figures 9.26 and 9.27. The names and distribution of these twigs are shown in Figure 9.28.

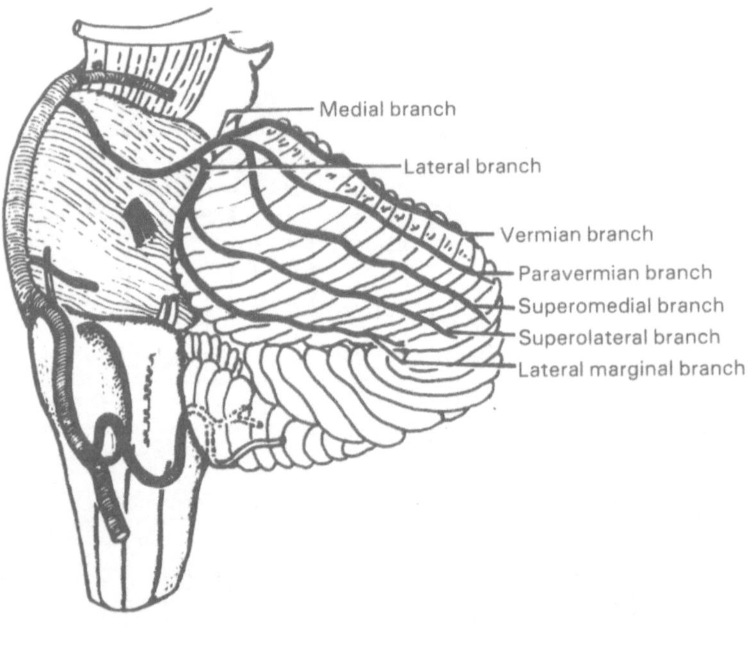

Figure 9.26 Course and branches of the superior cerebellar artery

Occlusion of the superior cerebellar artery may lead to lateral pontine syndrome which involves ipsilateral cerebellar dysfunction and abnormal movements of the ipsilateral upper and lower limbs, and the loss of appreciation of pain and temperature over the contralateral half of the body.

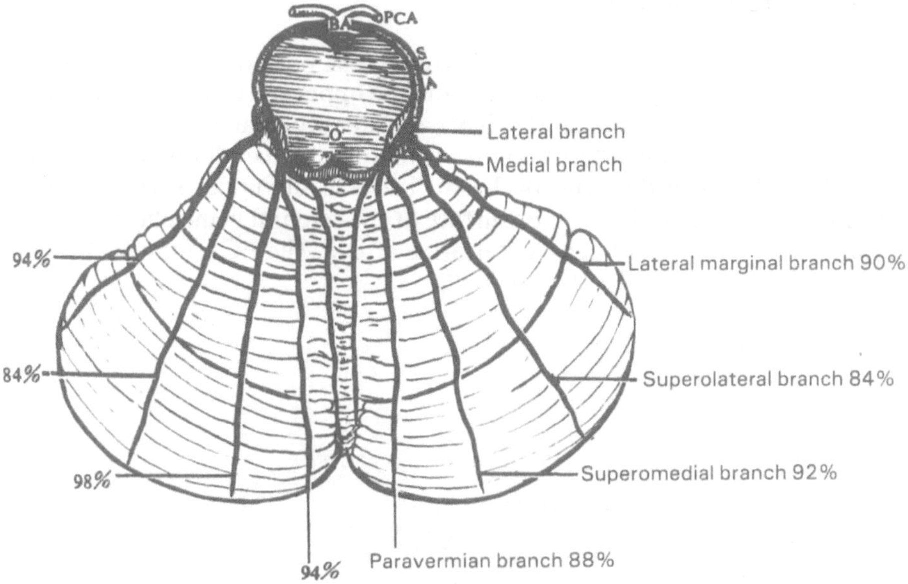

Figure 9.27 Incidence of the hemispheric branches of the superior cerebellar artery

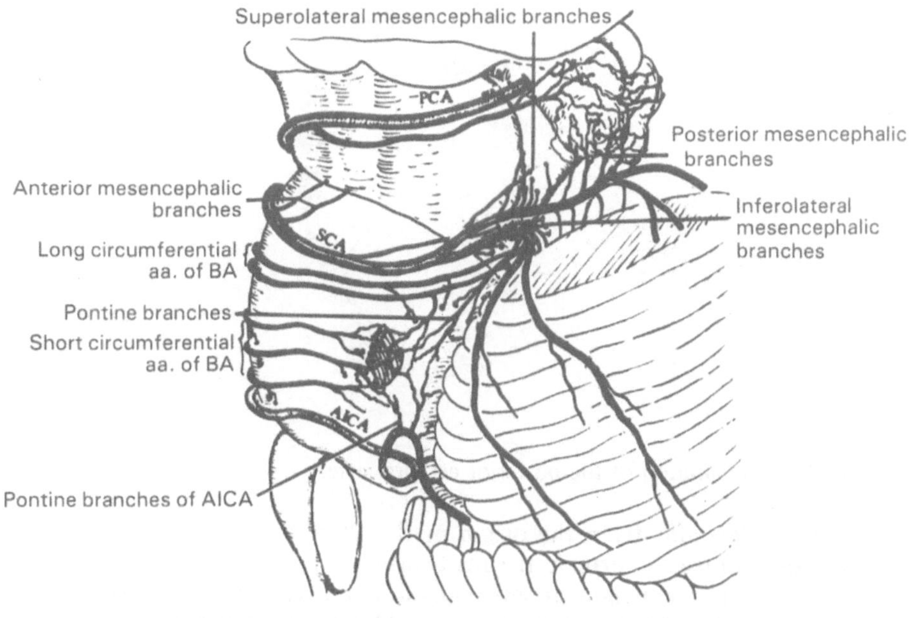

Figure 9.28 Branches to the brain stem from the superior cerebellar artery

Posterior cerebral artery (PCA)

Segmentation of the posterior cerebral artery The posterior cerebral arteries are the right and left terminal branches from the upper end of the basilar artery on the ventral surface of the pons. They pass laterally to anastomose with the posterior communicating artery and then wind round the midbrain to cross the tentorial notch. They then run backward between the upper surface of the tentorium cerebelli and the inferior surface of the cerebral hemisphere to enter the parieto-occipital artery and the calcarine artery. The PCA may be divided into three segments (P_1–P_3) (Figure 9.29).

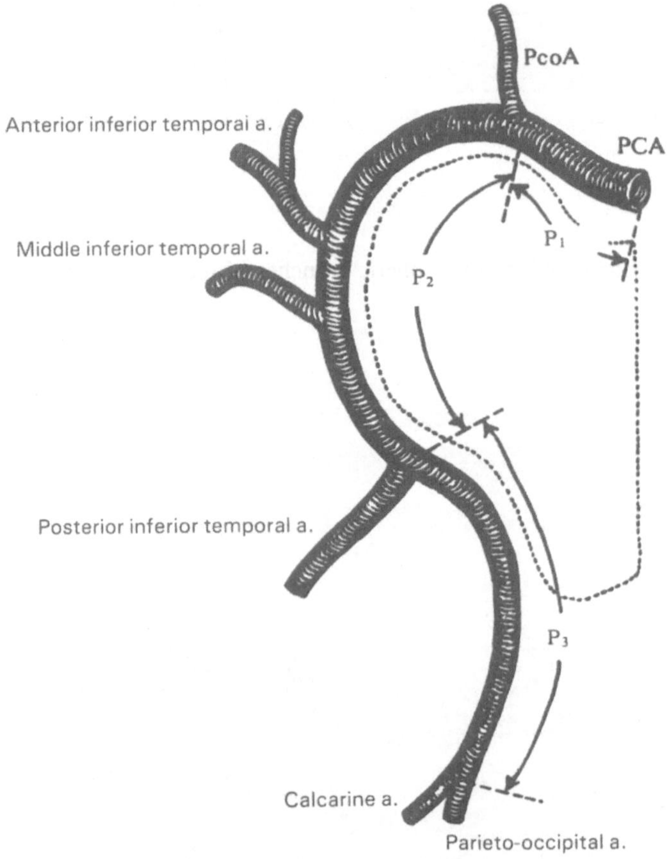

Figure 9.29 Segmentation of the posterior cerebral artery

Segment P_1 extends from the origin of the PCA to its junction with the posterior communicating artery. It runs transversely and laterally and bends slightly backward. The length of this segment averages 7.7 (5.2–16.8) mm on the left, and 7.2 (3.5–10.0) mm on the right. The outer diameter averages 2.4 (1.18–3.07) mm on the left, and 2.3 (0.79–2.88) mm on the right.

Segment P_2 extends from the origin of the posterior communicating artery to the posterior margin of the cerebral peduncle. It winds round the midbrain and runs posterolaterally. At the middle of the peduncle it first bends backwards and upwards and then turns posteroinferiorly at the posterior margin of the peduncle where it passes just posterior to the medial geniculate body and close to the pulvinar. The length of this segment averages 27.8 (20.9–40.6) mm on the left, and 29.4 (21.7–42.9) mm on the right. Its outer diameter on both sides averages 2.4 (1.75–2.83) mm. The calibre of P_1 is mostly equal to that of P_2 on the same side. However, in the rest of the cases, the calibre of P_2 is often larger than that of P_1. It is probable that where P_1 is smaller than P_2, the blood flow in P_2 is reinforced by that in the posterior communicating artery.

Segment P_3 extends from the posterior margin of the cerebral peduncle to the bifurcation of the posterior cerebral artery and divides into two terminal branches – the parieto-occipital and calcarine arteries. The length of this segment averages 26.6 (9.0–48.0) mm on the left, and 29.1 (10.5–52.3) mm on the right. The outer diameter averages 1.8 (1.24–2.13) mm on both sides.

Cortical branches of the posterior cerebral artery The PCA gives off five thick cortical branches from P_2 and P_3. They are the anterior, middle and posterior inferior temporal arteries, the parieto-occipital artery, and the calcarine artery. Of these, the posterior inferior temporal artery has many more variations. According to the number of stems and the combination of branches, they are divided into five types, which are shown in Figure 9.30.

1. The anterior inferior temporal artery, with an incidence of 100%, is the first cortical branch arising from the posterior cerebral artery. It first runs laterally across the hippocampal fissure into the collateral sulcus. It then continues forward to divide into the medial and lateral branches. It arises chiefly from P_2 (58%) and the common temporal artery (41%), and occasionally from the anterior choroid artery (1%). Its outer diameter averages 0.76 (0.39–1.43) mm on the left and 0.74 (0.48–1.28) mm on the right.
2. The middle inferior temporal artery, with an incidence of 88%, is the second cortical branch of the PCA. It arises just behind the anterior inferior temporal artery from P_2 (54.9%), P_3 (3.3%), the common temporal artery (40.7%), or the anterior choroid artery (1.1%). After arising from the stem of the PCA it runs posteriorly and laterally across the hippocampal fissure, the collateral sulcus and the anterior part of the fusiform gyrus to the middle part of the inferior temporal sulcus to be distributed to the middle part of the lower half of the inferior temporal gyrus and the anterior part of the fusiform gyrus, or rarely to the posterior part of the lower half of the inferior temporal gyrus and the middle part of the fusiform gyrus. The outer diameter of this artery averages 0.77 (0.47–1.71) mm on the left and 0.88 (0.62–1.48) mm on the right.
3. The posterior inferior temporal artery, with an incidence of 100%, is the third cortical branch of the PCA. It arises from P_2 (40%), P_3 (28%) and the common temporal artery (32%). It runs laterally across the hippocampal fissure and collateral sulcus, and then passes the middle and

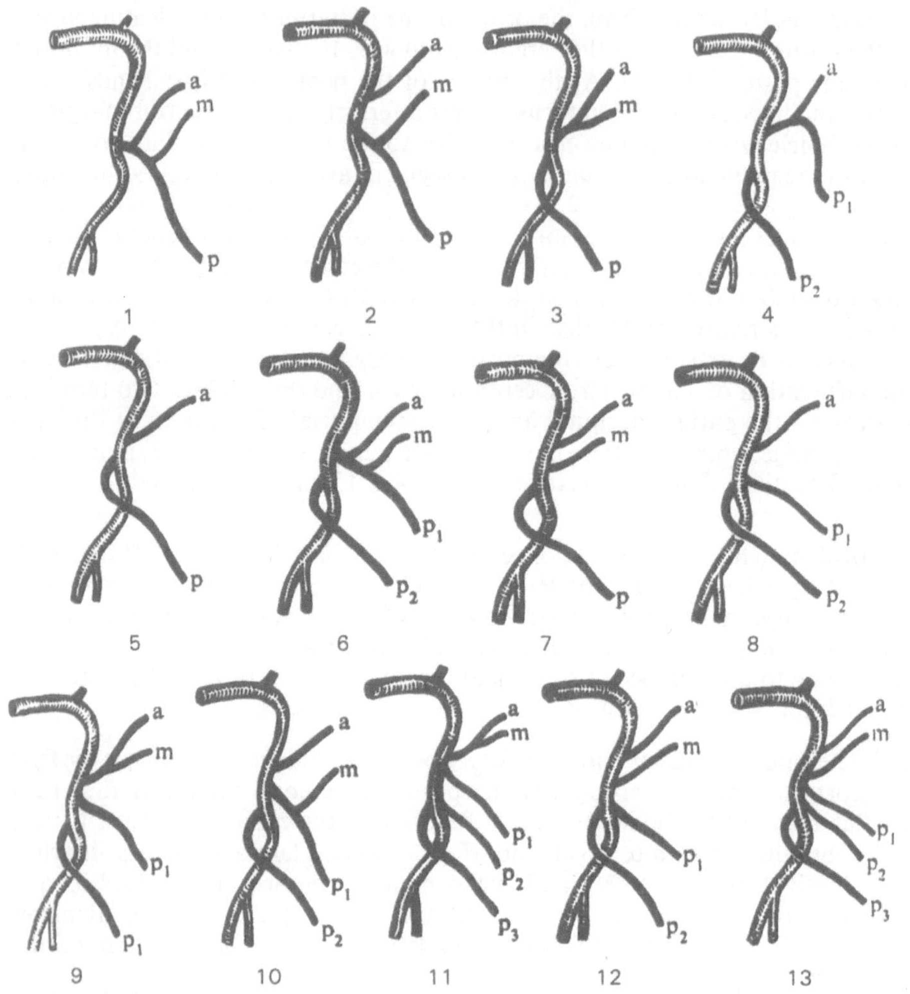

Figure 9.30 Types of stems of the cortical branches of the posterior cerebral artery. **1**: single-branched type; **2–6**: double-branched type; **7–10**: triple-branched type; **11, 12**: quadruple-branched type; **13**: quintuple-branched type. **(a)** Anterior inferior temporal a.; **(m)** middle inferior temporal a.; **(p)** posterior inferior temporal a.

posterior parts of the fusiform gyrus, where it gives off four secondary cortical branches to supply the fusiform gyrus, lingual gyrus, lateral occipital gyrus and the area of the occipital pole. The outer diameter of this artery averages 1.48 (0.68–2.11) mm on the left and 1.40 (0.70–2.18) mm on the right.

4. The calcarine artery, with an incidence of 97%, is one of the two terminals of the PCA. It originates from P_3 in 98%, and from P_2 in 2%. It is usually given off by the PCA and divides into the superior and inferior branches in the calcarine sulcus to supply the lower part of the cuneus and the posterior part of the lingual gyrus. The outer diameter of this artery averages 0.98 (0.50–1.67) mm on the left and 0.99 (0.58–1.44) mm on the right.

5. The parieto-occipital artery, with an incidence of 100%, is one of the two terminals of the PCA. It usually arises from the calcarine artery in the parieto-occipital sulcus, and divides into two trunks. The upper trunk sends its branches to the posterior part of the precuneus, the posterior margin of the inferior parietal lobule and the superior occipital gyrus. The lower trunk divides into several branches to supply the upper part of the cuneus and the posterior margin of the lateral occipital gyrus. The outer diameter of this artery averages 1.41 (0.96–1.82) mm on the left and 1.30 (0.74–1.84) mm on the right.

In addition to the above-mentioned five large cortical branches, the PCA also gives off another three secondary cortical branches, i.e. the hippocampal artery and the arteries to the dentate gyrus and the splenium, which supply the corresponding portions of the brain.

Since there are rich anastomoses between the cortical branches of the PCA and those of the middle cerebral artery on the anterior part of the hippocampal gyrus, the inferior temporal gyrus and the area of occipital pole, occlusion of the cortical branches of the PCA rarely produces any clinical signs. If the anastomosis is inadequate or absent, signs of occlusion will occur. Occlusion of hippocampal artery leads to amnesia. Occlusion of the posterior inferior temporal artery on the dominant side may cause nominal aphasia and visual agnosia, and that of the calcarine artery may cause contralateral homonymous hemianopia.

Perforating branches of the posterior cerebral artery The perforating branches of the PCA may be classified into two groups, i.e. the truncal and ventricular perforating branches. According to their length, the former may be subdivided into direct perforating and circumferential branches. These are tabulated as follows (see Figure 9.31):

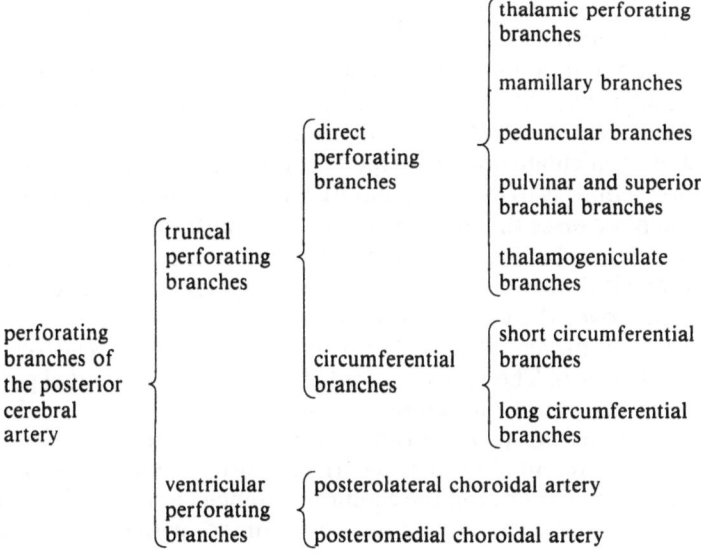

- perforating branches of the posterior cerebral artery
  - truncal perforating branches
    - direct perforating branches
      - thalamic perforating branches
      - mamillary branches
      - peduncular branches
      - pulvinar and superior brachial branches
      - thalamogeniculate branches
    - circumferential branches
      - short circumferential branches
      - long circumferential branches
  - ventricular perforating branches
    - posterolateral choroidal artery
    - posteromedial choroidal artery

All of the thalamic perforating branches arise from the posterior wall of the proximal part of P_1. The incidence is 100%. They are usually two in number. The outer diameter of the largest thalamic arteries averages 0.63 mm. They divide again into two to four small branches, piercing the posterior perforating substance to be distributed to the medial part of the thalamus, hypothalamus and subthalamus. They also supply the upper part of the midbrain.

The mammillary branches are mainly derived from the distal part of P_1 and the proximal part of P_2. The incidence is 58%. They course backward, upward and medialward, and terminate at the mamillary body and the posterior perforating substance. Most of them are single. Its outer diameter averages 0.3 mm.

The peduncular branches arise mostly from P_2. The incidence is 98%. They may be further divided into anterior, middle and posterior groups to terminate at the anterior, middle and posterior parts of the cerebral peduncle respectively. They are commonly four in number. The outer diameter averages 0.32 mm.

The pulvinar and superior brachial branches, most single, arise frequently from P_3. The incidence is 60%. They run upward to terminate at the pulvinar, the brachium of the superior colliculus and the lateral geniculate body. The outer diameter averages 0.38 mm.

Most of the thalamogeniculate arteries arise from P_2 and P_3. The incidence is 99%. The outer diameter averages 0.46 mm. The thalamogeniculate arteries arising from P_2 pass backward and medialward to terminate at the anterior part of the medial geniculate body, while those arising from P_3, usually four or five in number, run forward and medialward to terminate at the posterior part of the medial geniculate body and the inferior brachium of the inferior colliculus.

The thalamic perforating branches supply, in addition to the anteromedial part of the thalamus, such structures as the hypothalamus, subthalamus, cerebral peduncle, and upper end of the nucleus. Occlusion of these branches may lead to paramedian mesencephalic syndrome, which includes superior syndrome and inferior syndrome of the red nucleus. Since the former involves the upper part of the red nucleus, rubrothalamic tract and subthalamus, it may also cause kinetic tremor and ipsilateral hemiasynergia. The latter involves part of the pyramidal tract, red nucleus, and the nucleus and root of the oculomotor nerve, so that it causes hemiplegia oculomotoria alternans.

The thalamogeniculate branches chiefly supply the posterolateral part of the thalamus corresponding to the VPM and VPL nuclei of the thalamus. Occlusion of these branches causes thalamic syndrome. As both the spinothalamic tract and medial lemniscus project to the posterolateral part of the thalamus, it may lead to anaesthesia dolorosa, i.e. loss of pain, temperature and deep sensations and hyperpathia over the contralateral limbs.

The short circumferential branches usually arise from P_1 and/or the long circumferential branch. Their incidence is 62%. They are distributed posteriorly to the posterior margin of the cerebral peduncle, the tectum of midbrain and the medial geniculate body. Their outer diameter averages 0.38 mm.

The long circumferential branch is derived mostly from P_1. Its incidence is 100%. It winds backward round the cerebral peduncle, and usually divides into two branches to the superior collicullus to anastomose with the branches of the superior cerebellar artery on the surface of the quadrigemina. Its outer diameter averages 0.62 mm.

Most of the posteromedial choroidal arteries arise from P_2 and P_3. The incidence is 100%. The outer diameter averages 0.73 mm. The artery winds round the cerebral peduncle, runs backward, passing through the quadrigeminal cistern to the lateral side of the pineal body. It then enters the third ventricle to form the choroid plexus of the third ventricle. Finally, it passes through the interventricular foramen to enter the lateral ventricle. It gives off fine branches along its course to supply the cerebral peduncle, tectum mesencephali, medial and lateral geniculate bodies, pulvinar, pineal body and habenular trigone.

The posterolateral choroidal artery arises mostly from P_2 or P_3. The incidence is 99%. Its outer diameter averages 0.64 mm. It ascends close to the lateral surface of the thalamus and enters the lateral ventricle through the choroidal fissure. It sends off a lot of perforating branches to the lateral geniculate body, superior brachium and pulvinar. It also sends off a few perforating branches to the cerebral peduncle and the medial geniculate body.

The short and long circumferential arteries supply the median and posterior parts of the base of the cerebral peduncle, substantia nigra, the lateral portion of the tegmentum and the upper part of the midbrain and the tectum mesencephali. Occlusion of these arteries may involve the pyramidal tract, the nucleus and roots of the oculomotor nerve and the extrapyramidal system to cause the hemiplegia oculomotoria alternans (Weber's syndrome) as well as the posterolateral mesencephalic syndrome. The clinical features include homolateral cerebellar dysfunction and contralateral anaesthesia dolorosa. Contralateral impairment of hearing may sometimes occur.

COLLATERAL CIRCULATION IN THE BRAIN

ZHANG WEILONG AND ZHENG ZHILIANG

There has long been controversy about the existence of anastomoses between the cortical and central branches of the cerebrum and cerebellum, or among either of these branches. Since 1872, when Cohnheim proposed that cerebral arteries belong to the end artery it has generally been accepted that the cortical and central branches of cerebral arteries are two separate systems which do not communicate with each other. However, recent studies have proved that this is not the case. Morphologically the cortical branches of cerebral arteries divide in the pia mater into long and short branches. The long or medullary branches penetrate the grey matter to a depth of 3–4 cm to supply the white matter, while the short branches are confined to the cortex, forming a rich anastomotic network. The central branches arising from the internal carotid and the anterior, middle and posterior cerebral arteries enter the interior of the brain and anastomose to form numerous precapillary and capillary anastomoses. Therefore, in either the grey or white matter of the brain, all of the vessels form a continuous reticular anastomosis. Judging from clinical practice, occlusion or ligation of the major artery in the neck does not often result in ipsilateral cerebral ischaemia. A slight or slowly developed cerebral occlusion does not lead to the development of symptoms of cerebral ischaemia immediately. The infarcted area resulting from the occlusion of a cerebral artery is smaller than that supplied by the artery. The above-mentioned phenomena may be accounted for by the effect of cerebral collateral circulation. Rich collateral circulation provides the brain with an adequate blood supply. However, it must be pointed out that the calibres of the anastomotic vessels within the brain are usually too small to establish immediately an effective collateral circulation. Whether the collateral circulation can be directly established with or without the appearance of symptoms of cerebral ischaemia depends on various factors. Generally speaking, collateral circulation may play a compensatory role with cerebral obstructions of a slight degree and chronic onset, as well as large anastomotic channels and a good general condition on the part of the patient. On the contrary, it is not likely to set up or to compensate effectively. Cerebral anastomoses may be divided into the following categories in accordance with their locations.

Intracranial arterial anastomoses

Circle of Willis

The circle of Willis is formed at the base of the brain by the two anterior cerebral arteries joined to each other by the anterior communicating artery, the two posterior communicating arteries, the segment of internal carotid artery between the origins of the anterior cerebral artery and the posterior communicating artery, and the proximal segments of the two posterior cerebral arteries. It was first described by Willis in 1664. The circle may be divided into two portions. The proximal segment of the anterior cerebral artery and the anterior communicating artery constitute the anterior portion, while the remains make up the posterior portion. On the basis of variations in the posterior portion of the circle, and knowledge of phylogenesis, the circle can usually be divided into five types.

1. The late type: the calibres of the proximal segment of the posterior cerebral arteries are larger than those of the posterior communicating arteries. They serve as the chief source for the distal segment of the posterior cerebral artery. This type occurs more frequently (62%) and is also known as the 'normal type'.
2. The primitive type: the calibres of the proximal segment of the posterior cerebral arteries are smaller than those of the posterior communicating arteries. The blood in the distal segment of the posterior cerebral artery comes mainly from the internal carotid artery. This type occurs in about 5% of cases.
3. The transitional type: the posterior cerebral arteries are almost as large as the posterior communicating arteries. This occurs in about 4% of cases.
4. The mixed type: either side of the circle of Willis belongs to one of the types mentioned above, while the opposite side belonds to another type. The incidence of this type is about 29%.

5. The hypoplastic type: the posterior communicating artery is lacking in this type, which is, however, of rare occurrence.

Since the circle of Willis in the first four types is complete, they are collectively known as the closed type. The last one appears as an incomplete circle, and is thus called the open type (Figure 9.31).

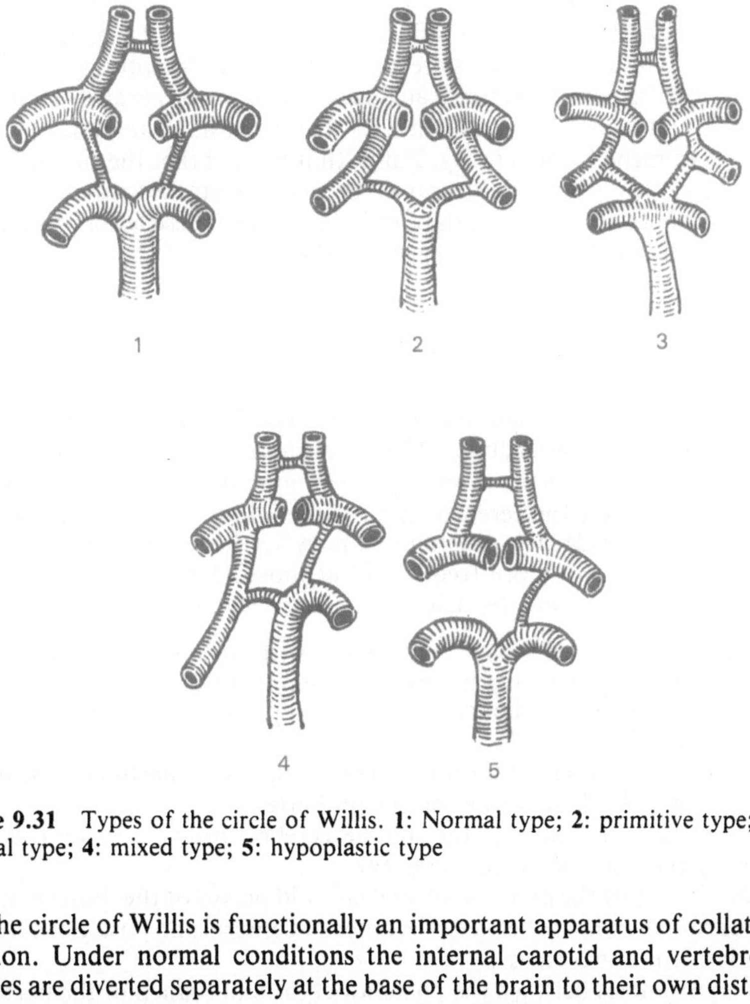

Figure 9.31 Types of the circle of Willis. **1**: Normal type; **2**: primitive type; **3**: transitional type; **4**: mixed type; **5**: hypoplastic type

The circle of Willis is functionally an important apparatus of collateral circulation. Under normal conditions the internal carotid and vertebrobasilar arteries are diverted separately at the base of the brain to their own distributing areas. The blood in the two systems does not mingle, so as to maintain a normal balance. If the carotid artery or any of the component arteries of the circle of Willis is occluded, the blood will be redistributed in order to restore a new balance. The effect of collateral circulation between the internal carotid arteries is more obvious than that between the internal carotid and the vertebrobasilar arteries.

Intracranial aneurysms occur most frequently near the circle of Willis, especially at the bifurcations or bends of its component arteries. This is due to the local intravascular haemodynamic changes exerted on these areas which are thus subject to the maximal pulse pressure. For instance, aneurysm of the basilar artery usually occurs at the site where it divides into the posterior cerebral arteries. This is related to the change in the vertical position of the basilar artery into the lateral direction of the posterior cerebral arteries. It is also proved by clinical data that the variations in the circle of Willis are responsible for the pathological changes in cerebrovascular disorders. Padget considered that the incidence of aneurysms in case of abnormal circle of Willis was twice that of the normal. Arutunova examined 100 cases of saccular aneurysm and found that 74% of aneurysm cases are accompanied by structural variations in the circle of Willis. Alpers demonstrated that in case of cerebral softening the circle of Willis remains normal only in 33%. On the basis of analysis of a large number of specimens from autopsy, Zang Xu indicated that the site of hypertensive haemorrhage, cerebral thrombosis as well as metastatic tumours of the brain was closely related to the variations in the circle. These lesions often first occur on the side of the circle with large calibre.

Arterial anastomoses over the surface of the brain

There are numerous arterial anastomoses in the leptomeninges over the surface of the cerebrum and cerebellum. These anastomoses are rich among the branches of major arteries but relatively few among those of the same artery. Moreover, arteries over the cerebellum cross the mid-line to anastomose with those on the opposite side. The anastomoses between the neighbouring branches of cerebellar arteries are more frequent than those of cerebral arteries. The superficial anastomoses mainly include (Figures 9.32 and 9.33):

1. The anterior cerebral artery anastomoses with the middle cerebral artery in a long and narrow area on the dorsolateral surface of the hemisphere from the frontal to the parietal lobes 2.5 cm lateral to the median longitudinal fissure.
2. The pericallosal artery of the anterior cerebral artery anastomoses with the callosal branch of the posterior cerebral artery.
3. The occipital branches of the middle cerebral artery anastomose with those of the posterior cerebral artery.
4. In the vicinity of the pineal body and choroid plexus of the third ventricle, there are anastomoses between the anterior cerebral and posterior cerebral arteries of the two sides.
5. The anastomosis between the posterior choroidal branch of the posterior cerebral artery and the anterior choroidal branch of the internal carotid artery.
6. The anastomosis between the posterior cerebral and superior cerebellar arteries.
7. The anastomosis between the posterior and anterior inferior cerebellar arteries.

8. The anastomosis between the anterior inferior and superior cerebellar arteries.
9. The anastomosis between the meningeal branches of the vertebral and anterior spinal arteries.
10. The anastomosis between the posterior spinal artery which comes from the vertebral or posterior inferior cerebellar artery, and the anterior spinal artery.

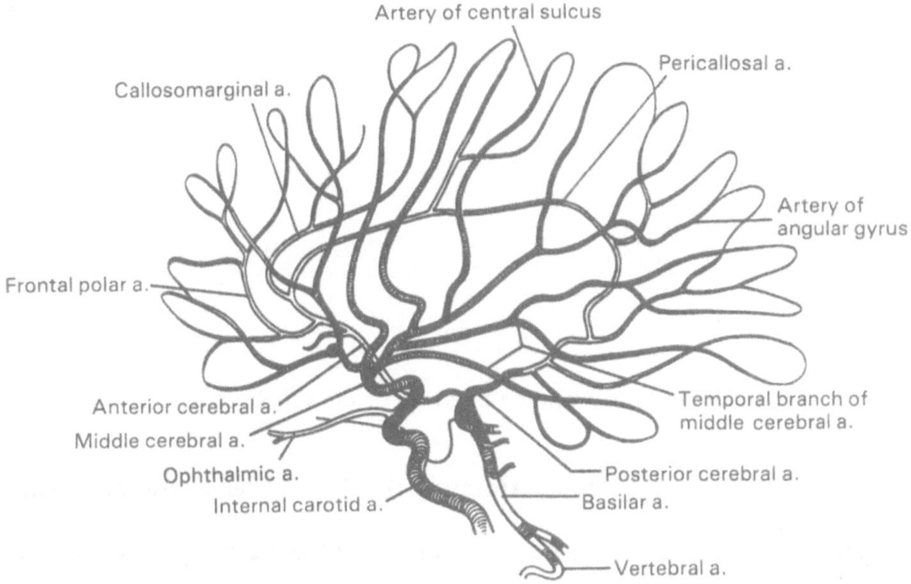

Figure 9.32 Anastomoses between the anterior, middle and posterior cerebral arteries

Anastomoses of the central arteries

The central arteries enter the brain through its base to supply the diencephalon, corpus striatum and internal capsule. Precapillary and capillary anastomoses are formed among these central arteries or between them and the medullary branches of the cortical branch. The calibre of these anastomoses is too small to undergo an effective collateral circulation. Anastomoses also exist between the central arteries of the cerebellum.

Anastomoses in the dura mater of the brain

1. The anterior meningeal branch of the opthalmic artery anastomoses with the middle meningeal artery of the maxillary artery and also with the posterior meningeal branch of the ascending pharyngeal artery.
2. The meningeal branch of the cavernous segment of the internal carotid artery anastomoses with the middle meningeal artery.

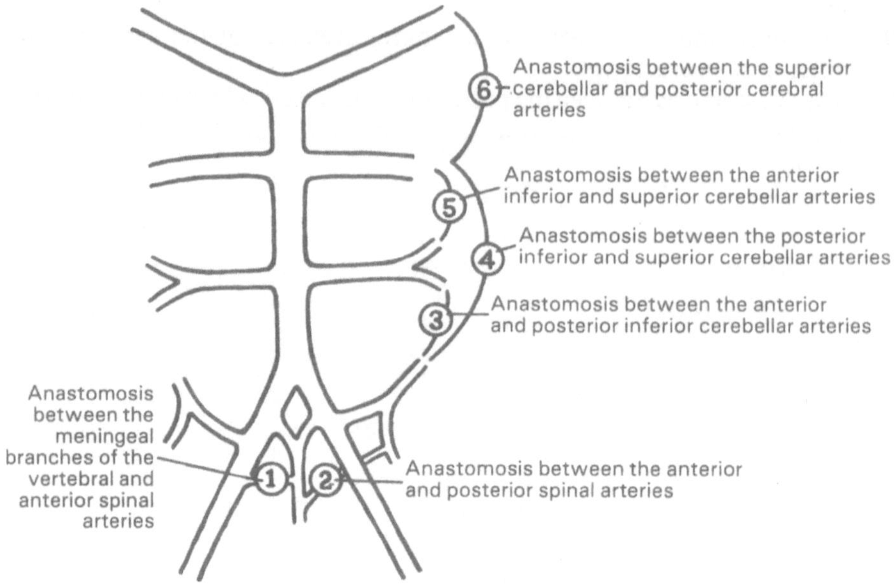

Figure 9.33 Anastomoses between the branches of the vertebrobasilar artery (After Leob, C.)

3. Some inconstant branches perforating the dura mater anastomose with arteries on the surface of the brain.
4. The anterior cerebral artery anastomoses with the meningeal artery of the falx cerebri.

Anastomosis between the intra- and extracranial arteries

Anastomoses between the intra- and extracranial external carotid arteries take place chiefly in three regions, namely, the eye, ear and nose (Figure 9.34).

1. The dorsal nasal artery of the ophthalmic artery anastomoses with the medial angular artery of the facial artery at the dorsum of the nose and the medial angle of the eye.
2. The lacrimal branch of the ophthalmic artery anastomoses with the zygomatico-orbital branch of the superficial temporal artery in the vicinity of the lacrimal gland.
3. The dorsal nasal and ethmoidal arteries of the ophthalmic artery anastomose with the infraorbital and sphenopalatine arteries of the maxillary artery in the maxillary region and the nasal cavity.
4. The caroticotympanic branch of the petrous portion of the internal carotid artery anastomoses with the anterior tympanic branch of the maxillary artery.
5. The pterygoid branch of the petrous portion of the internal carotid artery anastomoses with the corresponding branch of the maxillary artery.

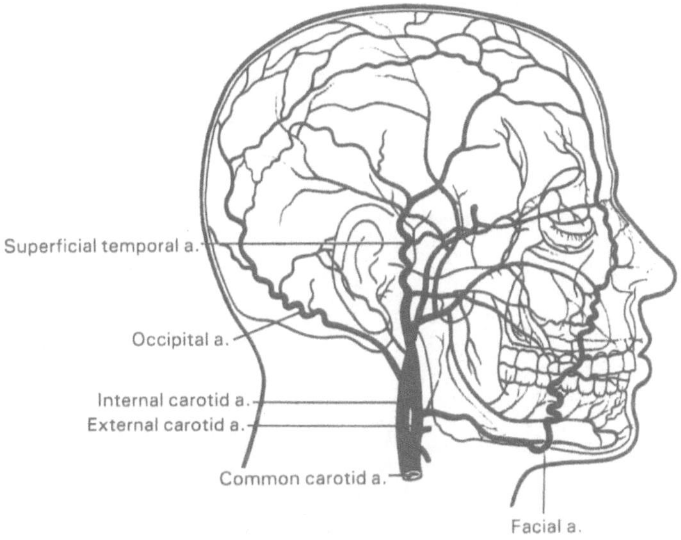

Figure 9.34 Collateral circulation in the brain (lateral view)

Anastomoses among extracranial arteries (Figure 9.35)

1. Anastomoses between the branches of the external carotid artery and between these branches (especially the facial, lingual and superior thyroid arteries) and their fellows of the opposite side.
2. The muscular branches of the vertebral, ascending pharyngeal and deep cervical arteries destined to the upper part of the neck anastomose with the occipital artery.
3. The muscular branches of the vertebral artery destined to the middle and lower parts of the neck anastomose with those of the thyrocervical trunk.
4. The inferior thyroid artery of the subclavian artery anastomoses with the superior thyroid artery of the external carotid artery.

Remnant of the embryonic internal carotico-basilar anastomosis

In the embryonic stage the anastomoses between the internal carotid and basilar arteries include the primitive trigeminal, otic and hypoglossal arteries. These used to disappear one after another in the 14 mm embryo. Persistance of these arteries may serve as important collateral routes between the internal carotid and basilar arteries.

CEREBRAL VEINS AND VENOUS SINUSES OF THE DURA MATER

ZHANG MINGXIAN

Cerebral veins

Most of the cerebral veins are not accompanied by arteries. They may be divided into superficial and deep groups according to the area they drain. The

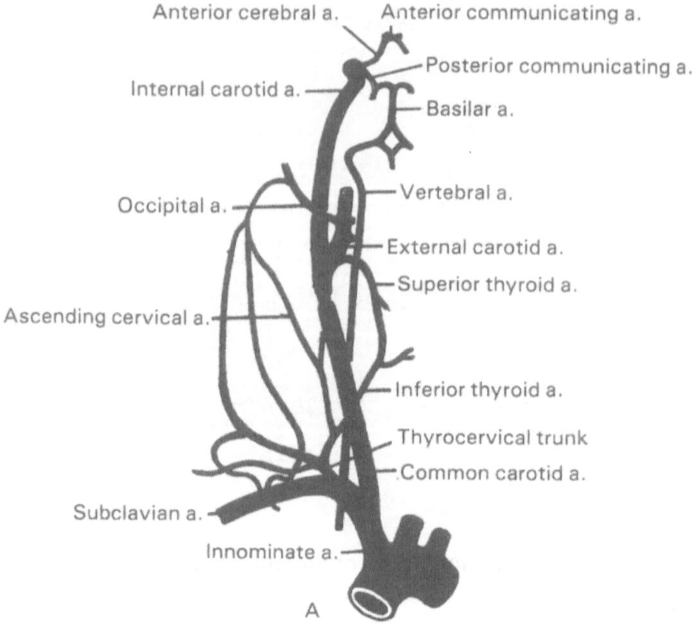

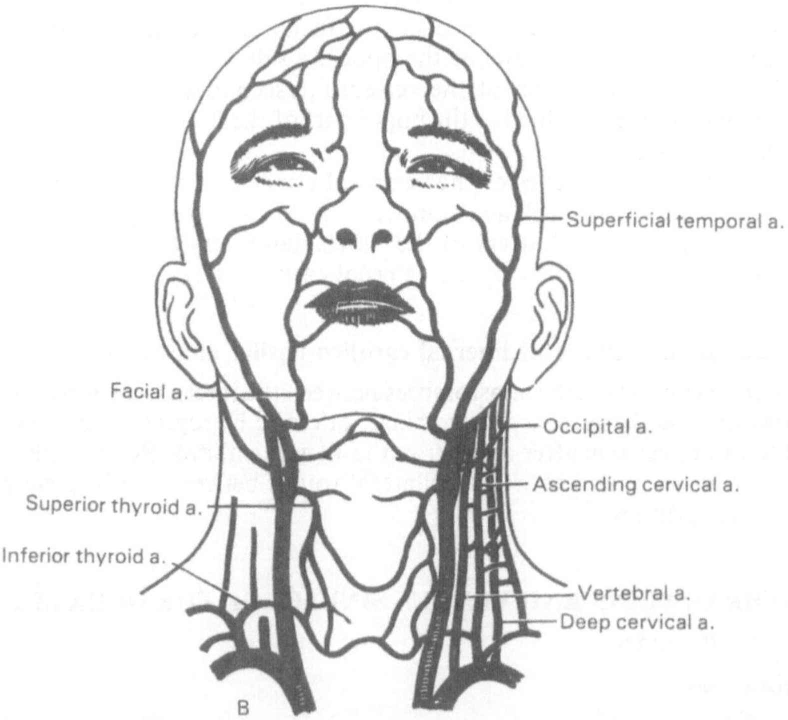

Figure 9.35 Collateral circulation in the brain (front view)

superficial group drains the veins of the cortex and the underlying white matter, and joins the adjacent venous sinuses of the dura mater. The deep group drains the veins from the deep part of the white matter, the basal ganglion and the thalamus, and opens into the straight sinus through the great cerebral vein. Anastomoses are abundant between these two groups.

Superficial cerebral veins

According to their courses, each of the superficial cerebral veins may be divided into five segments. The initial segment, small in calibre, is located in the grey and white matter. The pial segment runs for a short distance in the pia mater. The subarachnoid segment is bathed in the CSF. The subdural segment is located in the subdural space. As it looks like a bridge arching between the pia and dura maters, it is named the bridging vein. In head injury the brain may be shifted by the violence, while the dura mater remains still, so that the bridging veins may be lacerated and a subdural haematoma ensues. The dural segment is beside the venous sinuses and adheres closely to the inner plate of the dura mater.

The superficial cerebral veins fall into four main groups: the superior cerebral veins, the superficial middle cerebral veins, the inferior cerebral veins and the basal veins.

The superior cerebral veins

These collect blood from the dorsolateral and medial (above the corpus callosum) surfaces of the hemisphere and may be subdivided into the frontal, parietal and occipital groups. The tributaries of the frontal group, two to seven in number, ascend vertically to drain into the superior sagittal sinus. Those of the parietal group are one to three in number. The tributaries of the occipital group are the fewest, zero to two in number. Most of the tributaries of the parietal and occipital run forwards and medially and open into the venous sinus at an angle of 10–30 degrees. The superior cerebral veins enter the venous sinus in the direction against the blood flow within the superior sagittal sinus. This conduces to the elevation of the pressure within the sinus, which prevents the collapse of cerebral veins and accordingly ensures normal cerebral circulation.

The length of the bridging vein varies with different authors. Xu Yongzhao reported that most of them occur in the frontal, parietal and occipital lobes, being 5–20 mm in length. Perese reported from data gained in surgical operations that the lengths of the frontopolar veins were 6–18 mm, those of the frontal and parietal veins 30 mm and 2–5 mm respectively. The distance between the first bridging vein of the frontal lobe and the foramen caecum is nearly equal on both sides and measures 10–30 mm. Since the bridging veins are relatively short, they must be treated with care so as to avoid accidental haemorrhage when the brain is touched in operation.

The superficial middle cerebral vein

This vein, also called the superficial Sylvian vein, accompanies the middle cerebral artery. It runs forward and downward along the Sylvian fissure, winding round the temporal pole to the basal surface of the hemisphere, and terminates in the cavernous sinus, the superior petrosal sinus or the sphenoparietal sinus. It receives veins of the cortex and subcortical white matter of the frontal, parietal and occipital lobes in the vicinity of the Sylvian fissure. It anastomoses with the basal vein and the deep middle cerebral vein on the base of the brain. Adverse ligation of the stem of the Sylvian vein during operation will lead to congestion and oedema of the lower part of the precentral gyrus, which may increase to paralysis and spasm of the contralateral facial muscles.

The superficial middle cerebral veins are usually one to three in number (80.8%), and less frequently four (5.4%). They are sometimes very slender (9.6%) or absent (4.2%), and thus are compensated by the tributaries of the superior or inferior cerebral veins.

The bridging veins of the superficial middle cerebral vein are about 20–65 mm long and are not likely to be torn when the temporal pole is elevated during operation. However, if the head is injured they may be severed by the lesser wing of the sphenoid to cause haemorrhage.

The inferior cerebral veins

These are small veins, of which those draining the orbital and rectal gyri of the frontal lobe are called the frontopolar or orbital veins. They are three to seven in number, passing posteriorly into the basal vein as well as forwards into the superior sagittal sinus. Those draining the inferior surface of the temporal lobe open into the superior petrosal sinus, transverse sinus or the basal vein, and the others draining the occipital lobe are divided into medial occipital, suboccipital and lateral occipital veins, all of which flow into the transverse sinus. The bridging veins of the inferior cerebral vein are 20–65 mm in length.

The basal vein

This is formed by the union of the anterior and deep middle cerebral veins lateral to the optic chiasma. It runs posteriorly ventral to the optic tract, winding round the cerebral peduncle and superior colliculus, and joins the internal cerebral vein to end into the great cerebral vein. The anterior cerebral vein accompanies the artery and receives the blood from the medial surface of the frontal lobe. The deep middle cerebral vein drains the insula and neighbouring gyri. The basal vein also receives tributaries from the interpeduncular fossa, the inferior horn of the lateral ventricle, the hypothalamus and the ventral portion of the thalamus.

Important anastomotic veins of the superficial cerebral vein

1. The greater (superior) anastomotic vein (of Trolard) is one connecting the superficial middle cerebral vein with the superior sagittal sinus. It generally runs in the central sulcus or behind it. Its incidence is about 80%. Two

anastomotic veins of equal size may sometimes be seen. They are called the double veins of Trolard. That which extends along the posterior extremity of the lateral sulcus and joins the superior sagittal sinus is usually termed the Trolard's vein (Figure 9.32). This was first described by Trolard in 1870 and hence its name. The incidence of this vein is 13%.

2. The lesser (inferior) anastomotic vein (of Labbé) lies behind the lateral sulcus and connects the superficial middle and inferior cerebral veins (the occipital vein). It was first described by Labbé in 1879. Its incidence is about 10% (Figure 9.36).

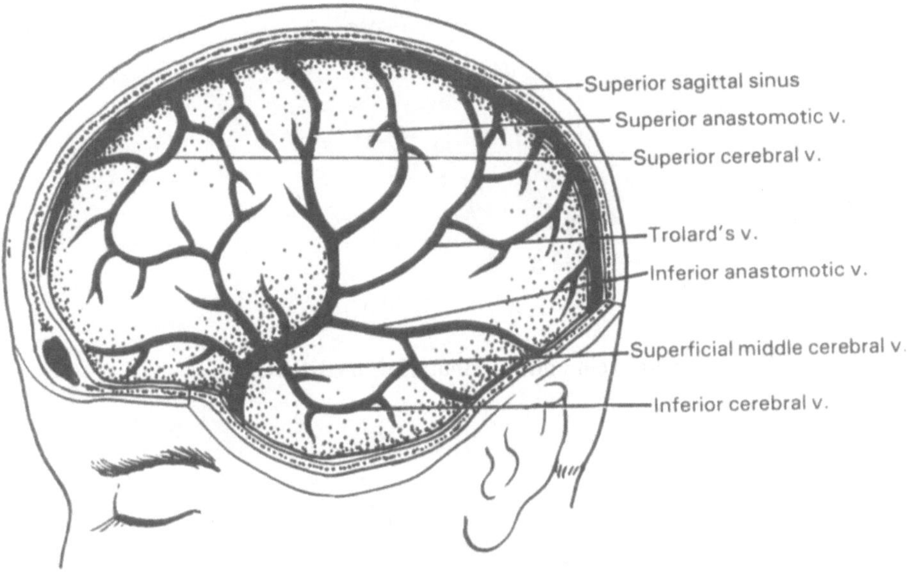

Figure 9.36 Veins on the lateral surface of the cerebral hemisphere

Deep cerebral veins

The most important of this group of veins are the internal cerebral and great cerebral veins.

The internal cerebral vein (or Galen's lesser vein)

These veins, one on each side, lie in the choroidal plexus on the roof of the third ventricle. Most of them are formed just behind the interventricular foramen by the union of its tributaries (80%), a few of them at the anterior two-thirds (12%) or one-third (8%) of the thalamus; they then run backward along the superomedial surface of the thalamus, and enter the great cerebral vein above the corpora quadrigemina (Figures 9.37 and 9.38).

1. The thalamostriate vein runs in the terminal sulcus between the thalamus and caudate nucleus. Its tributaries are the anterior terminal vein draining

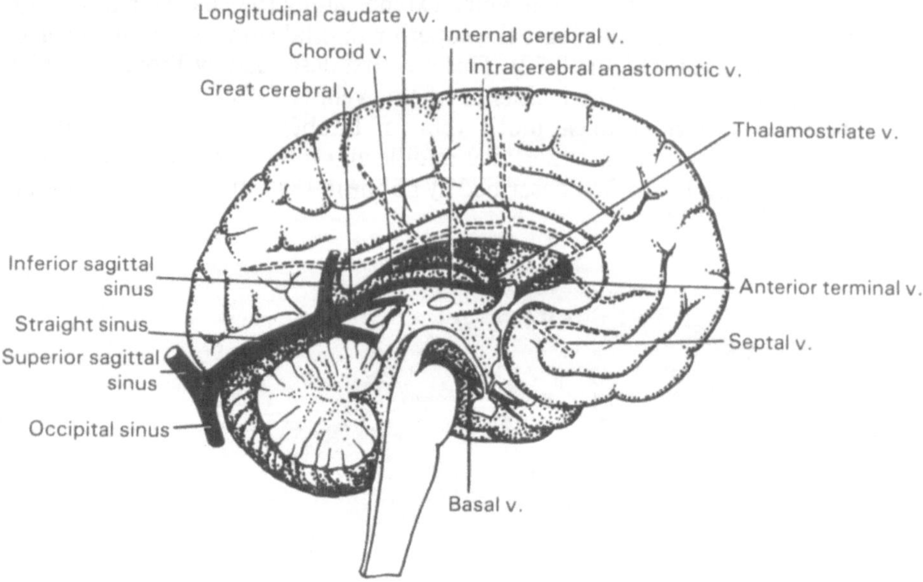

Figure 9.37 Great cerebral vein and its tributaries, medial view

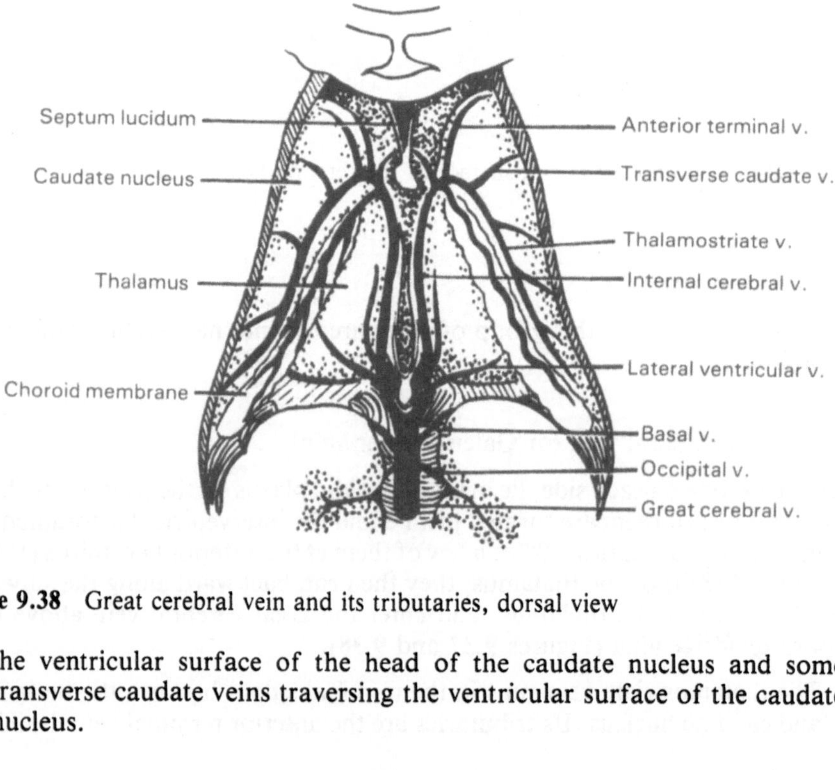

Figure 9.38 Great cerebral vein and its tributaries, dorsal view

the ventricular surface of the head of the caudate nucleus and some transverse caudate veins traversing the ventricular surface of the caudate nucleus.

2. The choroid vein runs along the lateral margin of the choroid plexus and drains the choroid plexus and the neighbouring hippocampus.
3. The septal vein receives tributaries from the rostrum of the corpus callosum and the septum lucidum.
4. The superior thalamic vein is a small vein which drains the dorsal portion of the diencephalon and enters the great or internal cerebral vein.
5. The lateral ventricular vein begins from the choroid plexus and runs on the upper surface of the caudal part of the thalamus to enter the internal cerebral vein.

The great cerebral vein (or Galen's great vein)

This is a short and thin-walled vein. It runs backwards and upwards below the splenium of the corpus callosum, and joins the inferior sagittal sinus to form the straight sinus. The great cerebral vein receives the right and left internal cerebral, basal and occipital veins. Since the deep cerebral veins are far more constant than the superficial veins, angiography of the internal cerebral veins, especially the thalamostriate vein, is conducive to recognizing the changes in their neighbouring structures.

Venous sinuses of the dura mater

Superior sagittal sinus

The superior sagittal sinus lies along the superior margin of the falx cerebri. It commences from the foramen caecum anteriorly, and flows backwards to the internal occipital protuberance, where it joins the straight sinus to form the confluence of sinuses. It deviates to the right to be continued as the right transverse sinus in 58% or to the left in 19%, or remains in the median line to connect the transverse sinuses on both sides in 23%. The cross-sectional area of the superior sagittal sinus is triangular and measures about 18.1 mm^2.

The superior sagittal sinus receives most of the venous blood from the surface of the cerebrum as well as from the dura mater and the skull. It communicates with the extracranial veins by means of the emissary veins of the parietal and occipital bone.

The straight sinus

This is situated at the junction of the falx cerebri and tentorium cerebelli. It can be divided into a single and a double type. The single type is more frequent. The so-called double straight sinus possesses a septum in its lumen, which may be divided partially or wholly. In the latter case, if it is divided sagittally, a left and a right sinus will be formed; where it is divided transversely, an upper and a lower sinus would be formed.

Most of the straight sinuses are the continuations of the inferior sagittal sinus. The great cerebral vein is the largest vein flowing into the straight sinus. From the end of the inferior sagittal sinus to the opening of the great cerebral vein there is a distance of 6 (2–13) mm. Of the double straight sinuses, the upper (or the left) one is the continuation of the inferior sagittal sinus, while the lower (or the right) is the continuation of the great cerebral vein. At the confluence of sinuses the bifurcated single straight sinus enters the right and left transverse sinuses mostly by two openings. The non-bifurcated single straight sinus ends at the centre of the confluence or into the left or right transverse sinus by a single opening. Of the double straight sinuses with complete partition, the upper (or left) straight sinus ends into the left transverse sinus, while the lower (or right) terminates in the right sinus.

The whole length (from the end of the inferior sagittal sinus to the opening of the straight sinus) of the straight sinus averages 55 (40–70) mm. The floor of the straight sinus looks like a gradually widened band from anterior backwards. The anterior margin of the floor averages 2.1 (1.0–3.4) mm, while the posterior margin measures 4.0 (2.2–8.8) mm. The cross-sectional area of the straight sinus averages 7.2 mm^2.

Transverse sinus

The transverse sinuses are situated on the posterolateral margin of the tentorium cerebelli. Each transverse sinus passes along the transverse groove laterally and anteriorly to be continued as the sigmoid sinus.

The transverse sinus is the thickest of the venous sinuses. Its size is influenced by the direction of the superior sagittal sinus. When the latter flows into the right, the cross-sectional area of the right transverse sinus is larger than the left, and vice-versa. The cross-sectional areas of the right and left transverse sinuses average 29.1 and 17.0 mm^2 respectively. In about 62% of cases the right one is larger than the left. If the left transverse sinus is too small, sudden occlusion of the right transverse sinus or surgical resection or ligation of the right internal jugular vein may obstruct the venous return from the brain.

Occipital sinus

The occipital sinus occupies the attached margin of the falx cerebelli. It commences from the posterior margin of the foramen magnum and ascends to the confluence of sinuses. Its calibre varies from 0.2 to 6.0 mm, being more than 1.0 mm in about 47%. It is generally believed that large occipital sinus has the same significance in collateral circulation as the transverse sinus. The variations in the occipital sinus are frequent. The incidence of the occipital sinus is 64.5%, of which the median occipital sinus occurs in 35%, double occipital sinus in 22.5%, left occipital sinus in 4%, and right occipital sinus in 3%. All of them connect with the confluence of sinuses. Those connected with the right transverse sinus amount to 10%; those with the left transverse sinus 8%; with the right sigmoid sinus 6%, with the left sigmoid sinus 3%, with the superior sagittal sinus 8%, and with the straight sinus 6%.

MICROSURGICAL ANATOMY OF SOME INTRACRANIAL REGIONS

ZHOU JIABAO AND ZHANG MINXIAN

Sellar region

The sellar region comprises the sella turcica and its adjacent structures. A thorough knowledge of the microsurgical anatomy of this region, such as the morphology of the sella turcica and sphenoid sinus, the relationship between the pituitary gland and the diaphragma sella, the topographical variations in the optic chiasma and nerve, the variations in the internal carotid artery and intercavernous sinus, is of great significance to clinical diagnosis and for deciding whether the transfrontal or trans-sphenoidal approach should be adopted in pituitary surgery.

Sella turcica

The deepest part of the sella turcica is also called the hypophyseal fossa, in clinical practice. The posterior boundary of the sella is a square plate of bone, the dorsum sellae, the tubercle on either side of which is termed the posterior clinoid process. There is a small elevation, termed the tuberculum sellae, on the anterior boundary. The sella turcica in the Chinese is frequently oval (69.6%), but less frequently round (24.6%) and flattened (5.8%). The sella takes shape in childhood, and bears no relation to age. The dimensions of the sella turcica measured in adult skulls are as follows: the length averages 11.2 (8.0–14.5) mm, the width 14.7 (8.0–19.0) mm, and the depth 8.7 (6.5–12.0) mm. These are in agreement with those measured on X-ray films. The volume of the sella varies greatly. Calculated by the mathematical formula for the volume of an ellipsoid, namely, volume (mm^3) = ½ (length × width × depth) suggested by Dichiro and Nelson (1962), the volume of the sella in Chinese adults averages 722 (371–1359) mm^3, which is larger than those recorded by Renn and Rhoton in 1975 (621 mm^3) and Dichiro *et al.* (594 mm^3), but approximates that measured by the 'casting method' (754 mm^3). It is believed that the sella turcica in acromegaly is comparatively large and shaped like a balloon. However, in case of chromophobic adenoma it is cup-shaped and its volume may reach 4500 mm^3. Normally, the jugum sphenoidale and the anterior wall of the sella turcica are almost at right angles. If the sella is enlarged it will become an acute angle.

The floor of the sella turcica varies in shape; it may be flat, concave or convex. It appears as a strip of compact bone in lateral film. Its thickness is frequently less than 1 mm and rarely attains 4.5 mm. A thin floor facilitates the trans-sphenoidal approach to the pituitary gland. Osteoporosis and destruction of bone are frequently seen in acromegaly and are even more obvious in chromophobic adenoma.

Diaphragma sellae

The diaphragma sellae forms the roof of the sella turcica and may be regarded as a barrier between the sella and the cranial cavity. In the centre of the diaphragm is a round or oval opening, called the diaphragmatic opening, which transmits the pituitary stalk. The longitudinal dimension of the diaphragma averages 11.7 (7–15) mm; the transverse dimension is 20.2 (15–24.5) mm. The diameter of the diaphragmal opening is more than 6 mm in 58%. Renn and Rhoton recorded that it was usually more than 5 mm, yet Bu Guoxuan (1979) maintained that it was often less than 2 mm and rarely over 8 mm. The diaphragma is thinner around the diaphragmal opening and thicker on the periphery. The thickness of the diaphragm and the size of the diaphragmatic opening affect not only the development of a pituitary tumour but also the process of trans-sphenoidal hypophysectomy.

Generally, the diaphragm extends from the posterior clinoid processes to the tuberculum sellae. The tumour may occur above or below the diaphragm. When the diaphragm is not intact the arachnoid may protrude into the sella turcica with the subarachnoid space and press the pituitary gland to the bottom of the sella, resulting in empty sellar syndrome or intrasellar arachnoidal cyst.

Pituitary gland

Owing to the different shapes of the sella turcica, that of the pituitary gland varies greatly. However, it is generally oval. When it is pressed laterally by the internal carotid arteries it loses its round contour and sends out tongue-like protrusions above and below the artery. The pituitary gland averages 9.9 (7–13) mm in the anteroposterior diameter, 13.9 (10–17) mm in the transverse diameter, and 5.5 (2.5–9.0) mm in the vertical diameter. The inferior surface of the pituitary gland usually conforms to the contour of the sellar floor. The growth of intrasellar tumours compresses the pituitary gland, or part of the gland may be squeezed into its surrounding structures, so that some of the gland may be left unremoved in total hypophysectomy.

The pituitary gland usually occupies only part of the sella turcica, the remainder of the space being filled with veins. The size of the gland, especially the degree of filling of the pituitary gland in the sella turcica, is of practical significance in the assessment of the course of signs of pituitary tumours.

Sphenoid sinus

The sphenoid sinus is the pneumatic cavity in the body of the sphenoid bone. It occupies the centre of the base of the skull. It usually serves as the portal of approach to the pituitary gland in transnasal hypophysectomy. The size and shape of the sphenoid sinus vary. According to the degree of pneumatization, it may be divided into three types:

1. The conchal type occurs in 2.5% of cases. It is very small and does not extend into the body of the sphenoid bone. The bony wall separating the sinus from the sella turcica is about 10 mm in thickness. This type is more common in children, and is not suitable for trans-sinusal surgery.

2. The presellar type is found in 11–13% of cases. The sinus is moderate in size. Its posterior wall is in front of the sella and thus adds difficulties to trans-sphenoidal operation.
3. The sellar type is found in 76–86% of cases. The sinus of this type is well developed and is in touch with the base of the sella. It is very suitable for trans-sphenoidal intrasellar hypophysectomy.

Bu Guoxuan reported that in 21% of cases the sphenoid sinus may be very large and extends into the occipital bone, so that only a very thin bony lamina exists between the clivus and the pons. If this lamina is inadvertently injured, blood may flow into the posterior cranial fossa so as to compress the brain stem to imperil life. Bateman (1972) found that in 60% of cases the sphenoid sinus intrudes into the occipital bone. However, it is not a contraindication to trans-sphenoidal operation.

The cavity and septum of the sphenoid sinus is of certain significance in operation. It is found that a single major septum separates the sinus into two cavities in 70%, two septa separate the sinus into three cavities in 10%, one vertical and one transverse septum separate the sinus into four cavities in 3.3%, an incomplete small septum exists in the cavity in 6.7%, and the septum is lacking in 10%. The major sagittal septum is located in the midline in 43.3%, or away from the midline in 46.7%. The remaining 10% comprise coronal septa or small incomplete ones. The major sagittal septum deviates from the midline as far as 4 cm and averages 0.81 mm in thickness. A posteroanterior film is essential to ascertain the relation between the septum and the floor of the sella for trans-sphenoidal approach.

In addition to the sellar floor and optic canal, which may bulge into the sphenoid sinus, the carotid arteries may also protrude into the superolateral wall of the posterior part of the sinus, being usually covered with a thin bony wall separating the artery from the mucosa of the sinus, which is more than 1 mm in thickness in about one-third of the cases. Nevertheless, it may be as thin as paper or even absent in 4%. Consequently, in trans-sphenoidal hypophysectomy, exposure of the optic nerve and carotid arteries in this region should be done with caution.

Optic chiasma

The topographical relation between the optic chiasma and the sella turcica and the hypophysis falls into three patterns (Figure 9.39).

Normal chiasma

This type of chiasma is located above the diaphragma sellae and the hypophysis with an incidence of 87%. The distance from the tuberculum sellae to the anterior margin of the optic chiasma averages 5.3 (2–8) mm.

Postfixed chiasma

The posterior margin of the chiasma reaches the dorsum sellae and covers it. The incidence is about 10%. The distance from the tuberculum sellae to the anterior margin of the chiasma averages 8.8 (7–11.5) mm.

Prefixed chiasma

The anterior margin of the chiasma reaches the tuberculum sellae and sometimes covers or even lies in front of it. This occurs in about 3% of cases. It is believed in clinical practice that if the distance between the tuberculum sellae and the anterior margin of optic chiasma is less than 2 mm, the operating field is too small to carry out transfrontal hypophysectomy. Consequently, a transtemporal or a combined transfrontal and transtemporal approach is advisable.

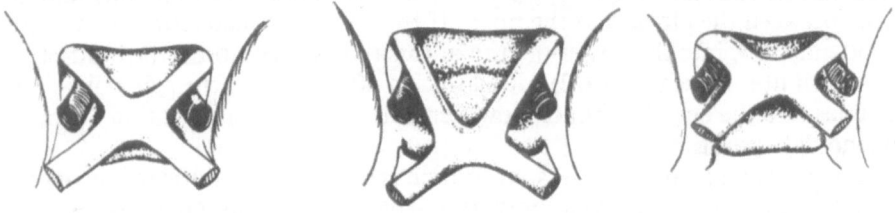

1: Normal type 87% 2: Postfixed type 10% 3: Prefixed type 3%

Figure 9.39 Topographical variations of the optic chiasma

Internal carotid artery

The distance between the intracranial portions of bilateral internal carotid arteries has a close bearing on whether hypophysectomy is difficult or easy to do. The distance between the two carotid arteries is the shortest at the anterior clinoid process (80%), the next being around the cavernous sinus (12%). In 8% of cases the distance between the two internal carotid arteries at the anterior clinoid process is equal to that around the cavernous sinus, the shortest distance averaging 11.9 mm.

The anterior clinoid process is anterosuperior to the internal carotid artery, while the posterior process is posterosuperior to it. The distance between the anterior and posterior clinoid processes averages 9.6 (6.0–12.5) mm. The oculomotor nerve may emerge from between the anterior and posterior clinoid processes, or lateral to or behind the posterior clinoid process.

Intercavernous sinus (Figure 9.40)

The cavernous sinuses of the two sides communicate with each other by the intercavernous sinus surrounding the hypophysis. According to its topographical relation with the hypophysis, the intercavernous sinus may be divided into anterior, posterior and inferior ones. The anterior intercavernous sinus lies in front of hypophysis (62%), the posterior intercavernous sinus behind the gland (60%), and the inferior intercavernous sinus beneath it (62%). Any of the intercavernous sinuses may be lacking, or they may vary. The anterior one is usually larger than the posterior, and may not be entirely within the diaphragma sellae, so that 10% of them may extend in front of the pituitary gland. A large anterior intercavernous sinus often makes trans-sphenoidal hypophysectomy more difficult.

In 94% of cases the basilar sinus is found on the posterior aspect of the dorsum sellae and the clivus of the sphenoid bone. It connects posterior ends of both cavernous sinuses, receives the superior and inferior petrosal sinuses, and communicates inferiorly with the vertebral venous plexus.

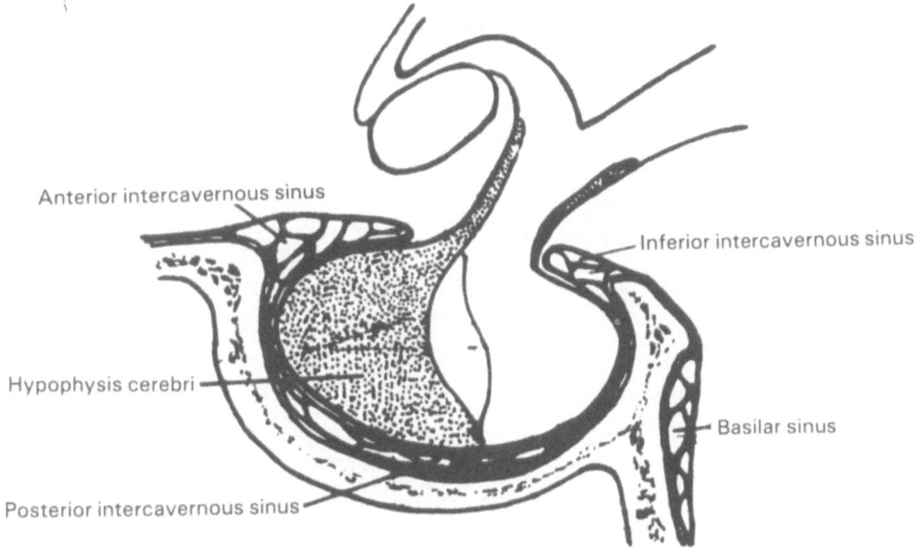

Figure 9.40 Position of the intercavernous sinus

Optic canal and its adjacent structures

In the course of progress in microsurgery, the intracranial approach for the decompression of the optic canal is replaced by the extracranial approach. The latter approach deals with a series of complicated structures. Besides the optic canal and the optic nerve and ophthalmic artery which pass through the canal, there are sphenoid and posterior ethmoid sinuses, which are adjacent to the medial wall of the optic canal, and the ethmoidal neurovascular bundle passing through the medial orbital wall.

Optic canal

The optic canal lies between the root of the lessor sphenoid wing and the body of the sphenoid bone. It has two openings and four walls. The internal opening is called the cranial opening, and the external one the orbital opening. These two openings are elliptical in shape. The transverse dimension of the cranial opening averages 6.9 (4.5–9.0) mm, and its height averages 4.1 (2.2–6.5) mm. The transverse dimension of the orbital opening averages 5.6 (4.5–7.0) mm, and its height 6.6 (5.5–8.0) mm. The four walls of the optic canal are different in length. By the length of the optic canal is generally meant the length of its upper wall, which averages 8.5 (4.0–13.0) mm.

The height of the orbital opening is greater than that of the cranial opening. The difference between them averages 2.5 mm. This is mainly because the inferior wall of the optic canal slopes downward from the cranial to the orbital opening with the result that the anterior margin of the medial wall is longer than that of the posterior margin (Figure 9.41). Attention should be paid to this morphological characteristic when the medial wall of the optic canal is excised for decompression.

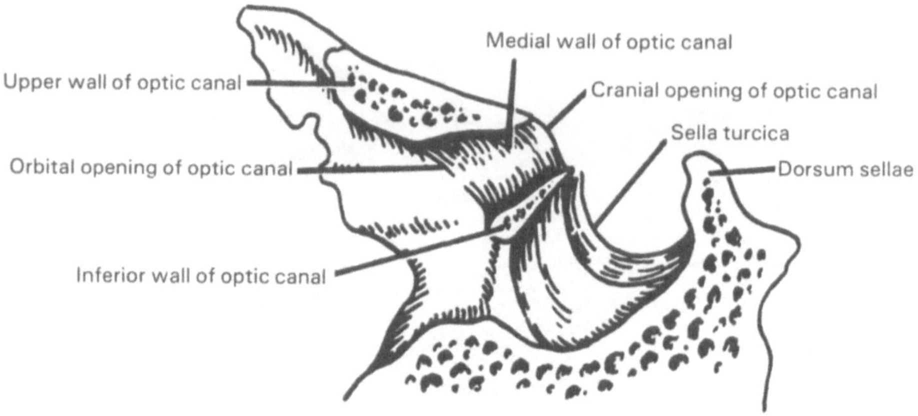

Figure 9.41 Optic canal (left side, sagittal section)

The optic canal is a passageway directing anterolaterally from behind and medially. The distance between the midpoints of the medial margins of bilateral orbital openings averages 26.1 (21.0–31.0) mm. That between the midpoints of the medial margins of two cranial openings averages 12.9 (9.0–19.0) mm.

At the upper margin of the cranial opening the dura mater forms a falciform fold (Figure 9.42). Its width (the widest part of the fold anteroposteriorly) averages 2.7 (0.7–8.8) mm. In a few cases the upper wall of the optic canal

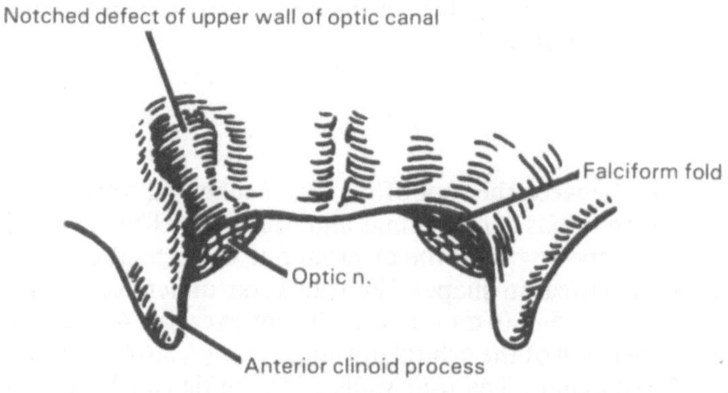

Figure 9.42 Falciform fold and the notched bony defect of the upper wall of the optic canal

presents a notched defect, so that the width of the falciform fold may reach 8.8 mm. In rare cases the fold may be very firm, tenacious and sharp-edged; it may damage the optic nerve during a closed-head injury. The optic nerve under cover of the fold has no bony protection. Caution should be exercised in intracranial operation.

Anterior and posterior ethmoidal foramina

The anterior and posterior ethmoidal foramina transmit the corresponding nerves and vessels respectively. These neurovascular bundles must be protected carefully in the extracranial approach for decompression of the optic canal. The posterior ethmoidal foramen is quite near the orbital opening of the optic canal, the distance averaging 6.3 (2.0–11.0) mm. That between the anterior and posterior ethmoidal foramina averages 13.6 (7.0–20.0) mm and the distance from the anterior ethmoidal foramen to the dacryon (the point of junction between the frontal, lacrimal and maxillary bones at the upper end of the lacrimal fossa) averages 3.2 (11.0–30.0) mm.

Prechiasmatic space and optic nerve

Prechiasmatic space

The prechiasmatic space resides between the anterior margin of the optic chiasma and the optic nerves. The field of operation in both hypophysectomy and decompression of the optic nerve will involve this area. The size of this space has a bearing on the length of intracranial segment of the optic nerve, the angle between the optic nerves, the distance between the two medial margins of the optic nerves at the cranial opening of the optic canal as well as the type of the chiasma.

Optic nerve

The optic nerve runs backward and medially from the eyeball into the skull through the optic canal and continues into the chiasma. It is ellipsoid in cross-section at the cranial opening of the optic canal. Its transverse dimension averages 5.2 (3.5–7.0) mm and the longitudinal dimension averages 2.7 (1.5–4.8) mm. The length of the intracranial segment of the optic nerve is equal to the distance between the anterior margin of the chiasma and the cranial opening and averages 11.5 (6.0–17.8) mm. At the cranial opening the distance between the medial margins of two optic nerves is 13.7 (6.8–17.2) mm. The angle between the two optic nerves averages 60.4 (10–85) degrees. It is believed that the smaller the angle, the narrower the operating field, which is unfavourable for transfrontal hypophysectomy (Figure 9.43).

Ophthalmic artery

The ophthalmic artery is one of the most important structures in the optic canal. In a few abnormal cases it passes through a small canal below the optic canal into the orbit.

Origin of the ophthalmic artery

The ophthalmic artery arises mostly singly from the internal carotid artery (91.2%). A few of them arise by two trunks from the middle meningeal and internal carotid arteries (7.5%) (Figure 9.44). Of these, the trunk from the middle meningeal artery is large and that from the internal carotid artery is very small. There are also 1.3% of cases in which the ophthalmic artery arises singly from the middle meningeal artery.

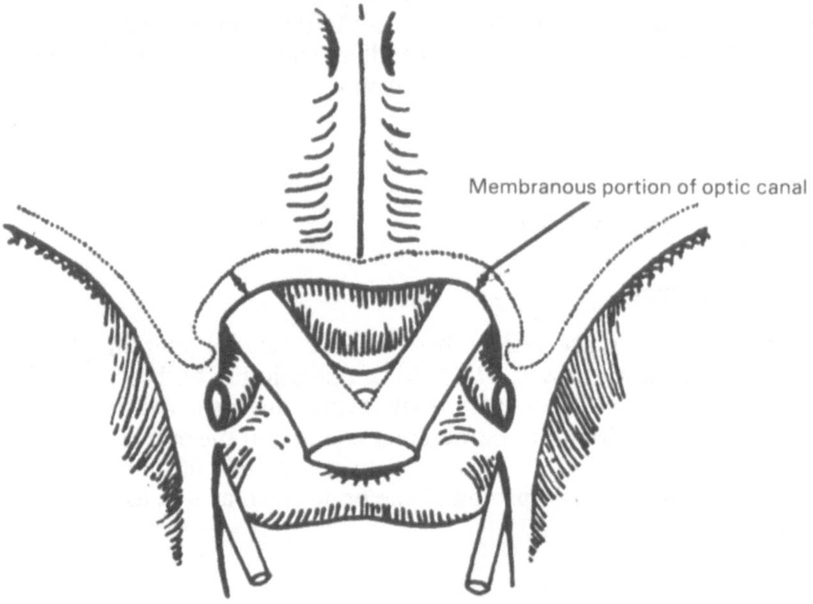

Figure 9.43 Angle between two optic nerves

The ophthalmic artery arising from the middle meningeal artery enters the orbit through the superior orbital fissure or a small foramen just lateral to the fissure (Figure 9.44). The ophthalmic artery originates mainly from the part of the internal carotid artery which emerges directly from the cavernous sinus. This is called the subdural origin and accounts for 84.8% of cases. A few of them arise from the cavernous segment of the internal carotid artery and are said to have an extradural origin; this amounts to 15.2%. Of the arteries of subdural origin, those arising from the medial one-third of the extracavernous portion of the internal artery account for 76.0%; from the middle one-third, 21.5%; and from the lateral one-third 2.5%.

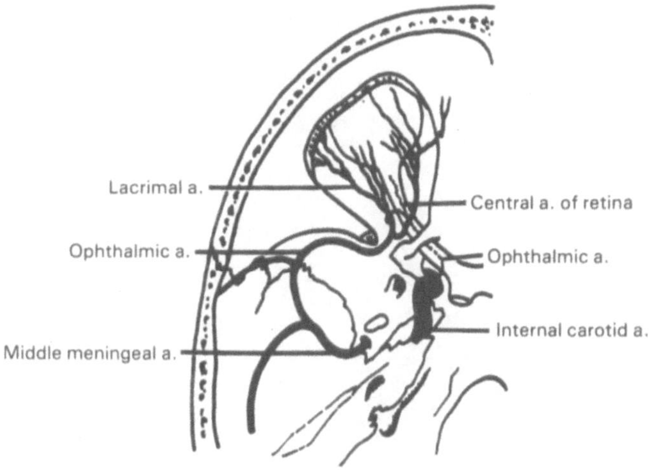

Figure 9.44 Abnormal origins of the ophthalmic artery

Divisions of the ophthalmic artery

Hayren *et al.* (1962) divides the intracranial and intracanalicular segments of the ophthalmic artery into the following parts: short limb, angle *a*, long limb, angle *b* and the distal part (Figure 9.45). The short limb is the part between the commencement of the ophthalmic artery and angle *a*, being 1.3 mm long (0.5–3.0) mm. The long limb is the part between angle *a* and angle *b*, 2.9 (1.4–5.2) mm in length. From angle *b* forward the artery is continued as the distal part.

The ophthalmic artery of subdural origin enters the inferior wall of the dural sheath of the optic nerve at or slightly distal to angle *b*, and then proceeds directly forward to the apex of the orbit. The site where it penetrates the dural sheath lies anterior to the free margin of falciform fold (in the optic canal) in 60.8%, posterior to the free margin (in the cranial cavity) in 27.5%, and inferior to this margin in 11.8%. The ophthalmic artery of extradural origin runs forwards in the inferior wall of the dural sheath of the optic nerve. That the walls of the artery within the dural sheath adhere firmly to the surrounding sheath makes the dissection of this artery very difficult.

If this part of the dural sheath is injured, the walls of the artery are liable to damage, and bleeding is hard to staunch.

Topographical relation between the ophthalmic artery and optic nerve

The site of origin of the ophthalmic artery lying inferomedial to the optic nerve accounts for 62.0%, that lying lateral to the nerve for 21.1%, and that lying directly beneath the nerve for 16.9%. Since the ophthalmic artery has a more marked lateral inclination during its course than that of the optic nerve, it deviates gradually to the inferolateral surface of the nerve. The distal part of the opthalmic artery is situated within the dural sheath inferolateral to the optic

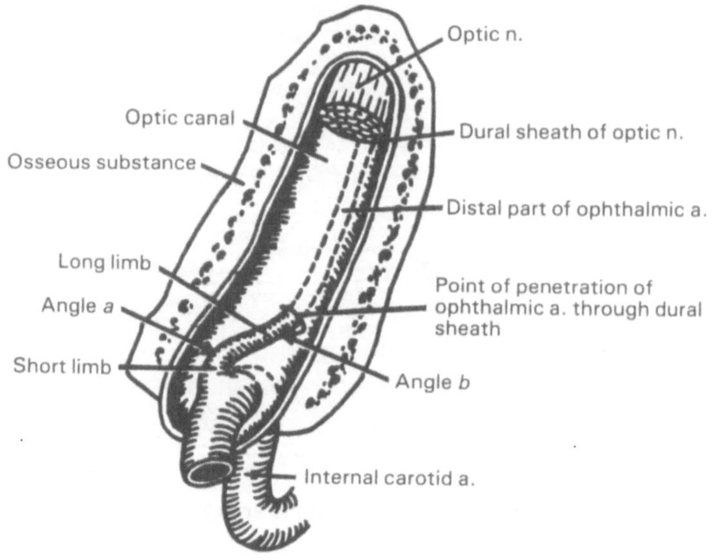

Figure 9.45 Division of the ophthalmic artery (right side)

nerve in 70.4%, directly beneath the nerve in 26.8%, and medial to the nerve in only 2.8%. In the removal of the medial wall of the optic canal for decompression, care should be taken not to involve the inferior wall, especially near the cranial opening, to avoid injury to the ophthalmic artery, which traverses in the dural sheath close to the medial part of the inferior wall of the optic canal.

Posterior ethmoid sinus

The medial wall of the optic canal is adjacent to the sphenoid sinus in most cases, being also close to the posterior ethmoid sinus which intrudes into the body of the sphenoid (Figure 9.46). In the extracranial approach for the decompression of the optic canal, attention must be paid to the variations in the sphenoid and posterior ethmoid sinuses.

The posterior ethmoid sinus may not only extend backwards into the body of the sphenoid to be adjacent to the medial wall of the optic canal in 47.2%, but also into the upper, lower and lateral walls of the optic canal. In other words, it may surround the optic nerve completely, so that the optic nerve is separated from the sinus only by a thin layer of bone. When decompression of the optic canal is to be performed by means of the intracranial approach, two thin layers of bone should be extracted during the removal of the upper wall of the optic canal.

Relations of the medial wall of the optic canal

The length of the medial wall of the optic canal averages 9.7 mm. Since the sphenoid sinus varies greatly, and the posterior ethmoid sinus usually extends into the body of the sphenoid, the relations of the medial wall of the optic canal are

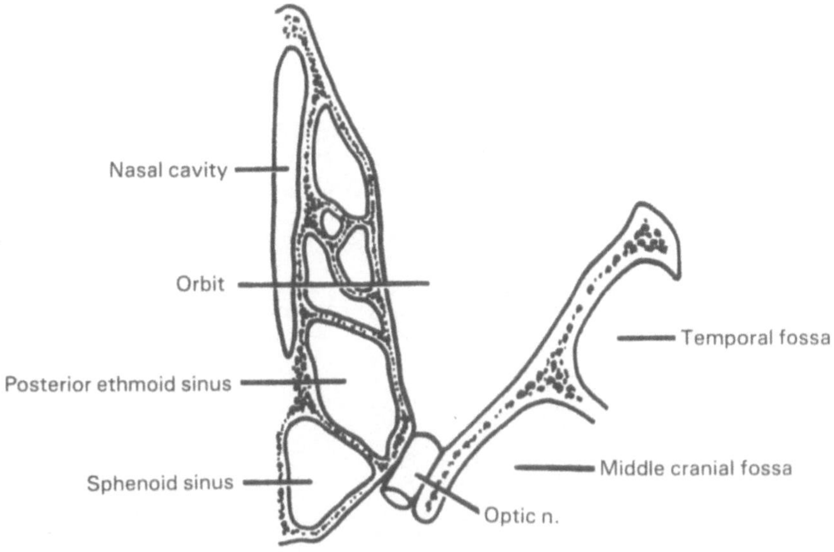

Figure 9.46 Posterior ethmoid sinus extending into the body of the sphenoid

complicated. The medial wall of the optic canal is close to the ipsilateral sphenoid sinus. However, if the latter is hypoplastic while the contralateral one is highly developed so as to cross the midline, the medial wall of the optic canal will be close to the contralateral sphenoid sinus. When the posterior ethmoid sinus extends backward, the medial wall of the optic canal is then adjacent to the posterior ethmoid sinus. In the conchal type of sphenoid sinus the medial wall of the optic canal is connected with the bony substance in the body of sphenoid. There are many other complex forms (Figure 9.47).

The more variations in the topographical relations between the medial wall of the optic canal and the sinuses, the more morphological changes in the linear attachment of the bony septa (including the partitions of the ethmoid cells) between the sinuses. The thickness of the medial wall of the optic canal is increased along the line of attachment of the septum. The thickness of the medial wall of the optic canal averages 0.2 mm, but it may reach 0.6 mm with compact bone on the attachment of the septum between the sphenoid and posterior ethmoid sinuses, where care must be taken during operation.

Cavernous sinus

The cavernous sinus is an irregular space between the two layers of the dura mater. Its name was first adopted by Winslow (1732). He found that there were many fibrous trabeculae which separated this space into numerous cells communicating with each other and gave the sinus a spongy appearance; hence its name.

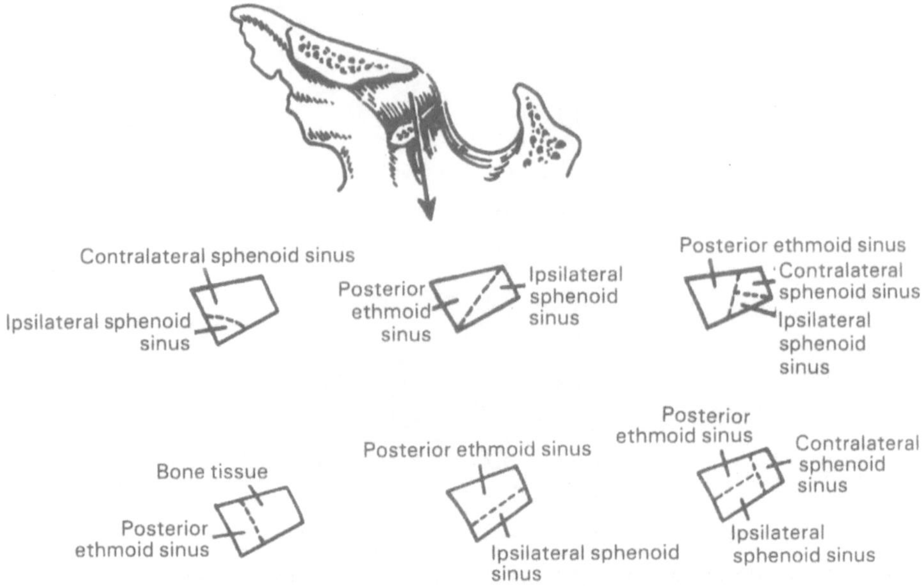

Figure 9.47 Topographical relations of the medial wall of the optic canal (left side)

The position and shape of the cavernous sinus

The cavernous sinuses are located on either side of the hypophysis and sella turcica. According to Chinese data the majority of cavernous sinuses extend anteriorly to the superior orbital fissure (83%), posteriorly to the apex of the petrous portion of the temporal bone (83%), superiorly to the line drawn from the medial to the posterior clinoid processes, inferiorly to 3–4 mm from the line joining the medial margins of the foramina rotundum and ovale (60.5%) and laterally to the maxillary nerve and trigeminal ganglion.

The cavernous sinus is irregularly shaped, being long and narrow antero-posteriorly. It looks somewhat like a right-angled triangle in frontal section through the mid-point of a line joining the anterior and posterior clinoid processes (Figure 9.48), with the right angle directed outward and upward, the hypotenuse near the hypophysis and sella turcica and the base parallel to the level of the diaphragm sellae. In this section the length of the lateral wall ranges mostly from 15 to 22 mm (79%), and those of the medial and upper walls are 15–22 mm (74%) and 7–12 mm (90%) respectively.

The distance between the bilateral cavernous sinuses varies with the form of the skull. In general, it is shorter in a dolichocephalic and longer in a brachycephalic. The mean distance is 13.2 mm.

Arteries within the carotid sinus

The internal carotid artery forms an anterior and a posterior bend in the cavernous sinus, which allows it to be divided into three corresponding

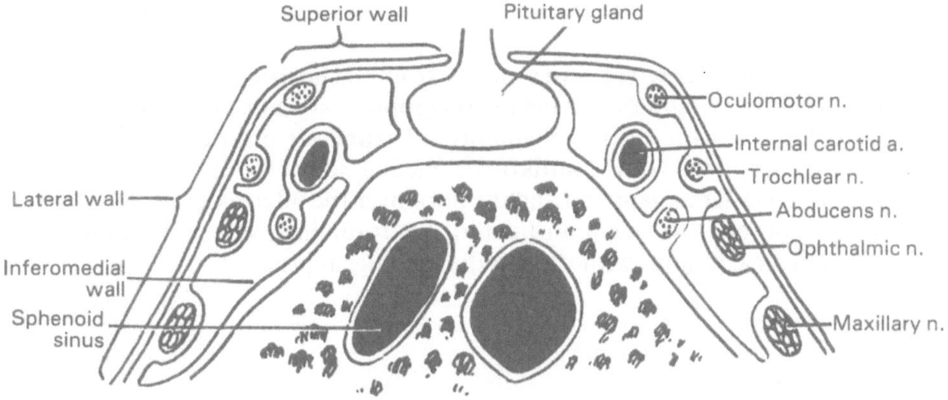

Figure 9.48 Frontal section of the middle part of the cavernous sinus through the mid-point of a line connecting the anterior and posterior clinoid processes

segments; namely, the posterior ascending, the horizontal, and the anterior ascending segments. There are three constant branches from the intracavernous portion of the carotid artery.

The meningohypophyseal trunk

This is the largest and most constant branch, which arises at the level of the dorsum sellae from the horizontal segment. It is approximately of the same size as the ophthalmic artery and divides immediately into the following branches (Figure 9.49).

Tentorial artery The tentorial artery is the most constant of the branches. It runs backwards and laterally to the roof of the sinus and then sends off branches along the free margin of the tentorium to the third and fourth cranial nerves to anastomose with the meningeal branch of the ophthalmic artery and the fellows of the opposite side. Its course is wavy, measuring 5-35 mm in length in normal angiography. If its length exceeds 40 mm, pathological lesions may be predicted.

Dorsal meningeal artery The dorsal meningeal artery usually arises from the meningohypophyseal trunk (90%). However, it may sometimes arise directly from the internal carotid artery (6%). It then runs backwards and divides into several branches to supply the dura mater over the roof of the sinus, the dorsum sellae, the clivus, and the abducent nerve. It anastomoses with its fellow of the opposite side.

Inferior hypophyseal artery The inferior hypophyseal artery arises mostly from the meningohypophyseal trunk (nearly 80%) or directly from the cavernous portion of the internal carotid artery. It runs medially and enters the bottom of the hypophysis. It supplies the dura mater over the bottom of the sella and the posterior lobes of the hypophysis, and anastomoses with its fellow of the opposite side.

Inferior cavernous artery

The inferior cavernous artery arises mostly from the horizontal segment about 5 mm distal to the origin of the meningohypophyseal trunk. Only 6% of the arteries come from the meningohypophyseal trunk. It passes first over the abducent nerve and then downwards on the medial side of the ophthalmic nerve to supply the semilunar ganglion and the dura over the inferolateral wall of the cavernous sinus and the neighbourhood of the foramina ovale and spinosum, where it may anastomose with the middle meningeal artery.

Capsular artery

The capsular arteries arise from the inferomedial side of the horizontal segment about 5 mm distal to the origin of the inferior cavernous artery. They may be divided into the inferior and anterior capsular arteries. The inferior capsular artery runs medially in the dura, which covers the sellar floor to supply the anterior lobe of the hypophysis and anastomoses with the inferior hypophyseal artery. The anterior capsular artery runs medially in the dura of the anterior sellar wall and anastomoses with its fellow of the opposite side.

In addition to these constant branches, the cavernous portion of the internal carotid artery may occasionally give rise to the ophthalmic artery. The latter enters the orbit through a small foramen on the floor of the optic canal or through its cranial opening. It must be ligated in surgical management of the caroticocavernous fistula.

The above-mentioned branches anastomose not only with their fellows of the opposite side but also with the external carotid artery via the meningeal branches, so that the collateral circulation of the cavernous portion of the internal carotid artery is comparatively rich and provides an important pathway in the occlusion of internal carotid artery below the cavernous sinus. In a case of caroticocavernous fistula these branches may be abnormally enlarged and are of diagnostic significance. In the surgical management of the caroticocavernous fistula, in addition to the ligature of the internal carotid artery, these branches have also to be ligated, lest it should be difficult to bring about a good result.

Venous tributaries of the cavernous sinus and their connections

The cavernous sinus connects directly or indirectly with the venous system of the orbit, brain and meninges by means of the superior and inferior ophthalmic veins, the middle and the inferior cerebral veins, and the sphenoparietal sinus respectively. The cavernous sinus also communicates with the transverse sinus via the superior petrosal sinus; with the internal jugular vein via the inferior petrosal sinus; with the v. angularis via the superior ophthalmic vein; with the pterygoid venous plexus by emissary veins passing through the foramen ovale, foramen lacerum, and foramen rotundum; and with the vertebral plexus by means of the basilar sinus.

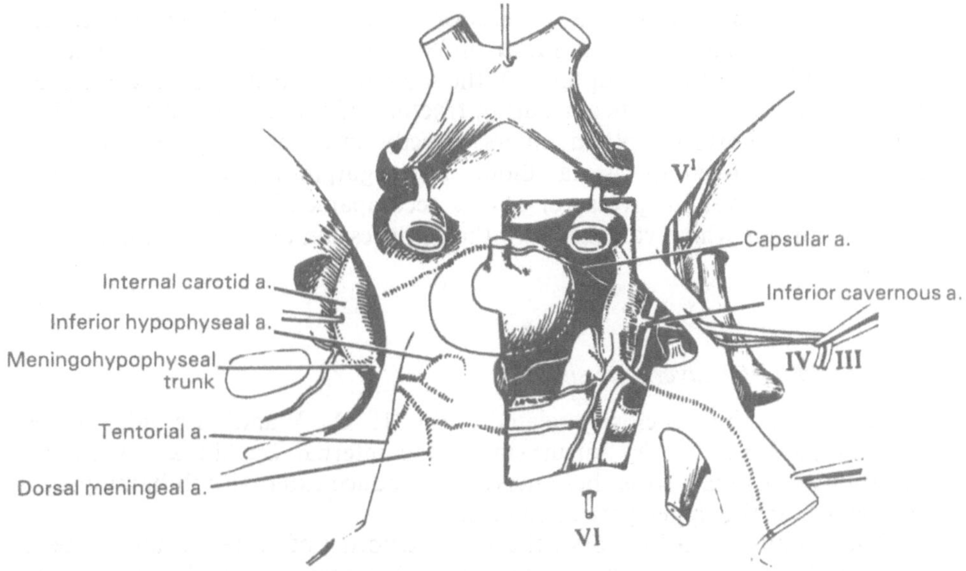

Figure 9.49 Internal carotid artery and its branches in the cavernous sinus

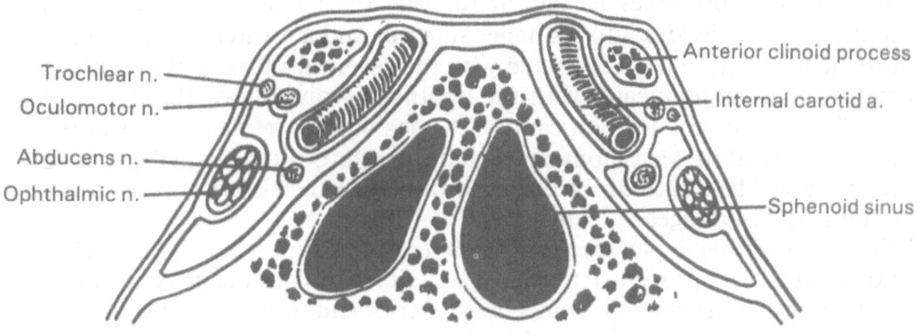

A. Frontal section through the anterior clinoid process

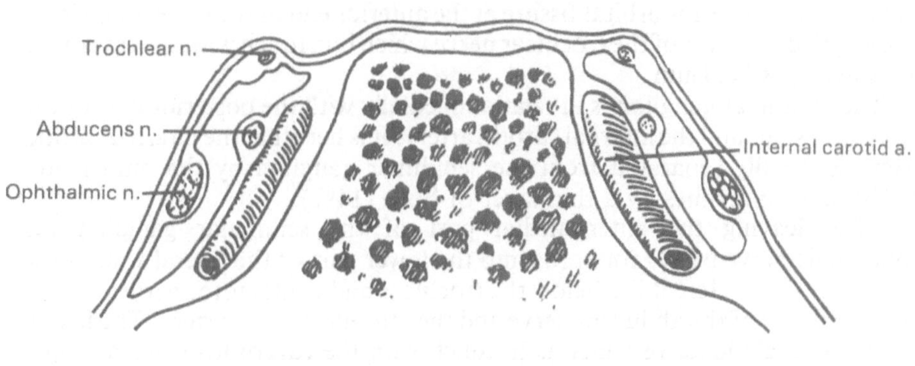

B. Frontal section through the posterior clinoid process

Figure 9.50 Frontal sections of the cavernous sinus

Owing to these extensive connections made by the cavernous sinus, inadvertent management of facial infections may lead to intracranial involvement. In case of rupture of the cavernous portion of the internal carotid artery and its branches during fracture of the middle portion of the base of skull, arterial blood enters directly into the sinus, resulting in cavernous arteriovenous fistula. Blood may regurgitate into the ophthalmic vein to raise its venous pressure. This is accompanied by exophthalmos and arterial murmur which vanishes with the compression of the common carotid artery.

Nerves within the cavernous sinus

The cavernous sinus is closely related to the III, IV, V and VI cranial nerves (Figures 9.49 and 9.50). Aneurysm of the internal carotid artery in the cavernous sinus may press these nerves to produce external ophthalmoplegia and pain over the upper part of the orbit.

The oculomotor nerve crosses the attached border of the tentorium cerebelli just lateral to the dorsum sellae. It pierces the inner layer of the dura mater just above the meningohypophyseal trunk midway between the anterior and posterior clinoid processes to the lateral wall of the cavernous sinus. The oculomotor nerve divides into a smaller superior and a greater inferior ramus. Before the bifurcation it is connected with the cavernous plexus by one or two filaments, and communicates with the ophthalmic division of the trigeminal nerve. The superior and inferior rami of the oculomotor nerve run forwards to the anterior end of the cavernous sinus, and enter the orbit through the superior orbital fissure. The length of the oculomotor nerve which is in contact with the cavernous sinus averages 9.3 mm.

The trochlear nerve pierces the inner layer of the dura mater a little behind the posterior clinoid process to reach the superior border of the petrous portion of the temporal bone where it enters the posterior end of the lateral wall of the cavernous sinus. It passes forward in the lateral wall below the oculomotor nerve and above the ophthalmic division of the trigeminal nerve. It then gradually ascends across the lateral side of the oculomotor nerve to its top side, and enters the superior orbital fissure at the anterior end of the cavernous sinus. The length of the part of the trochlear nerve which is in touch with the cavernous sinus averages 10.9 mm.

The semilunar ganglion is in relation medially with the posterior part of the cavernous sinus and the internal carotid artery. It is here that the internal carotid artery is usually separated from the semilunar ganglion by the dura mater (84%), and sometimes by a thin layer of bone (14%).

After leaving the anteromedial part of the semilunar ganglion the ophthalmic nerve passes forwards into the lower part of the lateral wall of the cavernous sinus. Here it lies below the trochlear and oculomotor nerves and on the lateral side of the abducent nerve and the internal carotid artery. The length of the ophthalmic nerve which is in touch with the cavernous sinus averages 15.8 mm. The ophthalmic nerve receives filaments from the cavernous plexus, and gives off the meningeal branch from its commencement, which runs backwards along the trochlear nerve to supply the tentorium cerebelli, and has three rami communicantes to connect with the oculomotor, trochlear and abducent nerves respectively.

The abducent nerve pierces the dura mater lateral to the dorsum sellae and proceeds close to the posterior surface of the apex of the petrous portion of the temporal bone. It crosses the inferior petrous sinus to its anterolateral aspect and then enters the cavernous sinus under the petrosphenoidal ligament. In the sinus it proceeds at first lateral to the ascending segment and then inferolateral to the horizontal segment of the internal carotid artery and enters the orbit through the superior orbital fissure. The length of the nerve in contact with the cavernous sinus averages 17.9 mm. Sometimes the abducent nerve is not a single trunk but splits into two to five filaments instead in the cavernous sinus.

Clinically the cavernous sinus may be divided into three parts: the anterior, middle and posterior ones (Figures 9.48 and 9.50). The anterior part is in front of the anterior clinoid process; the middle part resides between the anterior and posterior clinoid processes, and the posterior part behind the posterior clinoid process. The typical section of the cavernous sinus is made through its middle part. In the section are seen the oculomotor, trochlear, ophthalmic, and maxillary nerves arranged from above downwards on the lateral wall of the sinus. The maxillary nerve is close to the inferolateral corner of this section, and is formed by many small nerve bundles as is the ophthalmic nerve. The abducent nerve lies medial to the ophthalmic nerve and inferolateral to the internal carotid artery. The section of the anterior part of the sinus is similar to that of the middle part except for the fact that there is no maxillary nerve in this area and the trochlear nerve crosses the oculomotor nerve laterally from below to its upper side. In the section of the posterior part it can be seen that the trochlear nerve lies superiorly and the ophthalmic nerve lies below it in the lateral wall of the sinus, while the abducent nerve passes through the sinus and is attached to the lateral side of the internal carotid artery.

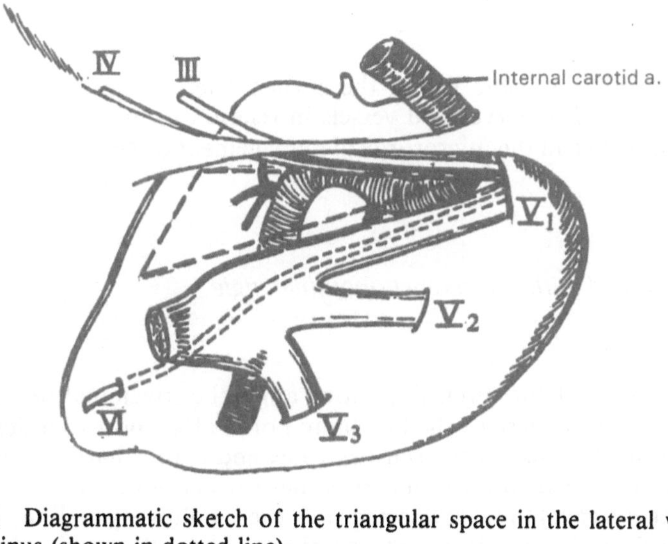

Figure 9.51 Diagrammatic sketch of the triangular space in the lateral wall of the cavernous sinus (shown in dotted line)

Parkinson (1965) described a triangular space (Figure 9.51) which is bounded above by the oculomotor and trochlear nerves, below by the abducent and ophthalmic nerves, and behind by the slope between the dorsum sellae and the clivus. According to the statistics made by Harris (1976), the superior margin of this space (formed by the inferior edge of the trochlear nerve) averages 13 (8–20) mm, the inferior margin (formed by the superior edge of the trigeminal nerve) averages 14 (5–24) mm, and the posterior margin averages 6 (3–14) mm. It is a favourable surgical approach to make an incision in this space for the exposure of the internal carotid artery and its branches without injury to the cranial nerves.

The intracavernous sympathetic nerves arise from the upper end of the superior cervical ganglion and surround the internal carotid artery to form the internal carotid plexus, which accompanies the artery to be continued as the cavernous plexus. In addition to the wall of the internal carotid artery, the cavernous plexus also supplies the pituitary gland. The cavernous plexus communicates with the oculomotor, trochlear, ophthalmic and abducent nerves and the ciliary ganglion.

Relationship between the cavernous sinus and the hypophysis

The cavernous sinus lies on either side of the hypophysis. The main distance between the medial margin of the intracavernous carotid artery and the lateral margin of the hypophysis is only 2.3 mm with a maximum of 7 mm. The carotid artery may sometimes protrude out of the medial wall of the sinus to be embedded in the hypophysis (28%) to alter the shape of the gland. Sometimes a tongue-like projection of the hypophysis extends above or below the carotid artery. These anatomical features may add difficulties to hypophysectomy.

Cerebellopontine angle

The cerebellopontine angle lies at the corner where the medulla, pons and cerebellum meet. The nerves and vessels in relation to this angle are of great clinical significance in the microsurgical management of acoustic tumours and the like.

Nerves concerned with the cerebellopontine angle

Trigeminal nerve

In the upper part of the cerebellopontine angle the trigeminal nerve emerges from the brain at the base of the brachium pontis. Its motor root lies superior to the anteromedial side of the sensory root, and is thus hardly visible in the suboccipital approach. Both roots cross the petrous ridge into the trigeminal cavity (Meckel's cave) to be connected with the semilunar ganglion. Not a few authors considered that trigeminal neuralgia may be the result of a mild or severe deformity of this nerve which is due to its compression by the superior cerebellar artery or its branches. The trigeminal nerve is in touch with the superior cerebellar artery in 51.5% of the case, with the middle inferior cerebellar artery in 27.3%, and with the anterior inferior cerebellar artery in 21.2%.

Stephen and his associates found at autopsy that in those who had suffered from trigeminal neuralgia, the nerve was in touch with the artery in 85%, of which 90% showed evidence of compression.

In about half of these cases a trigeminal artery may also be present. It arises from the upper or middle segment of the basilar artery and runs posterolaterally along the basilar part of the pons to the root of the trigeminal nerve. It then divides into branches running along the trigeminal nerve, some of which may anastomose with the trigeminal branches of the anterior, middle or posterior inferior cerebellar artery. Caution should be taken in severing the trigeminal nerve.

Abducent nerve

The abducent nerve emerges from the brain in the furrow between the lower border of the pons and the upper end of the pyramid of the medulla oblongata. The nerve sometimes has two roots: the superior and inferior ones (16.7%). After leaving the brain it proceeds forwards and superolaterally into the subarachnoid space, where it remains between the pons and clivus along the lateral side of the basilar artery. Here it is crossed ventrally (73%) or dorsally (23.5%) by the anterior inferior cerebellar artery. The artery passes between the two roots of the nerve only in 3.5%. When the artery lies behind the nerve it may press the nerve against the clivus.

Facial and vestibulocochlear nerves

The root of the facial nerve lies lateral to the root of the abducent nerve, and emerges from the surface of the brain between the lower border of the pons and the olive. The nervus intermedius of the facial nerve lies between the motor root of the facial nerve and the root of the vestibulocochlear nerve. The root of the vestibulocochlear nerve lies posterolateral to the facial nerve. The vestibular nerve lies medially between the olive and the inferior cerebellar peduncle while the cochlear nerve lies laterally and attached to the posterolateral aspect of the peduncle. The vestibulocochlear nerve accompanies the facial nerve closely to the internal acoustic meatus, where the facial nerve lies ventral to the vestibulocochlear nerve. In an occipital approach the facial nerve is not visible, being entirely hidden by the vestibulocochlear nerve. When the facial and vestibulocochlear nerves pierce the meninges, they are enclosed within a sheath formed by the arachnoid, and dura mater, which extends to the internal acoustic meatus together with the corresponding spaces.

The length of the facial and vestibulocochlear nerves from the brain stem to the internal acoustic meatus averages 10–13 mm. The length of the part within the meatus is about 9–12 mm. Most acoustic tumours originate from the part of the vestibular nerve that is within the meatus. Near the internal acoustic meatus the motor root of the facial nerve lies in a furrow just above and anterior to the vestibulocochlear nerve. The intermediate nerve is sandwiched between the root of the vestibulocochlear nerve and the root of the facial nerve. At the middle of the meatus the intermediate nerve joins the motor root of the facial nerve to form a common trunk, which crosses the anterior aspect of the vestibulocochlear nerve to its upper side at the distal end of the meatus (Figure 9.52). At the bottom of the meatus the facial nerve and the superior branch of the vestibular nerve are transmitted through the anterior and posterior parts of the superior vestibular area respectively, the cochlear nerve and the inferior branch of the vestibular nerve are transmitted through the anterior and posterior part of the inferior vestibular area, and the posterior part of the inferior area is transmitted by the posterior ampullar nerve of the vestibular nerve.

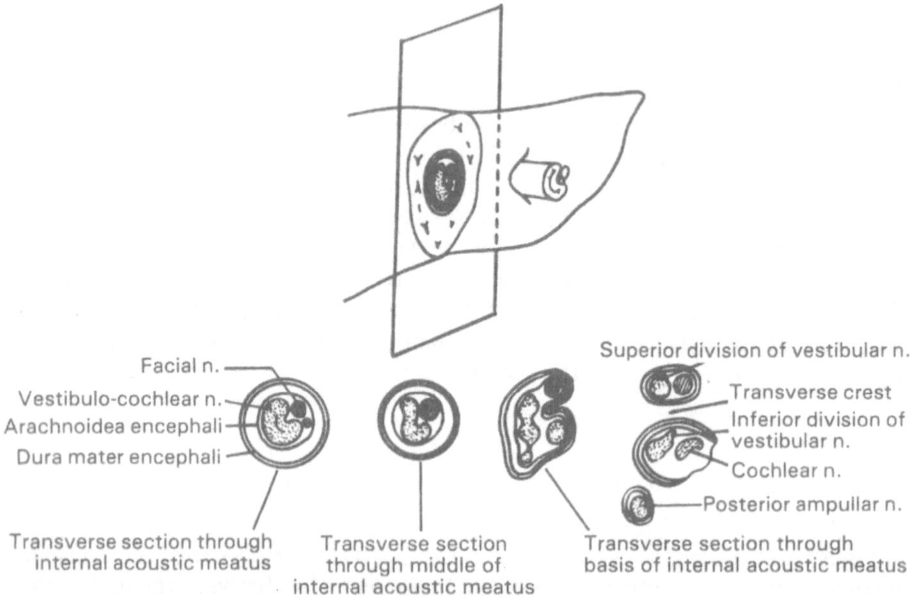

Figure 9.52 Topographical relations of the facial and vestibulocochlear nerves within the internal acoustic meatus

Glossopharyngeal nerve

The glossopharyngeal nerve emerges from a groove between the olive and the inferior cerebellar peduncle by five or six filaments just below the roots of the facial and vestibulocochlear nerves and above those of the vagus. The filaments of the glossopharyngeal nerve gather up laterally to form a trunk in front of the flocculus. It runs anterolaterally with the vagus and accessory nerves and leaves the skull through the jugular foramen. The jugular foramen may be divided into a smaller anteromedial part (neural part) and a greater posterolateral part (venous part). The former transmits the glossopharyngeal nerve; the latter transmits the internal jugular bulb and the vagus and accessory nerves.

These two parts are usually separated by a fibrous or bony partition in about 7% of cases. The dura mater covering the jugular foramen possesses two corresponding apertures. One is the glossopharyngeal aperture, which is funnel-shaped with its apex towards the outside of the skull. Through it the glossopharyngeal nerve enters the neural part. The other is the vagal aperture, through which the vagus and accessory nerves enter the venous part, and is located anteromedial to the jugular bulb. These two apertures are usually separated by a dural partition 0.5 mm thick, which is formed by the continuation of the inferior petrosal sinus or the adhesion of the walls of this sinus.

The length of the glossopharyngeal nerve from the brain stem to the dura mater averages 17.6 mm, its diameter being 0.4–1.1 mm. This nerve is usually fused by a dorsal and a ventral part. The ventral part is relatively small, representing motor fibres, while the larger dorsal part contains sensory fibres.

Vagus and accessory nerves

The vagus nerve emerges from the groove between the olive and the inferior cerebellar peduncle by 8–10 rootlets which lie below the roots of the glossopharyngeal nerve. The cranial roots of the accessory nerve are attached to the brain stem by four or five rootlets below the roots of the vagus nerve. The accessory nerve passes through the arachnoid and dura mater, and is enclosed with the vagus nerve by a dural sheath, in which the cranial and spinal roots of the accessory nerve join to form a short trunk passing through the posterolateral part of the jugular foramen (the venous part). The length of the vagus nerve from the brain stem to the dura mater averages 17.1 (12–22.9) mm. Its diameter is 0.1–1.5 mm.

Vessels in relation to the cerebellopontine angle

The posterior inferior cerebellar artery

This artery ascends tortuously to the ventral side of the roots of the glossopharyngeal, vagus and accessory nerves, loops dorsally at various levels between the anterior margin of the glossopharyngeal nerve and the posterior margin of the accessory nerve, and descends along the lateral surface of the medulla oblongata and the inferior surface of the cerebellum. The loop passing through the rootlets of the vagus nerve to turn backwards is more frequently observed and represents 52.7%; that located at the anterior margin of the roots of the glossopharyngeal nerve occurs in 20.0%, and that between the roots of the glossopharyngeal and vagus nerves accounts for 27.3% (Figure 9.53). The posterior inferior cerebellar artery sometimes possesses a low origin, that is, it passes from between the cranial and spinal roots of the accessory nerve to ascend close to the restiform body, and then descend to form a loop. This loop (the lateral loop of the medulla oblongata) is usually convex superolaterally within the boundary of the cerebellopontine angle. Therefore, great care must be taken to deal with the loop during operation. Moreover, in about 13.7% of cases this loop is in touch with the facial and vestibulocochlear nerves.

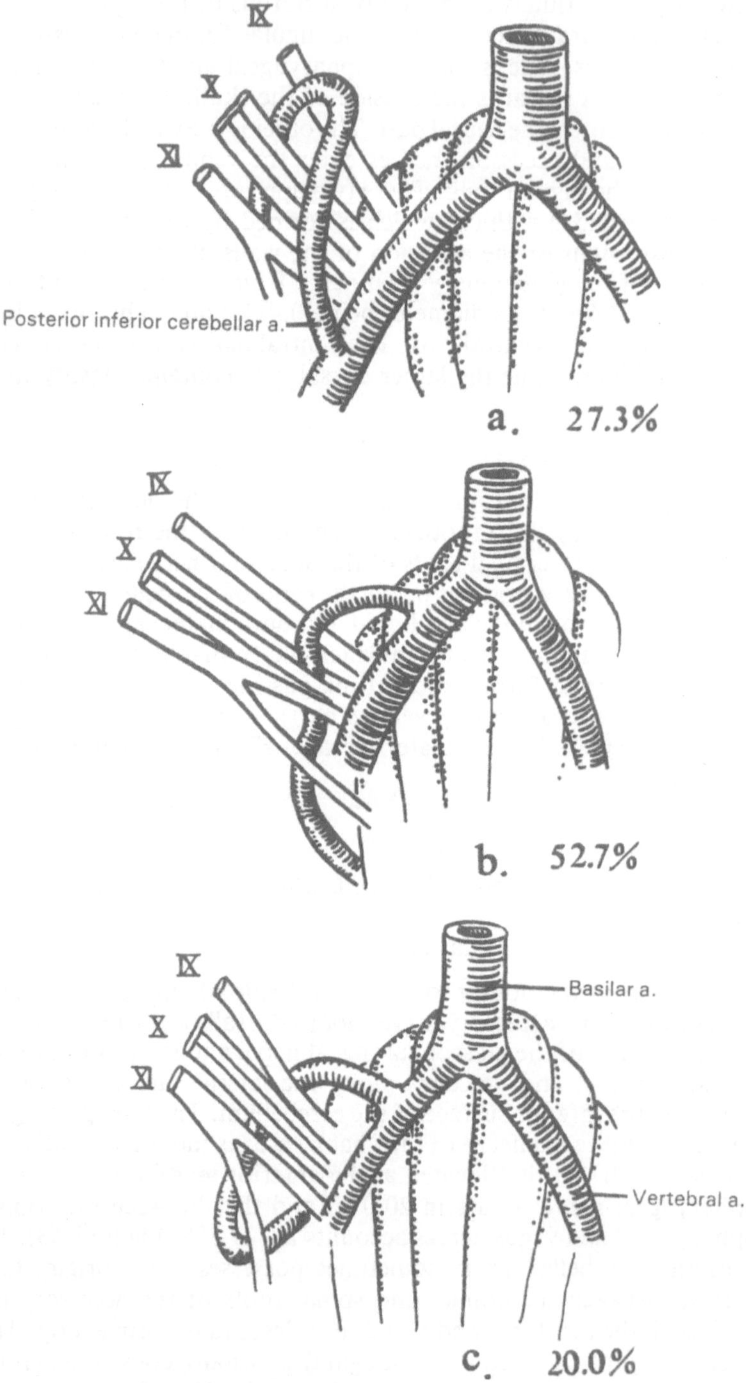

Figure 9.53 Topographical relations between the posterior inferior cerebellar artery and the IX and X cranial nerves

Ouaknine and his associates (1980) found a case in which the lateral loop of the posterior inferior cerebellar artery pressed the intermediate and vestibulocochlear nerves to cause neuralgia of the geniculate ganglion and disturbances of vestibular and auditory functions.

The outer diameter of the posterior inferior cerebellar artery at its commencement averages 1.6 mm, and most of them are equal on both sides.

The anterior inferior cerebellar artery

This artery runs backwards and laterally after arising from the lower one-third of the basilar artery. It lies usually ventral to the abducent nerve. A few of them pass dorsal to or from between the two roots of the nerve. The anterior inferior cerebellar artery or its anterolateral branch passes ventral (50.6%) or dorsal (10.5%) to the facial and vestibulocochlear nerves, or from between the two nerves (39%). Superolateral to the brachium pontis and flocculus, it forms loops of internal acoustic meatus and brachium pontis. The former is constant in position and its summit may extend to the internal acoustic meatus (22%) or even into it (14%) (Figure 9.54). The latter is in touch with the posterolateral surface of the root of the trigeminal nerve in 22%, the distance between them being 1-10 mm. Some held that the summit of this loop may serve as a mark in the angiogram for the localization of the trigeminal nerve. The summit of the loop is apart from the root of the trigeminal nerve within 6 mm in 67.4%. Owing to the close relationship between the anterior inferior cerebellar artery and the facial and vestibulocochlear nerves, reciprocal compressive symptoms may occur between the artery and nerves.

The outer diameter of the anterior inferior cerebellar artery averages 1.2 mm and is mostly equal on both sides (58.6%).

Labyrinthine artery (internal auditory artery)

The labyrinthine artery usually arises from the anterior inferior cerebellar artery. A few may arise from the basilar artery, the posterior inferior cerebellar artery or the common trunk of the anterior and posterior inferior cerebellar arteries. If it arises from the basilar artery it accompanies the facial and vestibulocochlear nerves into the internal acoustic meatus; if it arises from the anterior inferior cerebellar artery it usually commences from the summit of the loop within or near the internal acoustic meatus and passes between the facial and vestibulocochlear nerves to the bottom of the meatus where it sends some branches to the inner ear. Two labyrinthine arteries may be present on either side. One of them arises from the basilar artery and the other from the anterior inferior cerebellar artery.

Variations in the anterior inferior cerebellar and labyrinthine arteries are very important in operations on the cerebellopontine angle. Since the anterior inferior cerebellar and labyrinthine arteries are the main blood supply for the pons and upper part of the medulla oblongata, injury to these arteries even at the level of the internal acoustic meatus may lead to infarction of the brain stem.

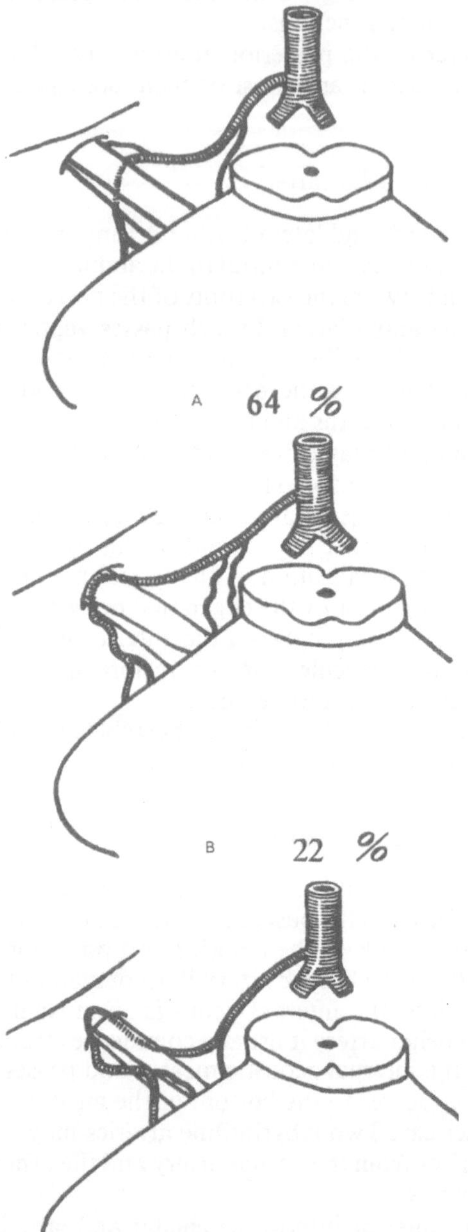

Figure 9.54 Topographical relation between the anterior inferior cerebellar artery and the internal acoustic meatus (after Salahs)

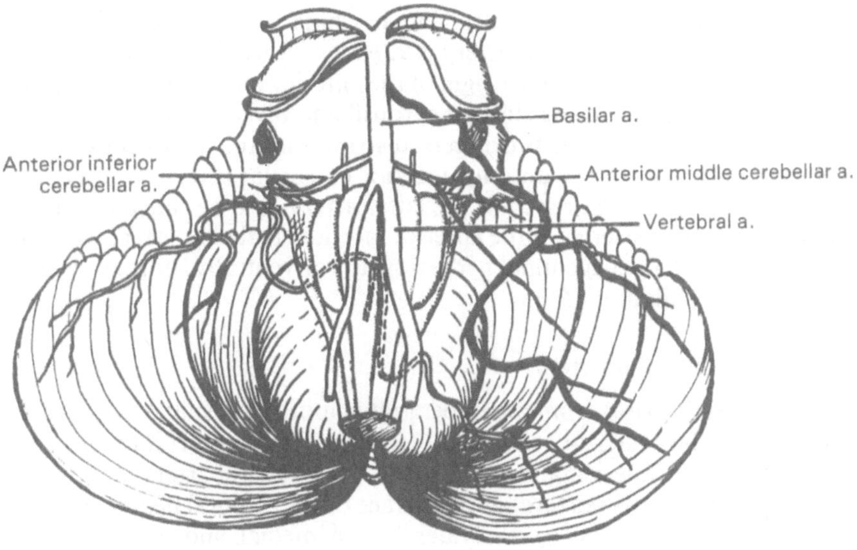

I. Middle inferior cerebellar artery in contact with the ventral surface of the trigeminal nerve

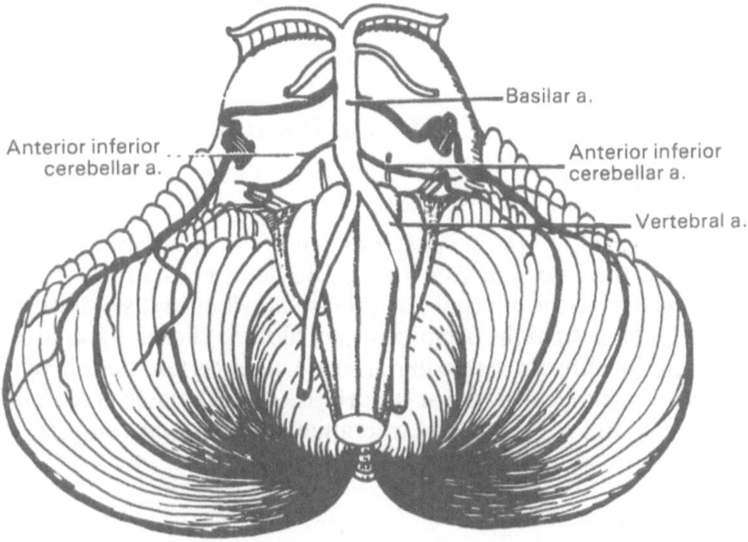

II. Middle inferior cerebellar artery in contact with the dorsal surface of the trigeminal nerve

Figure 9.55 Relation between the middle inferior cerebellar artery and the trigeminal nerve

Middle inferior cerebellar artery

A comprehensive study of anatomical data in China indicates that the incidence of the middle inferior cerebellar artery is 9.0% on either side. It arises from the basilar artery above or below the origin of the anterior inferior cerebellar artery, and sends off branches to the flocculus, tonsil and biventer lobule of the cerebellum. Judging from either its origin or distribution, the middle inferior cerebellar artery is a part of the anterior inferior cerebellar artery. Consequently, it may be considered as a branch of the latter artery, and be called the superior or inferior accessory arteries of the anterior inferior cerebellar artery. It is sometimes in touch with the trigeminal nerve dorsally or ventrally, or may even wind round the nerve (Figure 9.55).

The superior cerebellar artery

This artery mainly arises from the upper segment of the basilar artery proximal to the origin of the posterior cerebral artery. It usually winds round the cerebral peduncle below the lower margin of the posterior cerebral artery and then proceeds backward. On the posterolateral surface of the cerebral peduncle or in the lateral mesencephalic sulcus, it divides into a medial and a lateral branch (80.1%) or into three branches, i.e. the middle, intermediate and lateral branches. If there are two superior cerebellar arteries the upper one corresponds to the medial branch, while the lower one corresponds to the lateral branch. The lateral branch is usually smaller. It runs on the posterolateral surface of the root of the trigeminal nerve and gives off a twig to the root. The outer diameter of the superior cerebellar artery averages 1.5 mm. Most of them are equal in size bilaterally.

APPLIED ANATOMY OF THE INTRA-EXTRACRANIAL ANASTOMOSIS

ZHANG WEILONG AND ZHENG ZHILIANG

Recently the superficial temporal, posterior auricular or occipital artery has often been selected for anastomosis with the middle cerebral artery in surgical treatment of ischaemia in the internal carotid system, while in cases of ischaemia of the vertebrobasilar system the occipital artery alone is chosen for anastomosing with the posterior inferior cerebellar artery. Under certain definite circumstances the middle meningeal artery or the arteries of the greater omentum may also be used as the donor for intra-extracranial vascular anastomosis.

Arteries of the scalp

Superficial temporal artery

The superficial temporal artery is a terminal branch of the external carotid artery. It begins behind the neck of the mandible, lying deep to the parotid gland, and crosses over the root of the zygomatic process to ascend for about

20–30 cm above the zygomatic arch, where it divides into an anterior and a posterior branch. The site of bifurcation is above the level of the supraorbital margin in 65%, and below this in 35%. The stem of the superficial temporal artery directing anterosuperiorly forms an angle of 0–40° with the vertical line. The outer diameter of its initial segment averages about 2.6 mm.

Anterior or frontal branch

The anterior branch is larger than the posterior (67%). The outer diameter averages 1.8 mm. It arises mostly at an angle of 15–45° with the vertical line (58%), or at an angle of 0–15° (21%) or 45–90° (21%), to incline forwards and upwards. It curves upwards above the superolateral angle of the orbit or near the frontal eminence to the vertex of the skull. The degree of the angle is related to the level of the bifurcation. When the bifurcation is at a higher level the angle will be obtuse and the anterior branch tends to run horizontally. If the bifurcation is at a lower level the angle will be acute and the anterior branch will tend to run vertically. Most of the anterior branches cross superficial to the frontalis and galea aponeurotica (82%); few of them have a segment piercing deep to the frontalis (12%). The anterior branch gives off vertically two to five fronto-occipital branches, which pass backwards to supply the vertex of the skull. Of these some may have a diameter of over 1 mm and account for 82%. The anterior branch again gives off one to four small fronto-orbital branches directed downwards and forwards to the vicinity of the orbit to anastomose with branches of the ophthalmic artery.

The posterior or parietal branch

This is relatively small: its outer diameter averages about 1.7 mm. It arises at an angle to 0–70° (about 30° on average) with the vertical line and inclines backwards and upwards over the surface of the temporal fascia to reach the parietal eminence. In 67% of cases the posterior branch is of the main trunk type, running tortuously to the centre of the vertex and giving off fine branches to either side along its course to anastomose with the anterior branch of the superficial temporal artery, the branches of the occipital artery and the fellow of the opposite side. The dispersed type of the posterior branch occurs in 27%. They divide into the supra- and infraparietal branches above the level of the superior orbital margin; the former passes above or in front of the parietal eminence to the vertex of the skull, while the latter runs to the parietal eminence. The bifurcating type lacks the trunk of the posterior branch and occurs in 6%; its supra- and infraparietal branches arise directly from the superficial temporal artery, or the infraparietal branch arises from the superficial temporal artery, while the supraparietal branch arises from the anterior branch.

The postoperative angiogram of an intra-extracranial anastomosis demonstrates that the calibre of the branches of the anastomosed superficial temporal artery is enlarged. Kletter *et al.* (1976) studied sections of the aortic arch, the bifurcation of the common carotid artery, the siphon of the internal carotid artery, the middle cerebral and superficial temporal arteries from 50 cadavers. They also made histological observations of the segments of superficial temporal artery collected from more than 200 cases of craniotomy, and found that the arteriosclerotic changes in the superficial temporal artery differed from those of other vessels mainly in the increment of elastic laminae and thickening of the arterial wall, which was capable of dilatation. Calcification was present in only five out of 250 cases of superficial temporal artery. However, the rest of the arteries were accompanied by calcification and lipid deposition in their wall, which resulted in the constriction of the lumen and incapability of dilation. Thus, the superficial temporal artery is an ideal donor for intra-extracranial anastomosis.

Posterior auricular artery

The posterior auricular artery is a small branch of the external carotid artery arising at the level of the superior margin of the digastric muscle or sharing a common trunk with the occipital artery. It runs upwards and backwards, and divides between the auricle and the mastoid process into an auricular and an occipital branch to supply the cranial surface of the auricle and the scalp above and behind the ear. The outer diameter of this artery measured above the level of the supraorbital margin is over 0.8 mm in only 15% of cases.

Occipital artery

The occipital artery arises from the posterior wall of the external carotid artery and passes backwards and upwards deep to the lower border of the posterior belly of the digastric muscle to the occipital groove of the temporal bone. In most cases it pierces the fascia between the attachments of the sternomastoid and trapezius (61%), or passes through the fibres of the attachment of the trapezius (22%) or those of the sternomastoid (17%) to the subcutaneous tissue. It lies 2–3 cm below the external occipital protuberance and 3–4 cm apart from the mid-line. The artery gives off branches on the way to the sternomastoid and the muscles of the nape. It then ascends tortuously in the superficial fascia to supply the scalp. At the level of the supraorbital margin the occipital artery has mostly only one main trunk (76%); a few of them may divide into two (23%) or three (1%) branches. The calibres of these arteries are more than 1.1 mm.

Measurements of the calibres of the superficial temporal posterior auricular and occipital arteries where craniotomy performed

Chater *et al.* (1976) indicated that the diameter of the artery which is used for intra-extracranial anastomosis should not be less than 1.0 mm. In order to offer, for reference sake, values of the calibres of the arteries mentioned above, which are useful in craniotomy, Zhong Shizhen *et al.* designated several areas on the skull for measurement (Figure 9.56). The calibres of the anterior and posterior branches of the superficial temporal, posterior auricular and occipital arteries are shown in Table 9.1, from which it is thus clear that, above points A and B, the vast majority of calibres of the anterior and posterior branches

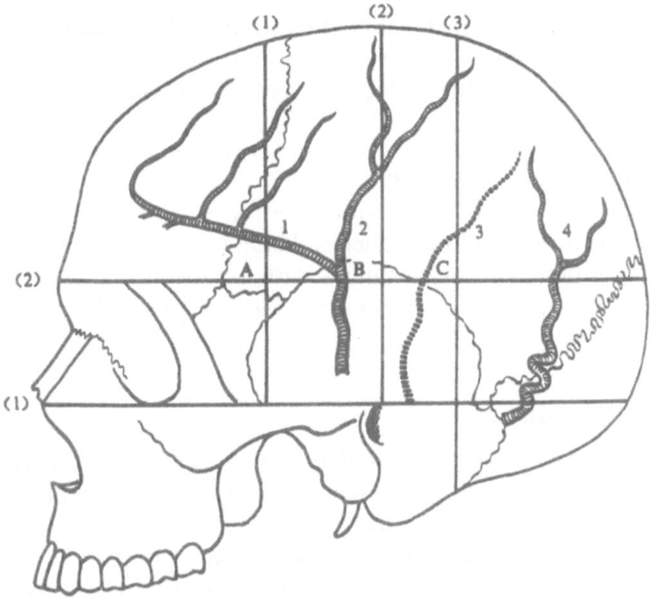

Figure 9.56 Areas for the measurement of the superficial temporal, posterior auricular and occipital arteries. **1**: Anterior branch of superficial temporal artery; **2**: posterior branch of superficial temporal artery; **3**: posterior auricular artery; **4**: occipital artery. *Horizontal lines*: (1) Line joining the infraorbital margin with the superior margin of the external acoustic meatus. (2) Horizontal line passing through the supraorbital margin and parallel with (1). *Vertical lines*: (1) Vertical line passing through the midpoint of the superior margin of the zygomatic arch. (2) Vertical line passing through the midpoint of the upper margin of the external acoustic opening. (3) Vertical line passing through the posterior basic point of the mastoid process

Table 9.1 The measurement of the calibres of 100 cases of the arteries of the scalp (percentage standard error)

Calibre (mm)	*Anterior branch of superficial temporal artery*	*Posterior branch of superficial temporal artery*	*Posterior auricular artery*	*Occipital artery*
0.8–1.0	4.0 ± 2.0	4.0 ± 2.0	2.0 ± 1.4	
1.1–1.3	19.0 ± 3.9	18.0 ± 3.8	10.0 ± 3.0	24.0 ± 4.3
1.4–1.6	25.0 ± 4.3	21.0 ± 4.1		26.0 ± 4.4
1.7–1.9	24.0 ± 4.3	35.0 ± 4.8	3.0 ± 1.7	30.0 ± 4.6
2.0–2.2	22.0 ± 4.1	17.0 ± 3.8		17.0 ± 3.8
2.3–2.5	3.0 ± 1.7	3.0 ± 1.7		3.0 ± 1.7
2.6–2.8	3.0 ± 1.7	2.0 ± 1.4		

of the superficial temporal artery are over 1.0 mm. These two branches are also constant in localization, and differ from other arteries histologically in being capable of forming a compensatory dilatation after anastomosis. Therefore they are good donors for intra–extracranial anastomosis. However, in rare cases they give off many branches, which are very divergent or are provided with small calibres. These may add difficulty to surgical manoeuvre or may result in inadequate compensation after anastomosis. A suitable artery in the adjacent area should then be used instead.

The posterior auricular artery is mostly too small to serve as a donor.

The occipital artery and its branches, being large in calibre and constant in position, are suitable for anastomosis with the posterior inferior cerebellar artery, the angular artery or the posterior temporal artery of the middle cerebral artery.

Middle meningeal artery

In the vast majority (94%), the middle meningeal artery arises from the first segment of the maxillary artery. It ascends between the lateral pterygoid muscle and the sphenomandibular ligament and enters the cranial cavity through the foramen spinosum. The length of its trunk averages 17 mm. The outer diameter is about 2.0 mm. After entering the skull it passes forwards to divide, within a range of 20 mm (51.8%) or 20–45 mm (48.2%), into a frontal and a parietal branch. The frontal branch, being larger, runs forwards and upwards from the mid-point of the zygomatic arch to assume a backward concave course. It crosses the greater wing of the sphenoid and the anteroinferior angle of the parietal bone, and then ascends for a short distance behind the anterior border of the parietal bone to ramify into several branches. Some of them reach the vertex of the skull, while others reach the occipital region. When the frontal branch passes near the pterion it ofen courses through a bony canal (60%), the length of which averages 10 mm. When the dura mater is to be separated from the skull in this region the middle meningeal artery may be torn, and bleeding ensues. The parietal branch, being slightly smaller than the frontal, runs backwards and upwards on the inner surface of the squamous part of the temporal bone. On reaching the posteroinferior angle of the parietal bone it divides into branches to supply the posterior part of the dura mater and the cranium (Figure 9.57).

An accessory meningeal artery sometimes arises from the middle meningeal artery before the latter enters the foramen spinosum, or directly from the maxillary artery. The artery enters the cranium through the foramen ovale, and supplies the trigeminal ganglion and the adjacent dura mater. Its outer diameter averages 1.0 mm.

The bifurcation of the middle meningeal artery is 1.2 cm above the midpoint of the zygomatic arch. The frontal branch runs upwards and forwards to the pterion and then turns backwards midway between the inion and nasion. Its main trunk is parallel to the paracentral gyrus. The parietal branch proceeds upwards and backwards to the lambda. The surface projection of the bony canal is within the range from 4 mm below to 19 mm above point A. In most cases its highest level is above point A.

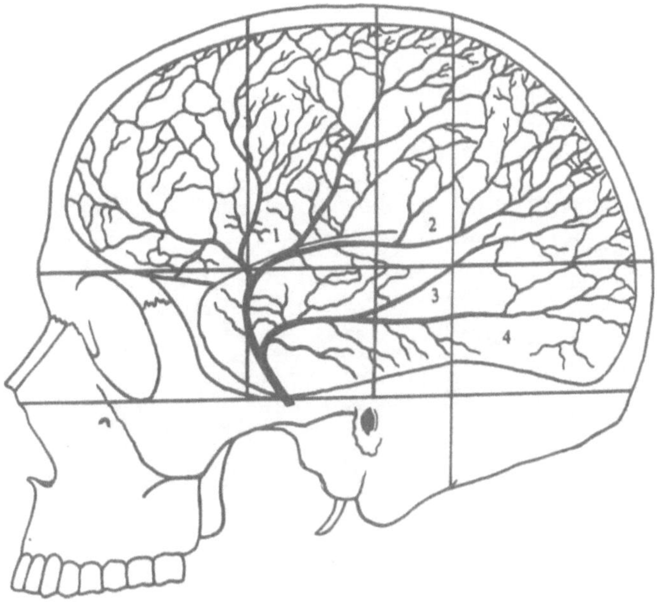

Figure 9.57 A schematic diagram showing the middle meningeal artery and the site for cranial fenestration. **1**: Frontal branch of middle meningeal a.; **2**: posterior ramus of frontal branch of middle meningeal a.; **3**: anterior ramus of parietal branch of middle meningeal a.; **4**: posterior ramus of parietal branch of middle meningeal a.

Cranial fenestration has been used over points A, B and C for observation of the calibres and branches of the middle meningeal artery. The results are as follows. Most of the posterior rami of the frontal branch of the meningeal artery (63%) can be met with within the fenestra 6 cm above the external auditory meatus, which measures 3 × 3 cm and is commonly used in clinical practice. The frontal branch and the anterior ramus of the parietal branch can be seen in the fenestrae over point A (65%) and point C (57%) respectively. The outer diameter of the arteries, which is more than 1.0 mm, accounts for 98%, 82% and 70% of the cases over points A, B and C respectively. Only in 1–8% of the cases can branches with a calibre less tha 0.6 mm be met with in these fenestrae. Generally, branches of the middle meningeal artery located in the above-mentioned fenestrae become gradually smaller from the front backwards. However, the vast majority of them are more than 1.0 mm in diameter.

Since the middle meningeal artery which arises from the external carotid artery keeps close to the dorsolateral surface of the cerebral hemisphere within the cranial cavity (Figure 9.58) and possesses a thin wall and a large calibre, it can also be used as a donor in intra-extracranial anastomosis under certain circumstances. Recently, the middle meningeal-middle cerebral arterial anastomosis (MMA-MCA) has been carried out with good results in China and abroad. Mishikawa indicated that if the superficial temporal or occipital artery is not suitable for a donor, the middle meningeal artery may then be adopted. The latter has some advantages: postoperative ischaemic necrosis of the scalp

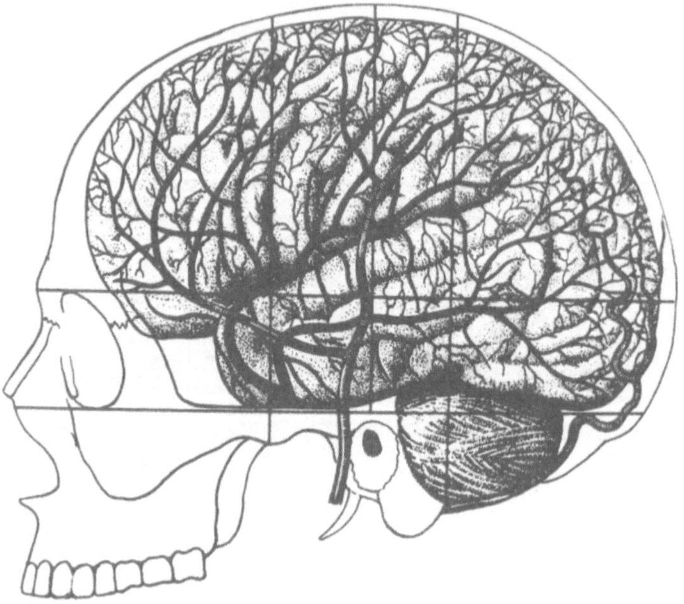

Figure 9.58 Diagram of the superficial temporal, occipital, middle meningeal and middle cerebral arteries

can be avoided; the middle meningeal artery can be more easily exposed and is nearer to the middle cerebral artery, so that anastomosis can readily be performed after dissecting a short segment of this vessel; the wall of the middle meningeal artery is thinner, being nearly equal to that of the middle cerebral artery. These add convenience to vascular anastomosis with no bad effect on cranioplasty. The only shortcoming is that the middle meningeal artery and its branches usually adhere firmly to the dura mater and are not easy to separate from it, so that they are often subject to injury during craniotomy.

Vessels of the greater omentum

In 1973 Goldsmith transplanted the pedicled greater omentum onto the surface of the cerebrum of a dog through a thoracocervical subcutaneous tunnel. When the dog was sacrificed 9 months later, vascular anastomosis between the vessels of the omentum and the brain had been established. Consequently, on the basis of animal experiments, in 1976 he performed the intracranial transplantation of pedicled omentum in three patients who suffered from ischaemic stroke with aphasia and improved in neurological functions. Since 1980 this operation has been carried out in China with satisfactory results.

Either the transference of pedicled omentum or the transplantation of free omentum by means of microsurgical technique is in close relation to the anatomy of the vascular distribution in the greater omentum.

Middle cerebral artery

Patterns of branches of the middle cerebral artery

The stem of the middle cerebral artery runs in the depth of the lateral cerebral sulcus and ramifies near the insula to supply the cerebral cortex. There are three types of branching: truncal, bifurcated, and trifurcated types. Of the latter two types the arteries supplying the temporal lobe and the angular artery usually arise from their inferior trunk. The distinctions between these types are concerned with the selection of cortical artery for anastomosis in case of occlusion or stenosis of the middle cerebral artery. For example, if occlusion or stenosis occurs at the superior trunk (or the middle trunk) or its branches, the donor must be anastomosed with the cortical arteries above the lateral cerebral sulcus or with those in the ischaemic area, but not those below the lateral sulcus in order to prevent the blood from flowing into the segment proximal to the occlusion or stenosis without proper effect. Consequently, when it is necessary to carry out an intra-extracranial anastomosis to relieve an occlusion or stenosis of the middle cerebral artery, one should first of all make a precise localization of the occlusion followed by the choice of an appropriate cortical artery as the recipient.

Number of cortical branches of the middle cerebral artery

The cortical branches of the middle cerebral artery emerge from the lateral cerebral sulcus to the dorsolateral surface of the cerebral hemisphere. Some of these cortical branches or their rami can be clearly seen on the surface of the hemisphere, while others are hidden in the depth of the sulci. Most of the temporal polar arteries distributed to the temporal pole are located in the shallow sulci of the temporal pole; only 20% of them appear on the surface of the hemisphere. Other arteries are relatively constant, being mostly visible near the lateral cerebral sulcus. Of these the orbitofrontal arteries distributed to the anterior part of the frontal lobe are usually one or two in number in 75%, and three in 18%; the anterior temporal arteries distributed to the temporal lobe are also frequently one or two in number in 82%, and three in 17%. Most of the precentral, central, postcentral and middle temporal arteries are one or two in number in about 95% of the cases, few of them being three in number (1–2%). The posterior parietal angular and posterior temporal arteries, which supply the posterior part of the parietal lobe, the occipital lobe and the posterior part of the temporal lobe, are mostly single, only a few of them being two in number or invisible on the surface. In brief, there are more cortical branches in the area anterior to the lateral cerebral sulcus and fewer in the area posterior to the sulcus. It must be pointed out that the central artery runs obliquely from behind forwards and crosses those gyri which shut up the central sulcus. It then enters the sulcus, coursing along the anterior or posterior margin. The angular artery assumes a curve convex downward when crossing the superior temporal gyrus. The posterior temporal artery emerges from the posterior end of the lateral cerebral sulcus and soon divides after descending obliquely across the posterior part of the superior temporal gyrus. Since these three arteries are constant in course and position, they are easily recognized during operation.

Outer diameter of the cortical branches of the middle cerebral artery

The calibre of the cortical branches is an important criterion in the selection of arteries in the donee. Chater *et al.* (1976) measured the calibres of the cortical branches of the middle cerebral artery and proposed that the angular artery be the thickest and best donee for intra-extracranial anastomosis. Based on Chinese data it has been found that of the cortical branches above the lateral cerebral sulcus the orbitofrontal artery is relatively small and only 59% of them have an outer diameter larger than or equal to 1.0 mm, so that it can seldom be chosen as a donee. The outer diameter of more than 80% of the precentral, central, postcentral and inferior parietal arteries exceeds or equals 1.0 mm. This is especially true of that of the central artery, which may exceed or be equal to 1.0 mm in about 90% of cases. These arteries are mostly thick and suitable for being a donee vessel. Of those arteries below the lateral cerebral sulcus the temporal polar artery is usually hidden in the sulcus and few of its small branches are visible, so that it cannot be chosen as the donee. The posterior temporal and angular arteries are very large, their outer diameter being 1.0 mm in more than 95% of cases; they are good donee vessels. The outer diameters of the anterior and middle temporal arteries are 1.0 mm in 63% and 85% respectively. They can be selected as the donee under certain circumstances. The angular and posterior temporal arteries have been chosen as donee vessels for a long time. From the point of view of their thickness they are reliable for this purpose. However, some authors hold that in a case of occlusion or stenosis of the internal carotid artery, the anterior temporal artery, which is near the proximal segment of the middle cerebral artery and below the lateral sulcus, is a better choice. The reason is that when the internal carotid artery is occluded the brain is supplied by the ophthalmic or the anterior and posterior communicating arteries, in which the blood flow is antegrade. When anastomosis is performed near the proximal segment of the middle cerebral artery the direction of the blood flow in the collateral circulation is the same as that from outside the skull. This will be in favour of the blood supply of the ischaemic area and the extension of the supplied area. Nevertheless, since the anterior temporal artery is deeply located and is difficult to manipulate, it may be selected depending on circumstances.

10

The microsurgical anatomy of peripheral nerves

ZHONG SHIZHEN, TAO XIANGLUO AND LIU MUZHI

INTRODUCTION

The traditional treatment for severed peripheral nerve was the epineural suture, but the result was unsatisfactory. Based on the anatomical studies on the internal structures of the peripheral nerve trunk, Langley (1917) and Sunderland (1953) suggested the idea of funicular suture, whence the possibility of raising the effect of operative treatment was recognized theoretically. Nevertheless, this idea could not be carried out until the microsurgical technique was developed. Subsequently, Smith, Kurze, and Michon (1964) first applied the microsurgical technique to the repairment of the peripheral nerve. Millesi *et al.* (1972) reported good results of funicular suture. Zhu Jiakai (1973–79) performed a funicular suture and nerve graft in China, and analysed its long-term effect. At the present day, thanks to the application of the surgical microscope and the improvement in suture materials, surgical treatment of peripheral nerve injury has yielded conspicuously better results.

Since the perineurium contains less connective tissue than the epineurium, the funicular suture, with the help of microsurgical technique, can prevent the rapidly growing connective tissue from entering the anastomosing gap, thus ensuring free passage of new axons in the funiculi through the gap in favour of their regeneration. The effect of the surgical treatment is thus greatly increased. When motor funiculi are separated from the sensory ones, end-to-end suture must be done accurately, since nervous functions cannot recover after a false suture. After the motor and sensory funiculi have been mixed, both kinds of new axons have equal chance of false growth after suture. However, in a mixed funiculus there is still a distinction between the motor and sensory components. Hence, functional recovery will be satisfactory, if mixed funicular groups with similar functions are sutured end-to-end.

At present, there are mainly three ways to distinguish the motor and the sensory funiculi, namely,

Electrophysiological diagnostic method

This was suggested by Haktian in 1968. When the motor funiculus is stimulated with an electrical stimulator the distal muscle contracts, but no pain is felt.

When the sensory funiculus is stimulated pain is felt and the distal muscle does not contract. However, the electrical stimulation method can only be used in cases of recent injuries. When the neurons have degenerated the response is not obvious. It is therefore unsuitable for the detection of old injuries.

Histochemical method

Grabb (1973) and Freilinger (1976) suggested this method on the basis of experimental and clinical practice. The amount of acetylcholine esterase contained in the axons was determined to identify the motor and sensory funiculi in a peripheral nerve. However, this method has its limitations in clinical practice because these enzymes are present only in fresh, healthy nerve fibres. It can be detected only within 72 hours of injury. Besides, tissue blocks must be sectioned and treated by histochemical methods, which requires 25–30 hours of incubation to draw any conclusion. It remains under theoretical discussion and of little practical value.

Method of anatomical localization of funiculi

This is based on the rule that the motor and sensory funiculi in a nerve trunk shift from the distal to the proximal end. Making a series of illustrated diagrams aids in identifying the property of an individual funiculus within the nerve at different levels of section. Sunderland mentioned the intraneural segmental funicular patterns of nerve trunks early in 1948. This set of topographical diagrams had been adopted by clinicians. As the distance of each segment is represented by an absolute value, the diagrams appear to be very complex and are not convenient for use. On the basis of previous research and from the microsurgical viewpoint, Zhong Shizhen (1977) made a design in terms of proportionate equidistance in the limb, and produced a topographical diagram of the nerve trunk through the funicular dissection method with stress on some significant funiculi for surgical anastomosis. Consequently, other anatomists have presented practical diagrams for anatomical topographies of some other nerve trunks. They are Si Xincheng (1980, on the obturator nerve), Wang Qihua (1981, on the recurrent laryngeal nerve), Zhou Chongman (1982, on the sciatic nerve). These studies have added to the anatomical data for the microsurgery of peripheral nerves, and have provided an important theoretical basis for the funicular suture.

Structure of the peripheral nerve

The basic component units of a peripheral nerve are the nerve fibres. Tens of thousands of nerve fibres aggregate into a funiculus, some of which are brought together to become a nerve trunk. A nerve fibre does not run along the course of a single funiculus, but shifts between the funiculi, from one to the other. The continuous and reciprocating shift of the nerve fibres among the funiculi makes the size, number and position of the latter change all the time, i.e. even within the range of 1 mm, the morphology of the funiculi would become quite different (Figure 10.1). The distribution of funiculi is also uneven in the cross-section of a nerve trunk, usually showing a dense or loose grouping.

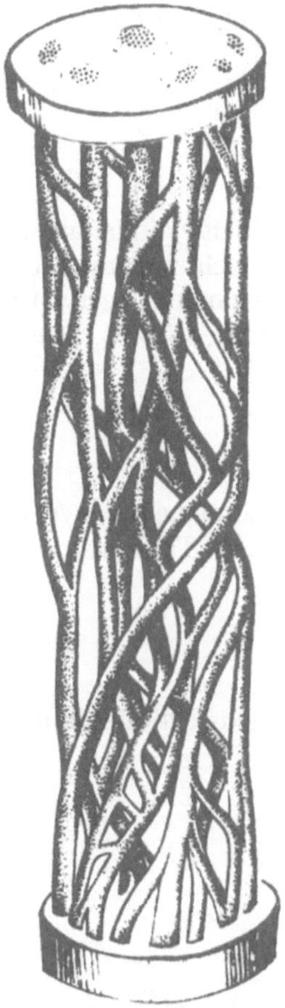

Figure 10.1 Diagrams of funiculi in the peripheral nerve trunk

There is a lot of interstitial tissue, besides the nerve fibres, in a peripheral nerve trunk. The interstitial tissue includes collagenous and elastic fibres, fatty tissue and nutrient and lymph vessels. It distributes mainly between, but rarely within, the funiculi. The amount of the interstitial tissue varies with different nerve trunks or in different parts of a trunk. According to Sunderland, the interstitial tissue accounts for about 30–75% of the cross-sectional area of a nerve trunk of the extremities. In general, there is less interstitial tissue near the nerve roots of the extremity.

As there is a fair amount of interstitial tissue in the nerve trunk and the position or arrangement of funiculi varies, the stumps of the funiculi, after a nerve is interrupted for even a short segment, may show different arrangements. Therefore, in repairing a nerve injury, suturing the epineurium alone cannot approximate the funiculi accurately, so that some of the funiculi have to touch the distal interstitial tissue. As a result the growing axons cannot get into the cords of Schwann cells of the distal stump but coil to form a pain-sensitizing neuroma which retards recovery of function. Eventually the basic studies on the funicular patterns in the cross-sections of nerve trunks are significant in guiding precise suture of nerve funiculi.

Nerve fibre

A nerve fibre is composed of an axis cylinder and an overlying Schwann sheath. The Schwann cell can produce myelin substance enclosing the axon. Depending on the presence or absence of the myelin, nerve fibres may be divided into two kinds: myelinated and unmyelinated fibres. Most of the peripheral nerves are composed of myelinated fibres.

Myelinated nerve fibre

The axis cylinder is enclosed by a segmental layer of myelin sheath. There is one Schwann cell around each segment. The constricted part between two segments is called the node of Ranvier.

Unmyelinated fibre

This is composed of very fine axis cylinder and the overlying Schwann cells.

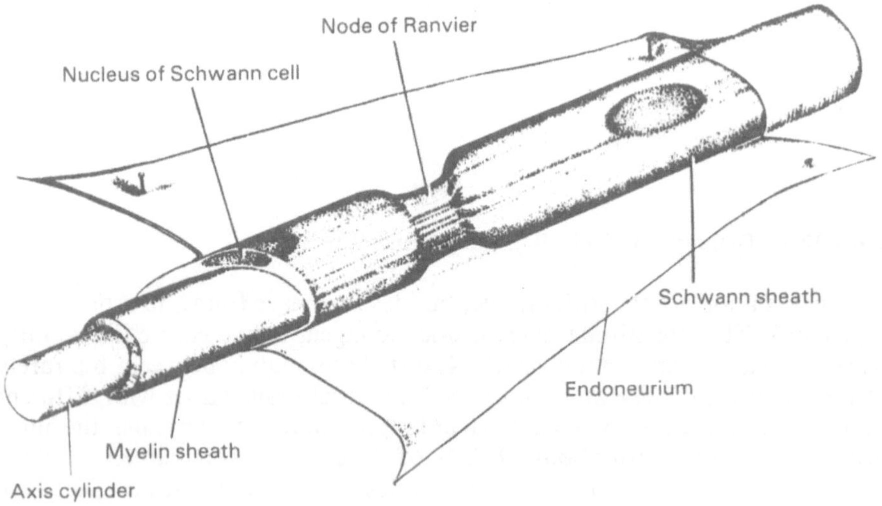

Figure 10.2 Diagram of a myelinated fibre

All spinal nerves contain sensory, motor and sympathetic nerve fibres. In the course of nerve regeneration the motor or sensory fibres must re-establish their connections with corresponding functional cells or tissues, i.e. the regenerating axon of a motor fibre has to connect itself with the muscle fibre in order to re-establish the motor endplate and that of a sensory nerve has to reach the original tissue in order to restore the sensory receptor, whence the function of the nerve can be properly recovered. If the nerve funiculi with different functions are wrongly sutured, it will hinder the recovery of functions. However, nerves cannot be divided purely into motor or sensory, for example, in the deep branch of the ulnar nerve there are 60% of sensory fibres ending in the Pacinian corpuscles.

Connective tissue membranes

Endoneurium

Each nerve fibre is enclosed by a thin delicate connective tissue membrane, called the endoneurium.

Perineurium

A funiculus composed of several nerve fibres is enclosed by the perineurium. The thickness of the perineurium varies from 2 to 100 μm, and is directly proportional to the diameter of the funiculus. The connective tissue of the perineurium is arranged as three concentric circular lamellae.

1. Internal lamina: the internal lamina is a single layer of the perineural cells, named the perineural epithelium. The inner surface of this layer is smooth, and there is a certain degree of mobility between it and the endoneurium. At the boundaries among the perineural cells, cytoplasmic processes congregate and overlap each other, forming a closely connected layer of cells. The basement membranes of the cells fuse together to form a layer of septum which acts as a barrier against the extension of infection.
2. Middle lamina: the middle lamina, also called the laminar layer, is composed of perineural cells arranged regularly in concentric circles, from several to more than 10 in number. As the collagenous fibres in the perineurium have the ability of contraction, the nerve fibres present a wavy and slack appearance. When a nerve is severed the perineurium appears to shrink.
3. External lamina: the external lamina is the site of transition between the perineurium and the epineurium. The collagenous fibres increase gradually in thickness and are arranged irregularly.

Membrane of the funicular group

In nerve trunks of the limbs, the number of funiculi varies enormously. There is only one funiculus in some of them, but others may have more than 100. Therefore, several funiculi usually collect to form a funicular or fascicular group. It is enclosed outside by a relatively thick connective tissue membrane which is a part of the perineurium. As it is of practical significance in microsurgery, it may be called the membrane of the funicular group. The perineurium and the membrane of the funicular group present strong resistance against tension, and internal pressure within the funiculi is higher. If there is a defect on the perineurium the nerve tissue will protrude through it, and if the funiculi are severed a colloid fluid will leak out in the shape of a mushroom. Where there is an abundance of funiculi they are very fine and delicate and are liable to damage during surgical manipulation. Excessive dissection, then, may destroy a lot of vascular networks of the membrane of the funicular group and induce a serious tissue reaction with bad effect. In the evaluation of the funicular suture some authors still dissent and consider the traumatic tissue reaction to be so great that the funicular suture is not superior to the epineural one. Therefore it is not necessary, or sometimes impossible, to dissect and suture the funiculi during operation, where the funiculi abound. At present the funicular group is usually considered as a unit for dissection and suturing, and the thickness of the membrane of the funicular group is taken advantage of in performing suture between funicular groups. The 'funicular suture' performed under the microscope includes, in fact, not only funicular and funicular group sutures, but also the epineural suture of small nerves, such as epineural suture of digital nerves.

Epineurium

The peripheral nerve is enclosed in the outermost layer by a thick lamina of loose connective tissue which can slide on the surface of the nerve, and which is called the epineurium. Some experiments showed that the antigen responsible for the rejection of nerve homograft is mainly in the connective tissue of the epineurium and perineurium.

Blood supply of the nerve trunk

The blood supply of a nerve trunk originates from the neighbouring arteries or their branches. They usually enter the nerve in a segmental manner. The connective tissue at the place where these arteries enter is called mesoneurium. The segmental vessels form a longitudinal epineural network along the epineurium. The network is probably composed of small vessels. The epineural artery of a relatively large peripheral nerve may be about 1 mm in diameter. When the mesoneurium is severed during operation, part of the segmental vessels will be destroyed. This can be compensated by freeing the nerve trunk for a certain distance and making a longitudinal anastomosis of the epineural vascular network. Although individual survival was reported after the nerve had been dissected for 15 cm, the optimal length seems to be less than 6–8 cm. If this range is exceeded the compensation of the blood supply will hardly be within the bounds of possibility.

Branches of epineural vessels enter the funiculi of funicular groups forming an interfunicular vascular network. A thick epineural arteriole is estimated to be able to supply five funiculi. Venules are alike in structure. They belong to the type of small vessel and occur between layers of the perineurium. Some of these vessels pass obliquely through the layers and communicate with those of the epineurium and endoneurium. The branches of interfunicular vessels pass through the perineurium and enter the funiculi to form the intrafunicular vascular network which consists mainly of capillaries but occasionally of pre- or post-capillary vessels as well. When nerve grafting or suture is performed with microsurgical technique, the intraneural tissue and vessels may be injured in extensive intraneural dissection. Owing to the protective action of the perineurium as a barrier, injury to the intrafunicular vascular network remains the least. Therefore, intraneural dissection can induce extensive cicatrix outside the perineurium but slight reaction within it. If the funiculus is dissected free for about 2 cm, the blood supply of the intrafunicular vascular network remains good.

The position of the large vessels in the mesoneurium and epineurium can be easily identified during operation. They serve as excellent marks for matching nerve stumps in end-to-end suture.

Lymph vessels of the nerve trunk

It is now generally thought that there are no lymph capillaries in nerve funiculi, so that the perineurium has an apparent action as a barrier. Lymph networks are present in the perineurium and epineurium. They drain into the local lymph nodes through the lymph vessels that accompany the arteries.

MEDIAN NERVE

Zhong Shizhen, Tao Xiangluo and Liu Muzhi

In the median nerve the number of sensory fibres is larger than that of motor fibres. According to Sunderland, the sensory fibres account for 67%, while the motor fibres account for 33%. Therefore, when funicular anastomosis of the median nerve is performed, the topographical localization of the funiculi of the muscular branches must be studied intimately. We studied the upper limb with anatomic dissection, and diagrams of the topography of the funiculi in the nerve trunk were made. For the sake of good memory and application, the forearm is to be divided into eight equal segments, and the arm into four. They are described from below upwards (Figures 10.3 and 10.4).

External form, dimensions and number of funiculi of the median nerve

The median nerve near the wrist is flattened anteroposteriorly and is approximately round between segments 2/8 and 5/8 of the forearm. As it ascends between the two heads of the pronator teres (between segments 5/8 and

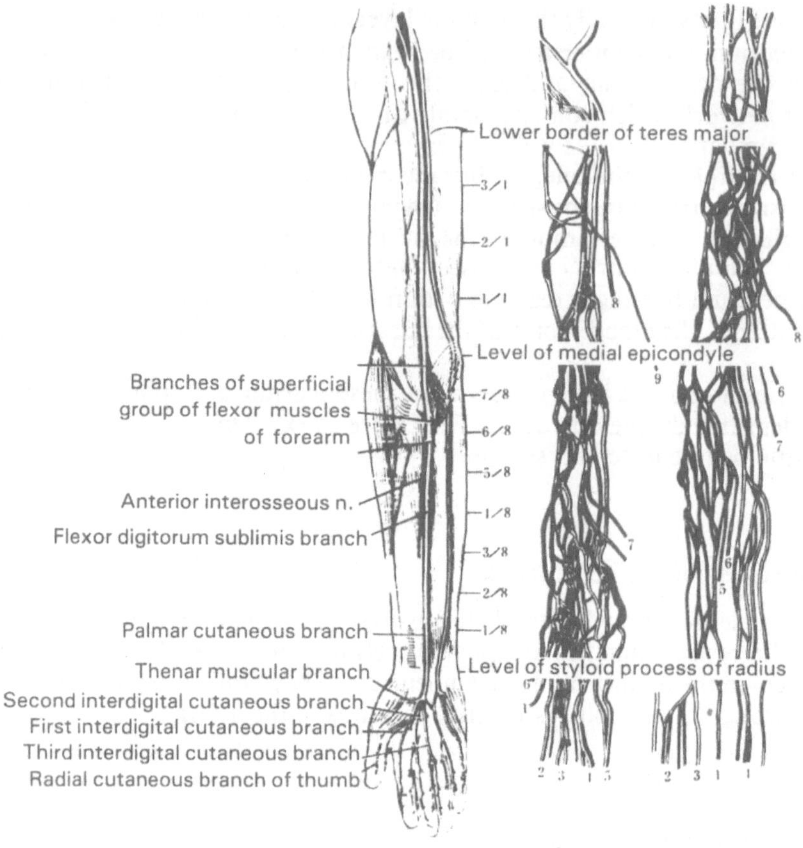

Figure 10.3 Sites for recording the median and ulnar nerves at different levels, and the dissected specimens

7/8 of the forearm) it is sagittally flattened due to compression by the muscle. When it reaches above the elbow the nerve returns to its oval or approximately round shape. The data and number of funiculi of the median nerve are shown in Table 10.1

The data shown in Table 10.1 indicate that the wrist and palmar portion of the median nerve is thick and contains more connective tissues, while the middle segment of the forearm is the thinnest. When it reaches the arm the median nerve becomes thicker again. In the arm it tends to be thinner. Since there are numerous terminal branches in the distal segment, the number of funiculi in the wrist and palmar portions is the largest. The higher the portion of the nerve, the lesser the number of funiculi. Near the cubital fossa the anterior interosseous nerve and the branches to the superficial group of the flexor muscles of the forearm join the main trunk, so that the number of funiculi increases moderately. The number of funiculi finishes again across the elbow joint.

Table 10.1 The mean value of the dimensions and number of funiculi of each segment of the median nerve

Levels	*Transverse dimension* (mm)	*Anteroposterior dimension* (mm)	*Area of cross-section* (mm^2)	*Number of funiculi*
Origin of thenar branch	7.1	2.2	12.3	27
Styloid process of radius	5.5	2.4	10.4	22
Forearm 1/8	4.5	2.5	8.7	19
Forearm 2/8	3.5	2.7	7.2	17
Forearm 3/8	3.1	2.7	6.6	15
Forearm 4/8	3.1	2.7	6.6	14
Forearm 5/8	3.0	3.0	6.9	14
Forearm 6/8	2.8	3.9	8.6	14
Forearm 7/8	2.9	4.8	10.9	16
Medial eipcondyle of humerus	2.9	5.3	11.8	17
Arm 1/4	2.8	4.9	10.5	13
Arm 2/4	2.9	4.5	10.2	12
Arm 3/4	3.1	4.3	10.3	8
Lower border of teres major	3.3	4.0	10.1	5

Terminal branches of the median nerve

Branches to the muscles of the thenar eminence

In all of the specimens there is a large branch to the muscle of the thenar eminence; and in 50% of cases there is, in addition, a small branch. Occasionally there happen to be two small muscular branches in individual cases.

Large muscular branch (or bulbar muscular branch)

This arises from the median nerve 40 mm below the styloid process of the radius. It contains about 1.3 funiculi. The mean transverse diameter is 1.0 (0.7 to 1.5) mm. After entering the nerve trunk, it can be dissected separately for 60 (52–88) mm before it mixes with other sensory funiculi. The topography of this nerve is as follows. The site of its entrance into the trunk is along the anterior portion of the radial border, whence it ascends to segment 1/8 of the forearm. In most cases it mixes with the sensory funiculi from the radial side of the thumb. In the course of mixing it shifts from the radial side to the posterolateral quadrant. On reaching segments 2/8 to 4/8 of the forearm each funicular group, already mixed with the fibres of the muscular branches of the thenar eminence, lies in the posterior part. This mixed funicular group turns out to lie in the centre of the trunk above the 6/8 segment of the forearm.

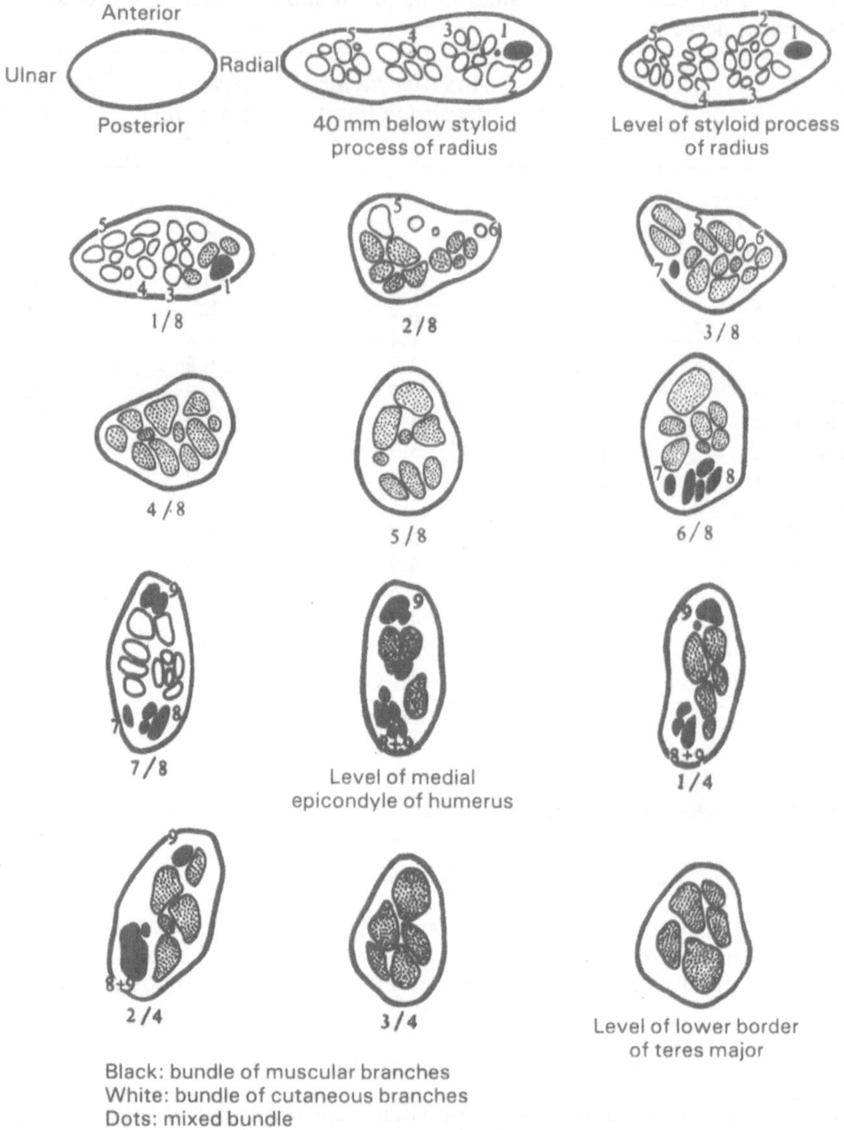

Figure 10.4 Diagram of the topographical localization of funiculi in the median nerve trunk

Small muscular branch

This contains about 1.2 funiculi, the transverse diameter being 0.5 (0.3–0.9) mm. Most of them supply the deep head of the flexor pollicis brevis only. This funiculus can only be dissected separately for 9 (5–20) mm before mixing with the large muscular branch or the funiculus arising from the first digital space.

Branches to the adductor pollicis and the lumbricales manus

In all of the specimens there are branches to the first and second lumbricales. In 60% of the cases there is, in addition, a branch to the third lumbricalis. In 50% of the specimens there is another branch to the adductor pollicis. These branches, being fine, can be dissected separately only for a short distance (5–17 mm).

The sensory branches of the fingers

Of the terminal branches of the median nerve, the sensory nerves from the fingers attain to an enormous proportion. The radial cutaneous branch of the thumb contains 1.2 funiculi on average, the transverse diameter being 1.3 mm. There are 7.2 funiculi in the cutaneous branch of the first digital space, the transverse diameter being 2.0 mm; 7.4 funiculi in the cutaneous branch of the second digital space, the transverse diameter 2.1 mm, and 6.9 funiculi in the cutaneous branch of the third digital space, the transverse diameter 1.8 mm.

After entering the trunk, those sensory branches are arranged from the radial to the ulnar side as follows: the radial cutaneous branch of the thumb, the cutaneous branch of the first, second and third digital spaces. In the ascending course these funicular groups mix gradually with the neighbouring funiculi. The order of arrangement remains unchanged after mixing. What mixes first is the radial funicular group of the thumb, which interweaves with the large muscular branch of the thenar eminence at segment 1/8 of the forearm. Then comes the funicular group of the first digital space, which mixes with the muscular branch of the thenar eminence and the radial cutaneous branch of the thumb between segments 1/8 and 2/8 of the arm. The last to mix is the funicular group of the second and third digital spaces. Near the middle segment of the forearm all of the funiculi have got mixed, so that the funicular group of the third digital space is the longest one capable of being dissected separately, the available length being about 100–140 mm.

The four sensory funicular groups mentioned above, in their course of ascent and mixing, change their internal configuration gradually in conformation to the transformation of the contour of the nerve trunk from a flattened to a round one. The funicular groups on both the radial and ulnar sides are pressed to the anterior, and the two in the middle are crowded to the posterior. Above segment 3/8 of the forearm the funicular group of cutaneous branch of the third digital space, originally lying anteriorly on the ulnar side, moves anteriorly to the radial side (Figure 10.4).

Ramification of the median nerve

The palmar cutaneous branch

This consists of one or two small funiculi. The available length for separate dissection is 59 mm and the transverse diameter is 0.8 mm. Between segments 1/8 and 2/8 of the forearm it enters the nerve trunk, first lying anterolaterally and then turning gradually to the radial side.

Branches to the flexor digitorum sublimis

This may arise from the median nerve or the anterior interosseous nerve. There are 2.2 (1–4) branches on average arising from the nerve trunk. The distal branch arises between segments 2/8 and 4/8 of the forearm and the intermedius branch arises between segments 4/8 and 5/8. These two kinds of branches are fine and contain only one funiculus, the transverse diameter of which is 0.5 mm. It usually leaves the trunk posteriorly on the ulnar side. The available length for separate dissection is less than 15 mm. The proximal branch arises between segments 6/8 and 7/8 of the forearm and contains 1.9 funiculi, the transverse diameter being 0.7 mm. It leaves the trunk from the ulnar or posterior part, and immediately mixes with the funicular group of the anterior interosseous nerve.

Anterior interosseous nerve

This nerve averages 1.8 mm in diameter and contains 4.5 funiculi. It arises at segment 6/8 of the forearm where the contour of the nerve trunk changes rapidly from a nearly round to a flat one. This funicular group lies at first posterior to the trunk and then turns posteromedially. In the course of ascent it mixes with the proximal branch of the flexor digitorum sublimis and the distal branch of the superficial group of the flexor muscles of the forearm. The available length for separate dissection of these branches measures 102 mm. At the level of segment 1/4 of the arm it begins to mix with neighbouring sensory funiculi.

Branches to the superficial group of the flexor muscles of the forearm

Generally, there are two to four branches supplying the superficial group of the flexor muscles of the forearm arising from the medial epicondyle of the humerus. The muscles supplied by these branches are not constant. The regular pattern is that the distal branch usually contains the components supplying the pronator teres; it may also supply the flexor carpi radialis, the palmaris longus and the flexor digitorum sublimis, but occasionally it may send branches to the pronator teres. The proximal branch supplies mainly the pronator teres. The observational data of the funiculi supplying the superficial flexor muscles of the forearm are listed in Table 10.2.

Table 10.2 The dimensions, number of funiculi and level of origins of the branches supplying the superficial group of the flexor muscles of the forearm

Branch	*Transverse dimension*	*Number of funiculi*	*Level of origin*
Distal branch	1.0	2.1	forearm 6/8–7/8
Intermediate branch	0.9	2.1	forearm 7/8–8/8
Proximal branch	0.7	1.6	forearm 8/8–arm 1/4

Although all the branches mentioned above arise from the posterior part (or the ulnar part) of the nerve trunk, in their ascending course within the trunk they usually collect into two groups lying in the anterior and posterior parts of the nerve trunk respectively. The funiculi destined for the posterior part usually pass through the medial superficial layer and reach the anterior end immediately. The funicular groups collected into the anterior group mostly belong to the distal and proximal branches, while those collected into the posterior group mostly belong to the intermedial branches. Most of the components of the pronator teres occupy the anterior portion of the nerve trunk. The posterior funicular groups immediately mix with the neighbouring motor funiculi and begin to mix with the neighbouring sensory funiculi until they reach over segment 1/4 of the arm.

Localization and application of the main motor funicular groups of the median nerve

In the forearm and arm the internal structures of the median nerve present a shift of lateral rotation from below upward. Mastering the regular pattern of these changes will aid in surgical applications.

The main large muscular branch of the thenar eminence enters the nerve trunk from the radial or anterior side. It can be dissected separately from the palm to segments 1/8 or 2/8 of the forearm. Its position is shifted from the radial side to the posterolateral quadrant. In the course of ascent it mixes with the neighbouring sensory funicular group. Above segment 6/8 of the forearm, due to the addition of the funiculi of the superficial flexor muscles of the forearm both posteriorly and anteriorly, the mixed funiculi, blended with the muscular branches of the thenar eminence, remain ascending in the central part of the nerve trunk and mostly join the medial root of the median nerve after all.

The funiculi of the superficial group of the flexor muscles of the forearm and the anterior interosseous nerve arise in succession between the upper portion of the arm and the cubital fossa. These funicular groups lie separately in the anterior and posterior parts of the nerve trunk, which assumes a flattened band-like profile in the sagittal direction. The posterior part, being larger, occupies nearly the posterior one-quarter of the nerve trunk, while the anterior part is smaller, occupying about the anterior one-fifth. The intermediate part between the anterior and posterior parts is mainly filled with the mixed funicular groups related to the terminal branch. Though the motor funicular groups of the anterior and posterior parts mix with the neighbouring sensory funiculi gradually above segment 1/4 of the arm, these parts are still mixed funicular groups with motor fibres as the main components, which can be recognized and utilized during operation. After reaching the upper part of the arm the mixed funicular groups of the anterior part deviate laterally and most of them join the lateral root of the median nerve; while the mixed funicular groups of the posterior part pursue medially and the majority join the medial root.

Parts of the median nerve trunk susceptible to injury by compression

Carpal tunnel

The walls of the carpal tunnel consist of firm tissues, i.e. the scaphoid and trapezium for the radial side; the pisiform and hamate for the ulnar side; the scaphoid, lunate, capitate and trapezoid for the dorsal side; and the ligamentum carpi transversum for the palmar side. There are altogether nine tendons passing through the carpal tunnel in company with the median nerve. They are so closely packed that any cause which may raise the pressure within the canal will compress the median nerve, thus initiating the carpal tunnel syndrome. Clark (1979) analysed 561 cases of decompression operation for the fibro-osseous tunnel of the upper limb and reported that the compression of the median nerve in the wrist accounts for 73%. Generally the transverse carpal ligament is to be resected in order to relieve the syndrome. In case of apparently thickened nerve sheath and atrophy of thenar muscles, neurolysis should be performed under the microscope after the nerve sheath has been cut open.

Tunnel of the pronator teres

When the median nerve passes through the pronator teres the muscular tunnel formed from its superficial and deep heads does not, in general, much compress the median nerve, so that clinical symptoms are apparently rare. Only when an abnormal fibrous band appears deep to the superficial head of the pronator teres does the compression of the median nerve become obvious, especially during pronation.

ULNAR NERVE

ZHONG SHIZHEN, TAO XIANGLUO AND LIU MUZHI

In the ulnar nerve trunk, the numbers of motor and sensory fibres are nearly equal. According to Sunderland the motor fibres account for 46% and the sensory fibres 54%.

External form, dimensions and number of funiculi of the ulnar nerve trunk

The end of the ulnar nerve trunk, where the superficial and deep branches unite, appears to be oval. As it passes over the superficial surface of the transverse carpal ligament the trunk gradually becomes triangular with the tip of the triangle facing medially and backward. When the ulnar nerve trunk passes through the superficial carpal tunnel, a bony fibrous canal which is surrounded by the pisiform bone, the pisochamate ligament and the volar carpal ligament, it is covered in part on the anterolateral aspect by the ulnar vessels. In segments 1/8 and 2/8 of the forearm the trunk inclines medially. It is oblate in the sagittal plane because it is pressed tightly by the tendons of the flexor digitorum sublimis and the flexor carpi ulnaris, whereas it is oval between segments 2/8 and 7/8 of the forearm. From segment 7/8 to the medial epicondylar segment of the humerus the trunk lies in the cubital tunnel and is pressed superficially by the arcuate ligament and by the flexor digitalis profundus on its deep side. It is slightly flattened in the sagittal plane, but returns to oval or nearly round shape on reaching the arm. The observational data and the number of the funiculus of the ulnar nerve are shown in Table 10.3, which shows that the ulnar nerve is thicker in the carpo-

Table 10.3 The mean value of the dimensions and the number of funiculi of each segment of the ulnar nerve

Level	*Transverse dimension* (mm)	*Anteroposterior dimension* (mm)	*Area of cross-section* (mm^2)	*Number of funiculi*
Bifurcation into superficial and deep branches	4.3	2.9	9.8	19
Styloid process of radius	3.2	3.4	8.6	15
Forearm 1/8	2.6	3.7	7.6	14
Forearm 2/8	3.0	3.3	7.8	15
Forearm 3/8	3.4	2.9	7.7	17
Forearm 4/8	3.2	2.9	7.3	14
Forearm 5/8	3.2	2.8	7.0	11
Forearm 6/8	3.3	2.8	7.3	9
Forearm 7/8	3.1	3.2	7.8	8
Medial epicondyle of humerus	2.5	4.4	8.6	6
Arm 1/4	2.8	3.7	8.1	7
Arm 2/4	3.4	3.0	8.0	10
Arm 3/4	3.5	2.8	7.7	8
Lower border of teres major	3.3	2.8	7.3	7

palmar region and near the elbow but is thinner in the forearm and arm. The number of funiculi is largest in the palm and wrist, where many terminal branches join. It diminishes gradually during ascent. The number of funiculi increases at segment 2/8 of the forearm where the dorsal cutaneous branches of the hand join, and they diminish to the least near the posterior part of the elbow. In the lower part of the arm the funiculi slightly increase in number, but they diminish again near the axilla.

Terminal branches of the ulnar nerve

Deep branch

The level of bifurcation into the superficial and deep branches is 5 mm below the styloid process of the radius. The deep branch is purely muscular. It lies

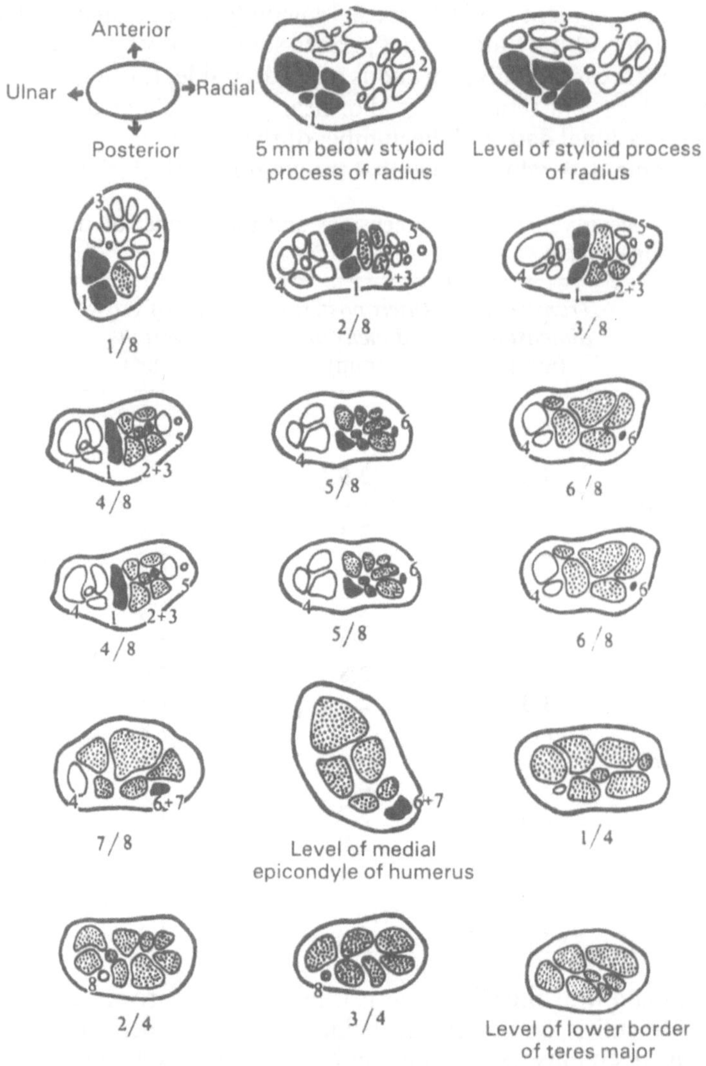

Figure 10.5 Diagram of topographical localization of funiculi in the ulnar nerve. Black = bundle of muscular branches; white = bundle of cutaneous branches, dots = mixed bundle

posteromedial to the lower end of the ulnar nerve trunk. When it passes through the superficial carpal tunnel in front of the wrist joint it is situated at the tip of the triangle, facing backward. In segments 1/8 and 2/8 of the forearm the deep branch remains posterior to the trunk. In segment 1/8 of the forearm the fibres of the cutaneous branch of the fourth digital space begin to mix with it and at segment 2/8 those of the ulnar cutaneous branch of the little finger join it. Still upward, the deep branch thus mixed sends some fibres to the neighbouring funicular groups. Near segment 2/8 of the forearm the relatively great funicular groups of the dorsal cutaneous branch join the trunk and push the mixed funiculi to the centre of the trunk. The observational data of the funiculi of the branches of the ulnar nerve are shown in Table 10.4.

Table 10.4 Related data of the branches of the ulnar nerve

Name of branch	*Transverse dimension* (mm)	*Number of funiculi*	*Dissectable length* (mm)	*Level of origin*	*Level of mixing*
Muscular branch of ramus profundus	1.4	4.2	46	Below styloid process of radius	Forearm 1/8
Cutaneous branch of fourth interdigital space	1.9	6.4	34	Below styloid process of radius	Forearm 1/8
Ulnar cutaneous branch of little finger	1.4	4.7	34	Below styloid process of radius	Forearm 1/8
Branch to ulnar artery	0.2	1.2	84	Forearm 2/8-6/8	Forearm 5/8-7/8
Dorsal cutaneous branch of hand	1.8	6.1	167	Forearm 2/8	Forearm 5/8-7/8
Distal branch of flexor carpi ulnaris	0.4	1.3	29	Forearm 4/8-6/8	Forearm 5/8-7/8
Proximal branch of flexor carpi ulnaris	0.7	1.8	41	Forearm 7/8-arm 1/4	Forearm 8/8-Arm 1/4
Flexor digitorum profundus branch	0.7	1.9	38	Forearm 7/8-arm 1/4	Arm 1/4
Branch to elbow joint	0.2	1.0	89	Forearm 8/8-arm 2/4	Arm 3/4-4/4

Superficial branch

Though the superficial branch is composed mainly of cutaneous branches, a few components of the muscular branches still exist such as the branch to the palmaris brevis. In some specimens there are occasionally branches to the adductor digiti quinti and the third and fourth lumbricals.

1. The cutaneous branch of the fourth digital space lies in the anterolateral part of the nerve trunk. Ascending to segment 1/8 of the forearm, it mixes with the ulnar cutaneous branch of the little finger. At segment 2/8 it sends fibres to the funicular groups of the deep branch.
2. The ulnar cutaneous branch of the little finger lies at first in the anterior part, while at the 1/8 segment it begins to mix with the funicular group of the fourth digital space. On reaching the segment 2/8 it mixes with the deep branch.

3. The cutaneous branch of the palm and the branch to the ulnar artery are smaller and mix immediately with the corresponding funicular groups.

Branches of the ulnar nerve

The branches to the ulnar artery

These branches also known as the cutaneous branches of the palm, are one or two in number and are small.

The dorsal cutaneous branch of the hand

This is the largest branch of the ulnar nerve in the forearm. It joins the nerve trunk at segment 2/8 of the arm, in which it lies in the medial part. This funicular group is surrounded by much connective tissue, and is easily separated from other funiculi. Near segments 5/8 to 7/8 of the forearm it merges into the neighbouring mixed funiculus.

Branches to the flexor carpi ulnaris

These are one to three in number.

1. The distal branch is present in about 30% of cases. It enters the nerve trunk near segments 4/8 to 6/8 of the forearm, ascends along the radial side and then turns posteriorly, mixing with the funiculus of the flexor digitorum profundus.
2. The proximal branches, one or two in number, arise between the segment 7/8 of the forearm and segment 1/4 of the arm, residing mostly in the posterolateral quadrant of the nerve trunk. However, there are a few small funiculi traversing the anteromedial quadrant in 25% of specimens. Near the elbow joint it merges into the neighbouring mixed funicular groups.

The branch to the flexor digitorum profundus

This consists mostly of one branch but two or three branches may occur in a few cases. Part of them may share a stem in common with the flexor carpi ulnaris. Most of them arise between segment 7/8 of the forearm and segment 1/4 of the arm and lie in the posterolateral quadrant of the nerve trunk. The branch first mixes with the funiculus of the flexor carpi ulnaris and then merges at the 1/4 segment into the mixed funiculi from the arm.

Branches to the elbow joint

These branches, one or two in number, arise mostly between the medial epicondyle of the humerus and segment 2/4 of the arm. About 25% of them arise below the medial epicondyle. The branches to the elbow joint lie in the posterior part or posteromedial quadrant of the nerve trunk, and merge into the neighbouring mixed funicular groups at segments 3/4 and 4/4 of the arm.

Localization of application of the main funicular groups of the ulnar nerve

Terminal branch

The number of deep branches is smaller than that of the superficial, the ratio being about 4 : 6. From the palmar part to segment 2/8 of the forearm the deep branch lies in the posterior part of the nerve trunk, and the superficial one in the anterior. Most of the funicular groups of the superficial and deep branches can be completely separated below segment 1/8 of the forearm. Though these two branches begin to mix between segments 1/8 and 3/8 of the forearm, when they are bluntly dissected in the specimens and observed under the operative microscope with 6–10 times magnification, the interruption of nerve fibres is usually not present, or is only mild. When dissected above segment 3/8 of the forearm, serious interrupted phenomena of nerve fibres appear. Therefore, the deep branch of the ulnar nerve below segment 3/8 of the forearm may be admitted for blunt dissection during operation.

Dorsal cutaneous branch of the hand

This funicular group is larger and occupies the medial one-third to one-quarter of the nerve trunk. It is surrounded apparently by connective tissue and is easily identified and isolated, the length available for individual separation being quite long (167 mm on average). It is closely approximated to the mixed funicular groups, which come from the deep branch and consist mainly of muscular branches and may be used as a guide during operation for the search for such groups.

Muscular branches to the forearm

Although the number of branches of the ulnar nerve to the relevant flexor muscles of the forearm and the site of their emergence are quite inconstant, the funicular group lies in the posterolateral part of the nerve and is easy to locate for practical purposes. This group mixes with the neighbouring funiculi at segment 1/4 of the arm, but its main component still runs upwards along the posterolateral part of the nerve trunk after mixing.

Sites susceptible to injuries by compression in the ulnar nerve

Superficial carpal tunnel

The superficial carpal tunnel is a bony fibrous canal surrounded by the pisiform bone and the pishamate and volar carpal ligaments. As the ulnar nerve trunk passes through it, the ulnar artery and vein remain anterolateral to the nerve.

About 60% of the deep branches of the ulnar artery cross obliquely over the superficial aspect of the ulnar nerve and then enter the deep part of it medially. Consequently, the ulnar nerve may suffer a certain degree of compression. However, as the overlying volar carpal ligament is thin and weak, the occurrence of nerve compression is rare. Clark (1979) reported the incidence rate of ulnar nerve compression in the wrist to be 3% after a statistical survey of 561 cases of decompression operation performed on the fibrous tunnel of the upper limb.

Cubital tunnel

The cubital tunnel is situated below the medial epicondyle of the humerus. The sulcus nervi ulnaris, the capsule of the elbow joint and the flexor digitorum profundus remain on its deep surface; the arcuate ligament deep to the flexor carpi ulnaris is to be on its superficial aspect. The clinical features manifested by the compression of the ulnar nerve in this region is known as the cubital tunnel syndrome. In Clark's 561 cases of decompression operation mentioned above, those performed on the cubital tunnel amount to 24%. The arcuate ligament is commonly resected in nerve decompression.

RADIAL NERVE

ZHONG SHIZHEN, TAO XIANGLUO AND LIU MUZHI

In the radial nerve trunk the motor nerve fibres are in more abundance than the sensory ones. According to Sunderland, the motor fibres amount to 71% and the sensory ones 29%. The muscle bellies of the extensors of the forearm innervated by the radial nerve are stout. They withstand the effect of atrophic degeneration due to denervation within a short time, therefore, the result of operative repairs after injury is fairly good.

External form, dimensions and number of funiculi of the radial nerve

The end of the radial nerve trunk, where the superficial and deep branches unite, is oval in the sagittal plane, the anteroposterior diameter being larger than the transverse one. It has two borders - the anterior and the posterior, and two surfaces - the radial and the ulnar. In the ascending course the nerve has a tendency to rotate laterally. Within the spiral sulcus it is slightly flattened and shifted from the sagittal to the transverse position, i.e. the anterior border becomes the radial; the posterior border becomes the ulnar. Before entering the axilla it resumes its oval contour, i.e. the radial border becomes the posterolateral one, and the ulnar border becomes the anteromedial. The observational data and the number of funiculi of the radial nerve are shown in Table 10.5, which shows that the radial nerve thickens gradually from below upwards. The number of funiculi is large in the upper and lower portions and smaller in the

Table 10.5 The mean value of the dimensions and the number of funiculi of each segment of the radial nerve

Level	*Transverse dimension* (mm)	*Anteroposterior dimension* (mm)	*Area of cross-section* (mm^2)	*Number of funiculi*
Lateral epicondyle of humerus	1.6	3.8	4.8	9.5
Arm 1/8	1.6	3.7	4.6	9.3
Arm 2/8	2.0	3.5	5.5	9.1
Arm 3/8	2.2	3.3	5.7	7.9
Arm 4/8	2.1	3.8	6.3	7.3
Arm 5/8	2.1	3.8	6.3	7.3
Arm 6/8	2.0	4.6	7.2	8.2
Arm 7/8	2.0	4.6	7.2	8.8
Lower border of teres major	2.2	4.6	7.9	9.4

middle. It is related to the number of branches; i.e. the more the branches of the lower portion of the radial nerve, the larger the number of the funiculi; the less the branches in the middle, the smaller the number of its funiculi. In the upper segment of the radial nerve the funiculi increase in number again, owing to the addition of the relevant cutaneous nerves of the arm and forearm and the branch to the triceps brachii.

Terminal branches of radial nerve

The site of bifurcation of the superficial and deep branches of the radial nerve is 2.2 mm above the lateral epicondyle of the humerus (Figures 10.6 and 10.7).

The superficial branch

This is mainly a cutaneous branch but in some specimens it may give rise to a branch to the extensor carpi radialis brevis. In very rare cases it may be absent, the region of innervation being thus replaced by the lateral cutaneous nerve of the forearm. The superficial branch lies in the anterior one-third of the nerve trunk at the end of the radial nerve. On reaching segments 1/8 to 3/8 of the arm it mixes gradually with the neighbouring posterior interosseous nerve and the funicular groups of the extensor carpi radialis and brachioradialis. After mixing, the main component of the sensory fibres, represented by the superficial branch, follows the lateral spiral course of the radial nerve to reach the radial side at the middle of the arm. Before entering the axilla it is situated in the posterolateral part of the nerve trunk. The relevant data of various branches of the radial nerve are shown in Table 10.6.

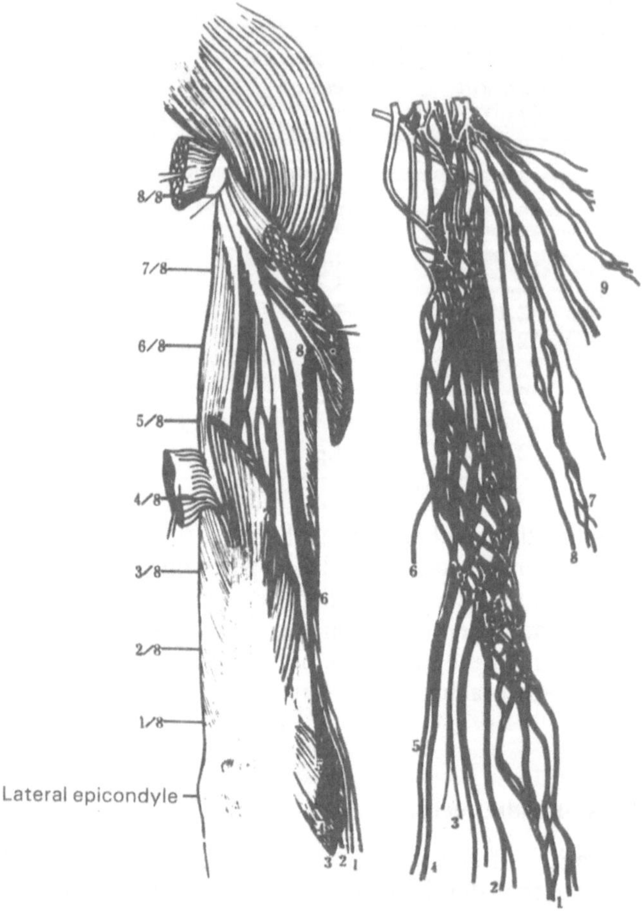

Figure 10.6 Level of recording and the dissected specimen of the radial nerve. **1**: Superficial branch of radial n.; **2**: deep branch of radial n.; **3**: fibres to extensor carpi radialis brevis; **4**: fibres to extensor carpi radialis longus; **5**: fibres to brachioradialis; **6**: branch to brachialis; **7**: posterior cutaneous n. of forearm; **8**: inferolateral cutaneous n. of arm; **9**: branch to lateral head of triceps brachii

The deep branch

The deep branch, also called the posterior interosseous nerve, consists of muscular branches. It resides in the posterior two-thirds of the radial nerve at the end of the trunk. On reaching segments 1/8 and 2/8 of the arm it first mixes with the fibres of the branches to the extensor carpi radialis and brachioradialis, and then with some of the fibres of the superficial branch. At the middle of the arm it shifts to the ulnar side. Before entering the axilla it comes to the anteromedial part of the nerve trunk.

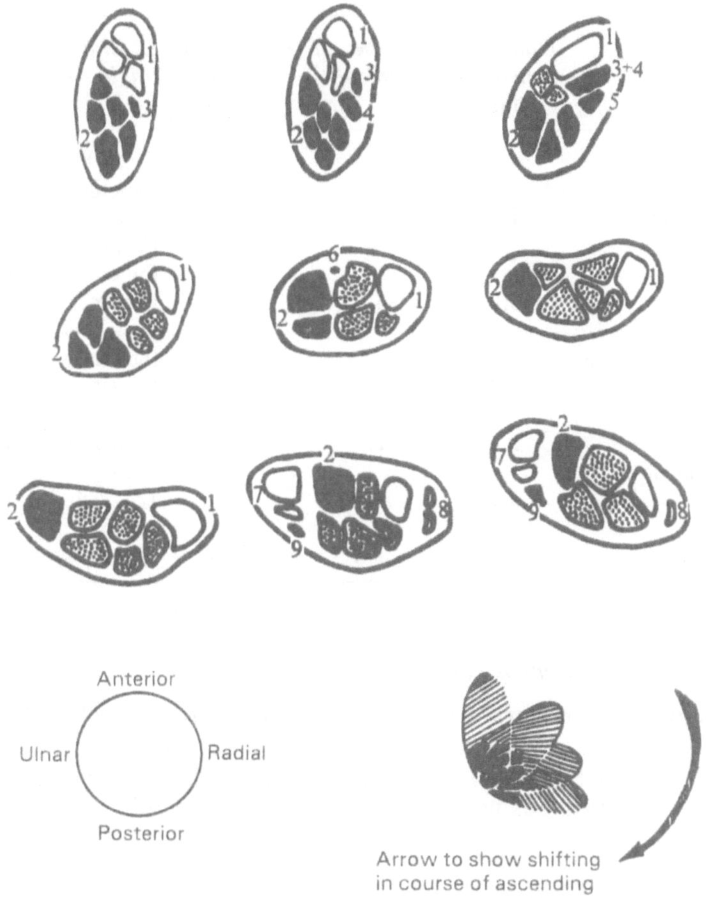

Figure 10.7 Diagram of topographical localization of the funiculi in the radial nerve trunk. Black = fibre bundle of muscular branch; white = fibre bundle of cutaneous branch; dots = mixed bundle

Branches of the radial nerve

The branch to the extensor carpi radialis brevis

This branch usually arises from the posterior interosseous nerve, but sometimes it appears as a branch of the superficial branch. Above the level of the lateral epicondyle of the humerus it lies between the funicular groups of the superficial and deep branches of the radial nerve, and is located in the lateral portion of the nerve trunk. At segment 2/8 of the arm it mixes at first with the funiculus of the extensor carpi radialis longus and then with the funicular group of the posterior interosseous nerve.

Table 10.6 The mean value of related data of the branches of the radial nerve

Name of branch	*Transverse dimension* (mm)	*Number of funiculi*	*Dissectable length* (mm)	*Level of origin*	*Level of mixing*
Superficial branch	1.7	2.8	52	From below the elbow to arm 1/4	From arm 1/4–2/4
Deep branch	3.0	4.6	61	From below the elbow to arm 1/4	From arm 1/4–2/4
Extensor flexor brevis branch	1.0	1.2	36	From below the elbow to arm 1/4	Arm 1/4
Extensor flexor longus branch	1.3	1.8	18	Arm 1/4	Arm 1/4–2/4
Brachioradialis branch	0.9	1.2	21	Arm 1/4–2/4	Arm 1/4–2/4
Brachialis branch	0.7	1.0	7	Arm 1/4–2/4	Arm 1/4–2/4

The branch to the extensor carpi radialis longus

This lies in the posterolateral part of the radial nerve trunk, the length available for separate dissection being fairly short. After mixing with the funiculi of the extensor carpi radialis brevis and brachioradialis it joins the funicular group of the posterior interosseous nerve and continues to ascend.

The branch to the brachioradialis

This consists mostly of one branch; a few may involve two. At segment 3/8 of the arm it mixes with the neighbouring motor funicular groups.

The branch to the brachialis

The level of origin of this branch is rather diverse, i.e. from segments 2/8 to 6/8 of the arm. The length available for separate dissection is very short. It mixes with neighbouring funicular groups almost immediately.

The posterior cutaneous nerve of the forearm

This is a relatively large cutaneous branch, its transverse diameter being 2.2 (1.5–3.0) mm. It contains four funiculi on average, about half of which arise near the uppermost part of the radial nerve trunk and the other half from the axilla. It can be dissected separately in the whole arm, because it is surrounded by thick connective tissue and is not mixed with the neighbouring funicular groups.

The lateral cutaneous nerve of the arm

This arises mostly from the axilla, except for a few which may arise from the uppermost part of the arm. The mean transverse diameter is 1.1 (0.8–1.5) mm and the average number of funiculi is 1.7. It can be dissected separately in the whole arm and does not mix with any other funicular group.

Branches to the triceps brachii

These arise mostly from the axilla. They are numerous and dispersed. Only a few of them arise from the uppermost part of the arm. They do not mix with other funicular groups in the arm.

Localization and application of main funicular groups of the radial nerve

The radial nerve follows a spiral course laterally from below upwards in the arm and the funicular groups in the nerve trunk assume a corresponding shifting. For the sake of better comprehension, memory and clinical application, this is illustrated by Figure 10.7 and Table 10.7. According to Figure 10.7 the funicular groups in the radial nerve trunk of the right upper limb are shown to undergo a clockwise shift.

Table 10.7 The topographical localization of the main funicular groups in the radial nerve trunk

Different levels in the arm	*Arm 1/8*	*Arm 4/8*	*Arm 6/8*	*Arm 8/8*
Funicular groups with predominance of sensory fibres	Anterior to the trunk	Anterolateral to the trunk	Lateral to the trunk	Posterolateral to the trunk
Funicular groups with predominance of motor fibres	Posterior to the trunk	Posteromedial to the trunk	Medial to the trunk	Anteromedial to the trunk

Sites susceptible to injuries by compression in the radial nerve

The chief motor branch of the radial nerve, the posterior interosseous nerve of the forearm, is liable to injury by compression at the lower part of the cubital fossa. The anatomical structures that may cause compression of the nerve are: the arch of the supinator (Frohse arch), the arch of the extensor carpi radialis brevis, branches of the radial recurrent artery and the fibrous membrane connecting the Frohse arch. The proximal border of the superficial fibres of the supinator presents itself as a semicircular arch, the transverse diameter of which is about 10–12 mm, and as a semitendinous structure. A firm, sharp and tendinous medial border exists at the origin of the extensor carpi radialis brevis.

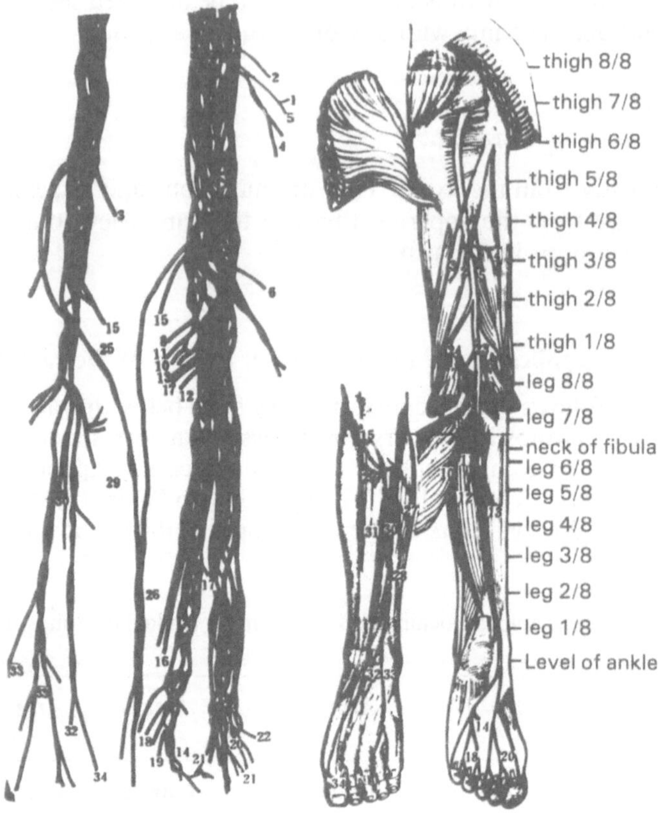

Figure 10.8 Level of recording and the dissected specimen of the sciatic nerve. **1**: Proximal branch to long head of biceps femoris; **2**: distal branch to long head of biceps femoris; **3**: branch to short head of biceps femoris; **4**: branch to semimembranosus and adductor magnus; **5**: branch to semitendinosus; **6**: branch to medial head of gastrocnemius; **7**: branch to lateral head of gastrocnemius; **8**: branch to popliteus; **9**: proximal branch to soleus; **10**: distal branch to soleus; **11**: branch to tibialis posterior; **12**: branch to flexor hallucis longus; **13**: branches to flexor digitorum longus; **14**: deep branch of lateral plantar n.; **15**: branch to knee joint; **16**: calcanean branches; **17**: vascular branches; **18**: superficial branch of lateral plantar n.; **19**: branch to flexor digiti minimi brevis; **20**: cutaneous branches of medial plantar n.; **21**: branches to lumbricales; **22**: branches to flexor digitorum brevis; **23**: medial cutaneous n. of calf; **24**: lateral cutaneous n. of calf; **25**: sural communicating branch; **26**: sural n.; **27**: branch to peroneus longus; **28**: branch to peroneus brevis; **29**: branch to tibialis anterior; **30**: branch to extensor digitorum longus; **31**: branches to extensor hallucis longus; **32**: branches to short extensor of digits; **33**: dorsal cutaneous n.; **34**: dorsal digital n. to lateral side of hallux and medial side of second digit.

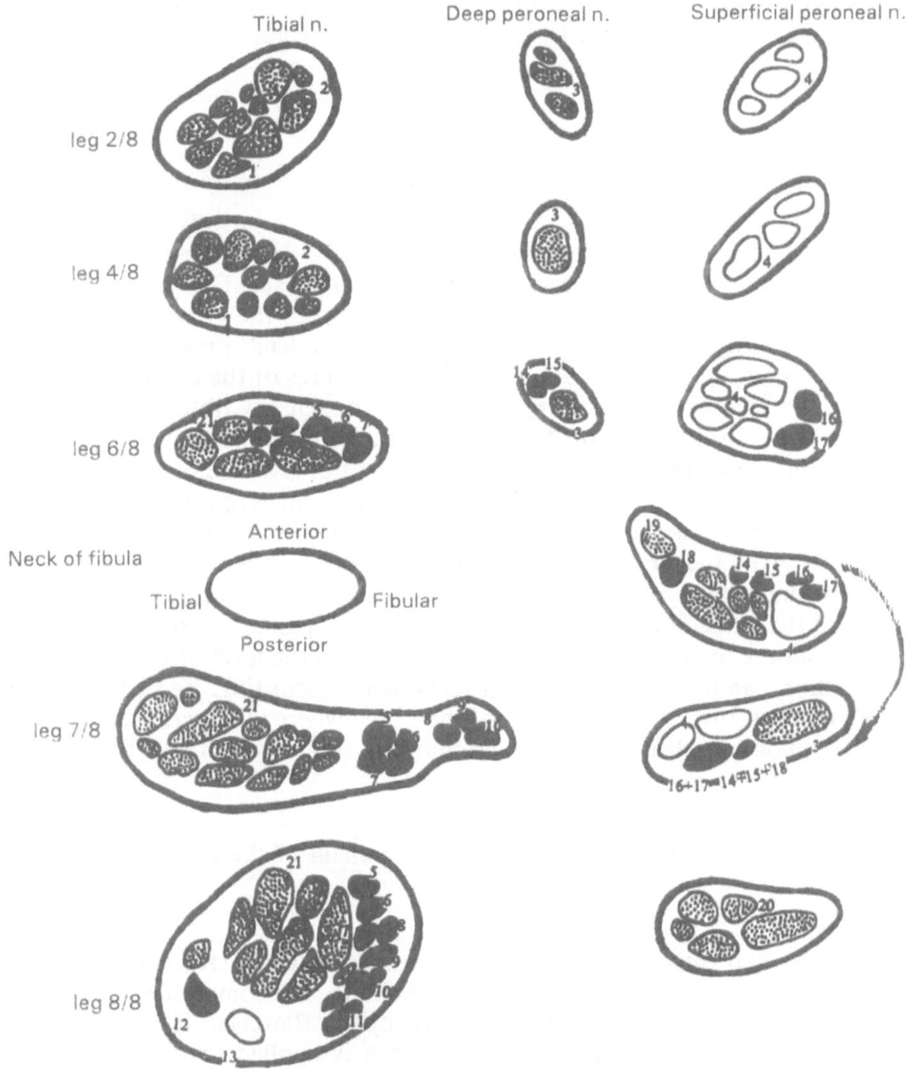

The arch of the supinator and the medial border of the extensor carpi radialis brevis often form a continuous arch and, in about one-third of cases, there is a thin and tough fibrous membrane connecting the tendon of the brachialis at the free border of the arch. When the forearm is pronated these structures are set in special tension, thus pressing the posterior interosseous nerve and leading to the dynamic type of entrapment neuropathy. Consequently, surgical resection of the arch of the extensor carpi radialis brevis and that of the supinator, together with the fibrous membrane connected to the tendon of the brachialis, will be the effective means of nerve decompression.

SCIATIC NERVE

ZHOU CHANGMAN AND ZHONG SHIZHEN

The sciatic nerve is the largest in the human body. Upon dissection the tibial and common peroneal divisions are found remaining separately enclosed in the thick epineurium-like connective tissue. Thus, from the viewpoint of microsurgical practice, these may be regarded as two completely independent entities. According to Sunderland's analysis the motor fibres of the common peroneal nerve, in the popliteal fossa, represent 34%, the sensory fibres, 66%; and the motor and sensory fibres of the tibial nerve amount to 32% and 18% respectively, the remaining 50% consisting of mixed fibres of the plantar nerves. In lower limb nerve injuries, functional rehabilitation is given priority to the groups of large muscles in contrast with the upper limb, the functional rehabilitation is given the first place to the small muscles of the hand.

For the sake of better memory and application, the distance between the level of the malleoli of the ankle and that of condyles of the femur, as well as that from the upper border of the sciatic notch to the level of the condyles of the femur, can be divided into eight sections for recording. Records have also been taken at the level of the neck of the fibula where the internal structure of the common peroneal nerve changes abruptly (Figures 10.8 and 10.9).

External form, dimension and number of funiculi of the sciatic nerve

Common peroneal nerve

The deep and superficial peroneal nerves combine to form the common peroneal nerve at the level of the neck of the fibula. The common peroneal nerve here has a greater transverse diameter and appears flattened. It contains a considerable amount of connective tissue which is applied to the anterolateral aspect of the neck of the fibula. The common peroneal nerve rotates laterally for about 180 degrees from the neck of the fibula to the popliteal fossa, the most abrupt rotation occurring mainly within 20–30 mm above the neck of the fibula. During the course of ascent, both the number of fascicles and the amount of connective tissue become lessened, so that the trunk gets slender. The common peroneal nerve, in segment 7/8 of the leg, is situated between the tendon of the biceps femoris and the upper margin of the lateral head of the gastrocnemius and has an elliptical profile in cross-section. In segment 2/8 of the thigh the lateral cutaneous nerve of the calf and the sural communicating nerve join the common peroneal nerve from behind, thus adding to the anteroposterior diameter and giving the latter an almost circular contour. The observational data relevant to the common peroneal nerve are as shown in Table 10.8.

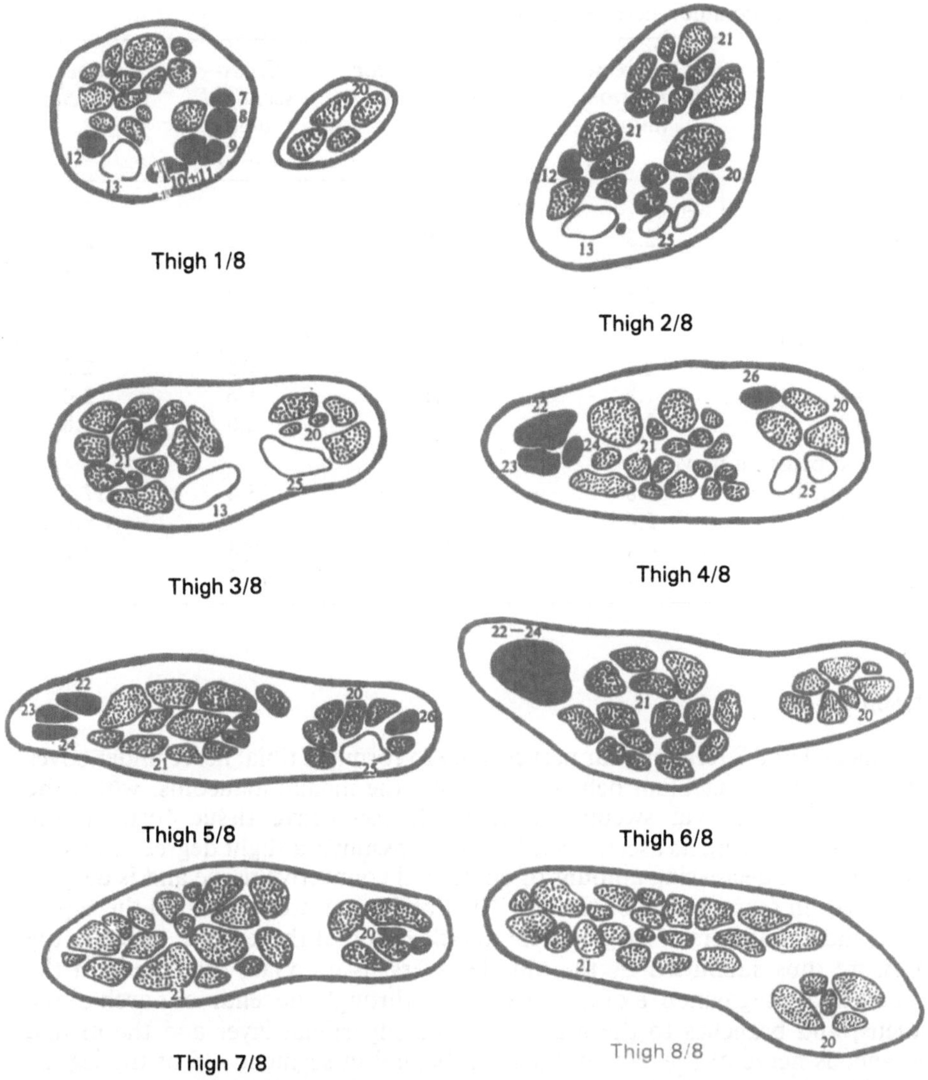

Figure 10.9 Internal topographical localization of the sciatic nerve. Black: fibre bundle of muscular branch; white: fibre bundle of cutaneous branch; dots: mixed bundle. **1**: medial plantar n.; **2**: lateral plantar n.; **3**: deep peroneal n.; **4**: superficial peroneal n.; **5**: branches to flexor digitorum longus; **6**: branches to flexor hallucis longus; **7**: proximal branch to soleus; **8**: branch to tibialis posterior; **9**: branch to popliteus; **10**: distal branch to soleus; **11**: branch to lateral head of gastrocnemius; **12**: branch to medial head of gastrocnemius; **13**: medial cutaneous n. of calf; **14**: branch to extensor hallucis longus; **15**: branches to extensor digitorum longus; **16**: branch to peroneus brevis; **17**: branch to peroneus longus; **18**: branch to tibialis anterior; **19**: branches to tibialis anterior and knee joint; **20**: $=3+4$; **21**: $=1+2$; **22**: branches to semimembranosus and adductor magnus; **23**: branch to long head of biceps femoris; **24**: branch to semitendinosus; **25**: lateral cutaneous n. of calf and sural communicating branch; **26**: branch to short head of biceps femoris.

Table 10.8 The mean value of the dimensions and number of fascicles in various segments of the common peroneal nerve

Level of segment	*Transverse dimension* (mm)	*Anteroposterior dimension* (mm)	*Cross-sectional area* (mm^2)	*Number of fascicles*
Superficial peroneal nerve				
leg 2/8	2.3	1.0	1.8	2.5
leg 4/8	2.1	1.0	1.7	2.4
leg 6/8	2.8	1.4	3.2	3.6
Deep peroneal nerve				
leg 2/8	1.7	1.1	1.5	2.0
leg 4/8	1.8	1.1	1.6	2.0
leg 6/8	2.5	1.4	2.8	3.8
Common peroneal nerve				
neck of fibula	6.8	2.9	15.4	12.0
leg 7/8	5.6	2.7	11.8	9.9
leg 8/3	4.4	2.8	9.8	6.5
thigh 1/8	3.1	4.6	11.3	7.6

Tibial nerve

The medial and lateral plantar nerves unite to form the tibial nerve under cover of the flexor retinaculum behind and below the medial malleolus, where the nerve forms an oval swelling with much connective tissue forming the epineurium. During its ascent the tibial nerve assumes a slight degree of medial rotation with decreasing amount of epineurial connective tissue and is deep to the soleus in segment 3/8 of the leg. The tibial nerve proceeds amid the superficial and deep layers of the posterior muscle group of the leg and, owing to the pressure thus submitted by the muscle layers, is coronally flattened. In the course above segment 6/8 of the leg it passes through the tendinous arch of the soleus, and branches to the muscles of the superficial layer and the medial cutaneous nerve of the calf join it from behind in segment 7/8 of the leg, so that the anteroposterior dimension increases, which together with the increment in connective tissue makes its cross-section appear oval and assume the maximum area. In segment 8/8 of the leg the nerve trunk gradually takes on a circular profile with an increasing number of fascicles. The observational data in relation to the posterior tibial nerve are listed in Table 10.9.

Sciatic nerve

Morphologically, the tibial and common peroneal nerves unite to form the sciatic nerve around the junction of the middle and lower thirds of the thigh. Based on the data obtained from the Chinese, the common type amounts to

Table 10.9 The mean value of the dimensions and number of fascicles in various segments of the tibial nerve

Level of segment	*Transverse dimension* (mm)	*Anteroposterior dimension* (mm)	*Cross-sectional area* (mm^2)	*Number fascicles*
Leg 2/8	3.1	4.9	11.7	14.7
Leg 4/8	4.8	2.8	10.5	12.8
Leg 6/8	5.8	2.8	12.5	15.7
Leg 7/8	5.8	3.5	15.6	17.7
Leg 8/8	4.9	6.2	23.9	20.1
Thigh 1/8	4.4	5.9	21.2	15.3

about 60.5–61.6%, while the highly branching type and the miscellaneous ones account for approximately 38.4–39.5%. The cross-section of the trunk of the sciatic nerve is oval, but the anteroposterior dimension of the medial part is greater than that of the lateral. During its ascent it assumes a slight medial rotation, and above segment 7/8 of the thigh the increment in connective tissue becomes prominent, leading to the rapid broadening of its transverse dimension and thickening of the nerve fascicles with the result of assuming a flattened tape-like conformation which is broad above and narrow below.

Table 10.10 The mean value of the dimensions and number of fascicles in various segments of the sciatic nerve

Level of segment	*Transverse dimension* (mm)	*Anteroposterior dimension* (mm)	*Cross-sectional area* (mm^2)	*Number of fascicles*
Thigh 2/8	7.5	5.5	32.3	23.9
Thigh 3/8	8.7	4.6	31.4	26.4
Thigh 4/8	9.7	4.4	33.8	28.4
Thigh 5/8	10.6	4.9	41.5	33.1
Thigh 6/8	10.1	5.0	41.7	31.8
Thigh 7/8	10.6	4.5	37.3	31.3
Thigh 8/8	16.9	4.2	54.9	29.6

Common peroneal nerve

The number of fascicles in individual branches of the common peroneal nerve, the level of origin of these branches and their individual dissectable length and the level of mixing are shown in Table 10.11.

Table 10.11 The mean value of individual branches of the common peroneal nerve

Name of individual branch	*Transverse dimension* (mm)	*Number of fascicles*	*Level of origin*	*Level of mixing*	*Dissectable length* (mm)
Peroneus longus branch	1.6	1.1	Neck of fibula	Thigh 1/8	107.7
Peroneus brevis branch	1.8	1.4	Leg 5/8–6/8	Thigh 1/8	147.0
Tibialis anterior middle branch	1.8	1.0	Neck of fibula	Leg 7/8–8/8	50.7
Tibialis anterior proximal branch and common branch to the knee joint	2.2	1.0	Neck of fibula	Leg 8/8	48.2
Extensor hallucis longus branch	1.2	1.2	Leg 5/8–6/8	Leg 7/8–8/8	72.2
Extensor digitorum longus branch	1.0	1.1	Leg 6/8–neck of fibula	Leg 7/8–8/8	52.5
Extensor digitorum brevis branch	1.9	1.5	Below zero	Zero	10.4
Short head of biceps femoris branch	1.9	1.0	Thigh 4/8–5/8	Thigh 6/8–7/8	123.8
Lateral cutaneous nerve of the calf and sural communicating branch	2.7	2.4	Thigh 1/8	Thigh 5/8–6/8	198.1
Proximal branch to the knee joint	0.9	1.0	Thigh 1/8–2/8	Thigh 4/8–5/8	80.4

Superficial peroneal nerve

Muscular branches

Mostly the peroneus longus has a thicker distal as well as a thinner proximal muscular branch, both mixing to form a single bundle behind the head of the fibula. The muscular branch to the peroneus brevis, being single, gives off in succession three to four twigs to the muscle.

Cutaneous branches

The superficial peroneal nerve, being the chief sensory nerve of the dorsum of the foot, has been formed by the combination of the medial and lateral branches below the ankle joint. It is subcutaneous below segment 3/8 of the leg but ascends past the intermuscular septum to join the lateral portion of the common peroneal nerve.

Deep peroneal nerve

The deep peroneal nerve is formed by the combination of the cutaneous branch to the web of the great toe and the branch to the extensor digitorum brevis 35 mm below the ankle.

Branch to the tibialis anterior

Most of the tibialis anterior has three twigs, namely, the distal, middle and proximal; a few have only middle and proximal twigs. The middle twig is thicker; the proximal one, being slender, often has a stem common to the branch of the knee joint and they enter the medial border of the stem at the level of the neck of the fibula.

Branches to the extensor hallucis longus and the extensor digitorum longus

These enter the deep peroneal nerve separately through its lateral side and readily combine into one bundle in segment 7/8 of the leg. In some cases they unite to form a common stem before entering the deep peroneal nerve.

Lateral cutaneous nerve of the calf and sural communicating nerve

These two nerves combine into one, each containing a nerve bundle, and enter the posterior aspect of the common peroneal nerve in segment 1/8 of the thigh.

Branch to the short head of biceps femoris

This branch enters the anteromedial aspect of the common peroneal nerve in segment 4/8 of the thigh.

The localization of the main groups of nerve fascicles in the common peroneal nerve

1. Branches to the muscles of the lateral group of the leg occupy the anterolateral portion of the common peroneal nerve at the level of the neck of the fibula. With the rotation of the common peroneal nerve, these are shifted to the posteromedial portion when approaching the popliteal fossa.

2. Branches to the muscles of the anterior group of the leg enter in succession the deep and common peroneal nerves anteriorly. These occupy the centre of the anterior portion of the common peroneal nerve and, following the lateral rotation of the common peroneal nerve, shift to the centre of the posterior part.

Tibial nerve

The number of fascicles in individual branches of the tibial nerve, the level of origin of these branches and their individual dissectable length and the level of mixing are shown in Table 10.12.

Table 10.12 The mean value of individual branches of the tibial nerve

Name of individual nerve	*Transverse dimension* (mm)	*Number of fascicles*	*Level of origin*	*Level of mixing*	*Dissectable length* (mm)
Flexor hallucis longus branch	1.5	1.0	Leg 5/8–7/8	Thigh 1/8	107.4
Flexor digitorum longus branch	1.5	1.0	Leg 6/8–7/8	Thigh 1/8	107.5
Tibialis branch	2.1	1.0	Leg 7/8–8/8	Thigh 1/8	81.9
Distal soleus branch	1.9	1.2	Leg 7/8–8/8	Thigh 1/8	86.6
Proximal soleus branch	2.5	1.05	Leg 7/8–8/8	Thigh 1/8–2/8	89.4
Popliteus branch	2.3	1.1	Leg 7/8–8/8	Thigh 1/8	78.2
Medial head of gastrocnemius branch	2.3	1.3	Leg 8/8–thigh 1/8	Thigh 2/8	82.1
Lateral head of gastrocnemius branch	2.2	1.2	Leg 8/8–thigh 1/8	Thigh 1/8–2/8	79.3
Distal long head of biceps branch	2.1	1.0	Thigh 5/8–6/8	Thigh 7/8	74.7
Semitendinosus branch	1.7	1.1	Thigh 4/8–5/8	Thigh 7/8	121.0
Semimembranosus adductor magnus branch	2.5	1.0	Thigh 4/8–5/8	Thigh 6/8–7/8	97.3
Medial cutaneous nerve of the calf	1.9	1.1	Leg 8/8–thigh 1/8	Thigh 2/8–3/8	112.4
Knee joint branch	1.6	1.0	Thigh 1/8–3/8	Thigh 4/8–5/8	89.4

Medial plantar nerve

The medial plantar nerve has a transverse diameter of 4.1 mm and contains 8.2 nerve fascicles on average. It gives off the abductor hallucis branch 31 mm below the ankle, the latter having a transverse diameter of 1.2 mm and containing one fascicle. The terminal branches consist of three cutaneous twigs: the medial twig has a transverse diameter of 2.9 mm and contains 1.8 nerve fascicles; the middle twig with a transverse diameter of 3.1 mm contains 3.4 fascicles and gives off the flexor hallucis brevis branch and the first lumbrical branch; the lateral twig contains two fascicles with a transverse diameter of 2.2 mm and gives off the second lumbrical branch.

Lateral plantar nerve

The lateral plantar nerve contains 5.9 fascicles and has a transverse diameter of 3.2 mm. The abductor digiti minimi branch which contains 1.4 fascicles and has a transverse diameter of 1.2 mm, springs from its base. It divides into two terminal branches; namely the deep and superficial twigs 66 mm below the ankle. The superficial one, being the lateral plantar cutaneous branch, gives off the flexor digiti minimi branch. The deep one, being known as the deep plantar muscular branch, contains 2.7 fascicles and has a transverse diameter of 2.8 mm. Its dissectable distance upward is 30 mm.

In the stem of the tibial nerve the lateral plantar nerve is situated in the posterolateral portion, while the medial plantar nerve in the anteromedial portion stays until segment 6/8 of the leg where the two nerves combine.

Flexor hallucis longus and flexor digitorum longus branches

The flexor digitorum longus branch passes over the anterior aspect of the stem of the posterior tibial nerve from its medial side to the lateral. In some of the specimens these two branches enter the tibial nerve in the form of a common stem. In a few specimens a minute distal flexor hallucis longus branch exists in segment 4/8 of the leg.

The tibialis posterior branch, the popliteus branch and the soleus branch

These ascend lateral to the tibial nerve in segments 7/8–8/8 of the leg.

The medial cutaneous nerve of the calf

This nerve mostly enters the tibial nerve from the posterior aspect as a single fascicle.

The medial head of the gastrocnemius branches

These consist of two branches that unite into one containing a thicker fascicle.

The lateral head of the gastrocnemius and proximal soleus branches

These mostly enter the tibial nerve posterolaterally in the form of a common stem. Still a few of the lateral heads of the gastrocnemius branch get into the nerve 21 mm above the proximal soleus branch. Individual medial heads of the gastrocnemius branch mix with the proximal soleus branch before entering the tibial nerve.

The semitendinosus, semimembranosus, adductor magnus and the long head of the biceps femoris branches

These join the medial portion of the sciatic nerve above segment 4/8 of the thigh and mix altogether in segment 6/8.

Localization of main groups of nerve fascicles in the tibial nerve

Branches to the muscles of the posterior group of the leg

Though the sites of emergence of the muscular branches of the posterior group muscles vary in height from segment 6/8 of the leg upwards until segment 1/8 of the thigh, their topography in the tibial nerve remains rather constant, i.e. their fascicles occupy the lateral and posterolateral portions.

Branches to the muscles of the posterior group of the thigh

With the exception of the short head of biceps femoris branch the nerve fascicles of this group reside constantly in the medial section of the tibial nerve in segments 4/8–6/8 of the thigh. Muscular branches still predominate in the mixed fascicles of the medial section of the tibial nerve though fusion with other mixed ones has taken place above segment 7/8 of the thigh.

Sites where the nerves are vulnerable to injury

Gluteal region

The sciatic nerve usually reaches the gluteal region as a single main trunk under cover of the lower border of the piriformis. Where the sciatic nerve passes through the piriformis (1.0%), or the common peroneal nerve passes through instead (34.9%), it is apt to be compressed during the spasm of the piriformis leading to neurological symptoms.

Neck of the fibula

The common peroneal nerve winds round the neck of the fibula posterolateral to the head, being here wrapped in a fibrous tunnel known as the peroneal canal. This segment of the common peroneal nerve becomes applied tightly to the bony surface, against which the nerve is prone to be knocked or pressed with the highest incidence of nerve injury. As a result, particular attention should be paid to the arrangement of the fascicles in the repair inside the nerve trunk, since it has undergone a kind of rapid change due to an abrupt turn of 180 degrees of the nerve with a rather short range.

The ankle region

The tibial nerve takes up a position deep in the leg and shallow in the ankle. It is bound down together with the tendons by the flexor retinaculum behind the medial malleolus and is liable to manifest a series of symptoms simulating the carpal canal ones and known as the ankle canal syndrome.

VAGUS NERVE

WANG ZIHUA, XIAO SHANGYING, WANG ZHINAN AND HAN FENGYUE

The vagus nerve is a pair of mixed nerves that have the longest course and the most extensive distribution and contain mainly the parasympathetic fibres. The parasympathetic fibres, or the general visceral efferents, originate from the dorsal motor nucleus of the vagus. The cells in the dorsal motor nucleus of the vagus in man have been estimated to be more than 9000 on either side. The nucleus consists of mainly smaller fusiform cells as well as those large cells containing coarser Nissl granules and diffused cells enclosing melanoid pigment. Their function is not yet fully known. It has been assumed that the large cells supply the smooth muscle of the visceral wall, especially the stomach, while the smaller ones innervate the heart and the smooth muscle of the vessels of the mucosa in the head.

The vagus and glossopharyngeal nerves are so closely related in respect to the topography of their attachment to the brain and exit from the skull that it is difficult to separate the rootlets of the vagus from those of the glossopharyngeal nerve, as on the lateral surface of the medulla oblongata. The glossopharyngeal and vagus nerves, after rising from the posterolateral sulcus of the medulla oblongata, pass jointly through the jugular foramen to the outside of the skull. Within the first few centimetres from the cranial cavity the vagus and glossopharyngeal nerves are closely adjacent to the internal jugular vein and are surrounded by regional lymph nodes. Such intimate topographic relationship remains until the level of the mastoid process is reached. The glossopharyngeal nerve then turns anteroinferiorly from behind the stylopharyngeus, while the vagus descends directly. Owing to such specific topographical relationship, the vagus must always be involved in the characteristic jugular foramen (Vernet's) syndrome.

Within the foramen there is an enlargement on the vagus trunk which is called the jugular or the superior ganglion, and another oval one called the nodose or the inferior ganglion is located just below the foramen. These ganglia consist mainly of pseudounipolar neurons. It has been demonstrated, however, that there are also multipolar neurons in the inferior ganglion, of which the functions remain unknown.

It has been reported that, at the level of the cricoid cartilage, the total number of the nerve fibres in the cervical segment of the vagus is 82 379 (45 110–111 807) on the left, of which the unmyelinated fibres amount to 80.9%, and 105 375 (69 951–153 123) on the right, with 81% of unmyelinated fibres.

Recurrent laryngeal nerve (Figure 10.10)

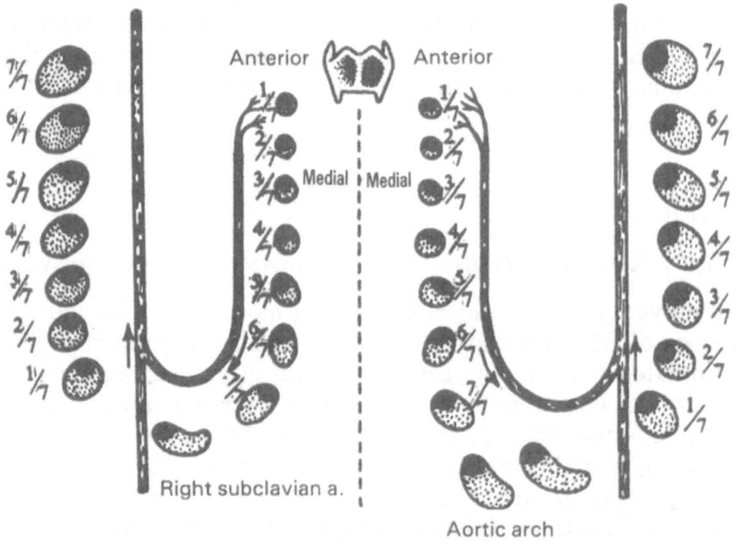

Figure 10.10 A schematic representation of the topography of the recurrent laryngeal nerve

One of the important branches of the vagus is the recurrent laryngeal nerve which has its origin in the ambiguous nucleus of the medulla oblongata. It has been reported that the number of the cells in the left ambiguous nucleus is 1942, while the right amgibuous nucleus has 1836 neurons. About half of the axons emerging from the ambiguous nucleus leave the vagus trunk anterior to the aortic arch on the left side, or in front of the right subclavian artery on the right, to form the recurrent nerves. The left recurrent laryngeal nerve winds below the aortic arch and then ascends in the groove between the oesophagus and trachea while the right nerve does the same below the right subclavian artery and takes the same course as the left. The course of the nerve on either side is closely related to the inferior thyroid artery. It lies either superficial or deep to the artery or its branches, or passes through these branches. At or above the level of the inferior horn of the thyroid cartilage, the recurrent nerve divides into the anterior ramus (to the lateral and posterior cricoarytenoids) and the posterior ramus (pharyngeal branch). In 55% of cases the recurrent nerve divides into an anterior and a posterior ramus at the level of the inferior horn of the thyroid cartilage. If the division takes place above the level of the inferior horn, the position of bifurcation varies between 2 and 7 mm; while where it is below the horn the bifurcation will be within the first 2 mm. The site of emergence of the pharyngeal ramus is always below the common stem of the two muscular branches, i.e. the anterior branch.

Because of the extremely intimate topographic relation between the recurrent nerve and the inferior thyroid artery, it is not rare to cause damage to the nerve during thyroid operations. It has been reported that bilateral paralysis of the vocal cord in adults due to thyroid surgery reaches 58%. Bilateral lesion of the recurrent nerves leads to the paralysis of both vocal cords with dyspnoea and disturbance in vocalization. Surgical repair of these injured nerves will bring subsequent relief to the suffering.

The average length of the left recurrent nerve from the inferior horn of the thyroid cartilage to the aortic arch is 82 (60–101) mm. If it is divided into seven equal parts the length of every part will be 11.7 mm. The average length of the right nerve from the inferior horn of the thyroid cartilage to the right subclavian artery is 63 (51–71) mm, so that every one-seventh part is 9 mm.

The ramus to the lateral cricoarytenoid appears to be the direct continuation of the recurrent nerve and mostly passes into the middle of the muscle. The ramus to the posterior cricoarytenoid gives off a series of twigs, which enter the muscle one after another from below upwards, if it sprouts below the inferior horn of the thyroid cartilage. When it springs above the horn its twigs enter the deep surface of the muscle superiorly from the upper half of the lateral border. In most cases a sort of loop is first formed by those twigs above and at the lateral edge of the muscle, whence ramuscules are again brought forth and enter the muscle.

The recurrent laryngeal nerve gives off ramuscules to the oesophagus and the trachea in each of the seven parts mentioned above. Two of the ramuscules are more constant; one of them is the pharyngeal ramus that arises from the site of union of two muscular rami and ascends superoposteriorly, while the other is the cardiac ramus that arises from the lowest seventh part, i.e. the part bordering the aortic arch or the right subclavian artery and thus winding below it. The cardiac ramus comprises one to three twigs directing toward the cardiac plexus.

When dissecting proximally from the rami to the lateral and posterior cricoarytenoid muscles, one may observe the recurrent laryngeal nerve being covered by the cricopharyngeus muscle near the inferior horn of the thyroid cartilage, which is more constant. Therefore, undoubtedly the inferior horn is a reliable mark for the recognition of the recurrent nerve. In view of the fact that the function of the lateral cricoarytenoid is to narrow the slit of glottis, while the posterior cricoarytenoid widens it, it would be helpful to carry out the apposition suture of the nerve fascicles within the recurrent nerve where the topographic arrangement of the fibres is clarified. From the anatomical point of view, however, it is rather difficult to distinguish them clearly. After forming a common trunk the fibres from the two rami begin to intermingle; yet according to the course of the fibres directed proximally from the muscular rami in the uppermost seventh part, it is still possible to distinguish the fibres to the lateral cricoarytenoid located anterolaterally from those to the posterior cricoarytenoid located deep to the former. It is also possible to distinguish the course of the fibres only in the upper half of the uppermost seventh part, provided that the union of the two muscular rami takes place above the inferior horn of the thyroid cartilage. Beginning from the second one-seventh part, the oesophageal and tracheal rami join the recurrent nerve and intermingle continually. Any attempt to distinguish the fibres to the lateral cricoarytenoid from those to the posterior cricoarytenoid becomes rather difficult. Beginning from the third or fourth one-seventh part, the fibres in the recurrent nerve are usually found to be grouped into two fascicles which, however, do not pertain to the muscular rami and the oesophagotracheal twigs respectively but are simply the result of reconstruction after intermingling. However, judging from their course and direction, the two muscular rami are mainly located anterolaterally, while the oesophageal and tracheal rami are prominently situated postomedially.

The outer diameter (transverse dimension times longitudinal dimension) of the left recurrent laryngeal nerve is 0.7×0.8 mm at the level of inferior horn of the thyroid cartilage, or 1.2×1.9 mm at the level of the aortic arch, while those of the right are 0.5×0.9 mm at the level of the inferior horn, or 1.0×2.1 mm at the level of the right subclavian artery.

The recurrent laryngeal nerve becomes gradually thicker from the point of union of both muscular rami to the site where it springs from the vagus and assumes a nearly cylindrical appearance. This distinct change in the appearance of the nerve is to be clearly seen where the nerve is winding below the aortic arch or the right subclavian artery. From the distal end proximally, the recurrent nerve appears almost like an irregular cylinder, its transverse dimension exceeding the longitudinal, and then assumes a curvature that is concave upward with the longitudinal dimension over the transverse, and finally resumes approximately the cylindrical contour. From the distal end to the aortic arch or the right subclavian artery, the two muscular rami are located anterolateral to the oesophageal and tracheal rami, then descend along their lateral side, and finally pass in front of them. After they enter the vagus nerve the average length of the left vagus is 109 (91–125) mm from the level of the aortic arch to the superior horn of the thyroid cartilage, also divided into seven equal parts, each being 16 mm. The average length of the right vagus from the level of right subclavian artery to the superior horn of the thyroid cartilage is 75 (60–92) mm, and each of the seven parts is 11 mm. From the level of the aortic arch or the right subclavian artery to the superior horn of the thyroid cartilage the topography of the recurrent nerve has essentially been as follows: anteromedial (or anterolateral) → anterior → anteromedial. In view of the whole course, it appears that the topography of the recurrent nerve within the vagus trunk is relatively constant.

The cross-sectional area of the recurrent nerve in the vagus and their percentages are shown in Table 10.13. Quoted from the reference, the number of fibres in the recurrent laryngeal nerves is 7496 (4392–15 697) on the left, the

Table 10.13 The cross-sectional areas (mm^2) of the vagus (CAV) and the recurrent (CAR) nerves, and the percentage of the area of the recurrent nerve

	Left			*Right*		
Level	*CAV* (mm^2) *(range)*	*CAR* (mm^2) *(range)*	*Recurrent n.* (%)	*CAV* (mm^2) *(range)*	*CAR* (mm^2) *(range)*	*Recurrent n.* (%)
Superior horn of thyroid cartilage						
7/7	5.07 (3.72–6.38)	1.24 (0.71–1.65)	24.46	4.51 (2.55–5.52)	1.26 (0.87–1.54)	27.94
6/7	4.25 (3.41–5.52)	1.15 (0.64–1.54)	27.06	4.12 (3.77–4.68)	1.07 (0.71–1.43)	25.97
5/7	3.60 (2.54–5.11)	1.13 (0.64–1.54)	31.39	4.27 (3.45–5.94)	0.99 (0.71–1.23)	23.19
4/7	3.29 (2.27–4.91)	0.88 (0.71–1.13)	26.74	3.45 (2.41–4.10)	0.98 (0.63–1.23)	28.41
3/7	3.29 (2.14–4.52)	0.93 (0.71–1.13)	28.27	3.40 (2.41–4.15)	0.87 (0.71–1.23)	25.59
2/7	3.12 (2.41–4.52)	0.88 (0.71–0.99)	28.21	3.29 (2.41–4.41)	0.81 (0.64–1.23)	24.62
Aortic arch or right subclavian artery						
1/7	3.15 (2.24–4.52)	0.88 (0.71–0.99)	27.94	3.32 (2.54–4.26)	0.87 (0.71–1.23)	26.20

unmyelinated fibres of which represent 66.7%, and 8003 (3651–16 806) on the right, the unmyelinated fibres representing 65.3%.

Blood supply of the recurrent laryngeal nerve

The blood vessels supplying the recurrent nerve arise from the branches of the vessels to the neighbouring organs and are usually rather small. The diameters of vessels are all less than 1 mm. The origins of the vessels are different on either side.

The left recurrent laryngeal nerve

This nerve has the sources of blood supply shown in Figure 10.11.

(1) Branch of the bronchial artery. The bronchial artery, the external diameter of which is 2 mm, arises from the descending thoracic aorta opposite

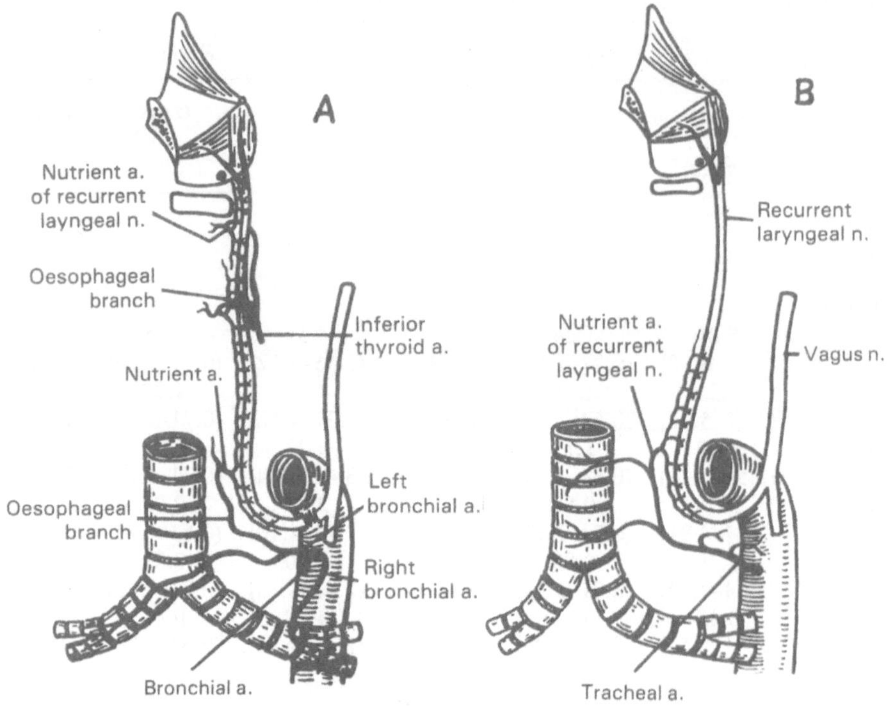

Figure 10.11 Blood supply of the left recurrent laryngeal nerve

the fifth thoracic vertebra, ascends between the aorta and the oesophagus and divides into the left and right bronchial arteries at the level between the fourth and fifth thoracic vertebrae. The right bronchial artery runs to the right and, when crossing the left recurrent laryngeal nerve, gives off branches which ascend in company with the recurrent nerve to enter the oesophagus at the level between the second and third thoracic vertebrae. The oesophageal branch gives off a ramus that subdivides medial to the recurrent nerve into an upper and a lower twig which enter the nerve.

(2) The branch of the tracheal artery that originates from the posterior wall of the thoracic aorta. Opposite to the level between the fifth and fourth thoracic vertebrae the tracheal artery springs from the thoracic aorta. The outer diameter of the artery is 1 mm. It ascends superomedially behind the aortic arch and in front of the trachea, giving off some branches to the aortic arch. The branch to the trachea gives off a ramus that subdivides medial to the recurrent nerve into an upper and a lower twig which enter the recurrent nerve.

(3) The branch from the inferior thyroid artery.

(4) The branch from the oesophageal branch given off by the inferior thyroid artery.

(5) The branch from the arterial plexus of the oesophagus.

(6) The branch continuing from the nutrient artery to the vagus nerve.

Right recurrent laryngeal nerve (Figure 10.12)

(1) Small branch from the right common carotid artery. A small branch with an outer diameter of 0.6 mm arises from the medial wall of the right common carotid artery, descends along the artery, and ends by bifurcating into an upper and a lower twig to enter the recurrent nerve from the site medial to it.

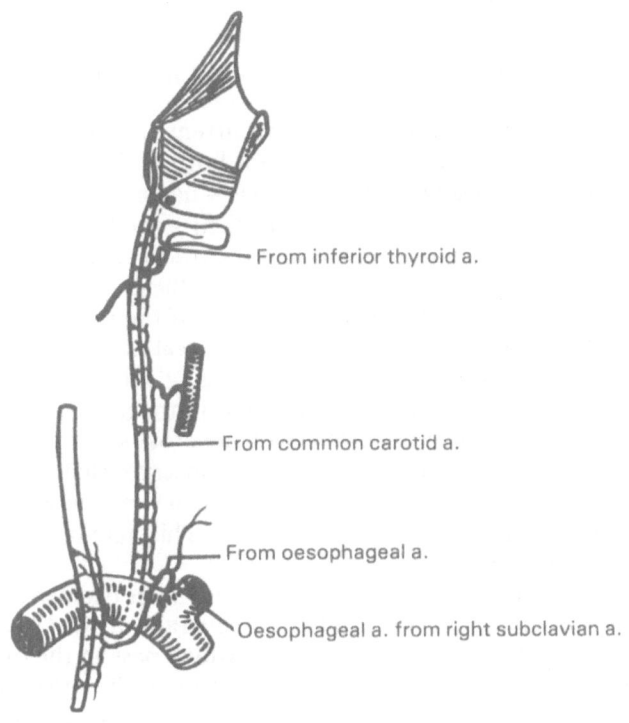

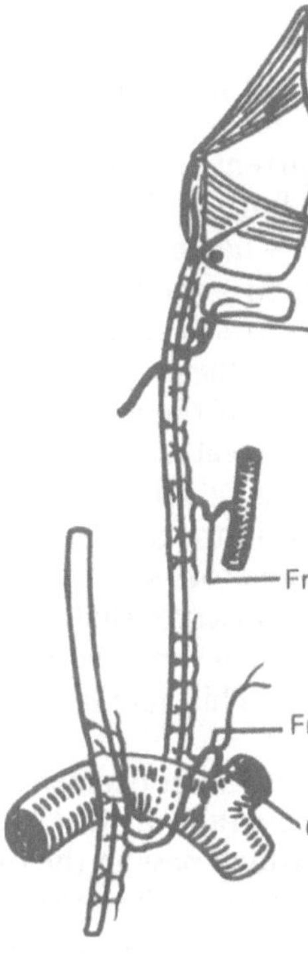

Figure 10.12 Blood supply of the right recurrent laryngeal nerve

(2) The branch originating from the posterior wall of the brachiocephalic trunk. The small branch with an outer diameter of 0.7 mm proceeds medially in a tortuous way to where the right recurrent nerve winds below the right subclavian artery, then passes upwards and medially, and finally subdivides into an upper and a lower twig to enter the recurrent nerve from the side medial to it.

(3) The small branch from the inferior thyroid artery.

(4) The small branch arising from the oesophageal artery. The cesophageal artery is given off from the posterior wall of the right subclavian artery at its commencement which corresponds to the site posterior to the initial portion of the vertebral artery, and proceeds medial to the posterior wall of the oesophagus, passing through the side posterior to the recurrent nerve. The oesophageal artery gives off some small branches to the vagus and the recurrent laryngeal nerves before reaching the oesophagus. The latter branch ends by bifurcating into an

upper and a lower twig on the side medial to the recurrent nerve and the lower one passes down to the point of origin of the recurrent nerve, while the upper ascends along the nerve and anastomoses with related arteries.

In addition, there are usually small veins on either side of the vagus trunk, which descend longitudinally between the recurrent nerve and the trunk of the vagus nerve and may be used as a sign marking the boundary between the recurrent and vagus nerves.

Essentials in the practical anatomy of the recurrent laryngeal nerve

(1) It is emphasized in the topography of the recurrent laryngeal nerve that the nerve gives off two muscular rami at the inferior horn of the thyroid cartilage, and after the nerve winds below the large vessels - namely, the aortic arch on the left and the right subclavian artery on the right - the left recurrent nerve lies in the groove between the oesophagus and the trachea, while the right one lies medial to the line connecting the point medial to the commencement of the right common carotid artery with the inferior pole of the thyroid gland. This is a mark available to identify the recurrent laryngreal nerve.

(2) The course of the fibres of the recurrent nerve within the vagus trunk is relatively constant, i.e. these fibres are situated in the anteromedial part of the vagus trunk, thus occupying one-fourth of the cross-sectional area of the vagus. After cutting through the carotid sheath it is observed that there is a small vein on the vagus trunk directing longitudinally downwards between the fibre bundle of the recurrent nerve and the vagus trunk. This may be used as a sign marking the boundary between them.

(3) The arterial supply of the recurrent nerve is rather extensive, but there is a characteristic in common; i.e. the arteries are generally divided into an upper and a lower twig medial to the recurrent nerve, which pass in the direction of the nerve fibres within the epineurium. The apposition of the vessels within the epineurium is of great significance in the surgical anastomosis of the nerve. As all the vessels supplying the nerve lie on the side medial to the recurrent, it is important to avoid stretching the recurrent nerve laterally, lest the blood supply of the nerve should be damaged.

Branches of the vagus to the lower part of the oesophagus and the stomach

The right and left vagus nerves enter the posterior mediastinum through the superior aperture of the thorax, pass downward to the posterior surface of the corresponding pulmonary root and give off bronchial and oesophageal rami. The bronchial rami join to form the pulmonary plexus, whence nerve twigs pass into the lung along the bronchus and its branches, while the oesophageal rami take part in the formation of the oesophageal plexus, which resumes the form of an anterior and a posterior vagus trunk below the level of the pulmonary root, that passes to the abdomen through the oesophageal hiatus of the diaphragm. The total number of nerve fibres in the oesophageal plexus is 578 253 (16 013–101 492), of which the non-myelinated fibres amount to 97%.

The composition of the anterior and posterior vagus trunks, and their topography through the oesophageal hiatus of the diaphragm

Below the level of the tracheal bifurcation the oesophageal plexus resumes the anterior and posterior vagus trunks. The former is composed mainly of the fibres from the left vagus, while the latter consists chiefly of those from the right vagus. The distance between the point of formation of the anterior and posterior vagus trunks and the diaphragm is varied. In 50% of cases the anterior trunk is formed 31 mm above the diaphragm, while the posterior trunk which is formed within 0–30 mm above the diaphragm represents 85%. The level where the posterior trunk is formed is usually lower than that where the anterior trunk is formed. The appearance of the trunks is oval or like a flat cylinder, and their breadth is varied. At the oesophageal hiatus the breadth of the anterior trunk varies mostly from 0.5 to 2.0 mm, which represents 80%, while that of the posterior trunk generally varies from 1.1 to 3.0 mm, which accounts for 75.6%. It is clear that the posterior trunk is wider than the anterior.

The topographic relationship between the right and left trunks and the oesophagus is rather constant as they pass through the hiatus. The anterior trunk usually lies anterior to and to the left of the oesophagus (95.7%), while the posterior is located to the right of and posterior to the oesophagus (99.0%) (Figure 10.13).

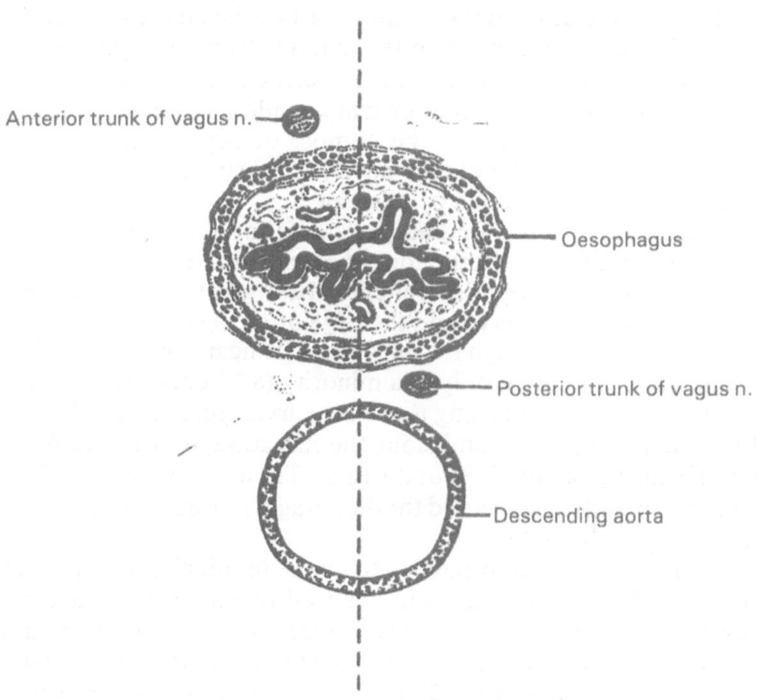

Figure 10.13 Topographic relationship of the vagus nerve with the oesophagus during its passage through the oesophageal hiatus

According to the number of rami from the trunks through the oesophageal hiatus the anterior and posterior trunks are divided into four types: type I is the unitrunk type, in which there is only one anterior or one posterior trunk, accounting for 65.5%. Because the site of the anterior and posterior trunks of the vagus through the oesophageal hiatus remains constant, it is easy to carry out vagotomy successfully near the oesophageal hiatus, where the anterior trunk usually borders tightly on the anterior wall of the oesophagus, yet the posterior trunk does not adhere closely to the posterior wall of the oesophagus, but rather lies against the aorta that is behind and to the right of the oesophagus. Being well acquainted with these topographic relations, one will be able to find out the vagus with facility during vagotomy.

Branches from the anterior trunk (Figure 10.14)

The main branches from the anterior trunk are the hepatic ramus and the anterior gastric nerve. Ninety per cent of the hepatic rami come from the anterior vagus trunk; only a few come from the posterior trunk or the common stem formed by the two trunks, and consist of one to two branches. In most cases the hepatic ramus arises from the anterior trunk at the level of the angle of His (or the cardiac notch), passes from the left to the right, entering the porta hepatis through the hepatogastric ligament, and gives off some rami to be distributed to the liver, pancreas and the bulbous part of the duodenum. The site of emergence of the hepatic ramus from the anterior trunk is higher, which is a distinct feature of the hepatic ramus. It is not difficult to identify precisely the hepatic ramus given off by the anterior trunk while the fibres of the anterior gastric branches are being cut. As the number of hepatic rami varies, they should not be cut at random until they have been clearly identified in order to avoid injury to the hepatic ramus by mistake.

The anterior gastric nerve, or Laterjet's anterior nerve, is the downward continuation of the anterior trunk along the lesser curvature of the stomach after it has given off the hepatic branches. In a great majority (92%), the distance between Laterjet's nerve and the edge of the lesser curvature is about 10 mm. The nerve passes through the hepatogastric ligament between the lesser curvature and its arterial arch; only in a minority (8%) does the nerve descend closely against the gastric wall along the lesser curvature. Laterjet's nerve gives off two to five anterior gastric rami along the curvature, of which three or four are the most frequent, making 84% of the total. The distance between the origin of the first anterior gastric ramus and the diaphragm is usually from 1 to 30 mm, which amounts to 92% of cases.

The anterior pyloric antrum ramus, being the terminal one of the anterior gastric nerve, is distributed to the anterior wall of the pyloric antrum like a crow's claw near the angular notch. The distance between the point of entrance of the anterior pyloric antrum ramus into the anterior wall of the stomach and the midpyloric point varies from 21 to 80 mm, most frequently from 31 to 50 mm (70.1%). This datum has been a significant reference in surgery. While performing hyperselective vagotomy the anterior pyloric antrum rami have to be saved from damage, lest the emptying power of the stomach should be affected. From anatomical observations the extent of distribution of the anterior pyloric antrum rami varies. Is it necessary to mark out this scope of innervation during operation? And what is its significance in clinical practice? Different authors have put forward various opinions. However, the distance from the entrance of the anterior pyloric antrum rami into the wall of the stomach to the midpyloric point varies from 60 to 90 mm. This is significant for reference.

In 59% of cases the anterior pyloric antrum rami form the terminal branches of the anterior gastric nerve, and in another 41% the ramus arises as a single stem from the hepatic ramus, and passes to the pyloric antrum directly as the anterior pyloric antrum ramus.

Branches of the posterior vagus trunk (Figure 10.14)

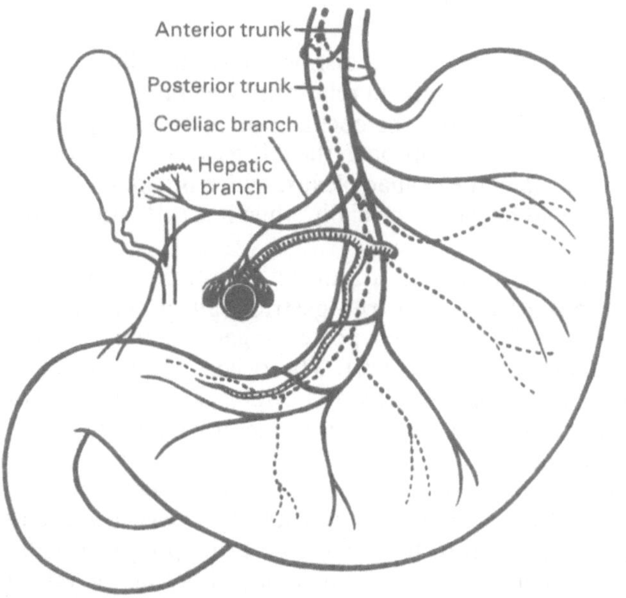

Figure 10.14 Branches of the vagus nerve

The posterior gastric nerve and the coeliac ramus are the main branches of the posterior vagus trunk.

The coeliac ramus is rather constant and consists of two-thirds of the total fibres of the posterior vagus trunk so that it may be looked on as the direct extension of the posterior trunk. The coeliac ramus arises from the posterior trunk at the transitional zone between the oesophagus and the cardia, where the left gastric artery turns to the lesser curvature. Therefore, a triangle is usually formed by the coeliac ramus, the posterior gastric nerve, and the left gastric artery, with the left gastric artery as the base line of the triangle, the distance from the base line of the triangle to its apex being about 22 mm (Figure 10.15).

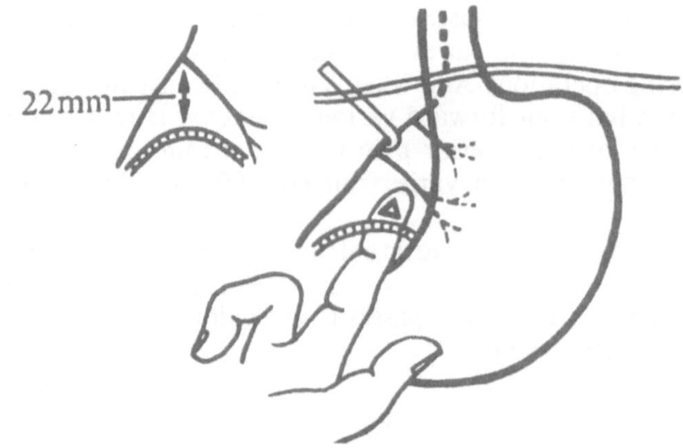

Figure 10.15 Triangular relationship among the coeliac ramus, the posterior gastric nerve and the left gastric artery

Since the left gastric artery is a distinct mark, it will be advantageous to be acquainted with the topographical relations in seeking for the posterior gastric nerve as well as in protecting the coeliac ramus during operation. Sometimes the coeliac ramus does not approach the left gastric artery, but descends along the diaphragm to end in the coeliac plexus, which is a kind of variation to which due attention should be paid, especially when it is difficult to find the posterior gastric nerve.

The posterior gastric nerve, or Laterjet's posterior nerve, generally keeps a distance of about 12 mm from the gastric wall at the middle of the lesser curvature. It gives off one to seven posterior gastric rami, of which two or three branches are more frequent (73%). The origin of the first posterior gastric ramus is usually 11–40 mm away from the diaphragm, which accounts for 82%. In addition there remain two conditions, one of which is the anastomosis existing between the anterior and posterior gastric branches, while the other is the 'recurrent' posterior gastric ramus which is given off less frequently by the coeliac ramus and passes in company with the left gastric artery to the lesser curvature of the stomach to be distributed to its posterior wall.

The posterior pyloric antrum ramus may either be the terminal branch of the posterior gastric nerve or may arise directly from the coeliac ramus. It is mostly single, but double branches may arise directly from the posterior vagus trunk or from the coeliac ramus. Generally, the posterior pyloric antrum ramus is not as constant as the anterior one, yet it also assumes the form of a crow's claw and is distributed to the posterior wall of the pyloric antrum.

It has been demonstrated that the cardio-fundus rami distributed to the oesophagus and cardia arise from the anterior and posterior vagus trunks at the lower part of the thorax or just below the oesophageal hiatus of the diaphragm. Their number varies from one to four, yet it is mostly single (66% from the anterior trunk, 70% from the posterior). Though the incidence of cardio-fundus ramus is quite constant, its origin and number often vary. It is thus imperative to expose fully the lower part of the oesophagus in order to make a complete resection of the cardiofundus ramus.

Essentials in applied anatomy of the lower segment of the vagus nerve

(1) Hyperselective vagotomy demands the section of the gastric rami and the preservation of Laterjet's nerves and the pyloric antrum branches in order to maintain the normal function of the pyloric antrum. It is not difficult to identify the anterior and posterior pyloric antrum rami, i.e. the 'crow-claw' nerves according to the topography of Laterjet's nerve. It is thus possible to start dissection at a point above the 'crow-claw', and then to cut the gastric rami one by one along the lesser curvature upwards until the level below the origin of the hepatic or coeliac ramus is reached. In the minority of cases, when it is difficult to identify the 'crow-claw' nerve of the posterior Laterjet's nerve, special attention should be paid to the triangular relationship among the left gastric artery, the posterior gastric nerve and the coeliac ramus, which is helpful when searching for the posterior gastric ramus.

(2) As it is a histological feature that the parietal cells or gastric oxyntic cells lie mainly in the fundus and the body of the stomach, this is another key leading to a successful hyperselective vagotomy to cut off whatever branches are directed to the cardio-fundus. If an operating microscope can be used to differentiate the cardio-fundus ramus before sectioning, the possibility of 'missing' will be greatly reduced.

It has been suggested by Holle that the Harkin's nerve which usually arises from the anterior vagus trunk 2–3 cm above the cardia, and enters into the muscular layer of the oesophagus in company with an arteriole, should be preserved, lest cardiospasm and dysphagia should result.

(3) Though the following two variations in the branching and course account only for 3%, they are important clinically: (a) the anterior vagus trunk is simply distributed to the anterior wall of the gastric fundus; both the hepatic rami and

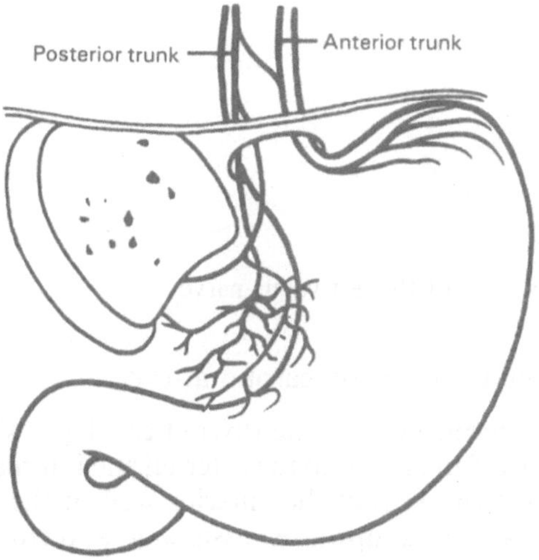

Figure 10.16 Anterior and posterior trunk of the vagus nerve (the anterior trunk ends in the gastric fundus; the anterior gastric nerve and the hepatic ramus arise from the posterior trunk)

the anterior gastric nerve arise from the posterior trunk (Figure 10.16); (b) the coeliac ramus gives off a branch that winds round the angle of His from the posterior gastric wall, passes in front of the cardia, and proceeds to the porta hepatis as the hepatic ramis.

Blood supply of the vagus nerve

Left vagus nerve

The blood supply of the left vagus originates from the following sources (Figure 10.17).

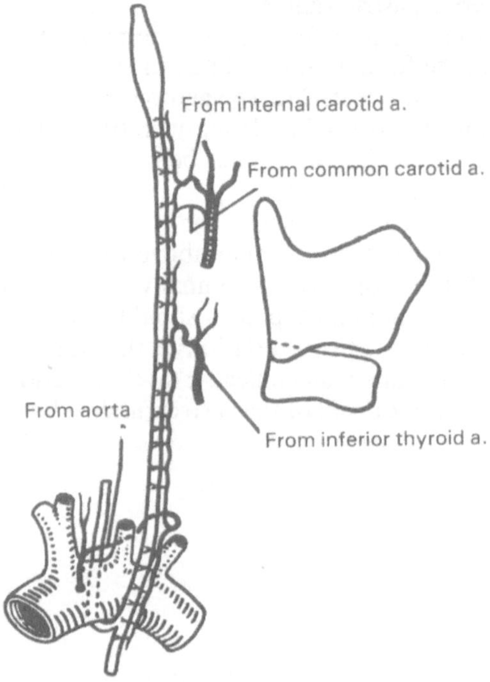

Figure 10.17 Blood supply of the left vagus nerve

Branches arising from the common carotid artery

At the level of the superior horn of the thyroid cartilage, where the common carotid artery ends by bifurcating into the external and internal carotid arteries, there arise two minute twigs from the anterior wall of the common carotid, which proceed laterally and upwards assuming a tortuous course along the medial side to the vagus and then bifurcate into an upper and a lower twig to enter the vagus. The ascending branch can be traced to the inferior ganglion of the vagus, and the descending one to the level of the cricoid cartilage.

(2) A branch from the aortic arch. This branch, with a diameter of 1.0 mm, arises from the anterior wall of the arch between the origin of the brachiocephalic trunk and the left carotid artery. It passes obliquely upwards and to the left until the back of the left common carotid artery, where the branch bifurcates into an upper and a lower twig to enter the vagus through its medial side. The ascending twig can be traced to the level of the cricoid cartilage, where it anastomoses with the descending twigs from the common carotid artery. The descending twig may be traced downwards along the vagus nerve to the origin of the recurrent nerve, which is seen to be supplied by minute twigs.

Blood supply of the right vagus nerve (Figure 10.18)

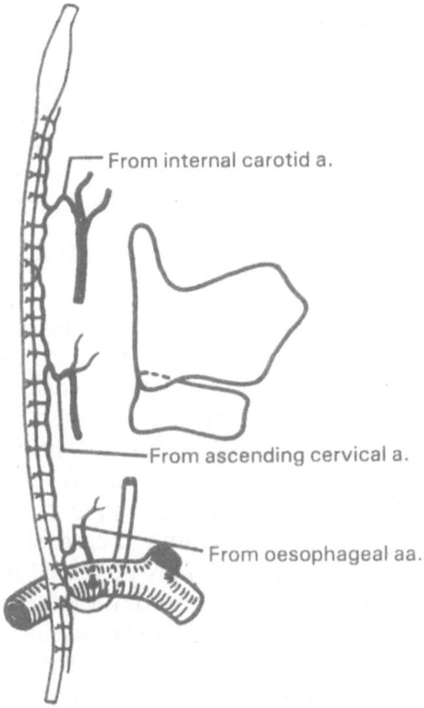

Figure 10.18 Blood supply of the right vagus nerve

Branch originating from the internal carotid artery

This branch arises from the lateral wall of the internal carotid artery at the level where the inferior ganglion of the vagus gives rise to the superior laryngeal nerve. It passes laterally in a tortuous manner and divides medial to the nerve into an upper and a lower twig to end in the inferior ganglion and the vagus nerve.

Branches from the commencement of the internal carotid artery

Two branches arise from the anterior wall of the commencement of the internal carotid artery at the level of the superior horn of the thyroid cartilage. They pass laterally to the side medial to the vagus tortuously, and bifurcate into an upper and a lower twig to enter the nerve.

Branch given off by the common carotid artery

The common carotid artery gives off this branch at the level of the inferior horn of the thyroid cartilage. It passes laterally and divides into an upper and a lower twig to enter the vagus through its medial side.

Branches from the oesophageal artery

The oesophageal artery, with a diameter of 1.4 mm, arises from the posterior wall of the commencement of the right subclavian artery. It passes medially through the back of the recurrent laryngeal nerve to the posterior wall of the oesophagus. Before reaching the posterior wall of the oesophagus the artery gives off two branches, one of which supplies the vagus while the other goes to the recurrent nerve and the cardiac plexus. The branch to the vagus ascends along the nerve and is seen to anastomose with the nutrient branches supplying the vagus, which arise from the ascending cervical artery.

Branches from the ascending cervical artery

At the level of the fifth and sixth cervical vertebrae the ascending cervical artery gives off a short stem, the diameter of which is 0.4 mm. It passes forward and upward and soon subdivides into three twigs, which proceed medialward, superomedially and downward respectively. The descending twig proceeds to the medial aspect of the vagus and then bifurcates into an upper and a lower ramuscule entering the vagus. The upper ramuscule can be traced to the level of the superior horn of the thyroid cartilage, where its supplying area overlaps that provided by the branches of the common carotid artery, but no anastomosis can be seen; the lower ramuscule may be traced to the level of the subclavian artery, and is seen to anastomose with the nutrient artery of the vagus nerve from the oesophageal artery. The twig passing medially reaches the posterior wall of the common carotid artery, while the twig proceeding upward and medially arrives at the prevertebral connective tissue.

11

The microsurgical anatomy of the lymphatic system

AUTHORS

INTRODUCTION

The study on the lymphatic system began in the 17th century, Aselli (1627) first described the lacteals of the small intestine, Pacquet (1651) reported observations on the cisterna chyli and thoracic duct, Rudbeck (1655) described the valves of the lymphatic vessels, and Wharton (1656) and Malpigh (1659) started the study on the histological structure of the lymphatic system.

Since the lymphatic vessels have small calibres and thin walls with colourless contents, observation on the lymphatic system is rather difficult to carry out. It follows that innovation and improvement in the research methods play a very important role in the study on this system. Nuck (1692) was the first to adopt the method of mercury injection, and then followed Cruihank (1786), Mascagni (1787), Teichmann (1909), Hyrtl (1865), Sappey (1885), Gerota (1896), Bartels (1909), Eosifov (1930), Rouviere (1932) and Zhdanov (1952), who made continuous improvements in methodology. They made use of various water- or fat-soluble dyes and advanced the polychrome injection method. They had gone deep into the study on the structural pattern of the lymphatics inside or outside the organs, and yielded good results. Along with the appearance of radioisotopes, Hahn (1952) introduced them into the experimental and clinical study on the lymphatic system.

Funaoka (1930) began direct radiography of the lymphatic vessels and achieved successful results, Kinmonth *et al.* (1952) employed the method of demonstrating lymphatic vessels with dyes prior to lymphangiography by means of direct puncture. They achieved good results and laid the foundation for its clinical application, which have successively been carried out by Liu Shiyi, Dong Jiping, and others in China since 1960.

The lymphatic-venous anastomosis in its early stage of development could only be performed between large lymphatic trunks and veins in the treatment of chyluria (Cockett, 1962; Zheng Kangqiao, 1965) and varicose lymphatics of the intestine (Mistitis, 1966). In 1974 O'Brien first succeeded in applying lymphatico-venous anastomosis to the treatment of the obstructive lymphatic oedema of limbs. In China since 1979 Zhu Jiakai, Yu Guozhong and others have performed such operations to control chronic erysipelas and the accompanying oedema with satisfactory results.

Chinese anatomists Wang Yunxiang and Yang Chunlin (1962–80) have been engaged in the study on the morphology of the lymphatic system and a great deal of information has been accumulated. Yuan Lian (1957), Song Jingqi (1957) and others have started experimental investigations in this field. In 1979 Liu Muzhi and Zhong Shizhen did research on the microsurgical anatomy of the lymphatic system of the limbs, and abundant basic theoretical data were thus furnished.

Introduction to the lymphatic system

The lymphatic system is one of the components of the circulatory system. It is composed of lymphatic capillaries and vessels and lymphatic organs (lymph nodes, spleen, etc.). The lymphatic capillaries collect the tissue fluid and convey it to the lymphatic vessels. These pass through the lymphatic nodes and gather into large lymphatic trunks and ducts, which finally end in the venous angle between the subclavian and internal jugular veins.

As the blood reaches the arterial end of the capillaries, part of the fluid filters through the wall of the capillary into the tissue space to form the tissue fluid. Following exchange of substances, most of the fluid is absorbed into the venous end of the capillaries and postcapillary veins, while a small part of it is absorbed by the lymphatic capillaries to form the lymph. The lymphatic channel is thus an important accessory pathway in the return of tissue fluid. The lymphatic vessels are connected with the lymph nodes, which filtrate the lymph and produce lymphocytes, participating in body immunization and constituting the important defensive apparatus of the body.

Lymphatic vessels

The lymphatic vessels comprise lymphatic capillaries, lymphatics, lymphatic trunks and lymphatic ducts.

Lymphatic capillaries

The lymphatic capillaries begin as slightly enlarged blind ends and anastomose with one another to form a meshwork. They are widely distributed and may be found elsewhere in the body except sites such as the epithilium, cornea, lens, cartilage, bone marrow, internal ear, placenta, central nervous system, nerve bundles and the endomysium of skeletal muscles. The lymphatic capillaries consist of a single layer of endothelial cells. The characteristics of capillaries are as follows. The lumen is large and irregular; the wall is very thin, being made up of overlapping layers of endothelial cells; some of the spaces between the cells may exceed 0.5 μm and the free overlapping margins of the cells drop into the lumen, serving as valves to permit the tissue fluid to flow into the lymphatic capillaries only.

Owing to the above characteristics the lymphatic capillaries have higher permeability than the blood capillaries. Therefore large molecules such as proteins, fats, bacteria, foreign bodies and cancer cells can enter the lymphatic capillaries without difficulty.

The lymphatic capillaries anastomose with one another to be distributed to the skin or mucous membrane of hollow organs, forming a superficial and a deep capillary network respectively. The calibres of the lymphatic capillaries may be enlarged to as much as three times. No valve has been found in the lymphatic capillaries.

Lymphatics

The lymphatics are formed by the confluence of lymphatic capillaries. On the way they usually pass through one or several lymph nodes, or a few organs or regions occasionally do not connect with any node but empty directly into the thoracic duct. The diameters of lymphatics vary from 0.1 to 1.2 mm (more frequently less than 0.5 mm). The lymphatics are numerous and communicate very profusely with one another. They have numerous valves, thus assuming a beaded appearance.

Lymphatic trunks

There are nine main lymphatic channels: the jugular trunk (paired), formed by the lymphatics of the head and neck; the subclavian trunk (paired), formed by the lymphatics of the upper limb and part of the thoracic and abdominal walls; the bronchomediastinal trunk (paired), formed by the lymphatics of part of the thoracic and abdominal viscera; the intestinal trunk (single), formed by those of the gastrointestinal tract and spleen; and the lumbar trunk (paired), formed by the lymphatics of the lower limbs, abdominal wall and the pelvic and abdominal viscera.

Lymphatic duct

The right jugular, bronchomediastinal and subclavian trunks join to form the right lymphatic duct. The rest of the trunks unite to form the thoracic duct. These two ducts empty respectively into the right and left venous angles.

Problems concerning the lymphatic system

Regeneration of lymphatics

Lymphatics have a great capacity for undergoing repair, and the construction of new vessels after damage is rather rapid. During regeneration, cells of the original endothelium of the lymphatics divide by mitosis to produce solid cellular sprouts. Subsequently, these connect with one another to form true deep lymphatic channels.

The role of body function and age on the growth of lymphatics

The lymphatic vessels present some characteristics in respect to age. In the fetus and infant the lumen of the lymphatics is relatively large with profuse anastomosis, which results in a dense network. With advancing age, lymphatics become thinner and fewer. In old age, lymphatic capillaries and vessels decrease in number, the size of meshes being enlarged and the network getting loose, and part of them may disappear or become deformed. The patterns of lymphatic channels are closely connected with their functions. For example, in the pregnant uterus the lymphatic capillary network proliferates markedly, its meshes becoming dense and the constituent vessels increasing both in number and calibre. In lactating breasts the lymphatic capillaries and vessels dilate. In cancer of the breast and carcinoma of the female reproductive organs at old age, as lymphatics become atrophied or disappear, metastases are not so frequent. On the contrary, in young patients, owing to the fact that the morphologic structure of the lymphatic system keeps pace with the active physiologic activities, metastasis occurs easily.

Factors for lymphatic drainage

Normally, human lymph returns to the blood at a speed of 120 ml per hour. The main factors for lymphatic drainage are: the pressure maintained by the continued addition of new lymph; the rhythmic contraction of the lymphatics themselves; the presence of lymphatic valves, which open with the blood stream and close against it; the pulsation of neighbouring arteries; the contraction of the surrounding muscles; the changes in the intrathoracic pressure during respiration, etc.

Collateral lymphatic circulation

Anastomoses exist among lymphatics, forming an abundance of collateral pathways. Under ordinary conditions these passages usually remain in a state of closure, being a kind of potential channel not participating in normal circulation. When the lymphatic pathway is obstructed due to inflammation, tumour or parasites, or when the lymph nodes are excised or the lymphatics severed, the main stream of the lymph will be blocked. As a result the pressure of the stream becomes increased, so that originally collapsed vessels are gradually enlarged, establishing a collateral circulation, which is governed by internal and external factors. It has been proved experimentally that such factors as movement, temperature and infection can promote the establishment of collateral circulation, while nerve injury, radioactive irradiation and immobilization delay it.

Aetiology of lymphatic oedema

Hypoplasia of the lymphatic system, obstruction of the lymphatic pathway, break in lymphatic circulation, the disturbance in lymphatic metabolism, and overproduction of lymph are among the factors responsible for the accumulation of fluid and proteins in the tissue spaces and retardation of lymph in the lymphatics, leading finally to lymphatic oedema.

Significance of lymphaticovenous anastomoses

With the aid of microsurgical technique, lymphatic vessels have been anastomosed to veins for shunting the stagnant lymph, thus alleviating the excessive accumulation of protein and tissue fluid in the limbs, and improving the system of lymphatic oedema. This technique has grown to be the method of treatment for lymphatic oedema.

Methods which have been used in lymphaticovenous anastomosis are as follows:

1. End-to-end anastomosis between the lymphatic trunk and the tributaries of a vein, such as that between the lumbar trunk and the testicular vein.
2. End-to-end anastomosis between the lymphatic vessels and veins of the right size.
3. End-to-side anastomosis between the broken end of a lymphatic vessel and the lateral wall of a thick vein.
4. The lymph node–vein anastomosis, i.e. the anastomosis between truncated surface of a lymph node and the lateral wall of a vein.

Of these methods it has been proved experimentally and clinically that end-to-end anastomosis between the lymphatic vessel and the vein has achieved good results. End-to-side anastomosis is not so good in the long term, because the implanted broken end of the lymphatic vessel is apt to constrict due to the pressure set up by the contraction of the wall of the vein, resulting in stricture or even obstruction. Lymph node–vein anastomosis is not very effective but is simple and convenient to manipulate.

Injection methods used in the study of lymphatic system

Indirect injection method

The indirect injection method consists of the introduction of pigments into the tissue spaces of the skin, subcutaneous tissue or organs of various depths. As the structure of the wall of the lymphatic capillary differs from that of the blood capillary, particles of pigment, which are unable to enter the blood capillary, may get into the lymphatic capillary and thence via the lymphatics to the regional lymph nodes.

Direct injection method

On the basis of demonstrating lymphatic vessels by the indirect method, the needle is introduced directly into the lymph vessel or node to demonstrate lymph nodes and efferent lymph vessels with developers.

Choice and application of the site of injection

If the site of injection is selected to conform to the principle of lymphatic distribution, good results will be obtained, or else worse outcome and even failure will follow. Each site has its own characteristics.

Sites frequently used in the limbs

In the lower limb the injection site selected is on the dorsum of the foot (the toes, metatarsophalangeal joints, and the webs of the toes), or its medial and lateral borders. In the case of upper limb it is on the back of the hand (the fingers and webs) or on its medial and lateral borders. The injections are to be carried out intradermally or subcutaneously and, according to clinical demands, a direct lymphangiography can be made on the dorsum of the wrist or around the medial malleolus after an indirect injection.

Methods for injecting the lymphatics of the spermatic cord

There are two ways of visualizing the testicular lymphatics. One is to inject the pigment into the parenchyma of the testis, followed by making an incision in the inguinal area and cutting through the coverings of the spermatic cord layer by layer to isolate the pigmented lymphatic vessels. Another method is to make an incision in the inguinal area and uncover the spermatic cord. The lymphatic vessels of the spermatic cord, being five to seven in number, have a fairly large diameter amounting to 1.2 mm in the adult. A temporary block can dilate these vessels and a direct injection that follows may demonstrate the lumbar lymph nodes, lumbar trunk, cisterna chyli and thoracic duct.

Method of regional injection

When regional intradermal injections are made in the limbs, numerous thin lymphatics may be visualized. If hypodermic injections are to be adopted, fewer yet larger collective lymphatic vessels may be seen. Generally, better results can be achieved using combined methods of intradermal and hypodermic injections.

Regional injection method is usually employed in lymphatico-venous anastomosis for the treatment of obstructive lymphatic oedema of the limb. Such patients present with pathological changes in the lymphatic system, resulting in obstruction and tortuosity of the lymphatic vessels and thus slowing down the lymph flow, so that pigment or radio-opaque substance can hardly reach the desired operative area. The appropriate distance between the site of injection and the surgical incision is about 10 cm. The site of injection should not be too far away, lest the pigment should fail to demonstrate the lymphatic vessels in the incision. However, it should not be too near to the incision and the pigment must not be given in excess, so as not to form a diffuse pigmentation over the site of the incision and make it difficult to define various structures.

Differentiation of lymphatics from small blood vessels and nerves

Lymphatics are located in the subcutaneous tissue with the arterioles, venules and small nerves. It is important to distinguish them correctly during operation.

(1) Lymphatics are surrounded by adipose tissue which glistens yellowish under the operating microscope or the magnifier and is enclosed with the lymphatics by a thin membrane. The adipose tissue is thick on either side of the lymphatics, but thin over their superficial and deep surfaces. In well-demonstrated cases the blue-tinged lymphatics are easily recognized by blunt dissection with curved mosquito foreceps. The unstained lymphatics are, however, difficult to visualize, being transparent and colourless tubules with very thin walls and transparent liquid columns in their interior. If the lymphatic vessel is gently held up and let down and the central end of the lymphatic vessel is slightly pressed to block the lymph stream temporarily, while its distal end is gently massaged to move the lymph to the obstructed portion, the lymphatic vessel can be seen expanded, giving a clearly beaded appearance, which vanishes when the obstruction is released. Those lymphatics which have had inflammation have thicker walls and more fibrous tissues around them. They are believed to have large diameter at the first glance. Once the fibro-adipose tissue is removed they become as thin as threads, which, when cut, will curl up into ball-like masses and are difficult to identify. They can then be recognized only when they are filled with blue-stained lymph on being squeezed gently from their distal end.

(2) Small veins (venules) are surrounded by scattered fibrous connective tissues. Their walls are relatively thick and may be distinguished into three coats. The inner coat is a layer of endothelium. The medium coat consists of one or more layers of smooth muscular fibres. Outside the medium coat are scattered fibroblasts and elastic and collagenous fibres. The small veins appear slightly pink but not shiny. They sometimes have twigs, from which blood may ooze on being dissected. If the fibrous coat is peeled off, a red blood core can be seen through the small vein. The blood column can be seen shifting when the venule is gently lifted and then let down, and the blood flows out when the vessel is incised.

(3) Arterioles are narrower than the companion veins. Their wall presents three coats. The inner coat consists of the endothelium and elastic membrane. The medium coat has smooth muscles. The outer coat is composed of longitudinal collagenous and elastic fibres as well as some fibroblasts. They exhibit pulsation and are rarely found in the superficial layer of the subcutaneous tissue.

(4) Small nerves glisten and are smooth in profile. They are composed of small fibre bundles arranged regularly, when seen under the microscope. The epineurium encloses small blood vessels and is surrounded by a small amount of loose adipose tissue. They exhibit no lumina or fluid columns on close examination. Sometimes, small branches can be seen. Nerve fibre bundles are clearly seen in cross-section.

Choice of the site for sectioning of lymphatics

The number of lymphatic valves bears close relation to the calibre and position of lymphatic vessels, e.g. in human extremities it averages 33.7 (28–42),

23.7 (15–29), 11.4 (8–16), 10.3 (9–14) and 7.4 in each centimetre of the lymphatics with diameters of 0.1, 0.2, 0.3, 0.4 and 0.5 mm respectively.

Sections should be made at the site without valves. Although valves vary in number and position, when the lymphatic is full and assumes a beaded appearance the site of attachment of the valves correspond to the base of the bead. The valve occupies only the lower part of the bead. In severing a lymphatic vessel it is necessary to choose the upper, but not the lower, part of the bead, lest a 'casing' of lymphatics should occur and add difficulty to suturing.

LYMPHATIC SYSTEM OF THE LOWER LIMB

Superficial lymphatics of the lower limb

The superficial lymphatics of the lower limb begin in the intradermal and hypodermic lymphatic plexuses. They are distributed in the fatty layer of the superficial fascia and may be subdivided into two groups. The superficial group is greater in number and smaller in diameter (0.1–0.2 mm). The deep group consists of fewer and larger vessels located superficial to the deep fascia, where some unite to form the collecting lymphatic vessels. The diameters of the latter amount to 0.3–0.6 mm. Although the superficial lymphatics of the lower limb are numerous, only a few of them - i.e. the collecting lymphatic vessels - are of practical significance for surgical purposes. These vessels have a definite concomitant relationship with the long and short saphenous veins, so that it is possible to find them in the light of the position of the venous trunks. The superficial lymph vessels of the lower limb may be distinguished into three groups (Figure 11.1).

(1) The medial group is the most numerous. The lymph vessels originate from the first, second and third toes, the medial border of the foot (7–15 in number with a diameter of 0.1–0.2 mm), and the dorsum of the foot. These ascend in the same direction as the long saphenous vein, consisting of 4–16 lymphatic vessels, among which there are two to four collecting vessels accompanying the long saphenous vein. Most of the lymphatics of this group drain into the medial members of the inferior group of the superficial inguinal lymph nodes and a few may end in the deep nodes.

(2) The posterior group, being fewer in number, consists of three to five lymph vessels, among which one to three large collecting vessels ascend in company with the short saphenous vein to the upper one-third of the back of the leg where they pass through between the two heads of the gastrocnemius, pierce the investing fascia into the popliteal fossa, and end in the superficial group of the popliteal lymph nodes. Occasionally there is a collecting lymph vessel which does not end in the superficial nodes but rounds to the thigh and finally ends in the medial ones of the inferior group of the superficial inguinal lymph nodes.

(3) The lateral group are again fewer in number. They begin respectively from the dorsal surfaces of the fourth and fifth toes, the lateral border of the foot (5–22 lymphatics with a diameter of 0.1–0.3 mm), the dorsum of the foot, and the lateral portions of the leg (about 13 lymphatics) and thigh (one to eight

lymphatics). Collecting lymph vessels are rare in this group. Most of the lymphatic vessels of the lateral group join the medial group and ascend with them. Some of them arise from the lateral part of the thigh and drain directly into the lateral members of the lower group of the superficial inguinal lymph nodes.

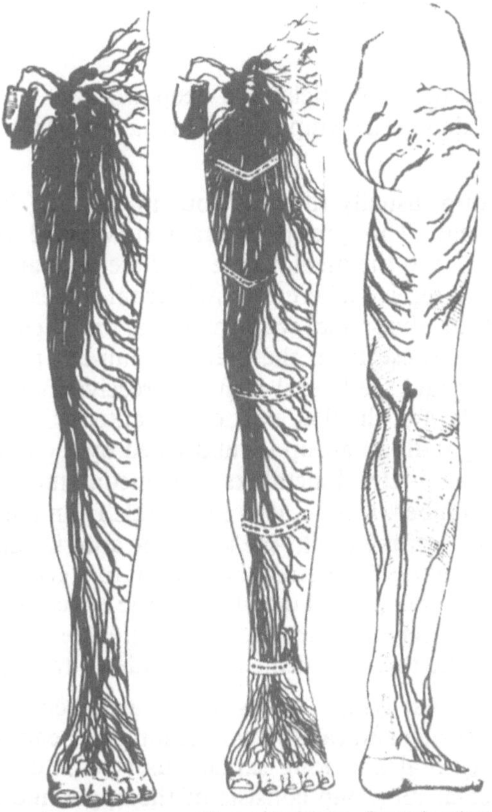

Figure 11.1 Distribution of the superficial lymphatics of the lower limb

Choice of the site of incision for lymphaticovenous anastomosis of the lower limb

Multiple lymphaticovenous anastomoses through segmental incisions are employed to relieve obstructive lymphatic oedema. The incisions are to be selected along the course of the long saphenous vein because thick collecting lymph vessels usually accompany subcutaneous venous trunks, i.e. the long and short saphenous veins (for the site of incision, see Figure 11.1).

The collecting lymph vessels of the lower limb vary from one to seven in number. They are distributed as follows: in the leg there are mostly one to three vessels within a range of 1 cm from the trunk of the long saphenous vein and two to four vessels within a range of 5 cm from it; while in the thigh there are usually one or two vessels within a range of 1 cm from the trunk of the long saphenous vein and two to four vessels within 5 cm from it.

Lymph nodes of the lower limb

The inguinal lymph nodes

These can be divided into superficial and deep groups.

(1) The superficial inguinal lymph nodes are arranged into upper and lower groups.

(a) The upper group, usually three or four in number, lies parallel to the inguinal ligament. This group is again subdivided by the superficial epigastric artery into the medial, intermediate and lateral members. The medial members receive afferent vessels from the external genitalia, the perineum and the abdominal wall below the umbilicus; the intermediate members receive those from the iliac and lumbar parts of the anterior abdominal wall; and the lateral members receive those from the lumbar region, the back, and the iliac part of the anterior abdominal wall.

(b) The lower (longitudinal) group is subdivided by the long saphenous vein into the medial and lateral members. The medial members of the group, one to five in number, receive afferent vessels from the posterior, medial and anterior sides of the thigh, the knee, the anterior and medial sides of the leg, and the ankle. The perineum and external genitalia also drain into the medial nodes. The lateral members of the lower group, two to five in number, receive afferent vessels from the gluteal region, the posterior and lateral sides of the thigh, and the lateral side of the leg.

(2) The deep inguinal lymph nodes are located beneath the fascia lata, usually in the femoral ring and canal, near the long saphenous vein. This group is divided by the femoral and long saphenous vein into medial and lateral subgroups. The medial subgroup consists of the upper and lower nodes. The upper ones are situated in the femoral canal, and the lower ones on the medial side of the femoral vessels. The lateral subgroup is lateral to the vessels.

(3) There are connections between the groups of the inguinal lymph nodes. Members of the upper group of the superficial inguinal lymph nodes are connected by lymph vessels with one another and send their efferents to the pelvic nodes. The medial and lateral members of the lower group of the superficial inguinal nodes are interconnected with each other and with the external iliac nodes by their efferents. Connecting vessels exist between the superficial and deep nodes. Following repeated confluence (three times) between the efferents of the medial and lateral groups, about half of the large efferents traverse the femoral nodes to connect with the external iliac and obturator nodes, while the other half are accompanied by the femoral vessels through the femoral canal to connect with the external iliac nodes (Figure 11.2).

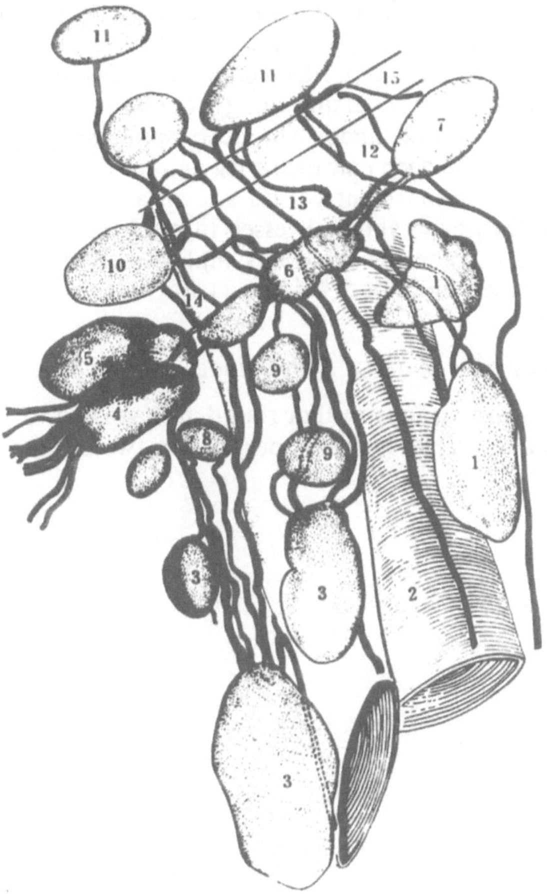

Figure 11.2 Inguinal lymph nodes and their connections. **1**: Lateral members of lower group of superficial inguinal lymph nodes; **2**: femoral a.; **3**: medial members (lower part) of lower group of superficial inguinal lymph nodes; **4**: medial members (upper part) of lower group of superficial inguinal lymph nodes; **5**: medial members of upper group of superficial inguinal lymph nodes; **6**: intermediate members of upper group of superficial inguinal lymph nodes; **7**: lateral members of upper group of superficial inguinal lymph nodes; **8**: medial group of deep inguinal lymph nodes; **9**: lateral group of deep inguinal lymph nodes; **10**: lymph node of femoral ring; **11**: external iliac lymph nodes; **12**: lateral group of deep lymphatics of thigh; **13**: intermediate group of deep lymphatics of thigh; **14**: medial group of deep lymphatics of thigh; **15**: inguinal ligament

The popliteal lymph nodes

The popliteal lymph nodes can be divided into the superficial and deep groups. The superficial group contains one or two nodes located around the popliteal vein and in the groove between the heads of the gastrocnemius. The deep nodes, two to six in number, are embedded in the fat around the popliteal vessels. The lymph nodes of the superficial group receive afferent vessels of the posterior group of the leg, and drain into the deep popliteal nodes. Sometimes there happens to be a lymphatic vessel coursing along the communicating vein to connect with the perforating lymph node. The deep popliteal lymph nodes receive afferent vessels from the deep part of the leg and the deep lymph vessels of the popliteal fossa and send efferent vessels known as the popliteal lymphatics, which pass along the popliteal blood vessels through the adductor hiatus to the thigh, where they become the femoral lymph vessels that connect with the inguinal lymph vessels and nodes (Figure 11.3).

The anterior and posterior tibial lymph nodes

These are small in size, usually oval or round in shape and vary in number and position. The anterior tibial lymph nodes, one or two in number, are situated

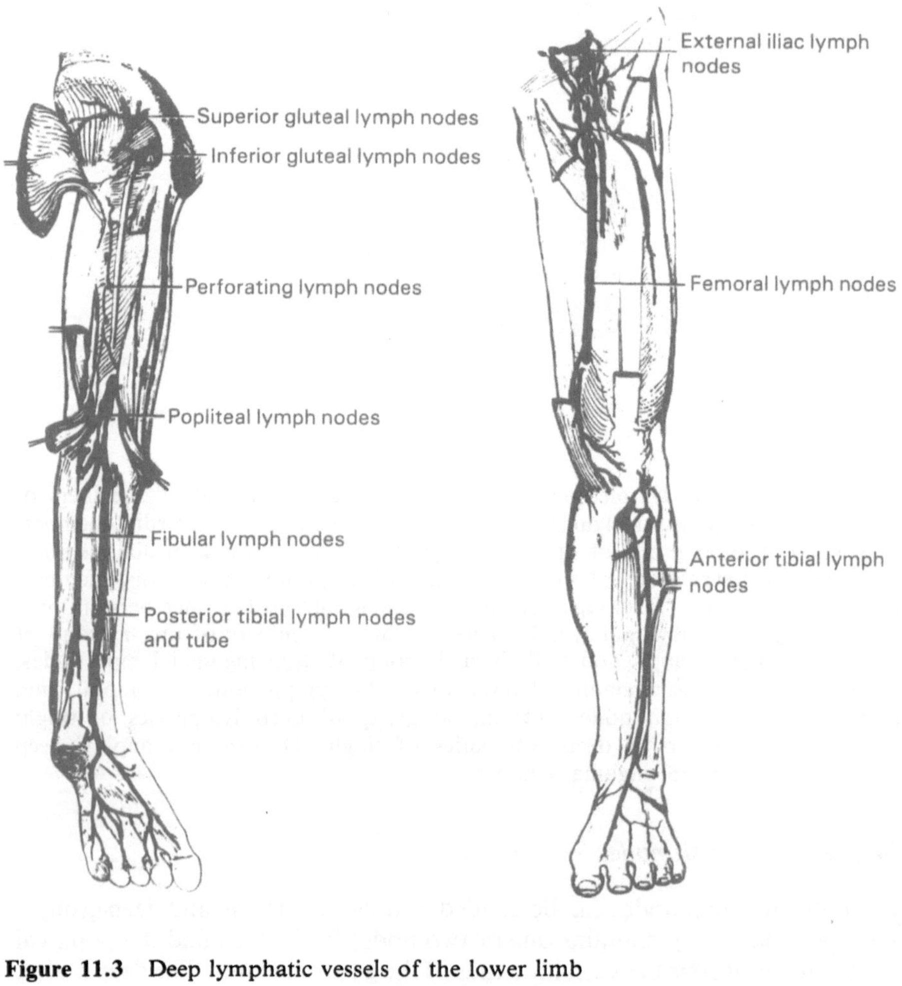

Figure 11.3 Deep lymphatic vessels of the lower limb

in front of the crural interosseous membrane around the anterior tibial vessels, the superolateral one being more frequently seen (Figure 11.3). The posterior tibial lymph nodes, one to three in number, are inconstant in position, being distributed along the posterior tibial vessels. They receive afferent vessels from the sole of the foot, the posterior crural muscles and tendons, joints, ligaments and periostea. The efferents of these nodes are connected with the deep popliteal lymph nodes.

The posterior deep femoral lymph nodes (perforating lymph nodes)

These are situated near the perforating arteries, one or two nodes often being seen around each perforating artery (Figure 11.3). They are interconnected by lymph vessels and link with the inguinal lymph nodes.

The deep gluteal nodes

These arrange themselves around the superior and inferior gluteal vessels and are called respectively the superior (two to five) and inferior (one to four) gluteal lymph nodes. They receive afferent vessels from the gluteal region and drain into the pelvic lymph nodes (Figure 11.3).

Deep lymphatic vessels of the lower limb

Anterior tibial lymph vessels

The deep lymph vessels of the dorsum of the toes join together to form those of the dorsum of the foot, which receive the arcuate and the medial and lateral tarsal lymph vessels to become the anterior tibial lymph vessels (Figure 11.3). The anterior tibial lymph vessels, one or two in number and 0.2–0.3 mm in diameter, begin by the union of the deep lymphatics of the dorsum of the foot near the transverse crural ligament and pass into the neurovascular sheath through the vascular foramen to the posterior part of the leg at the level of the tibial tuberosity. They join the posterior tibial lymph vessels below the tendinous arch of the soleus.

The posterior tibial lymph vessels

These begin from the lymph capillaries in the toes, the plantar muscles, tendons, ligaments and periosteum and pass through the lymphatic plexus to form the lymph vessels which accompany the venules and join repeatedly to form two to four medial and lateral plantar lymph vessels. After crossing the deltoid ligament they are called the posterior tibial lymph vessels (Figure 11.3), the diameter of which varies from 0.2 to 0.5 mm. It is usually 0.3 mm in the lower third of the leg, being 0.3 to 0.4 mm in the middle third and 0.4 to 0.5 mm in the upper third. Owing to the progressive confluence the posterior tibial lymph vessels tend to be thicker as they proceed.

Fibular lymph vessels

The lymph plexuses around the lateral malleolus and the muscle, tendon, joint, ligament and periosteum, as well as the fascia of the lateral part of the leg, combine to form the fibular lymph vessels, which are usually one or two in number and 0.1 mm in diameter and course along the synonymous neurovascular sheath from the lateral side obliquely toward the posterior median line to join the posterior tibial lymph vessel distal to the tendinous arch of the soleus (Figure 11.3).

The popliteal lymph vessels

These are four or five in number and 0.1–0.8 mm in diameter. However, there is a market variation in calibre, the range of 0.3–0.5 mm being the most common. In the popliteal region they receive the lymph vessels accompanying the tributaries of the popliteal vein. The popliteal lymphatic plexus, after several times of confluence, forms four or five lymph vessels, which pass through the inferior opening of the subsatorial canal to the femoral region, and are then known as the femoral lymph vessels (Figure 11.3).

The femoral lymph vessels

These consist of two to six thick lymph vessels surrounding the femoral artery. The deep femoral lymph vessels drain into them at the middle portion of the femoral triangle and are formed by 5–10 perforating lymph vessels converging at the anterior region of the thigh. The latter, being 0.2–0.4 mm in diameter, acccompany the perforating veins and are connected with perforating lymph nodes. They receive the medial and lateral femoral lymph vessels. The femoral lymph vessels may be divided in the upper portion of the femoral triangle into medial, intermediate and lateral groups. The lateral group consists of one to four lymph vessels, which pass deep to the inguinal ligament and are connected with the external iliac lymph nodes. The intermediate group consists of two to eight vessels, which course within the vascular sheath and are connected with the external iliac lymph nodes. The medial group is composed of two to four vessels, which pass beneath the inguinal ligament through the femoral canal to be connected with the external iliac and obturator lymph nodes (Figure 11.3).

The deep lymph vessels of the posterior femoral region

These vary in number and position. They are often seen near the perforating veins, one or two lymph nodes accompanying each perforating blood vessel. Two or three perforating lymph vessels connect these nodes with the deep femoral lymph vessels. Between the perforating lymph nodes themselves there are interconnecting lymphatics.

The deep lymph vessels of the gluteal region

These are formed by the lymphatics arising from the lymph nodes surrounding the superior and inferior gluteal vessels, the sciatic nerve, and the posterior cutaneous nerve of the thigh. They also receive afferent vessels from the gluteal muscles and tendons. These deep vessels pass through the supra- and infra-piriformis spaces to connect with the intrapelvic lymph nodes.

Deep lymph vessels and nodes of the lower limb

The deep lymph vessels of the lower limb are fewer than the superficial ones. However, they are larger, usually over 0.3 mm in diameter. At the base of the femoral triangle, just beneath the inguinal ligament, the femoral lymph vessels are 8–14 in number and larger in calibre, the thickest of these amounting to 1.5 mm in diameter. Their courses are apparently regular, i.e. accompanying the main neurovascular bundles. Hence they have provided a favourable condition for the performance of anastomosis between the deep lymph vessels and veins. The positions of the inguinal and popliteal lymph nodes are relatively constant, so that it is possible to puncture the lymph nodes directly in order to demonstrate the efferent lymph vessels, or to look for larger lymph vessels under the surgical microscope in the neighbourhood of these nodes.

LYMPHATIC SYSTEM OF THE UPPER LIMB

Grouping, course and direction of drainage of the superficial lymph vessels

The digital lymph vessels originating from the digital plexuses proceed along either border of the fingers to the webs where they join the lymphatics from the palm and the back of the hand, whence they continue forward in three directions and merge into the medial, lateral and intermediate groups respectively (Figure 11.4).

(1) The medial group consists of 6–16 lymph vessels from the little and ring fingers, a part of the middle finger, the ulnar border of the palm and the forearm. These vessels accompany the basilic vein and drain in the same direction. In the elbow some of these vessels end in the superficial cubital lymph nodes (supratrochlear lymph nodes) and the rest have one of two fates: some accompany the efferent vessels of the supratrochlear nodes and pierce the deep fascia with the basilic vein to end in the lateral group of the axillary lymph nodes; others (one to seven in number) have no connection with the supratrochlear nodes but run superficial to the deep fascia, in the medial bicipital groove. They pierce the axillary fascia to end in the lateral group of the axillary lymph nodes (Figure 11.4).

(2) The lateral group consists of less vessels (4–12) than the medial group. They come from the thumb, the index finger, a part of the middle finger, the lateral margin of the hand and the lateral side of the forearm. After passing

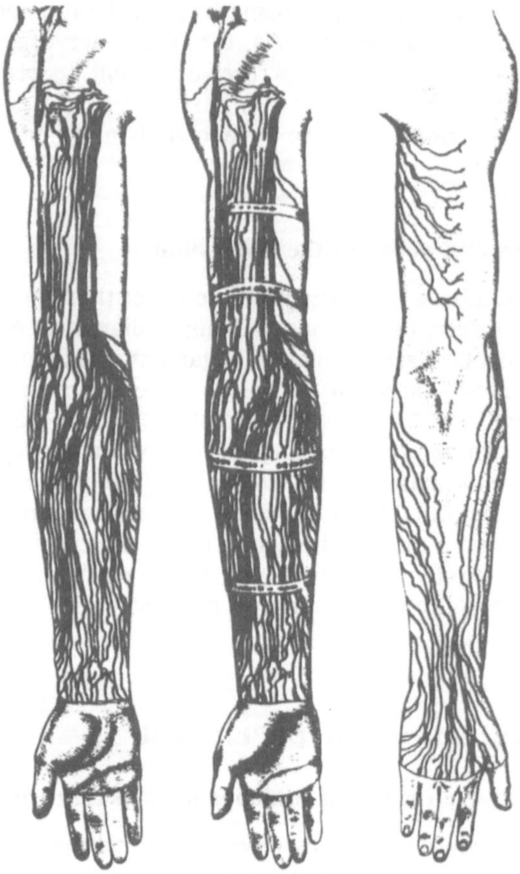

Figure 11.4 Distribution of superficial lymph vessels of the upper limb

through the lymph plexus on the back of the hand they merge into larger collecting vessels, and ascend together with the cephalic vein on the radial side of the forearm. In the cubital region they incline to the medial side of the arm, advancing in the medial bicipital groove, pierce the axillary fascia and end in the lateral group of the axillary lymph nodes. A few of them (one to three) run through the groove between the pectoralis major and the deltoideus and end in the pectorodeltoid lymph nodes or directly into the apical group of the axillary lymph nodes (Figure 11.4).

(3) The intermediate group, lying in the anterior aspect of the forearm, is composed of the vessels of the finger, palm and the intermediate part of the palmar aspect of the forearm. They are few in number (three to seven), accompanying the median vein of the forearm to the cubital region, whence they advance toward the medial side of the arm and ascend superficial to the deep fascia along the medial border of the biceps brachii. They eventually pierce

the axillary fascia to end in the lateral group of the axillary lymph nodes. A few of them cross the cubital region obliquely upward and medially to end in the supratrochlear nodes (Figure 11.4).

Choice of the site of incision for the lymphatico-venous anastomosis between the superficial lymph vessels and veins

Since the collecting lymph vessels of the upper limb course near the main superficial veins, it is possible to make two or three transverse incisions along the course of the latter in order to anastomose as many lymph vessels as possible and divert the obstructed lymph into the veins (Figure 11.4).

The number of collecting lymph vessels of the upper limb varies from one to 10. Their mode of distribution is as follows. In the upper part of the forearm there are one to three vessels within 1 cm from the main stem of the cephalic vein and three or four vessels within 5 cm from the vein; there are one or two vessels within 1 cm, and one to three vessels within 5 cm from the stem of the basilic vein. In the middle and lower parts of the forearm there are usually one or two vessels within 1 cm, and two to five vessels within 5 cm, from the stem of the cephalic vein.

Deep lymphatic vessels of the upper limb

The digital deep lymph vessels

These are formed from the digital lymph plexus. They follow the course of the digital blood vessels to the webs, where they pass to the palmar and dorsal aspects of the hand and connect with one another near the superficial and deep palmar arches to form the lymph plexus of the respective arch (Figure 11.5).

In the forearm, the deep lymph vessels

These fall into the radial, the ulnar and the anterior and posterior interosseous groups.

The radial lymph vessels proceed in the neurovascular bundle. They begin from the wrist and end in the cubital fossa to join the ulnar lymph vessels. They are mostly two in number (two to four) and 0.2–0.4 mm in diameter.

The ulnar lymph vessels are one to five in number and 0.1–0.5 mm in diameter.

The posterior interosseous lymph vessels are one or two in number and 0.1–0.2 mm in diameter. They pass through the vascular foramen at the upper part of the interosseous membrane to its anterior aspect, where they join the anterior interosseous lymph vessels to form the common interosseous lymph vessels.

The anterior interosseous lymph vessels, one to four in number and 0.1–0.2 mm in diameter, join the posterior interosseous lymph vessels in the cubital fossa 2–3 cm below its midpoint to form the common interosseous lymph vessels on the palmar surface of the interosseous membrane.

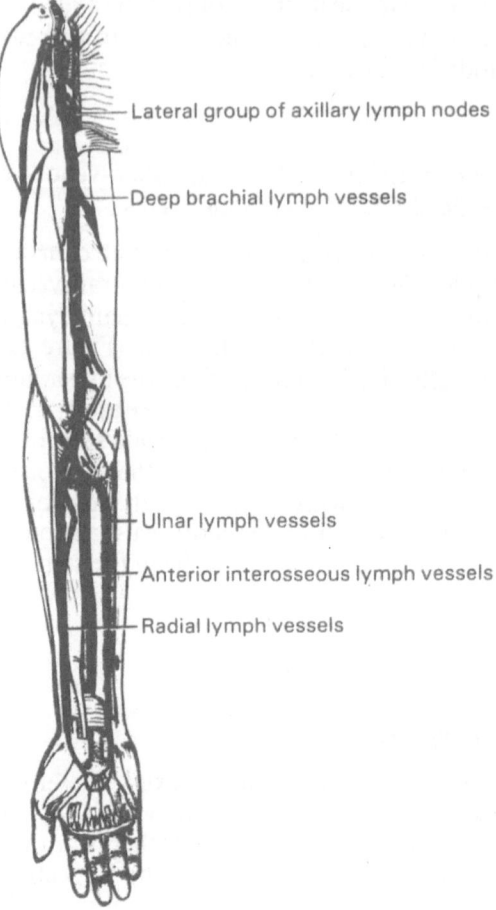

Figure 11.5 Deep lymph vessels of the upper limb

The common interosseous lymph vessels receive such lymphatics as those of the median nerve, as they ascend with the vascular bundle and thus become thickened. They drain into, or connect with, the ulnar lymph vessels at the level of the origin of the common interosseous artery.

The deep brachial lymph vessels

These are the continuations of those of the forearm. The collecting lymph vessels of the superficial group pierce the deep fascia over the medial bicipital groove and pass through the brachial neurovascular sheath. A few of them come from the efferents of the deep brachial lymph nodes. The lymph vessels originating from the distributing area of the branches of the brachial artery (such as the lymph vessels accompanying the ulnar, radial and middle collateral arteries, and the deep brachial lymph vessels coming from those of the triceps, etc.) also unite with the brachial lymph vessels to become gradually larger and end at length in the lateral axillary nodes.

The deep axillary lymph vessels

These are the continuations of the deep brachial lymph vessels. They originate from two groups. One of them consists of three to five superficial collecting lymph vessels, which pierce the axillary fascia to end in the lateral group of the axillary lymph nodes. The other group includes one or two deep lymph vessels, which proceed along the brachial artery and drain into the axillary lymph nodes. In the axillary cavity these two groups join the efferent vessels from the axillary nodes and a few from the arm to form a plexus around the axillary blood vessels. During repeated combination the vessels reduce in number. In the subclavian region they join near the root of the neck into one or two trunks called the subclavian trunks to enter the subclavian vein.

Lymph nodes of the upper limb

The lymph nodes of the upper limb fall into two categories. The superficial nodes comprise the superficial cubital lymph nodes (supratrochlear nodes), the superficial brachial lymph nodes, the deltoid–pectorial lymph nodes (vary in site and number), etc. The deep lymph nodes comprise the lymph nodes of the forearm (vary in site and number) and the deep cubital and axillary lymph nodes.

LYMPH VESSELS OF THE FEMALE EXTERNAL GENITALIA

Distribution and drainage of the lymph vessels of the female external genitalia

The lymph vessels of the vulva originate from the lymph plexus in the skin. They can be divided into superficial and deep layers. These unite to form lymph vessels, which pass to the superficial inguinal lymph nodes. The total number of the lymph vessels of the vulva varies from six to 10. Their diameter ranges from 0.1 to 0.5 mm, within the limit of 1 cm from the superficial external pudendal vein, three to seven lymph vessels may be found. Of these at least three have a diameter of more than 0.3 mm.

If the mons pubis and labia majora be divided roughly into three parts, i.e. the upper, middle and lower portions, the distribution and drainage of their lymph vessels are as follows (Figure 11.6).

1. The lymph vessels of the upper part, one to three in number, originate near the mons pubis and the clitoris. They ascend laterally, but some of them may first ascend above the inguinal ligament and then descend superficial to it. Most of them drain into the medial and intermediate members of the superior group of the superficial inguinal lymph nodes; a few drain into the medial ones of the inferior group.

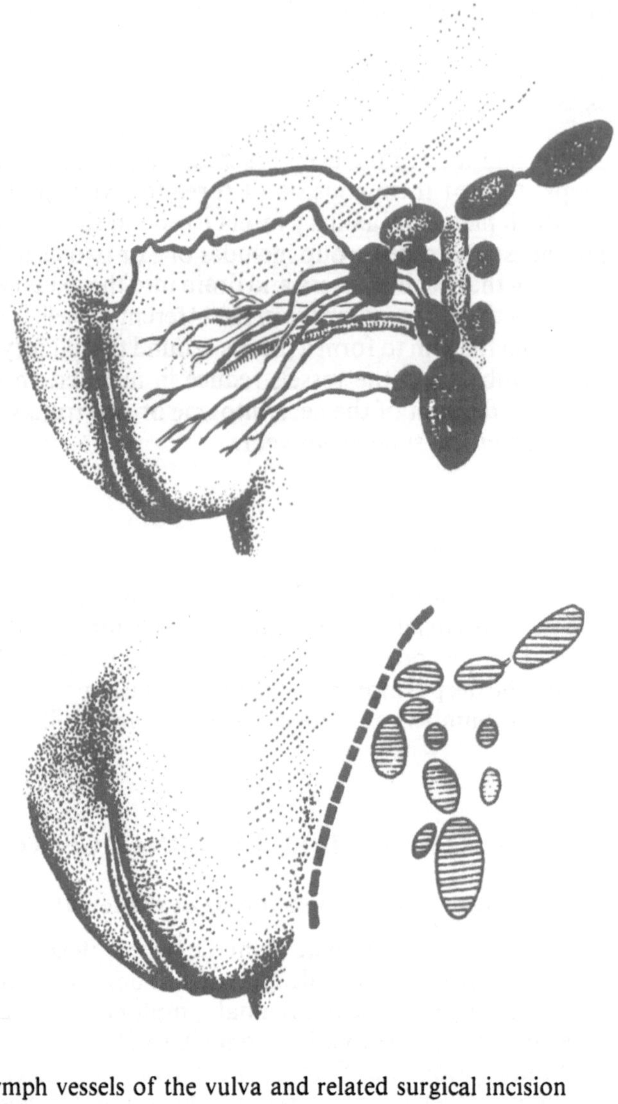

Figure 11.6 Lymph vessels of the vulva and related surgical incision

2. The lymph vessels of the middle part, one to four in number, originate from the upper half of the labia majora, run laterally, deep or superficial to the superficial external pudendal vein, and drain into the medial members of the inferior group of the superficial inguinal lymph nodes.
3. The lymph vessels of the lower part, one to five in number, originate from the lower half of the labia majora, proceed superolaterally from the inferomedial side to drain into the lower portion of the medial members of the inferior group of the superficial inguinal lymph nodes while part of them may drain into the upper portion.

Neighbouring veins and relevant surgical incisions

Veins of the vulva are called the superficial external pudendal veins, being one to four in number. In spite of some of their variations in drainage – that is, they may open into the long saphenous vein (71%) or may form a common trunk with the superficial epigastric vein before ending in the long saphenous vein (29%) – the collecting area of its upper and lower tributaries remains rather constant. In surgical treatment of obstructive lymphatic oedema of the vulva, the lymph vessels and veins from the vulva may be adequately exposed when a longitudinal curved incision between the vulva and the upper part of the thigh is made in accordance with the site indicated in Figure 11.6.

LYMPH VESSELS OF THE MALE EXTERNAL GENITALIA

Lymph vessels of the penis

In the skin and subcutaneous tissue of the penis there is an abundance of lymph capillaries. The lymph vessels originate from a circular plexus in the free margin of the prepuce. Every three to five adjacent lymph vessels combine to form a thicker vessel. Most of them deviate either to the left or to the right for a very short distance, and then advance in every aspect of the penis between the fascia penis and the proper fascia.

Number of lymph vessels of the penis and the site of drainage

The superficial lymph vessels of the penis are four to eight in number, five being more common. The lymph vessels of either side may overlap in the mid-line and divert to the opposite side. Having commenced from the root or either side of the penis, the uppermost lymph vessels assume a rather constant course, reaching the front of the symphysis pubis. They ascend first anterior to the superficial inguinal ring and then curve downwards across the superficial surface of the inguinal ligament to drain into the medial members of the superior group of the superficial inguinal lymph nodes. The lymph vessels on either side of the root of the penis pass laterally and horizontally, frequently accompanying the upper branch of the superficial external pudendal vein to end in the medial or intermediate members of the superior group of the superficial inguinal lymph nodes. Part of them end in the upper part of the medial members of the inferior group of the superficial inguinal nodes, being chiefly from the skin of the ventral side of the penis (Figure 11.7).

Diameter and valves of the superficial lymph vessels of the penis

The diameter of the superficial lymph vessels of the adult penis varies from 0.1 to 1.0 mm. About one-third of them are less than 0.2 mm, while two-thirds are more than 0.3 mm. In these vessels with a diameter of 0.5–1.0 mm there is a pair of valves in every 1.5 mm of the vessel.

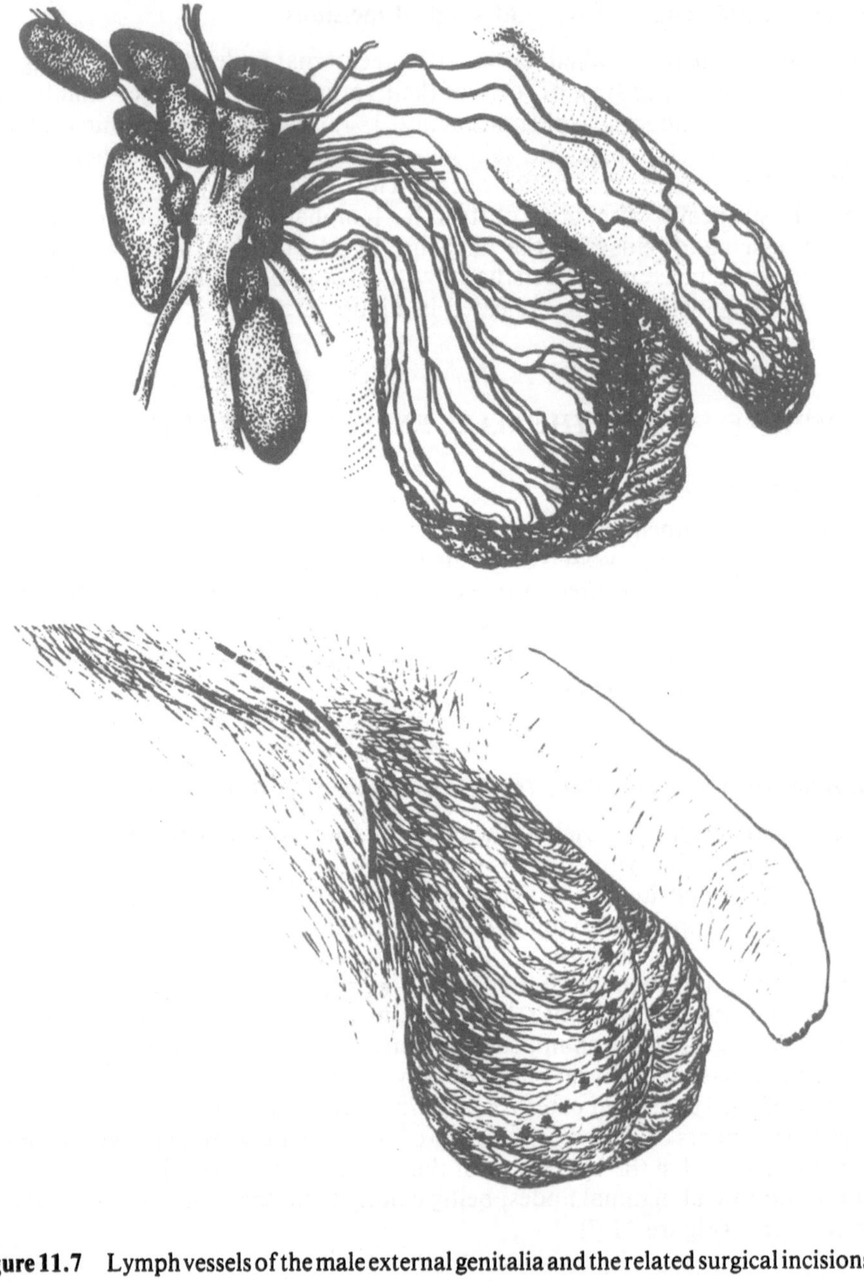

Figure 11.7 Lymph vessels of the male external genitalia and the related surgical incisions

Lymph vessels of the scrotum

The lymph vessels of the skin of the scrotum originate from the papillary layer of the dermis and the subcutaneous tissue. They can be found all over the scrotum in the form of a profuse lymph capillary network, from which fine lymph vessels are formed. After repeated confluence these reduce to 3–24 lymph vessels of larger calibre, which continue upward and laterally towards either side along the rugae of the scrotum. Near the raphe they can be seen decussating across the median line.

The lymph vessels of the upper part of the scrotum

These combine into two or three collecting vessels, which pass upwards and laterally to accompany or proceed above the upper branch of the external pudendal vein. When reaching the inguinal ligament these collecting vessels combine into a single vessel about 0.5 mm in diameter, which drains into the medial members of the superior group of the superficial inguinal lymph nodes or to the upper part of the medial members of the inferior group of the superficial inguinal nodes.

The lymph vessels of the median part of the scrotum

These form one to four collecting vessels, which ascend forwards and laterally to accompany the external pudendal vein and drain into the upper part of the medial members of the inferior group of the superficial inguinal lymph nodes.

The lymph vessels of the lower part of the scrotum

These unite to form one to four collecting vessels. They ascend laterally accompanying the inferior branch of the superficial external pudendal vein to end in the lower part of the medial members of the inferior group of the superficial inguinal lymph nodes.

Diameter and valves of the superficial lymph vessels of the scrotum

The diameter of the collecting vessels of the scrotum varies from 0.1 to 0.5 mm, the majority being 0.3–0.5 mm. One pair of valves occurs in every 1.5 cm of these vessels.

Veins of the male external genitalia and relevant surgical incisions

The lymph vessels of the male external genitalia accompany the superficial external pudendal vein and its tributaries. This vein usually has two branches, i.e. a superior and an inferior one. In surgical treatment of obstructive oedema of the male external genitalia the site for indirect injection of lymph vessels may be selected near the raphe of the scrotum and the root of the penis. If the incision is selected according to the position indicated in Figure 11.7, a longitudinal curved incision between the external genitalia and the upper part of the thigh may be used to expose the veins and lymph vessels simultaneously.

LYMPH VESSELS WITHIN THE SPERMATIC CORD

Origin and segmental distribution of lymph vessels

The lymphatic capillary network around the seminiferous tubules and under the tunica vaginalis serves as the origin of the lymph vessels within the spermatic cord. These begin as a lymphatic plexus between the testis and epididymis, from which are formed by repeated combination the efferent lymphatics of the testis that are more numerous in number (3–11).

The efferent lymphatics of the testis may be divided into four segments according to their position.

Scrotal segment

At the mediastinum testis the lymphatic plexus forms a number of efferents, which amount to 11 in adults. They ascend around the vas deferens and accompany the testicular vein within the spermatic fasciae. The outer diameter of the lymph vessel is 0.1–0.5 mm. In adults, vessels with diameters of 0.2–0.5 mm are more common, with a maximum of 1.5 mm. In infants and children most of the vessels are 0.1–0.3 mm in calibre.

Cordal segment

The cordal segment consists of three to seven vessels, which may change their positions on the way, i.e. they lie at first on the medial side of the spermatic cord, then on its lateral side and finally turn to its medial side again. They wind around the veins and within the cremaster and its fascia. The diameters of these vessels measure 0.2–0.7 (0.3–0.7 mm in the adult, and 0.2–0.5 mm in infants and children). Those with a diameter of 0.4 and 0.5 mm are frequently seen in adults. The largest amount to 1.5 mm (Figure 11.8).

Inguinal segment

The inguinal segment lies within the internal spermatic fascia, consisting of five to seven vessels. The outer diameters of these measure 0.2–0.7 mm, mostly 0.3–0.7 mm in adults and 0.3–0.5 mm in infants and children.

Abdominal segment

The internal spermatic lymph vessels ascend into the pelvis and unite repeatedly to form three or four collecting vessels. In the abdomen these vessels pass behind the peritoneum deviating slightly from the blood vessels and ascend along the lateral border of the psoas major between the ureter and the inferior vena cava. They finally drain into the regional lymph nodes beneath the renal vein.

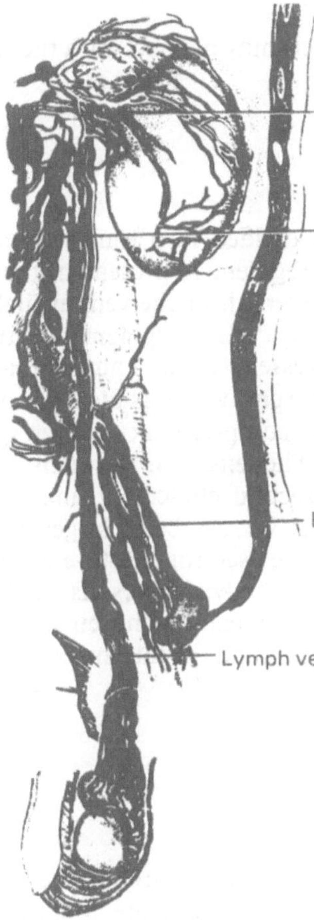

Figure 11.8 Lymph vessels and veins around the spermatic cord and kidney

On the right side they end in the nodes between the inferior vena cava and the abdominal aorta, the preaortic nodes. The diameter of these vessels varies mostly from 0.3 to 0.7 mm.

Connections between the internal spermatic lymph vessels and those in the environ

(1) When the internal spermatic lymph vessel reach the pelvic brim it has a short connection with the medial group of the external iliac lymph nodes. It is also connected with the pelvic segment of the lymph vessels of the vas deferens.

(2) At the deep inguinal ring are fine vessels connecting the internal spermatic lymph vessels with the hypogastric lymph glands.

(3) At the level of the lower pole of the kidney a lymph vessel can usually be seen to turn upward and laterally to connect the internal spermatic lymph vessels with those of the renal capsule.

(4) The internal spermatic lymph vessels may connect with the renal lymph vessels via the lumbar lymph nodes.

Internal spermatic vein

The internal spermatic vein can also be divided into four segments for the convenience of description. The scrotal segment is present in the form of a plexus, which is difficult to separate. The length of the vein available for dissection is too short to anastomose. The cordal segments of the internal spermatic veins consist of seven to nine vessels, about 1 mm in diameter, and the length capable of being separated is 1.5 cm, which is ideal for lymphaticovenous anastomosis. The inguinal segment comprises six or seven vessels, each of which has a diameter of about 1 mm. The length of the veins available for separation is nearly 1 cm, being of the second choice for anastomosis. The abdominal segment consists of two or three vessels, being larger in calibre and not easy to separate. Nevertheless they can be used for end-to-end anastomosis.

In attempts to relieve chyluria, most of the lymph vessels exposed around the kidney are about 1 mm in diameter. They can be chosen for anastomosis between the tributaries of renal capsular veins and the internal spermatic lymph vessels.

THORACIC DUCT

The variations of the thoracic duct are numerous. Since the criterion for classification varies with different investigators, there are countless shades of opinion.

Types of thoracic duct

The thoracic duct may be divided into six types. The form and incidence of each type are shown in Figure 11.9.

Occasionally the thoracic duct may originate from the cisterna chyli or the left lumbar trunk, going along the left side of the thoracic aorta, through the thorax to the neck, where it is situated on the left side. It empties finally into the junction of the left subclavian internal jugular veins. This kind of thoracic duct has been called the sinistral type. Yang Chunlin reported that either the sinistral or double type of the thoracic duct was found only in one out of 150 cases.

The thoracic duct is the largest vessel of the lymphatic system. Its length ranges from 14.3 to 37.0 cm. Its outer diameter varies with different locations and averages 3.8 (1.0–9.0) mm.

The thoracic duct runs such a long course through the abdomen, thorax and neck that it may be divided into three segments, i.e. the abdominal, thoracic and cervical segment.

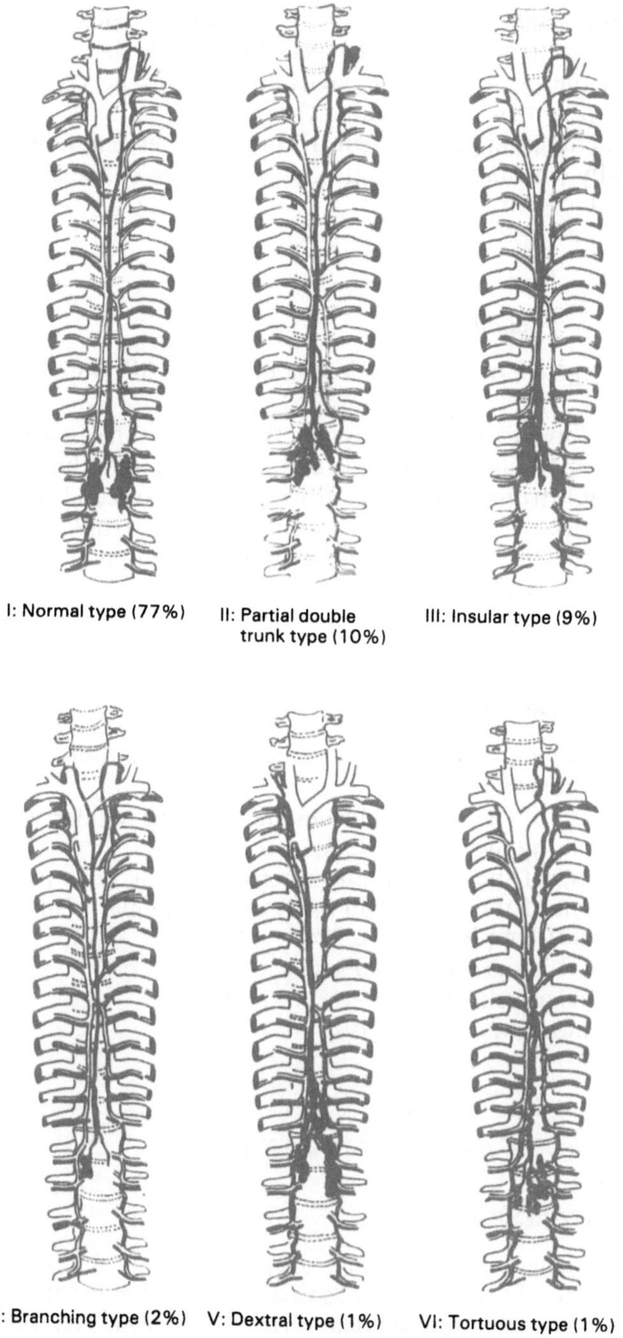

Figure 11.9 Types of the thoracic duct and their incidence

Cervical segment of the thoracic duct

The cervical segment of the thoracic duct begins at the level of the first thoracic vertebra and ascends along the lateral side of the oesophagus. It runs between the cervical portion of the oesophagus and the subclavian artery, then between the dome of the pleura and the vagus and phrenic nerves and the common carotid artery. It then passes behind the internal jugular vein, and ascends to the left of the internal jugular vein, forming the cervical arch of the thoracic duct. It finally descends to end into the confluence of the left subclavian and internal jugular veins.

Types of cervical segment

The cervical segment of the thoracic duct may be divided into four types (Figure 11.10).

There are three forms in the double trunk type. The first form consists of two trunks combining into a single one before draining into the vein, and is called the double trunk with single orifice (14%); the second is the double trunk with two orifices (3%); the third comprises one trunk draining into the confluence of the subclavian and internal jugular veins and another connecting with the deep cervical lymph nodes (2%).

The site of confluence

The site of confluence of the cervical segment of the thoracic duct has many variations. It may drain into

1. the junction of the left subclavian and internal jugular veins (78.6%);
2. the internal jugular vein (4.9%);
3. the junction of the internal and external jugular veins (6.8%);
4. the junction of the subclavian and external jugular veins (2.9%);
5. deep cervical lymph nodes (2.9%);
6. the external jugular vein (1.0%);
7. the subclavian vein (1.9%);
8. the left innominate vein (1.0%).

Types of the arch of the cervical thoracic duct

High-arched type (50%)

The cervical segment of the thoracic duct begins from the inlet of the thorax. After passing into the neck it ascends first to the left behind the internal jugular vein. At the level of the sixth cervical vertebra it descends lateral to the internal jugular vein and ends into the confluence of the subclavian and internal jugular veins.

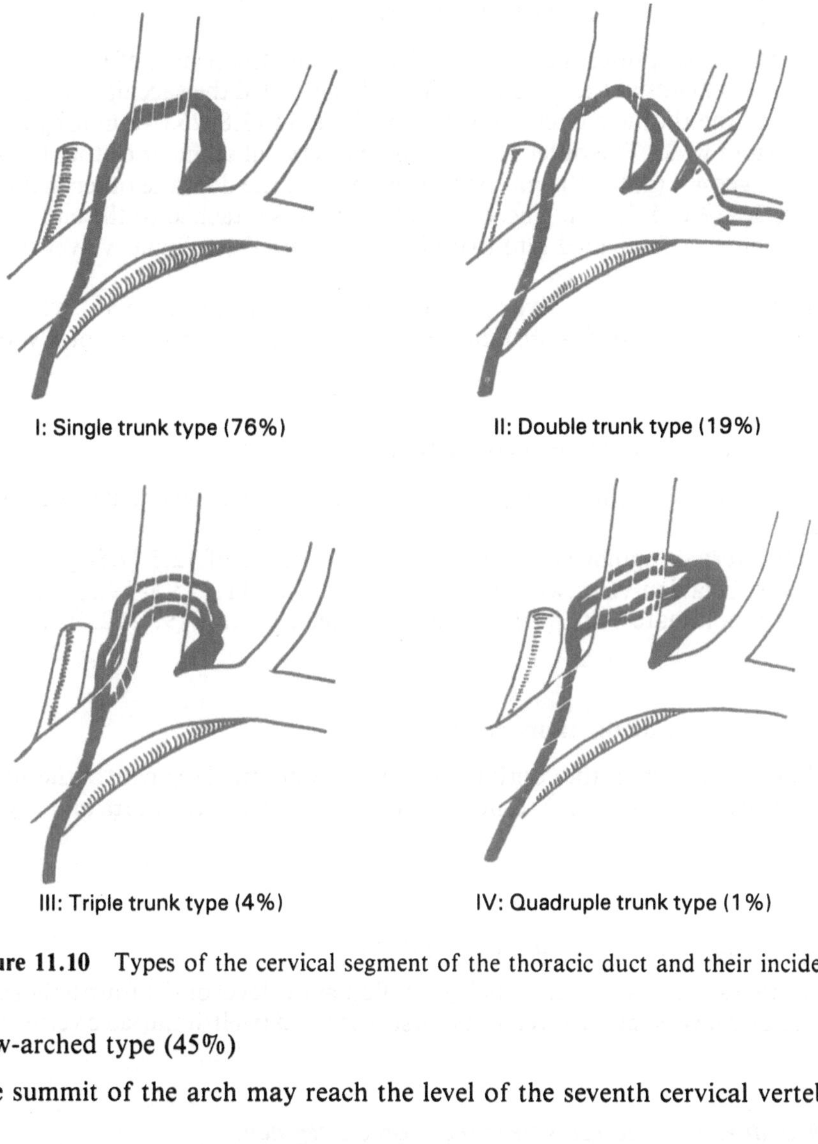

Figure 11.10 Types of the cervical segment of the thoracic duct and their incidence

Low-arched type (45%)

The summit of the arch may reach the level of the seventh cervical vertebra.

The oblique (non-arched) type (5%)

After entering the root of the neck the thoracic duct runs obliquely upwards and laterally to drain into the confluence of the subclavian and internal jugular veins.

In shunting the thoracic duct the high-arched type can be dissected for a wide range, while the low-arched type comes next. The surface projection of the high arch is about 3–5 cm above the clavicle. The position of the oblique type is lower, so that it is not easy to dissect, and demands special care. It will also increase the difficulty of anastomosis.

Saccular part (the ampulla) of the thoracic duct

The thoracic duct presents a dilatation between the lower part of the arch and where the duct ends in the venous angle, which is called the saccular part or the ampulla of the thoracic duct. This part is about 11 (3.8–25.0) mm long and 5 (1.5–9.7) mm wide. The outer diameter of the cervical segment of the thoracic duct averages 4.5 (2.4–8.9) mm. At the end part of the duct the outer diameter averages 3.3 (2.0–5.5) mm. There is a pair of valves attached to the end of the duct, which can be divided into two kinds: the paired semilunar valves (99%) and basilar valve (1%).

The right cusp of the valve averages 5.1 (2.0–6.0) mm in length, while the left cusp averages 3.0 (0.5–5.0) mm. Both of them are 1.5 (0.5–3.0) mm in width.

Veins relevant to the lymphaticovenous anastomosis

1. Left external jugular vein, with an outer diameter averaging 7.5 (3.0–13.0) mm.
2. Left internal jugular vein, with an outer diameter of 12.5 (7.8–23.7) mm.
3. Left subclavian vein, with an outer diameter of 11.0 (5.8–19.5) mm.
4. Left innominate vein, with an outer diameter of 15.6 (9.7–22.0) mm.

Thoracic segment of the thoracic duct

The thoracic segment is the continuation of the abdominal segment at the aortic hiatus of the diaphragm. It ascends in the sulcus between the aorta and azygos vein.

The outer diameter of the thoracic segment

This averages 3.8 (3.4–4.1) mm, being smallest at the level of the fourth thoracic vertebra and largest at the level of the first, fifth and twelfth thoracic vertebrae.

Outer diameter of the veins near the thoracic segment

The outer diameter of the azygos vein is 4.9 mm, becoming gradually larger from T_{12} to T_5. The outer diameter of the intercostal vein averages 3.6 (0.5–10.0) mm, the shifting range of the fourth to the twelfth intercostal veins being 12–17 mm.

Relationship between the thoracic segment and the greater splanchnic nerve

At the level of T_6–T_{12} the distance between the thoracic duct and the greater splanchnic nerve is gradually shortened. It goes from 32 to 6 mm and finally to zero. At the level of T_{12} the duct and the nerve become overlapped. This relationship indicates what should be noticed so as to avoid injury of the nerve during operation.

The valves of the thoracic segment

These may be divided into three types.

1. Double valve, semilunar in shape and arranged in pairs (78%).
2. Single valve, semilunar or saccular and arranged singly (12%).
3. Basilar valve, thick and stout and in pairs or singly (10%).

The thoracic segment has about 8.6 (6–21) valves, singly or in pairs. There is a great disparity in the distance between the valves. The average interval is 20 (8–60) mm.

The most common and complete double valves are 3.0 (1.0–5.0) mm long and 1.6 (0.2–8.3) mm wide (Figure 11.11).

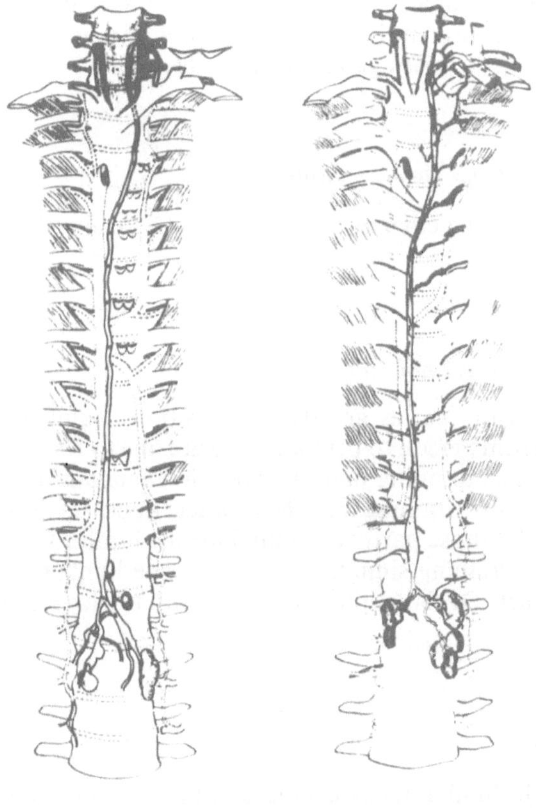

Figure 11.11 Diagram of the blood supply of the thoracic duct and the position of its valves

Abdominal segment of the thoracic duct

Origin of the thoracic duct

Thoracic ducts belong to two types in respect to their origin. The first type originate from the cisterna chyli; the second is formed by the union of the right and left lumbar trunks, the cisterna being absent.

Position of the cisterna chyli

The position of the cisterna chyli varies according to its length. It may be as high as the level of T_9–T_{10} and as low as L_2. It is located at the level of T_{12}–L_1 in 18%, of T_{11} in 2%, of T_{11}–T_{12} in 8%, of L_1–L_2 in 4%, of L_2 in 2%, of T_9–T_{10} and T_{11}–L_1 in 1%.

Formation of the cisterna chyli

The right and left lumbar trunks unite to form a saccular dilatation, called the cisterna chyli. It is present in 70% of the cases and absent in 30%. The shape of the cisterna chyli varies greatly (Figure 11.12).

Measurements of the cisterna chyli

The length of cisterna chyli averages 25.5 (7–62.5) mm; the width averages 6.7 (4–10) mm.

Drainage of the intestinal trunk

The intestinal trunk varies greatly. Its position, number and draining area usually differ from person to person. They are one to four in number but single in most cases. The draining patterns are miscellaneous and can be allotted to four types: (1) those draining into the thoracic duct; (2) those draining into the lumbar trunk; (3) those partly draining into the lumbar trunk and the cisterna chyli; (4) those draining simultaneously into the lumbar trunk, cisterna chyli and thoracic duct. Of these, those draining into the lumbar trunk are the most common.

Lumbar trunk

The length of the lumbar trunk averages 57 (36–72) mm. Sides are unequal. The outer diameter of this trunk averages 3.3 (1.0–9.4) mm, so that it is quite thick and long, and thus easy to mobilize.

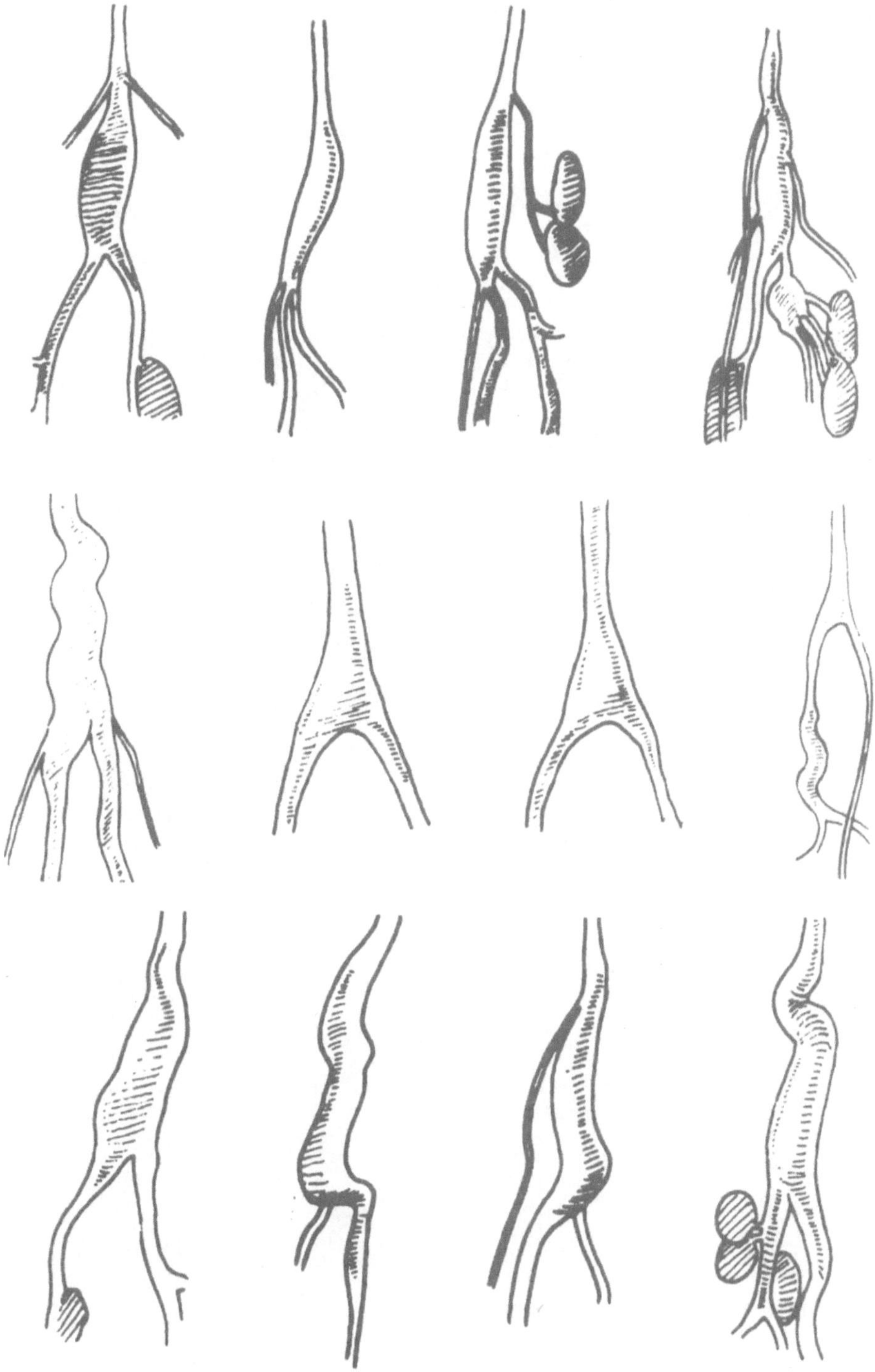

Figure 11.12 Profile of the cisterna chyli

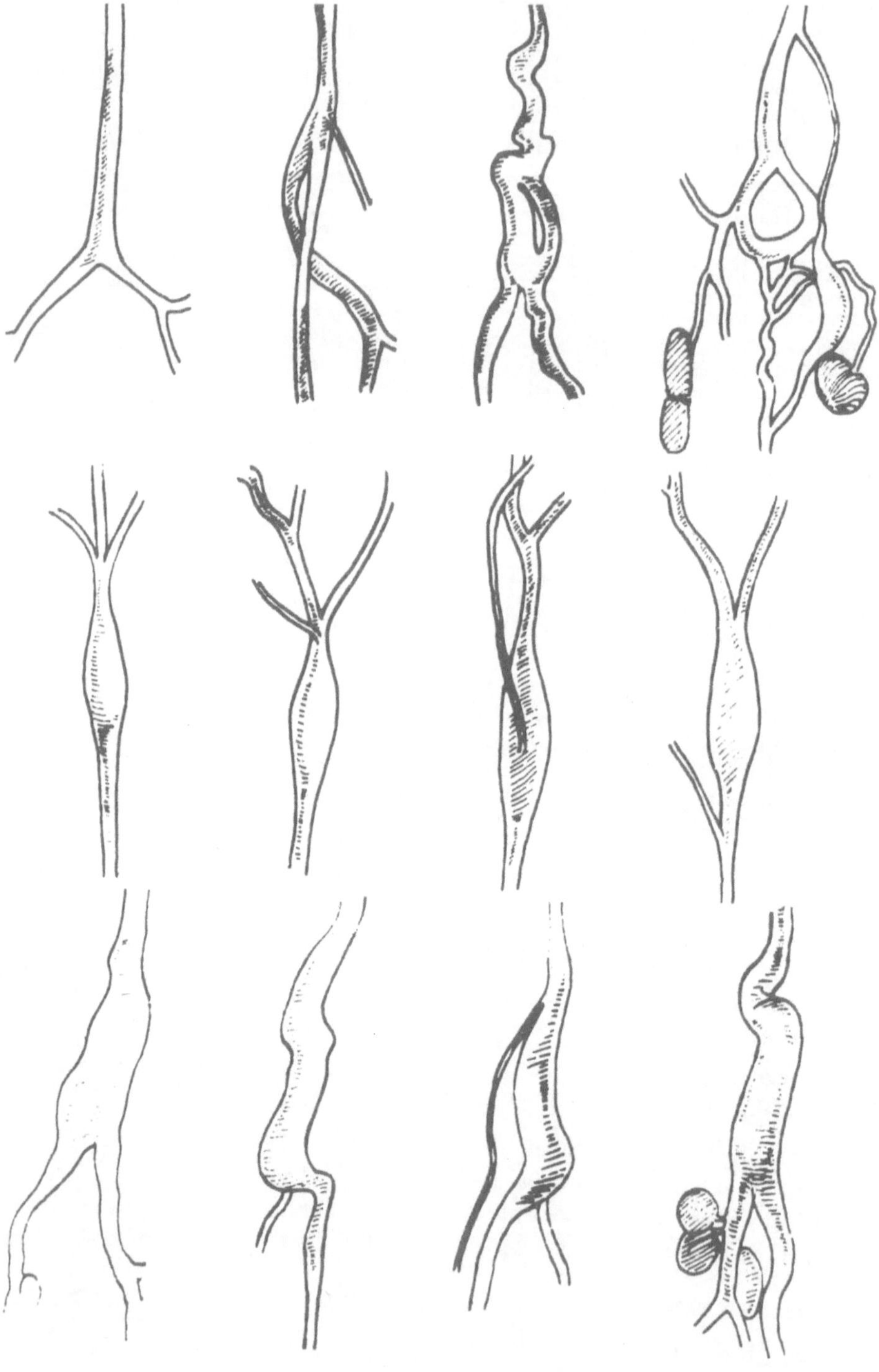

Figure 11.12

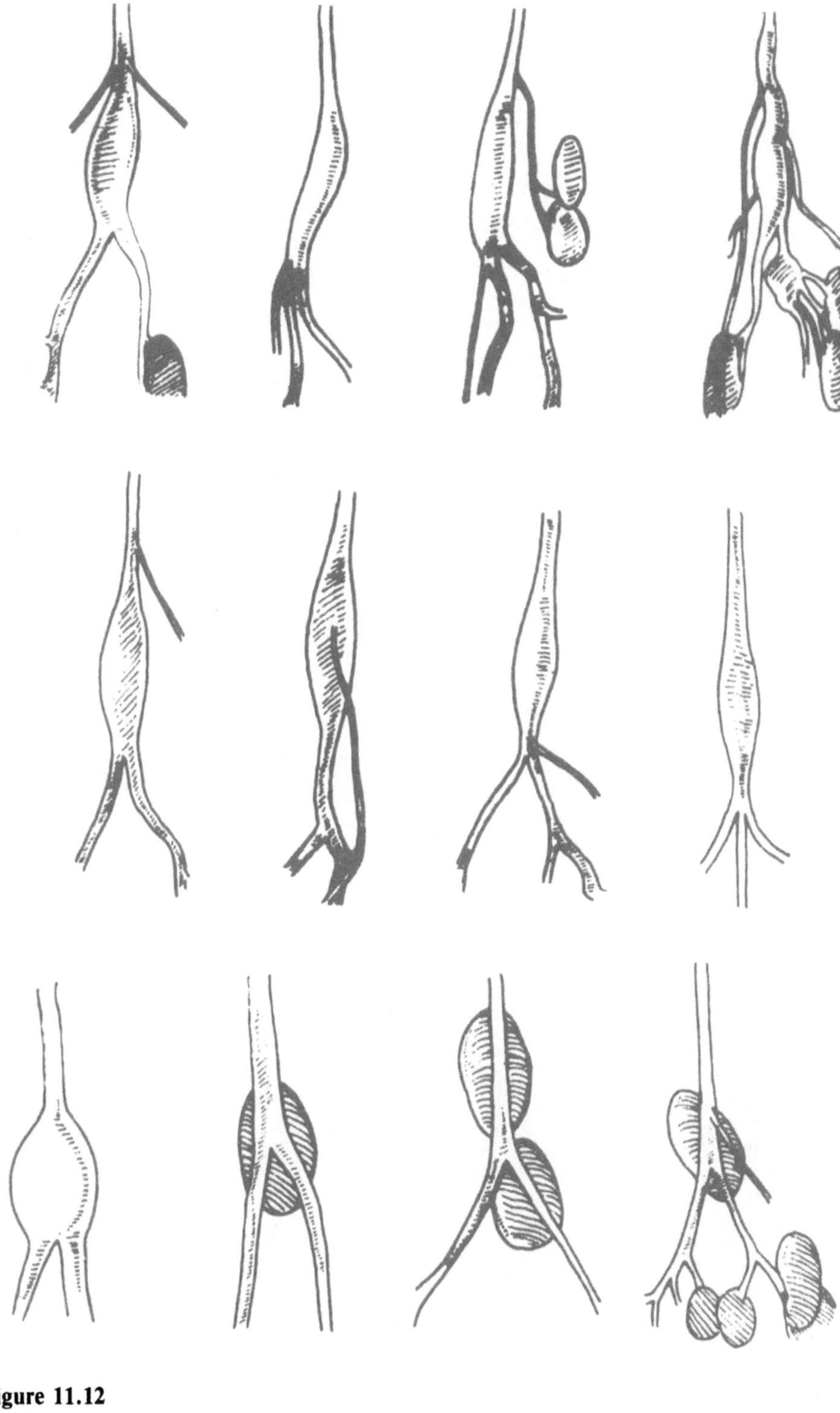

Figure 11.12

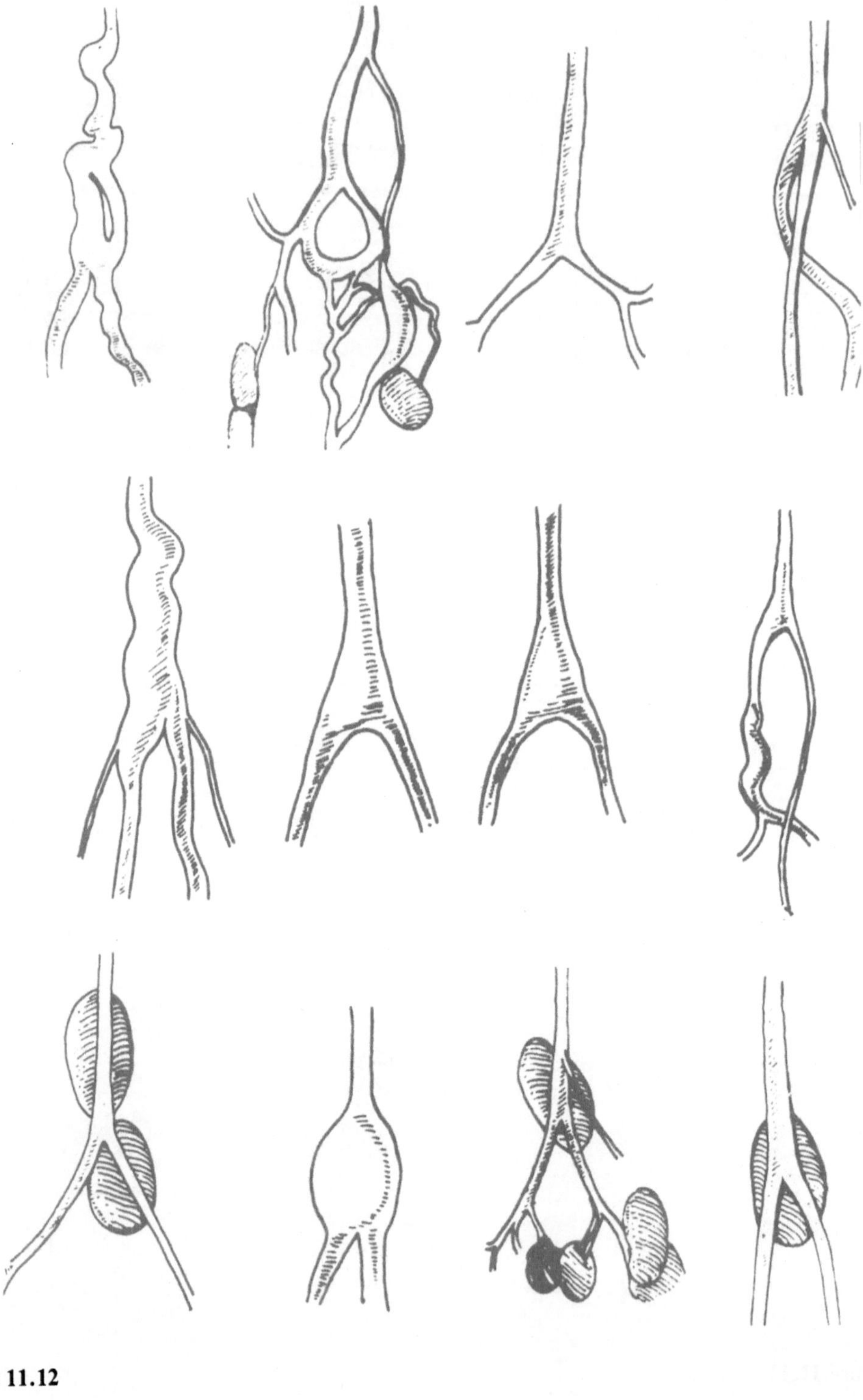

Figure 11.12

On either side of the abdominal aorta the lumbar lymph chain can be easily seen from the level of the renal vein down to the common iliac artery. When dye is injected into the lumbar nodes the entire trunk can be demonstrated. The internal spermatic, or ovarian, vein opens into the left renal vein. Although it varies markedly in diameter, its tributaries usually appear 1-3 cm below the renal vein and those near the mid-line have diameters similar to that of the lumbar trunk. Those tributaries, being near the trunk, are suitable for anastomosis between the lumbar trunk and the renal vein. The valves of the lumbar trunk vary from one to three pairs. They are triangular in shape but may sometimes be saccular or semilunar. Some of the lumbar trunks may have valves with single cusp and occasionally tricuspid valves may be seen. The interval between two valves is 10-15 mm.

Blood supply and nervous innervation of the thoracic duct

Blood supply of the thoracic duct

The arteries supplying the thoracic duct are derived from several sources and are generally 9-11 in number. The cervical segment of the thoracic duct is supplied by one or two branches from the inferior thyroid artery (Figure 11.11), the thoracic segment is often supplied by two (one to four) branches from the intercostal and oesophageal arteries and the abdominal segment by one or two branches from the first right lumbar artery.

Nervous innervation of the thoracic duct

Nerves of the thoracic duct are derived from the sympathetic, vagus and intercostal nerves. As the thoracic duct may be divided into three segments the origins of their nerve supply are correspondingly different. The nerves of the cervical segment are derived from the stellate ganglion, the left sympathetic trunk and the left recurrent laryngeal nerve. The nerves of the thoracic segment come from the greater splanchnic nerve, the aortic and oesophageal plexuses, the right fourth thoracic sympathetic ganglion and the ninth to eleventh intercostal nerves. The abdominal segment is innervated by the greater splanchnic nerve fibres arising from the left eleventh thoracic sympathetic ganglion. All of these fibres are distributed to the wall of the thoracic duct. Thus, in each layer of the wall of the thoracic duct are spread four kinds of nervous plexus.

The superficial plexus of the adventitia

This is composed of fine unmyelinated sympathetic fibres. These enter the wall of the thoracic duct alone or in company with blood vessels to form the plexus of adventitia. In this plexus there are clustered branching neurofibrillar laminae, end bulbs of Krause, Pacinian corpuscles, multipolar cells, small ganglia etc.

The supramuscular plexus

This is composed of a part of the branches of the superficial plexus and many unmyelinated axons. The plexus is distributed in the muscular layer and is connected with receptors in the adventitia.

The intermuscular plexus

The thin nerves of the superficial plexus enter the tunica media to form part of the nerve loops. They advance with or without blood vessels. Many axons are attached to the surface of muscular fibres in the form of a button.

The subendothelial plexus

This is made up of the thinnest fibres which get into the subendothelium and contain clustered or branched receptors.

The systalsis of the thoracic duct is a normal function under the control of the nerves mentioned above. After being isolated from the body for 1–3 hours the thoracic duct still has the spontaneous rhythmic contractibility with a frequency of two to six contractions per minute, and that of an oedematous patient is 6–12 per minute. In childhood the wall of the thoracic duct is more elastic and straight; while in old age it loses its elasticity and becomes curved.

12

The microsurgical anatomy of the middle ear

HAN YONGJIAN, ZHANG KEQU AND ZHANG MING

Otologic microsurgical operation was the first to be carried out and became more popular after the 1950s. The major otologic microsurgical operations performed were stapedectomy, laryngoplasty, the reconstruction of ossicular chain, the fenestration of semicircular canal, the operations of facial nerve, internal acoustic canal, etc. All of these operations are related to the anatomical structures of the middle ear. In this chapter the microsurgical anatomy concerning these operations will be briefly dealt with.

WALLS OF THE TYMPANIC CAVITY

Roof

The roof of the tympanic cavity, known as the tegmen tympani, is the roof of the tympanic cavity proper as well as the antrum. It is formed by the thinner part of the anterior surface of the petrous portion and the neighbouring squamous portion of the temporal bone. The suture between these two portions is called the petrosquamous fissure which does not close before the age of 2. Occasionally it remains open in the adult. This fissure transmits the veins from the middle ear into the superior petrosal sinus and may allow the passage of infection from the tympanic cavity to the middle cranial fossa. Therefore the fissure is one of the infective routes in otogenic intracranial complications.

Floor

The thickness of the floor of the tympanic cavity is inversely proportional to the size of the superior bulb of the internal jugular vein. In the case of small bulb the floor may be as thick as 10 mm and may contain air cells. However, it usually consists of a thin bony plate. It may be congenitally deficient, so that the jugular bulb bulges into the tympanic cavity. It is through neglecting this congenital anomaly during middle-ear operations that profuse bleeding results from injury to the bulb.

Anterior wall

The anterior wall of the tympanic cavity is rather short, being broad above and narrow below. At its upper part there are the canal for the tensor tympani and the opening of the pharyngotympanic tube. The latter faces the aditus to the tympanic antrum on the posterior wall, the level of which corresponds to the junction between the pars flaccida and pars tensa of the tympanic membrane. The lower part of the anterior wall is thinner or even absent. The anterior wall is vertical in position, while the floor slopes forward and downward, so that between them is formed an acute angle which is the hypotympanic recess where inflammatory exudates or secretions may accumulate. The recess corresponds to the cone of light seen on the tympanic membrane.

Lateral wall

The lateral wall of the tympanic cavity is formed mainly by the tympanic membrane, partly by the squamous portion of the temporal bone above the tympanic membrane and the downward part of the tympanic portion. The squamous portion, also known as the tympanic scutum, is the lateral wall of the epitympanic recess, and the tympanic portion separates the tympanic cavity from the medial part of the temporomandibular joint.

Posterior wall

The aditus ad antrum and the incudal fossa, that holds the short process of incus, occupy the upper half of the posterior wall. The features on the lower half are rather complicated, i.e. the styloid, pyramidal and chordal eminences together form the styloid complex and are derived from the cartilage of the second branchial arch. The styloid eminence is situated at the junction between the posterior and inferior walls, being formed by the root of the styloid process projecting into the tympanic cavity. The chordal eminence is situated below the pyramidal eminence and is medial to the tympanic ring. The aperture at the pointed end of the chordal eminence is the opening of the posterior canaliculus for the chorda tympani.

Medial wall

The medial wall features such structures as promontorium, fenestra vestibuli, fenestra cochleae and prominentia canalis facialis. The fenestra vestibuli is situated at the bottom of fossula fenestrae vestibuli and is closed by the foot plate of stapes. The fossula is also called stapes niche, the upper and lower limits of which are the horizontal part of the facial canal and the promontory respectively. Its superoinferior dimension and depth are influenced by the extent of prominence of the horizontal part of the facial canal and of the promontory. If the facial canal overhangs downward, in addition to a prominent

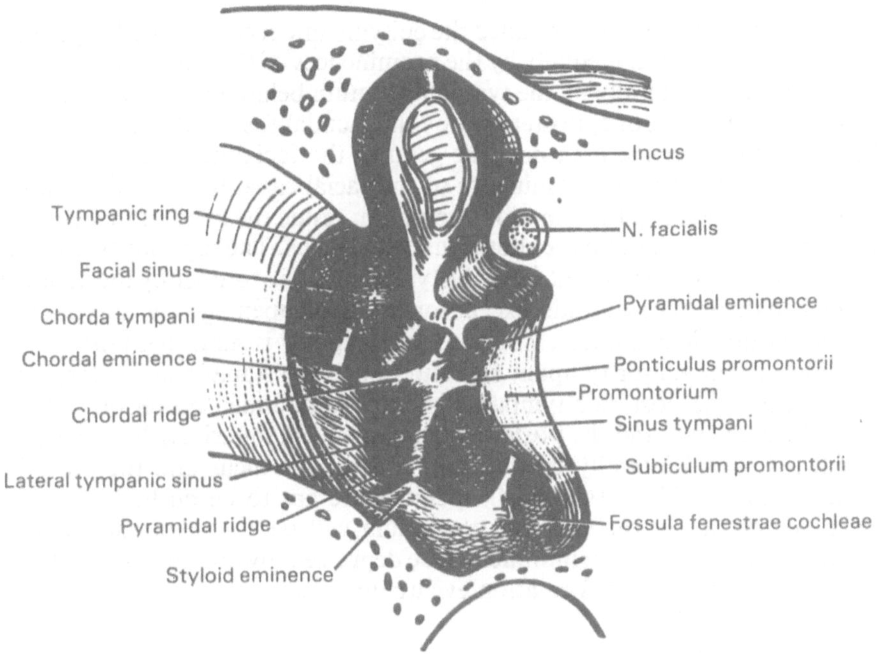

Figure 12.1 Posterior wall of the tympanic cavity

promontory, the inferior wall of the fossula becomes precipitous, so that its superior wall may be hidden deeply above and medial to the horizontal part of the facial canal. Such a deep, narrow fossula is the processus cochleariformis, around which winds the tendon of the tensor tympani, which is one of the important landmarks for identifying the facial nerve.

Posterior to the promontory, there are two constant bony ridges; namely, the subiculum and ponticulus promontorii. The former extends from the upper margin of the fossula fenestrae cochleae to the posterior wall of the tympanic cavity and the latter from the promontory to the pyramidal eminence.

THE TYMPANIC CAVITY

The tympanic cavity which faces the tympanic membrane is the tympanic cavity proper, or mesotympanum. The parts of the tympanic cavity above, below, anterior and posterior to the rim of the tympanic membrane are respectively called the superior, inferior, anterior and posterior tympanum. The depths of the anterior and inferior tympana vary greatly and the depths of the superior and posterior ones are constant and important in clinical practice.

Superior tympanum

The superior tympanum is also called the epitympanic recess, limited superiorly by the tegmen tympani, medially by the prominences of the lateral semicircular and facial canals, laterally by the tympanic scutum belonging to the squamous part of the temporal bone, posteriorly by the incudal fossa, which leads to the aditus, anteriorly by the area near the genu of the facial nerve and inferiorly by a line drawn from the prominence of the facial canal to the lower margin of the incudal fossa. In the superior tympanum reside the head of malleus, the largest part of the body and the short crus of the incus. The superior tympanum is almost completely separated from the tympanic cavity proper by the auditory ossicles and their mucosal folds, except for two small openings, i.e. anterior and posterior tympanic isthmuses. The anterior tympanic isthmus lies posterior to the tendon of the tensor tympani and anterior to the stapes and the long crus of the incus. The posterior tympanic isthmus is bounded posteriorly by the pyramidal eminence and the posterior tympanic wall, anteriorly by the medial incudal folds, and laterally by the short crus of the incus and the posterior incudal ligament. These two small openings are apt to be occluded in otitis media, so that air in the superior tympanum will be absorbed and the pars flaccida of the tympanic membrane will be depressed inward and perforated in due time. Cholesteatoma formation eventually results.

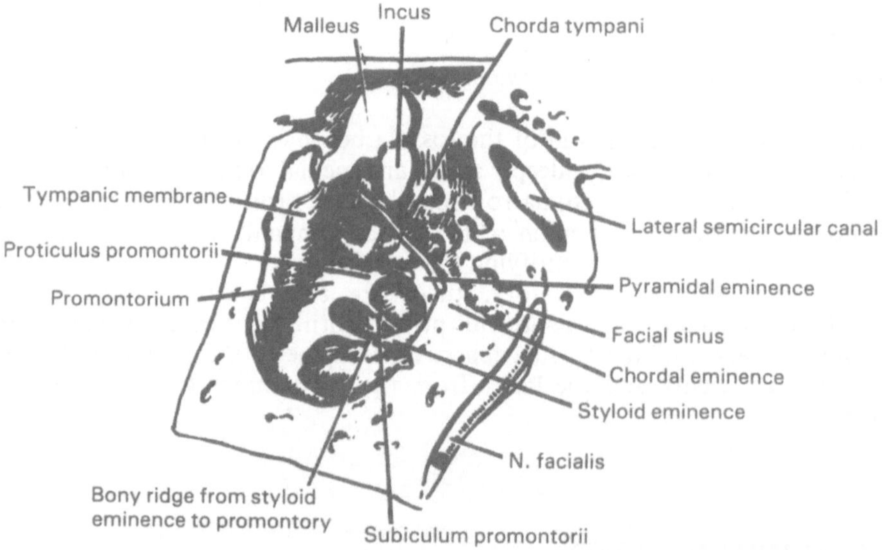

Figure 12.2 An oblique longitudinal section of the middle ear showing the facial sinus

Posterior tympanum

The posterior tympanum is the space left by the backward depression of the posterior wall of the tympanic cavity. It is limited laterally by the medial surface of the posterosuperior part of the tympanic ring, superiorly by the incudal fossa, inferiorly by the styloid eminence and medially by the bony labyrinth. Three bony ridges are related to the eminences of the posterior wall of tympanic cavity, i.e. the styloid ridge between the styloid and chordal eminences, the chordal ridge between the chordal and pyramidal eminences and the pyramidal and styloid eminences. The posterior tympanum is thus divided into four sinuses: tympanic, facial, posterior tympanic and lateral tympanic sinuses by these three ridges with the addition of another two, which arise from the medial to the posterior wall, namely, the subiculum and ponticulus promontorii. The inflammatory granulation or cholesteatoma may be hidden deep within these sinuses and the disease may linger due to incomplete elimination of diseased tissue in these sinuses. Of these, the tympanic and facial sinuses are large and deep-seated.

The tympanic sinus is bounded medially by the promontory, laterally by the pyramidal eminence and the facial canal, anteriorly by the ponticulus promontorii and anteroinferiorly by the subiculum promontorii. Posterolaterally it may extend to the posterior semicircular canal. The volume of the tympanic sinus measured by Papangelou averages 18.2 ml. Wang Ailian and others measured the maximal anteroposterior dimension of the sinus to be 3.0 mm, the maximal superoinferior dimension 2.1 mm and the maximal mediolateral dimension 1.8 mm. They also observed the mouth of the sinus to be occluded by a thin layer of bony plate, on the surface of which are some pits or small holes. The true cavum of the sinus is concealed medial to the plate, often extending backward, and is thus liable to be neglected. The cavum of the sinus can be approached only when the thin plate is removed and the focus of infection can then be eliminated completely.

The facial sinus or recess is more superficial than the tympanic sinus. It lies lateral to the latter sinus, being above the chordal ridge and posterosuperior to the pyramidal eminence. Moreover, it lies lateral to the vertical part of the facial canal, medial to the posterosuperior part of the tympanic ring and below the incudal fossa. It may serve as a guide of approach in posterior tympanotomy. The facial canal is usually situated deep to the medial wall of the facial sinus, but it may rarely reside in the lateral wall or the bottom (posterior wall) of the sinus. In case the facial canal is situated posterolateral to the facial sinus, the facial nerve is subject to injury in posterior tympanotomy. It is commonly thought that the facial nerve will not be damaged unless the facial sinus is exposed. It therefore seems necessary to pay serious attention to the presence of such variation.

THE TYMPANIC ANTRUM AND MASTOID AIR CELLS

The tympanic or mastoid antrum resides in the petrous portion of the temporal bone and its topographical relations claim utmost importance in otologic surgery. It leads forward through the aditus into the epitympanic recess and medial to the aditus is the lateral semicircular canal. Deep to the medial wall of the antrum is the posterior semicircular canal. Posteriorly the antrum is closely related to the sigmoid sinus. The roof of the antrum is the tegmen tympani. On the floor of the antrum are a number of apertures through which it communicates with the mastoid air cells. The lateral wall of the antrum is formed by the squamous portion of the temporal bone, which is very thin, only 2 mm thick, in the neonate. It is 12–15 mm thick in the adult. The lateral wall is the usual surgical route of approach to the middle ear. In the adult it corresponds to the suprameatal triangle. The volume of the antrum at birth has already attained that of the adult, and measures about 1 ml.

The mastoid cells are a group of intercommunicating air-containing compartments in the mastoid process, which lead to the tympanic cavity via the mastoid antrum. They vary considerably in number, size and form in different individuals. According to the degree of pneumatization of the cells the mastoid process can be divided into four varieties: pneumatic, diploetic, sclerotic and mixed types. In the course of development of the temporal bone the cells in its squamous portion may extend over the mastoid process so that they seem to be incorporated into it, but actually they lie superficial to the cells of the petrous portion. Between these two sets of cells a dense bony plate, the septum of Körner, may occasionally exist. If it is encountered in mastoidectomy it may be mistaken for the medial wall of the mastoid cavity so that the cells contained in the petrous portion deep to the septum fail to be opened and the diseased tissues cannot be completely exenterated.

After the mastoid process has been chiselled to exenterate the mastoid cells, a pyramid-shaped cavity is left. Its roof is the tegmen tympani. Its posterior wall is a bony plate separating it from the sigmoid sinus. The medial wall is called the dura plate, which separates the cavity from the dura mater of the posterior cranial fossa. The so-called Trautmann's triangle is a region on the medial wall of the cavity. Attention should be paid to the scraping of diseased mastoid cells and tissues in Trautmann's triangle, because its topographical relations are of great surgical importance. Thus, the superior limit of the triangle is the petrous portion of the temporal bone, keeping it from the superior petrosal sinus; the

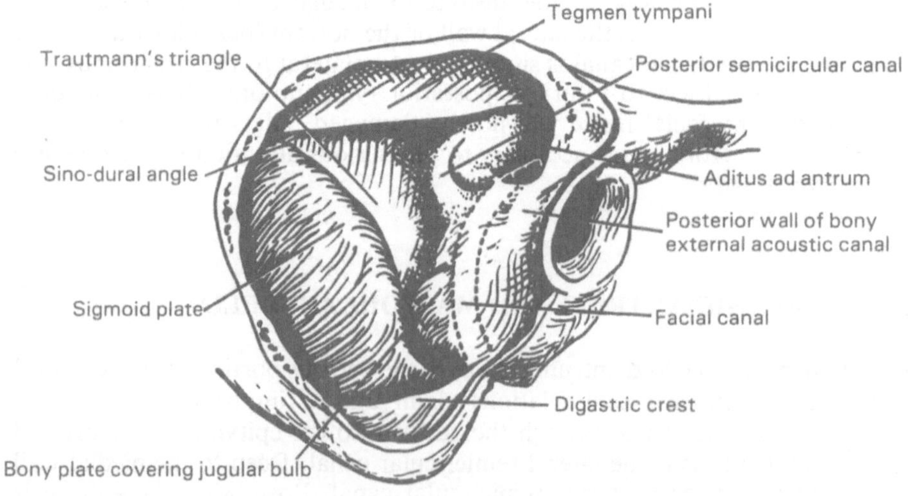

Figure 12.3 Structures seen after chiselling the mastoid process

posterior limit is the sigmoid plate, separating the sigmoid sinus, and the anterior limit is the bony labyrinth, separating it from the posterior semicircular canal. The bony wall anteroinferior to the mastoid cavity is convex, being closely related, from the outside inward, to the bony external acoustic canal, the tympanic ring, the facial sinus and the vertical portion of the facial canal successively. In the apical portion of the mastoid cavity can be seen the digastric ridge, which corresponds to the digastric groove and assumes an arched form bulging into the cavity. It is more distinct in the completely pneumatized mastoid process. The point where the digastric crest meets the bony wall which is anteroinferior to the mastoid cavity indicates the position of the stylo-mastoid foramen. It is due to lack of development of the mastoid process in infancy and childhood that the stylomastoid foramen remains superficial. This makes the facial nerve prone to injury by postauricular incision.

FOLDS AND COMPARTMENTS OF THE TYMPANIC CAVITY

The walls of the tympanic cavity are lined with the mucous membrane which invests the ossicular chain, the tendons of tensor tympani and stapedius, and the chorda tympani, forming the mucosal fold which contains blood vessels and ligaments of the ossicles and divides the tympanic cavity into several compartments. The inflammation in the tympanic cavity may be localized in a certain region or allowed to extend along a definite route according to the disposition of these folds and compartments.

Mucous folds

Mucous folds related to the malleus

(1) The anterior malleolar fold invests the anterior malleolar ligament and the anterior portion of chorda tympani and attaches to the bony surface near the petrotympanic fissure, the neck of malleus and the stria membranatympani anticus.

(2) The posterior malleolar fold attaches between the posteromedial aspect of the upper one-third of the handle of the malleus and the posterior tympanic spine. The posterior part of the chorda tympani is invested in the free border of this fold.

(3) The superior malleolar fold assumes a frontal position between the head of the malleus and the roof of the superior tympanum and invests the superior malleolar ligament.

(4) The lateral malleolar fold fans out superolaterally from the junction of the head and neck of the malleus to be inserted onto the entire rim of the tympanic incisure (notch of Rivinus), forming the roof of Prussak's pouch. It envelops the lateral malleolar ligament.

(5) The tensor tympani fold envelops the tendon of the tensor tympani and the anterior portion of the chorda tympani. It extends laterally from the

semicanal of the tensor tympani to the anterior malleolar ligament and separates the anterior part of the superior tympanum from the tympanic cavity proper.

(6) The interossicular fold is attached between the long crus of the incus and the upper two-thirds of the handle of the malleus.

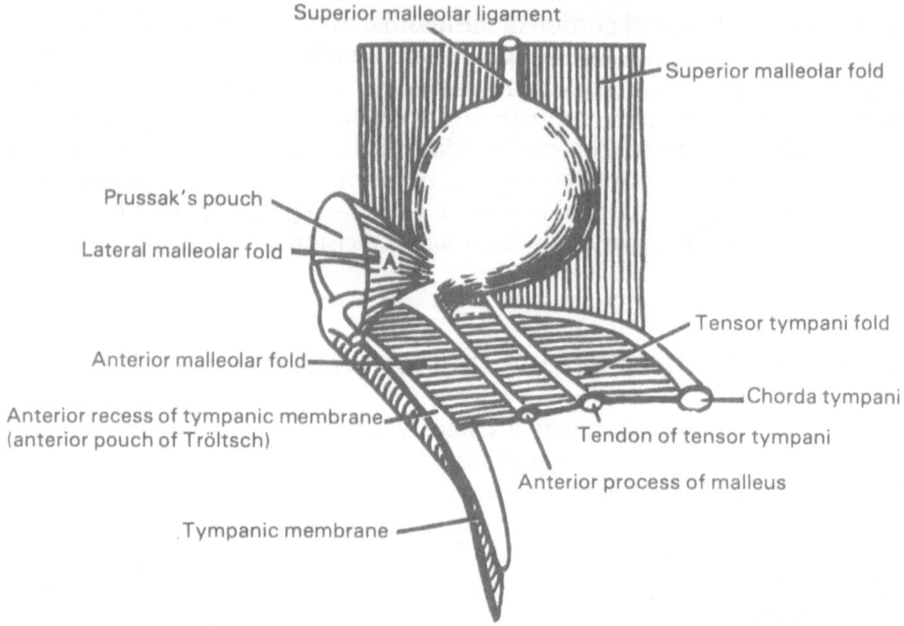

Figure 12.4 Mucosal folds and spaces in relation to the malleus (anterior view)

Mucous folds related to the incus

(1) The lateral incudal fold, extending from the lower margin of the short crus laterally to the lateral wall of the superior tympanus, invests the posterior incudal ligament and separates the superior tympanum from the tympanic cavity proper.

(2) The medial incudal fold is situated between the long and short crura of the incus and the pyramidal eminence. It envelops the tendon of the stapedius, separating the posterior part of the superior tympanum from the tympanic cavity proper.

(3) The superior incudal fold is situated between the body of the incus and the roof of the superior tympanum. It invests the superior incudal ligament.

Mucous folds related to the stapes

(1) The obturator fold closes the obturator foramen.

(2) The anterior stapedial fold is situated between the promontory and the anterior crus of the stapes.

(3) The posterior stapedial fold is situated between the promontory and the posterior crus of the stapes.

(4) The plica stapedis is situated between the pyramidal eminence and the medial border of the tendon of the stapedius, and the posterior crus of the stapes.

(5) The superior stapedial fold arises from the long crus of the incus or the horizontal part of the facial canal to the anterior or posterior crus of the stapes.

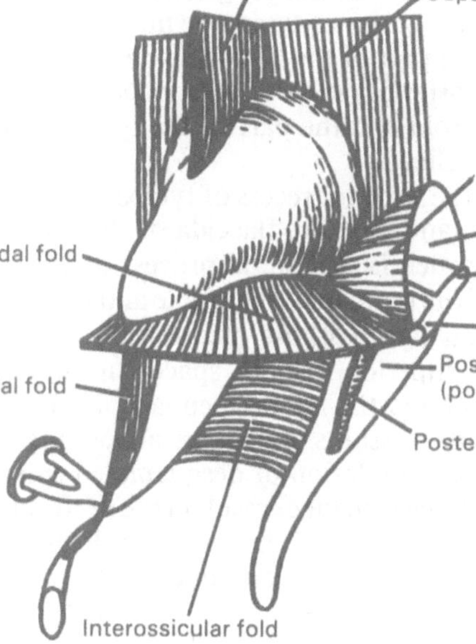

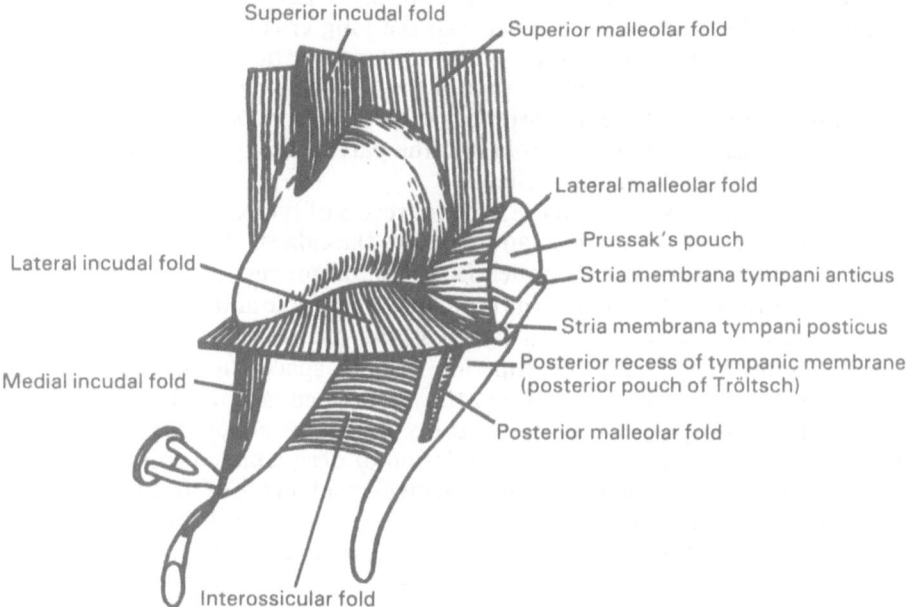

Figure 12.5 Mucosal folds and spaces in relation to the incus and malleus (posterior view)

Compartments

The superior tympanum is divided by the superior malleolar fold into the anterior malleolar compartment (anterior part of the superior tympanum) and the posterior malleolar compartment (posterior part of the superior tympanum). The anterior malleolar compartment is situated anterior to the superior malleolar fold and superior to the tensor tympani fold. It communicates inferiorly with the mesotympanum (tympanic cavity proper) by the anterior tympanic isthmus and posteriorly with the posterior malleolar compartment via the notch of the superior malleolar fold. The posterior malleolar compartment lies posterior to the superior malleolar fold and superior to the lateral incudal, the medial incudal and the lateral malleolar folds, and communicates with mesotympanum by the posterior tympanic isthmus.

The posterior malleolar compartment is further subdivided by the superior incudal fold into the superior incudal space (lateral to the fold) and the medial incudal space (medial to the fold). The superior incudal space leads into Prussak's pouch from between the lateral malleolar fold and the lateral incudal fold.

Beneath the floor of the superior tympanum, i.e. in the upper part of the mesotympanum, there are three compartments: the inferior incudal space, the anterior recess of tympanic membrane (anterior pouch or Tröltsch) and the posterior recess of tympanic membrane (posterior pouch of Tröltsch). The inferior incudal space is limited superiorly by the lateral incudal fold, medially by the medial incudal fold, laterally by the posterior malleolar fold and anteriorly by the interossicular fold which lies between the long crus of the incus and the handle of the malleus. The anterior recess of tympanic membrane lies between the anterior malleolar fold and the part of the tympanic membrane anterior to the handle of the malleus. The posterior recess of the tympanic membrane lies between the posterior malleolar fold and the part of the tympanic membrane posterior to the handle of the malleus.

Prussak's pouch, also called the superior recess of tympanic membrane, lies between the neck of the malleus and the pars flaccida of the tympanic membrane. The floor of Prussak's pouch is the lateral process of the malleus, its lateral wall is the pars flaccida of the tympanic membrane and its roof is formed by the lateral malleolar fold and ligament. As mentioned above, Prussak's pouch communicates with the superior incudal space through the fissure between the lateral malleolar fold and the lateral incudal fold. If this passage is obstructed, absorption of air in Prussak's pouch, retraction of pars flaccida of the tympanic membrane and accumulation of desquamated epithelium will subsequently develop. These prolonged changes result in the perforation of pars flaccida and the intrusion of squamous epithelium into Prussak's pouch. Primary acquired cholesteatoma is the usual consequence.

THE AUDITORY OSSICLES

The three pairs of auditory ossicles are the smallest bones in the human body. They are linked by joints and ligaments to form the ossicular chain so as to connect the tympanic membrane with the fenestra ovalis. Any injury to the ossicular chain will impair sound conduction.

Autologous auditory ossicles are ideal for the reconstruction of the ossicular chain because of the absence of necrosis or absorption of the ossicles or any other rejection phenomena. Based on the results of our study, the following data regarding the dimensions, malformation and variation in the ossicles as well as their blood supply are presented for reference.

Measurements and morphology of the auditory ossicles (Figure 12.6)

Malleus

The malleus is the longest of the auditory ossicles. Its average length is 7.9 mm and average weight 21.7 mg, being next to that of the incus. The facet on the posteromedial aspect of the head of the malleus articulates with that of the incus to form the incudomalleolar joint. The longitudinal depression on the anterior aspect of the head of the malleus is called the anterior fovea, the incidence of which is about 40%. In the remaining cases the anterior aspect of the malleus is smooth. The nutrient foramen is situated at the bottom of the anterior fovea or near the anterior crest of the malleus, which is a longitudinal bony ridge on the neck of the malleus located above the base of the anterior process of the malleus and gives attachment to the anterior malleolar ligament.

Table 12.1 Weight of ossicles (and range) (mg)

Ossicles	*Mean value*			*Standard deviation*			*Standard error*		
	Left	*Right*	*Total*	*Left*	*Right*	*Total*	*Left*	*Right*	*Total*
Malleus (200 cases)	21.6 (15.1–28.4)	21.8 (14.6–28.7)	21.7 (14.6–28.7)	2.9	2.9	2.9	0.3	0.3	0.2
Incus (224 cases)	24.2 (15.0–32.5)	24.3 (15.3–31.2)	24.2 (15.0–32.5)	3.9	3.5	3.9	0.4	0.3	0.3
Stapes (164 cases)	3.0 (1.3–5.2)	3.0 (1.4–5.2)	3.0 (1.3–5.2)	0.8	0.8	0.8	0.3	0.3	0.2

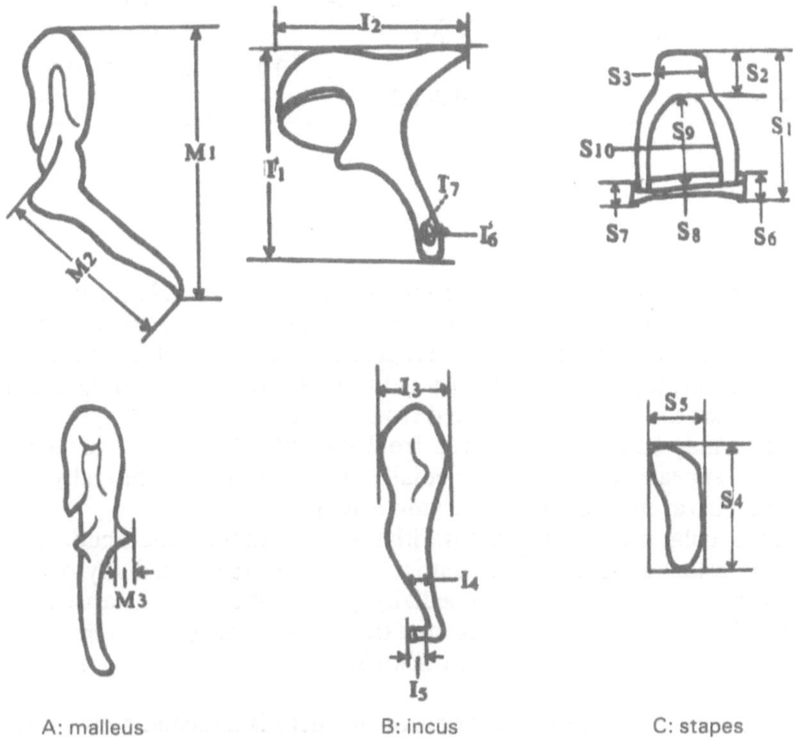

Figure 12.6 Method of measurement of the malleus (A), incus (B) and stapes (C)

The handle of the malleus averages 4.5 mm in length. It usually presents a forward curve in varying degrees when viewed from its lateral or medial aspect. The lateral edge of the handle of the malleus, which adheres to the tympanic membrane, bulges slightly in its middle portion in most cases. Occasionally it is straight or concave in its lower portion. The cross-sectional area of the handle is oval in shape, but its lower end is flattened and bends slightly laterally like a spade, so that it is called the spatula mallei, which corresponds to the umbo of the tympanic membrane (Figure 12.7).

The angle formed by the axis of the head and neck of the malleus with that of the handle averages 131°, ranging from 110° to 145°.

Table 12.2 Length of various parts of the malleus measured in 200 cases (and range) (mm)

	Mean value			*Standard deviation*			*Standard error*		
	Left	*Right*	*Total*	*Left*	*Right*	*Total*	*Left*	*Right*	*Total*
Whole length of malleus (M_1)	7.9 (6.9–8.7)	7.9 (7.0–8.8)	7.9 (6.9–8.8)	0.4	0.4	0.4	0.04	0.04	0.03
Length of handle (M_2)	4.6 (3.2–5.7)	4.6 (3.2–5.7)	4.5 (3.2–5.7)	0.4	0.4	0.4	0.04	0.04	0.03
Length of anterior process (M_3)	0.5 (0.2–1.2)	0.5 (0.2–0.8)	0.5 (0.2–1.2)	0.2	0.2	0.2	0.02	0.02	0.01

Incus

The incus weighs 24.2 mg on average and its body measures 1.9 mm in thickness. The long crus of the incus is well developed in most cases, the breadth measures 0.8 mm at its middle portion on an average. In a few cases (5.4%), it lags behind in development, tapering off toward its lower end with a very small lenticular process. When the long crus is viewed from its medial or lateral aspect it curves forward or may be straight. Viewed from the anterior or posterior aspect its upper part appears to be convex medially and its lower part laterally, so that a sigmoid curvature presents in varying extent.

The lenticular process articulates with the stapes to form the incudostapedial joint. The articular facet on the lenticular process faces medially or superomedially in most cases and inferomedially in 13% of cases. The articular facet is round or oval and its longitudinal and transverse dimensions average 0.6 and 0.5 mm respectively. The height (or thickness) of the lenticular process averages 0.3 mm.

The posterior end of the short crus of the incus is attached by the posterior incudal ligament to the incudal fossa. It is pointed in most cases, but may be round or flat. Sometimes it presents a notch on its lower border.

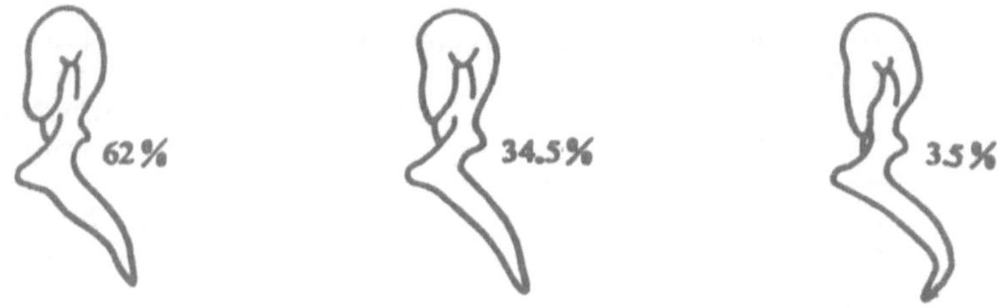

A. Morphological variations of the lateral edge of the handle of the malleus (anterior view)

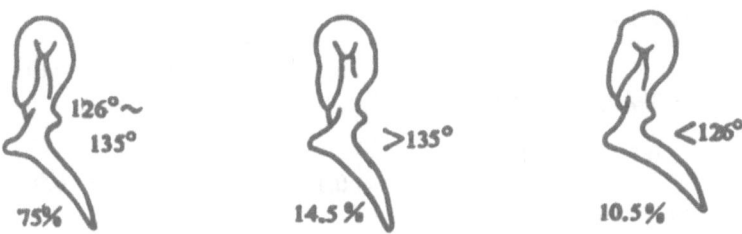

B. The angle formed by the head and neck of the malleus with the handle

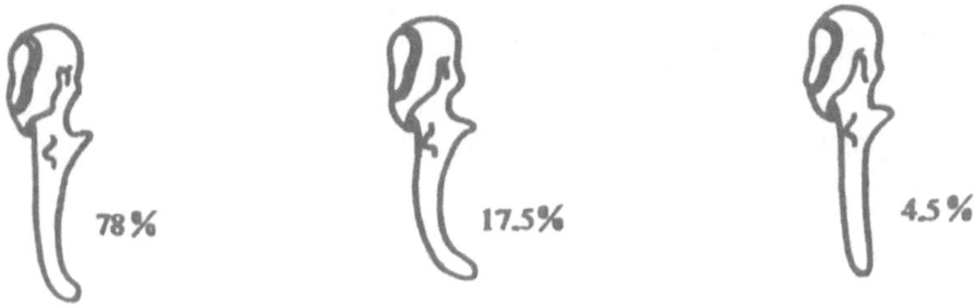

C. The variations of anterior curvature of the handle of the malleus (lateral view)

Figure 12.7 Morphological variations of the malleus

The longitudinal dimension of the incus is the total length of the long crus and the body of the incus and averages 6.8 mm, while the transverse dimension is that of the short crus plus the breadth of the body, averaging 5.0 mm. The angle formed by the tangents along the lower border of the short crus and the posterior border of the long crus averages 109°, ranging from 83–127°.

Stapes

The average length of the stapes is 3.3 mm, being about half of that of the malleus. Its average weight is 3.0 mg, which is one-seventh of that of the malleus or one-eighth of the that of the incus. This is because the periosteal bone over

Table 12.3 Length of various parts of the incus (and range) measured in 224 cases (mm)

	Mean value			*Standard deviation*			*Standard error*		
	Left	*Right*	*Total*	*Left*	*Right*	*Total*	*Left*	*Right*	*Total*
Longitudinal dimension of incus (I_1)	6.8 (5.7–7.7)	6.8 (5.9–7.7)	6.8 (5.7–7.7)	0.3	0.3	0.3	0.03	0.03	0.02
Transverse dimension of incus (I_2)	5.0 (3.9–5.8)	5.0 4.0–5.9)	5.0 3.9–5.9)	0.3	0.3	0.3	0.03	0.03	0.02
Thickness of body of incus (I_3)	1.9 (1.3–2.2)	1.9 (1.3–2.2)	1.9 (1.3–2.2)	0.2	0.2	0.2	0.01	0.01	0.01
Breadth of long crus at its middle point (I_4)	0.8 (0.5–1.0)	0.8 (0.5–1.1)	0.8 (0.5–1.1)	0.1	0.1	0.1	0.01	0.01	0.01
Thickness of lenticular process (I_5)	0.3 (0.2–0.6)	0.3 (0.2–0.6)	0.3 (0.2–0.6)	0.1	0.1	0.1	0.01	0.01	0.01
Transverse dimension of articular facet of lenticular process (I_6)	0.5 (0.1–0.9)	0.5 (0.1–1.0)	0.5 (0.1–1.0)	0.1	0.1	0.1	0.01	0.01	0.01
Longitudinal dimension of articular facet of lenticular process (I_7)	0.6 (0.1–1.0)	0.6 (0.1–0.9)	0.6 (0.1–1.0)	0.2	0.1	0.1	0.01	0.01	0.01

the obturator foramen has been absorbed in the course of development of the stapes, so that the primitive bone marrow becomes opened and the stapes becomes thinner and more fragile.

The head of the stapes faces laterally and articulates with the lenticular process of the incus to form the incudo-stapedial joint. Its neck is somewhat constricted with a transverse dimension of 1.1 mm. Nevertheless, the neck may be thicker than the head. The length of the neck also varies. In 26.8% of cases the neck is very short or even absent.

The thickness and curvature of the crura of the stapes also show much variation. In more than 95% of cases the crura are equal in thickness, or else the anterior crus is thinner than the posterior. A similar condition exists for the curvature of the two crura. According to the degree of bony absorption on the obturator surface of the crura of the stapes, the crura may present a shallow groove or trough-like appearance. If the bone is not absorbed the crura appear to be cylindrical and an infantile type of the stapes eventually occurs in four of 164 cases.

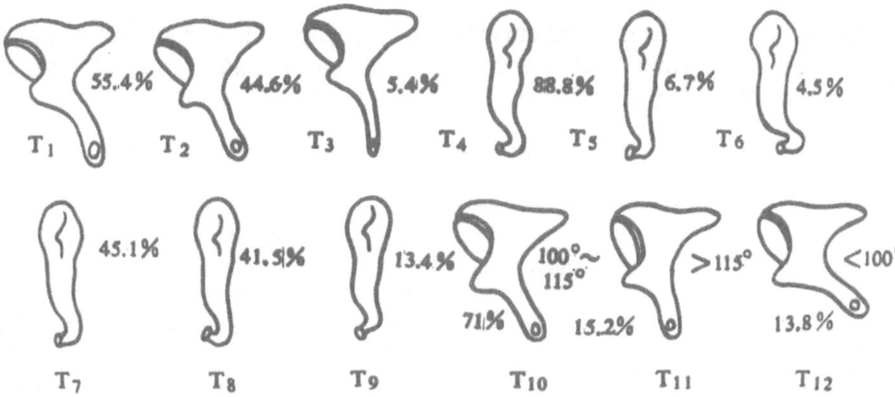

Figure 12.8 Morphological variations of the incus. $\mathbf{T_1}$–$\mathbf{T_2}$: forms of the long crus of the incus; $\mathbf{T_3}$: maldeveloped long crus of the incus; $\mathbf{T_4}$–$\mathbf{T_6}$: variations in the curvature of the long crus of the incus (viewed from the posterior aspect); $\mathbf{T_7}$–$\mathbf{T_9}$: variations in the direction of the facet on the lenticular process; $\mathbf{T_{10}}$–$\mathbf{T_{12}}$: variations in the angle between the long and the short crura of the incus

The longitudinal and transverse dimensions of the foot plate of the stapes average 2.8 and 1.3 mm respectively. The anterior portion of the foot plate is broader than the posterior, its upper border is slightly convex and the middle of the lower border a little concave or somewhat flattened. In consequence the basic form of the foot plate is the sole type, which accounts for 54.9% of cases. The second is known as the semilunar or sausage type in which the anterior and posterior parts of the foot plate are of equal breadth, in 39.6% of cases. In the third type the breadth of the anterior part of the foot plate is less than that of the posterior part, making up only 5.5% of cases.

When the foot plate is transilluminated it is found that its central part is thinner than the periphery, and the posterior margin is thicker than the anterior, the middle of the peripheral part being the thinnest (only 0.2 mm). Those which cannot be fully or basically transilluminated belong to the thick foot plate and account for 30% of cases, while those which can be transilluminated are known as thin foot plates and account for 70% (Figure 12.9).

The obturator foramen is encircled by the crura and the foot plate of the stapes. Its transverse and longitudinal dimensions average 1.6 and 1.7 mm

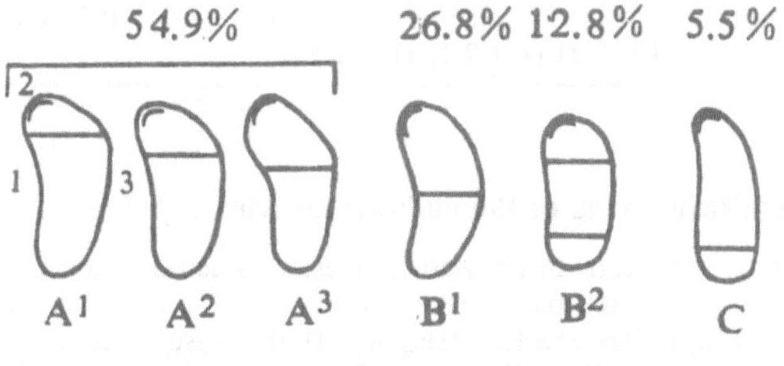

Figure 12.9 Morphological variations of the foot plate of the stapes (right stapes: A and B represent the anterior and posterior parts of the stapes respectively)

respectively. As the length and curvature of the stapes vary to a certain extent the obturator foramen may assume a somewhat triangular, round, ovoid, fusiform or even irregular form.

Table 12.4 Length of various parts of the stapes (and range) measured in 164 cases (mm)

	Mean value			*Standard deviation*			*Standard error*		
	Left	*Right*	*Total*	*Left*	*Right*	*Total*	*Left*	*Right*	*Total*
Total length of stapes (S_1)	3.3 (2.7–3.8)	3.4 (2.8–3.9)	3.3 (2.7–3.9)	0.2	0.3	0.3	0.03	0.03	0.02
Distance from head to upper margin of obturator foramen (S_2)	1.2 (0.7–1.5)	1.2 (0.8–1.4)	1.2 (0.7–1.5)	0.2	0.1	0.1	0.02	0.02	0.01
Transverse dimension of neck (S_3)	1.1 (0.6–1.7)	1.1 (0.8–1.4)	1.1 (0.6–1.7)	0.3	0.2	0.2	0.04	0.02	0.02
Longitudinal dimension of foot plate (S_4)	2.8 (2.4–3.2)	2.8 (2.0–3.4)	2.8 (2.0–3.4)	0.2	0.2	0.2	0.02	0.03	0.02
Transverse dimension of foot plate (S_5)	1.3 (1.1–1.6)	1.4 (1.6–2.5)	1.3 (1.0–2.5)	0.1	0.2	0.2	0.01	0.03	0.01
Thickness of posterior margin of foot plate (S_6)	0.5 (0.3–0.6)	0.5 (0.2–0.7)	0.5 (0.2–0.7)	0.1	0.1	0.1	0.01	0.01	0.01
Thickness of anterior margin of foot plate (S_7)	0.4 (0.2–0.5)	0.4 (0.2–0.5)	0.4 (0.2–0.5)	0.1	0.1	0.1	0.01	0.01	0.01
Thickness of middle portion of margin of foot plate (S_8)	0.2 (0.1–0.3)	0.2 (0.1–0.4)	0.2 (0.1–0.4)	0.1	0.1	0.1	0.01	0.01	0.01
Longitudinal dimension of obturator foramen (S_9)	1.7 (1.0–2.4)	1.7 (1.4–2.2)	1.7 (1.0–2.4)	0.2	0.2	0.2	0.03	0.02	0.02
Transverse dimension of obturator foramen (S_{10})	1.6 (1.0–2.1)	1.5 (1.0–2.1)	1.6 (1.0–2.1)	0.2	0.2	0.2	0.03	0.02	0.02

Congenital malformations of the auditory ossicles

Congenital malformations of the auditory ossicles usually coexist with those of the external ear or other parts of the body. Malformations of the ossicles without other anomalies are less frequent than those mentioned above. The congenital anomaly of the auditory ossicle is one of the aetiological factors of conductive deafness (Figure 12.10).

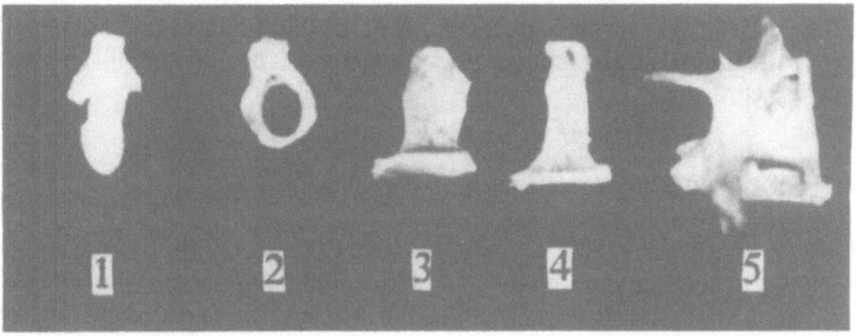

Figure 12.10 Congenital malformations of the auditory ossicles. **1**: Congenital fixation of the footplate of the stapes; **2**: ring form stapes; **3, 4**: columella (monopodal) stapes; **5**: osteoid tissue enclosing the stapes and connecting with the handle of the malleus and the long crus of the incus

Malleus

1. Fusion of the head of the malleus with the body of the incus and the fixation of the incudomalleolar joint.
2. Fixation of the head of the malleus to the tegmen tympani, or fixation of the lateral process of the malleus to the lateral wall of the epitympanic recess.
3. Small short handle of the malleus with inward curvature.

Incus

1. Fixation of the body of the incus to the medial wall of the epitympanic recess.
2. Absence of the body of the incus, only the long crus being present, or vice-versa.
3. The long crus of the incus is small and short or is replaced by fibrous tissue.
4. Absence of lenticular process.

Stapes

1. Congenital fixation of the foot plate of the stapes.
2. Columella (monopodal) stapes.
3. Ring form stapes, in which the anterior and posterior crura are connected at their basal ends but detached from the foot plate, forming a circle.
4. Absence of structures of the upper portion of the stapes (head, neck or a part of crura).
5. Fusion of the handle of the malleus, the long crus of the incus and the head of the stapes.
6. Absence of the stapes.
7. Absence of the oval window.

These malformations may appear singly or in combination, for example, the fusion of the incus and the malleus may coexist with the absence of the crus of the stapes, etc.

Arteries of the auditory ossicles

Arteries of the malleus and incus

The arteries of the malleus and incus mainly come from the anterior tympanic artery, which arises from the internal maxillary artery, passes through the petro-tympanic fissure or its vicinity into the tympanic cavity and divides into the malleolar and incudal arteries, the chorda tympani branch, the superior branch and the posterior branch. These are supplied to the malleus, incus, chorda tympani, the roof and lateral wall of the epitympanic recess (Figure 12.11). The stem common to the malleolar and incudal arteries is termed the ossicular artery or the incudomalleolar nutrient artery.

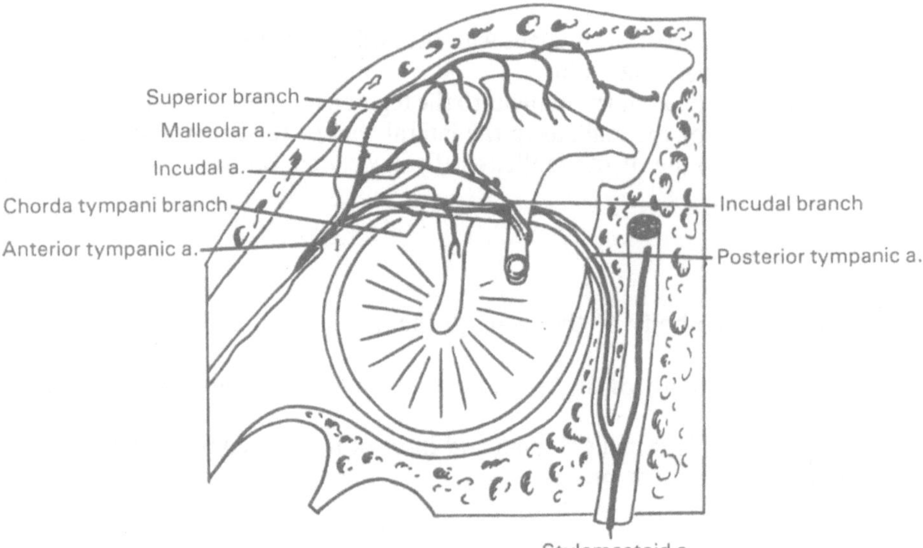

Figure 12.11 Lateral half of the right temporal bone showing the distribution of the branches of the anterior tympanic artery

(1) The malleolar artery passes into the bone through the nutrient foramen just above the base of the anterior process or at the bottom of the anterior fovea of the malleus. Prior to its entrance to the bone the malleolar artery gives off fine branches to the anterior malleolar ligament and the anterior and lateral processes of the malleus (Figure 12.12).

(2) The incudal artery passes medial to the neck of the malleus and inferior to the capsule of the incudomalleolar joint. It then continues from between the long crus of the incus and the handle of the malleus to reach the base of the

long crus, and finally enters the nutrient foramen, which is situated at the anteromedial aspect of the base of the long crus. The incudal artery also gives off fine branches to the inferior aspect of the incudomalleolar joint as well as the long crus of the incus.

(3) The superior branch, after arising from the anterior tympanic artery, courses upward and backward in the mucosa of the roof of the epitympanic recess, part of its course being through the bony substance. It gives off fine branches during its course above the malleus and incus to be distributed, via the superior malleolar and incudal folds, to the head of the malleus, the upper part of the capsule of the incudomalleolar joint, the body of the incus and sometimes the short crus of the incus.

(4) The chorda tympani branch arises from the anterior tympanic artery near the petrotympanic fissure. It accompanies the anterior part of the chorda tympani and gives off fine branches to the medial aspect of the neck of the malleus and its handle. The posterior part of the chorda tympani is supplied by the posterior tympanic artery, a branch of the stylomastoid artery, which also gives off a fine incudal branch to the long crus of the incus when the chorda tympani passes across it. Therefore, excessive traction of the chorda tympani during operation may impair the blood supply of the long crus. The anterior and posterior tympanic arteries form anastomosis along the chorda tympani, which is a component part of vascular anastomosis within the tympanic cavity.

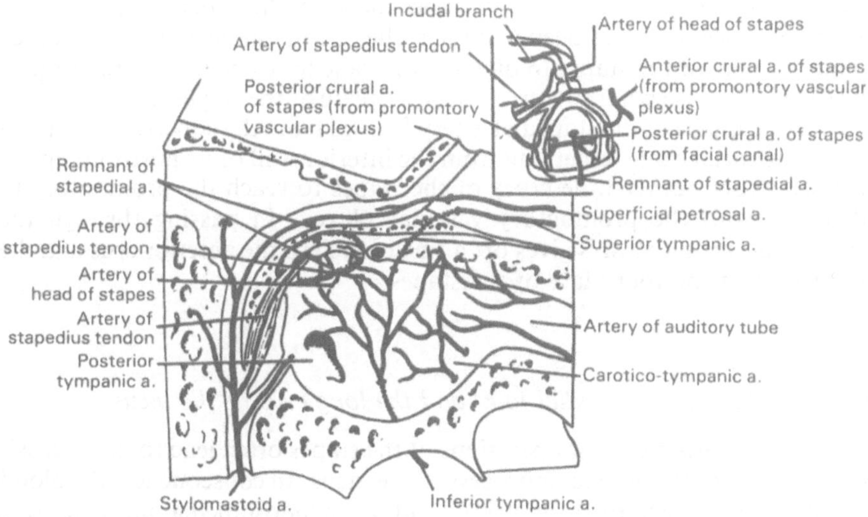

Figure 12.12 Medial half of the right temporal bone showing the distribution and anastomosis of the arteries on the medial wall of the tympanic cavity, the inset showing the arteries of the stapes

Arteries of the stapes

The stapes has no nutrient artery and is supplied mainly by mucosal arteries from various sources.

(1) The artery of stapedius tendon was previously called the stapedial artery, which is synonymous with the embryonic artery and thus leads to much confusion, so that it is advisable to use the present name. It is the largest branch of the stylomastoid artery, generally two in number, arising in the facial canal, passing out of the bony substance at the base of the pyramidal eminence, or above or below it, and then coursing close to the stapedius tendon to the neck and head of the stapes, the incudostapedial joint and the lower part of the long crus of the incus. It anastomoses, near the neck of the stapes, with the anterior and posterior crural arteries and the artery of the head of the stapes.

(2) The artery of the head of the stapes, usually single, arises from the promontory vascular plexus. It passes over the stapes niche and reaches the inferior aspect of the head of the stapes where it anastomoses with other arteries (Figure 12.13).

(3) The posterior crural arteries of the stapes come from two sources: one of them, arising from the superficial petrosal artery, a branch of the middle meningeal artery, emerges from the inferior wall of the horizontal portion of the facial canal to be distributed to the posterior crus and the posterior part of the foot plate of the stapes. The other originates from the promontory vascular plexus, entering the stapes niche to reach the middle portion of the posterior crus of the stapes where it divides into two branches to be distributed respectively to the neck of the stapes and the anterior part of the foot plate of the stapes.

(4) The anterior crural artery of the stapes stems from the anastomotic branch formed anteroinferior to the stapes niche by the superior and inferior tympanic arteries. It passes deeply to the niche, reaching the middle portion of the anterior crus of the stapes to divide into branches to be distributed respectively to the neck and anterior part of the foot plate of the stapes (Figure 12.14).

(5) The remnant of the stapedial artery springs from the superficial petrosal artery in the facial canal, emerging from the inferior wall of its horizontal part, and passes from between the crura of the stapes to reach the promontory to anastomose with the promontory vascular plexus. In passing through the obturator foramen it always gives off a fine branch to the anterior crus and the anterior part of the foot plate of the stapes.

Arteries of the incudostapedial joint and the long crus of the incus

Head trauma, otitis media or operations of the stapes often lead to the necrosis of the long crus or the lenticular process of the incus. In consequence, the blood supply of the lower end of the long crus and the incudostapedial joint has long been emphasized by otologic surgeons. By observing the injected specimen of the arteries it is seen that those supplying the incudostapedial joint are the artery of the stapedius tendon, the artery of the head of the stapes and the anterior and posterior crural arteries. These anastomose freely near the neck of the

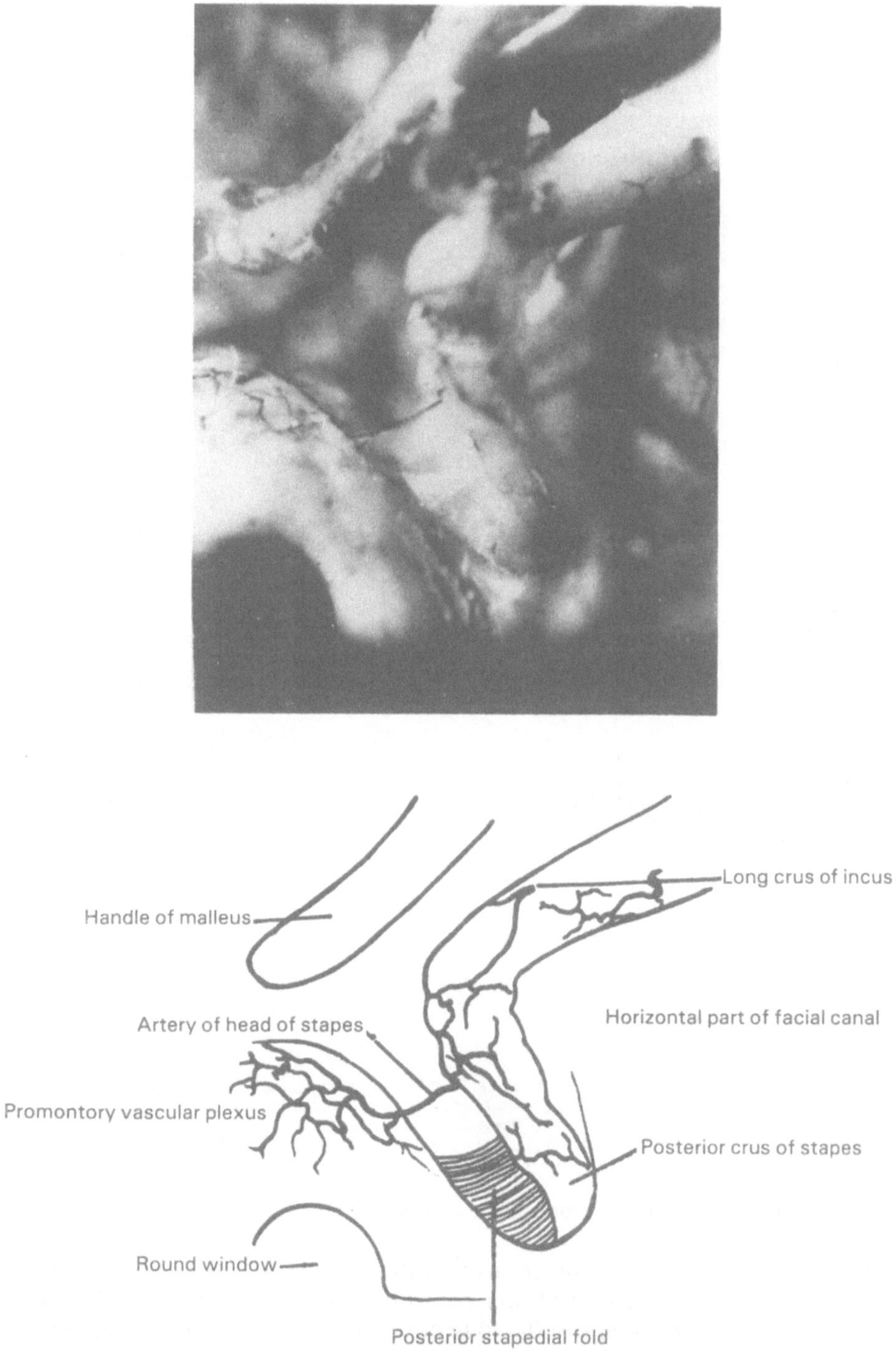

Figure 12.13 Artery of the head of the stapes

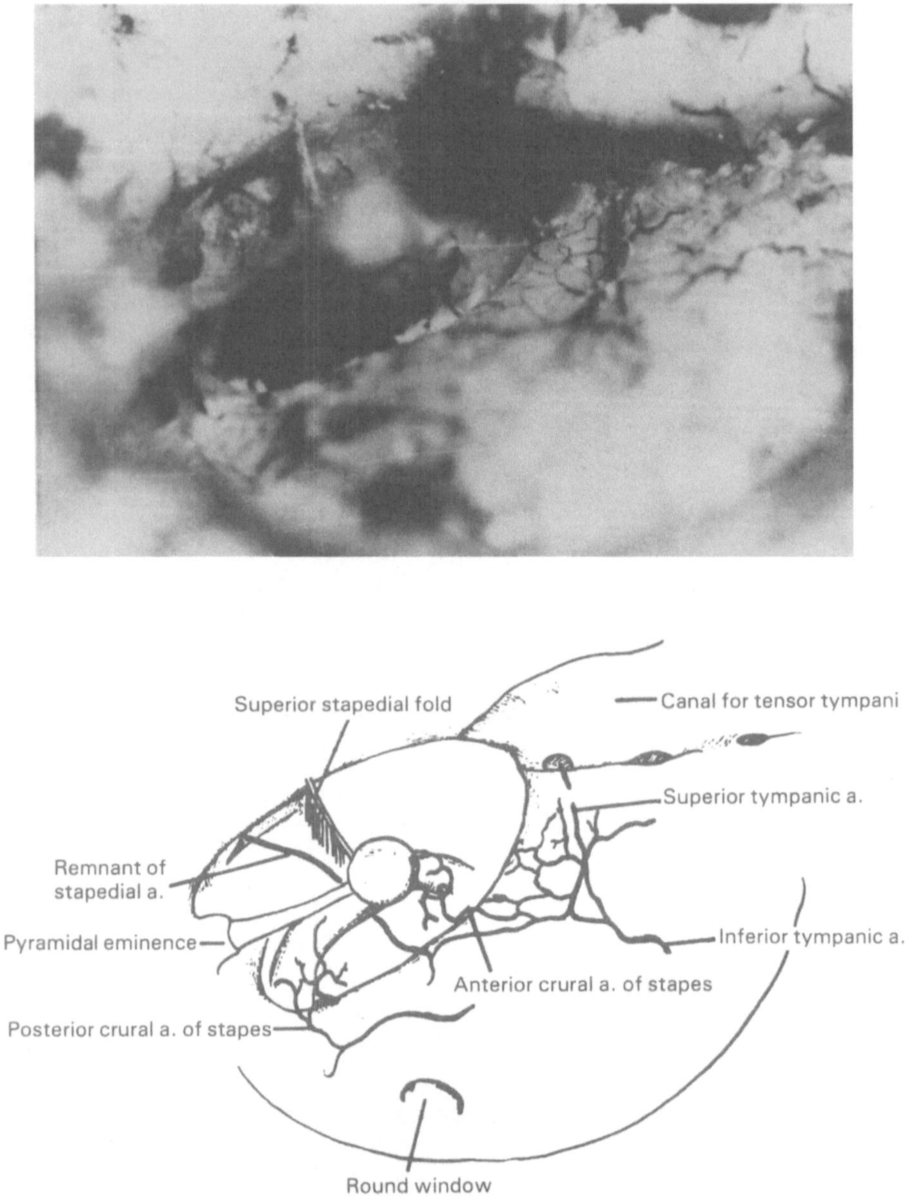

Figure 12.14 Arteries of the crura of the stapes

stapes and are further distributed around the capsule of the incudostapedial joint, continuing upward to the lower end of the long crus of the incus (Figures 12.15 and 12.16). Fine twigs to the long crus given off by the incudal and the posterior tympanic artery have become very minute on reaching the lower end of the long crus of the incus. Based on our observations it has been found that

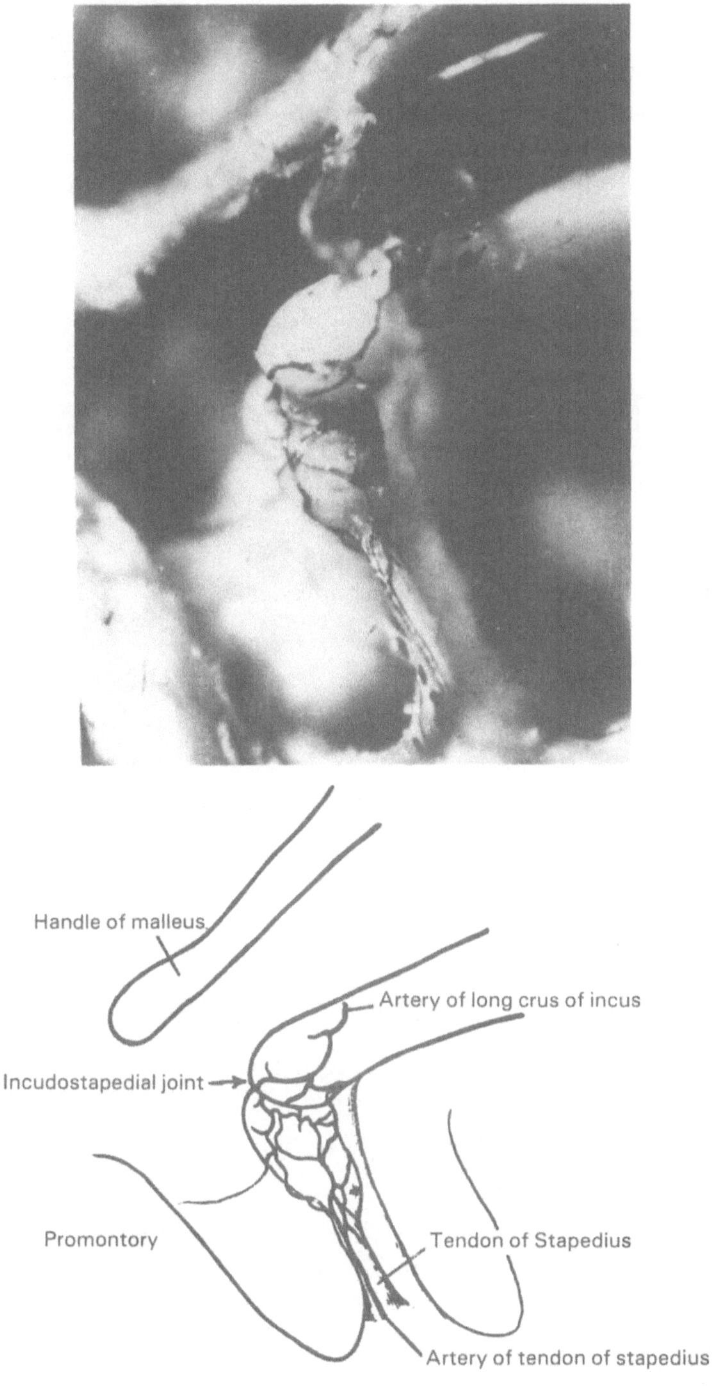

Figure 12.15 Arteries of the incudostapedial joint

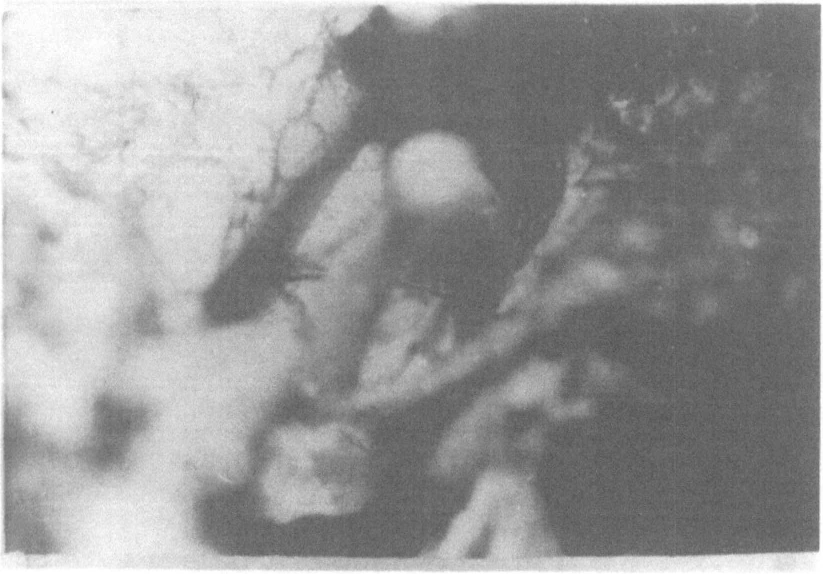

Figure 12.16 Remnant of the stapedial artery.

the incudostapedial joint and the lower end of the long crus of the incus are supplied by the arteries coming from the stapedial side, of which the artery of the stapedius tendon is the largest, which is usually double. Beales maintained that the tendon of the stapedius should be preserved during stapectomy to avoid necrosis of the incus.

Artery of the tympanic cavity

Although the tympanic cavity is a very narrow cleft the arterial supply is very profuse. There are plenty of vascular anastomoses on each wall of the tympanic cavity, particularly rich on the lateral and medial walls. The two nerves, chorda tympani and facial nerve, interposed between the two walls are also the sites of arterial anastomoses in the tympanic cavity. Figure 12.17 shows the sources and anastomoses of the arteries in the tympanic cavity.

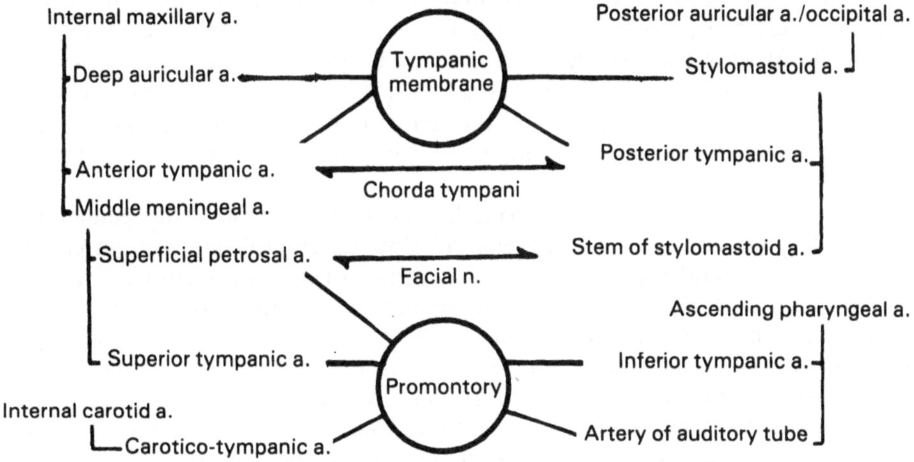

Figure 12.17 Arterial supply and anastomosis of the tympanic cavity

THE FACIAL NERVE

Division and course of the facial nerve

The facial nerve emerges from the brain stem through the lower border of the pons, passes across the cerebellopontine angle, and enters the internal auditory meatus with the statoacoustic nerve. The part of the facial nerve commencing from the brain stem to the internal auditory meatus is called the intracranial segment, about 10 mm in length. In the meatus the motor root of the facial nerve is situated in the concave gutter formed by the statoacoustic nerve facing antero-superiorly. The nervus intermedius is sandwiched between them. The part of the facial nerve from the level of the internal auditory meatus to the bottom of it is called the segment of the internal auditory meatus, about 13 mm in length. The facial nerve passes through the facial nerve area above the transverse (falciform) crest and anterior to the vertical bar (Bill's bar) of the bottom of the internal auditory meatus to the facial canal. It then runs lateralward and somewhat forward over the vestibule and between the cochlea and the semicircular canals to end in the genu of the facial nerve. The part of the facial nerve from the bottom of the internal auditory meatus to the genu of the facial nerve is named the labyrinthine segment; it is only about 4 mm in length and is the shortest and thinnest of the intratemporal facial nerves. Moreover, the facial canal of this segment is also the narrowest. Its diameter is 1.02 mm and that of the nerve is 0.85 mm. The difference between them is only 0.17 mm, so that this segment of the canal has less room for swelling of the facial nerve. At the anterolateral end of the labyrinthine segment the nerve bends backward at angle of 75–80°. The genu of the facial nerve is situated at the site of bending where the motor root of the facial nerve and the nervus intermedius unite to form an expansion, the genu of the facial nerve which holds the geniculate ganglion and gives off the greater superficial petrosal nerve. The geniculate ganglion and the greater superficial petrosal nerve may be separated from the middle cranial fossa by bony substance which, however, may be absent in about 15% of cases. The nerve sheath is then in direct contact with the dura mater. Therefore, care must be taken to avoid injury to the geniculate ganglion and the greater superficial petrosal nerve in the separation of the dura mater of the middle cranial fossa.

The facial nerve runs horizontally backwards from the geniculum immediately above the oval window and below the lateral semicircular canal. It then passes slightly downward and laterally to the fossa incudis. The part of the nerve from the genu to the fossa incudis is called the horizontal or tympanic segment of the facial nerve, and is about 11 mm in length. The diameters of the facial canal and nerve here are 1.53 and 1.12 mm respectively. The difference between them is 0.41 mm. A bony defect, known as the dehiscence of the facial canal, may often be found on the inferior wall of the horizontal segment of the facial canal just above the fenestra vestibuli. Its incidence is about 50%. It is of ovoid shape and its dimensions from 2 × 2 mm to 7 × 7 mm. As the wall of the horizontal segment of the facial canal is the thinnest and the neck of the malleus and the body of the incus lie just lateral to this segment, rupture of it may result from a blow which bumps the ossicles against the bony wall.

Below the lateral semicircular canal the facial nerve descends in the bony substance at the bottom of aditus ad antrum to the back of the pyramidal eminence, and continues downward in the mastoid process of the temporal bone to emerge from the styloid foramen. The part of the facial nerve from below the lateral semicircular canal to the stylomastoid foramen is named the vertical or mastoid segment, and is about 16 mm in length. The diameter of the corresponding segment of the facial canal is 1.48 mm and that of the facial nerve is 0.94 mm, the difference between them being 0.54 mm. The curved transitional part between the horizontal and vertical segments of the facial nerve is termed the pyramidal segment, which is more prone to damage in mastoid operation. The vertical segment inclines gradually from the front backward, so that it is nearer to the fenestra vestibuli than the round window. The vertical segment, viewed from the coronal plane, inclines gradually laterally, so that its lower part is more superficial and inclines slightly backward.

The lengths of the horizontal and vertical segments are 11 mm and 16 mm respectively, totalling 27 mm. The straight distance from the stylomastoid foramen through the medial wall of the tympanic cavity to the geniculate ganglion is 22 mm; therefore when the defected portion of the facial nerve is less than 3 mm the facial nerve may be removed from the facial canal, so that rerouting suture of the intratemporal facial nerve may be performed via the medial tympanic wall. The total distance from the geniculate ganglion through the stylomastoid foramen to the posterior border of the parotid gland is 61 mm, while the straight distance between the posterior border of the parotid gland and the geniculate ganglion is 44 mm. The latter can be further shortened by 6 mm by means of shifting upward the trunk of the facial nerve from the parotid gland. Thus the total length which can be shortened is 23 mm. When the defected portion of the facial nerve is from 15 to 20 mm the nerve can be sutured by the reroute method, i.e. it can be shifted from the geniculate ganglion via the medial toward the anterior tympanic wall, whence the nerve marks its exit. The above data serve as the anatomical basis for the extra- and intratemporal facial nerve rerouting suture.

Arteries of the facial nerve and its sheath

The arteries supplying various parts of the facial nerve are the anterior inferior cerebellar artery for the intracranial segments, the internal auditory (labyrinthine) artery for the segment of the auditory meatus, the superficial petrosal artery for the geniculate ganglion, and the superficial petrosal and the stylomastoid artery for the horizontal and vertical segments respectively. The latter two arteries anastomose with each other in the facial canal.

The sheath of the facial nerve is composed of the periosteum, the vascular layer (the arteries and venous plexus of the facial nerve) and the epineurium. At the fundus of the internal auditory meatus the sheath blends with the dura mater, while at the stylomastoid foramen it fuses with the adjacent fascia covering the posterior belly of the digastric muscle. The sheath is tough and shiny and is a valuable barrier against surgical trauma and infection. In the decompression operation of the facial nerve the sheath has to be incised so as to relieve the pressure and allow the expansion of oedematous contents.

Congenital anomalies of the facial nerve

It was held that congenital anomalies of the facial nerve were rarely seen. Nevertheless, current otological experience shows that an anomalous course of the facial nerve may exist in at least one-third of cases (Crabtree, 1974), especially in those patients with congenital malformations of the external or middle ear. The most frequently seen anomaly of the facial nerve is the overhang and anteroinferior displacement of its horizontal segment, which may protrude from the defect of the facial canal, or may lack the protection of the bony canal so as to be barely exposed in the tympanic cavity. The horizontal segment of the facial nerve may be divided into two branches passing above and below the stapes and enclosing it. The extremely displaced facial nerve may run across the promontory below the fenestra vestibuli. The pyramidal segment of the facial nerve may be humped or acutely angled so that it lies more superficially and posterior to the tympanic ring. The vertical segment may occasionally be divided into two branches, each of which occupies one bony canal. In short, the anomalous facial nerves mentioned above are vulnerable to damage during operation.

Localization of the intratemporal facial nerve

With the help of modern microsurgical techniques on the basis of constant landmarks of the facial nerve, any portion of the facial nerve may be approached.

Vertical segment of the facial nerve

This segment can be sought for by the following landmarks:

1. The relation between the facial nerve and the lateral semicircular canal can be used for this purpose. The former is situated below the latter. The distance between them averages 1.8 (1.0–2.3) mm.
2. The fossa incudis which holds the short crus of the incus is situated at the bottom of the aditus ad antrum and lies lateral to the junction of the horizontal and vertical segments of the facial nerve. The fossa incudis is an important landmark for operation on the middle ear. The shortest distance from the short crus of the incus to the facial nerve averages 2.4 (1.4–3.0) mm.
3. The junction of the digastric crest and the bony external auditory meatus marks the site of the stylomastoid foramen.

A line drawn from the prominence of the lateral semicircular canal to the anterior end of the digastric crest indicates the course of the vertical segment of the facial nerve.

Horizontal segment of the facial nerve

The landmarks for identifying the horizontal segment of the facial nerve are the processus cochleariformis, the fenestra vestibuli and the prominence of the lateral semicircular canal. The anterior end of this segment is situated just behind and very close to the processus cochleariformis. Posteriorly it is below the prominence of the lateral semicircular canal and above the pyramidal eminence.

Segment of the internal auditory meatus

In order to look for the segment of the internal auditory meatus in the middle cranial fossa, one should first search for the greater superficial petrosal nerve at the hiatus of the facial nerve canal, and then follow the nerve back to the geniculate ganglion, from which the tympanic cavity may be approached laterally and the labyrinthine segment medially. The landmarks for the segment of the facial nerve in the internal auditory meatus are the superior branch of the vestibular nerve and the vertical crest at the fundus of the internal auditory meatus. Having opened the mastoid cavity the lateral semicircular canal can be found. The exit of the superior branch of the vestibular nerve may be approached by eliminating the semicircular canals. Tracing the superior branch of the vestibular nerve, the vertical crest between the facial and vestibular nerves can be seen at the base of the internal auditory meatus and the facial nerve eventually identified.

13

The microsurgical anatomy of the transplantation of small organs

ZHANG WEILONG AND ZHENG ZHILIANG

INTRODUCTION

The history of the development of organ transplantation shows that the transplantation of some large organs had been successively reported from the fifties to the early part of the sixties of the present century. Of these, renal transplantation was the earliest and the most frequently done. In 1954 Murray first succeeded in clinical renal transplantation. The first case of the transplantation of liver was performed by Starzl in 1963. Barnard began transplantation of the heart in 1967. The transplantation of small organs was closely related to the microsurgical technique, and relevant reports increased gradually until the late sixties to the seventies of the present century. In hetero-transplantation the chief handicap is the rejection reaction, which is still far from being solved in spite of much progress gained recently. Once this is perfectly solved it will certainly begin a new era in which mankind will be endowed with enough means to combat disease.

Transplantation of small organs has been performed with microsurgical technique, since gross anatomical methods cannot meet the requirements. This chapter is a survey of information on the microsurgical anatomy of small organs. Though the kidney is one of the large organs, its nerves and segmental arteries are very delicate and require precise technique. In recent years infant kidney has been successfully used as a type of donor and a new scheme of supply of infant kidneys will be commenced soon. This chapter will deal with more microsurgical technique about the kidney, so that anatomical data concerning renal transplantation have also been here.

RENAL TRANSPLANTATION IN THE ADULT

ZHANG WEILONG AND ZHENG ZHILIANG

Renal graft is the most successful organ transplantation. Since Merrill and Murray (1954) first succeeded in performing a renal transplantation between uniovular twins, who survived for a long period, heterotransplantation, along with study of problems of rejection, has made much progress in China and abroad. After more than 20 years of experimentation both in animal and clinical practice, surgical techniques for renal transplantation have been perfected. Standardization has been followed regarding the choice of donor kidney, the site of transplantation, the method of vascular anastomosis and the management of the ureter. Renal transplantation at present is generally performed by an end-to-end anastomosis between the renal and internal iliac arteries, an end-to-side anastomosis between the renal and external iliac veins, and a ureteroureteral or ureterovesical anastomosis. The left kidney of the donor can be transplanted to the right iliac fossa of the donee, or the right kidney of the donor to the left iliac fossa of the donee. If necessary the kidney may be transplanted to the ipsilateral iliac fossa. When a child receives a kidney from an adult donor, as the iliac vessels of the child are relatively slender and the iliac fossa is too small to hold the adult kidney, an end-to-side anastomosis between the renal vein and the inferior vena cava (or the common iliac vein), an end-to-side anastomosis between the renal artery and the abdominal aorta (or the common iliac artery), and a ureteroureteral anastomosis or ureterovesical anastomosis are often performed.

Correct and skilful surgical manoeuvre is the key to successful renal transplantation in its early stage, and a thorough knowledge of the applied anatomy of structures such as the renal pedicle, the blood supply of the ureter and the iliac vessels is also indispensable for a successful operation. It will help surgeons remove the donor kidney and expose the iliac vessels successfully, select a suitable site for anastomosis, save on operating time, and reduce the complications of haemorrhage, lymphatic cyst, and urinary fistula.

Renal pedicle

The structures within the hilum of the kidney are the renal artery and vein, the renal pelvis and the lymphatic vessels and nerves, which collectively form the renal pedicle.

Renal artery

The renal artery, usually single (in about 85.8% of cases), arises from the abdominal aorta at the level of the intervertebral disc between the first and second lumbar vertebra. It passes laterally to enter the hilum of the kidney. The two-branched type represents 12.5%; the three-branched type 1.5%. Four- and five-branched types are very rare, each representing 0.1%. The incidence of the multi-branched type is nearly equal on either side. The origin of the accessory renal artery from the abdominal aorta varies between the upper margin of the first lumbar vertebra and that of the third, but is usually lower than that of the renal artery. In rare cases the accessory renal artery may be seen arising from the inferior phrenic artery, the gonadal artery, the bifurcation of the common iliac artery, the lumbar artery, the superior mesenteric artery or the inferior mesenteric artery. In taking the donor kidney the accessory renal artery arising from the aorta is easily identified, but those with rare origins may be neglected.

Careful inspection is therefore needed, so that once the accessory artery is present it must be dissected carefully for transplant. Inadvertent ligation of the artery will result in ischaemia of the renal segment and subsequent necrosis.

The renal artery usually divides into an anterior and a posterior branch or a superior and an inferior one. The length of renal artery averages 2.6 cm on the left and 3.5 cm on the right. Since the accessory renal artery may arise from the stem of the renal artery or its branches, the donor renal pedicle should be kept as long as possible to avoid injury to the potential accessory renal artery. The outer diameter (near its origin) of the renal artery averages 0.8 mm, and that of the abdominal aorta is about 2.7 times that of the renal artery.

Renal vein

The single-branched type is the most common of the renal vein and occurs in 88% of cases. The two-branched type occurs in 11% and the three-branched type in 1% of cases. The four-branched type is very rare, representing only 0.1%. The multi-branched type is usually present on the right side, thus having a marked difference in respect to sides. The renal vein of the single-branched type empties into the inferior vena cava at any level between the middle of the twelfth thoracic vertebra and the lower part of the second lumbar vertebra, but more frequently it ends at the level of the middle part of the first lumbar vertebra on the right side and of the upper part of the first lumbar vertebra on the left. The position of the left renal vein and the level of its termination into the inferior vena cava are usually higher than those of the right vein.

Separate polar veins are rare (5%). Most of them come from the upper extremity of the kidney and drain into the renal vein or its tributaries, except for a few which empty into the lumbar vein. Care must be taken to avoid injury to the vein in taking the donor kidney.

The length of the renal vein from the confluence of its tributaries to its termination into the inferior vena cava averages 6.5 cm on the left and 2.8 cm on the right. The left one is about 2.3 times longer than the right. Because the right renal vein is short and sometimes in duplicate, excision of the right kidney is more complicated. The outer diameter of the renal vein, measured while being pressed at its termination into the inferior vena cava, averages 15 (11–22) mm on the left, and 13 (10–16) mm on the right. That the left renal vein is wider than the right one is due to the fact that the former possesses more tributaries and a greater amount of blood flow and requires a longer course for draining into the inferior vena cava.

The left suprarenal and internal spermatic veins are tributaries of the left renal vein, but those of the right side are tributaries of the inferior vena cava. Only 10% of the internal spermatic veins empty into the right renal vein. The renal vein also anastomoses with the lumbar vein (63% on the left side and fewer on the right). In rare cases (1.5%) the left renal vein may have a superior and an inferior division to form a circumaortic venous ring around the abdominal aorta or may lie all behind it (Figure 13.1), so that in taking the donor kidney, especially on the left side, these tributaries and anastomosing branches must be dissected and ligated carefully, and variations of the renal vein noted.

It should be indicated that in about 20% of cases the gonadal arteries may arise from the abdominal aorta above the origin of the renal veins and descend just anterior to them. When the gonadal arteries arise below the origin of the renal veins they ascend behind the latter and then round the upper margin of the veins to descend in front of them. In taking the kidney from the donor the gonadal arteries must be protected from inadvertent injury or ligation (Figure 13.2).

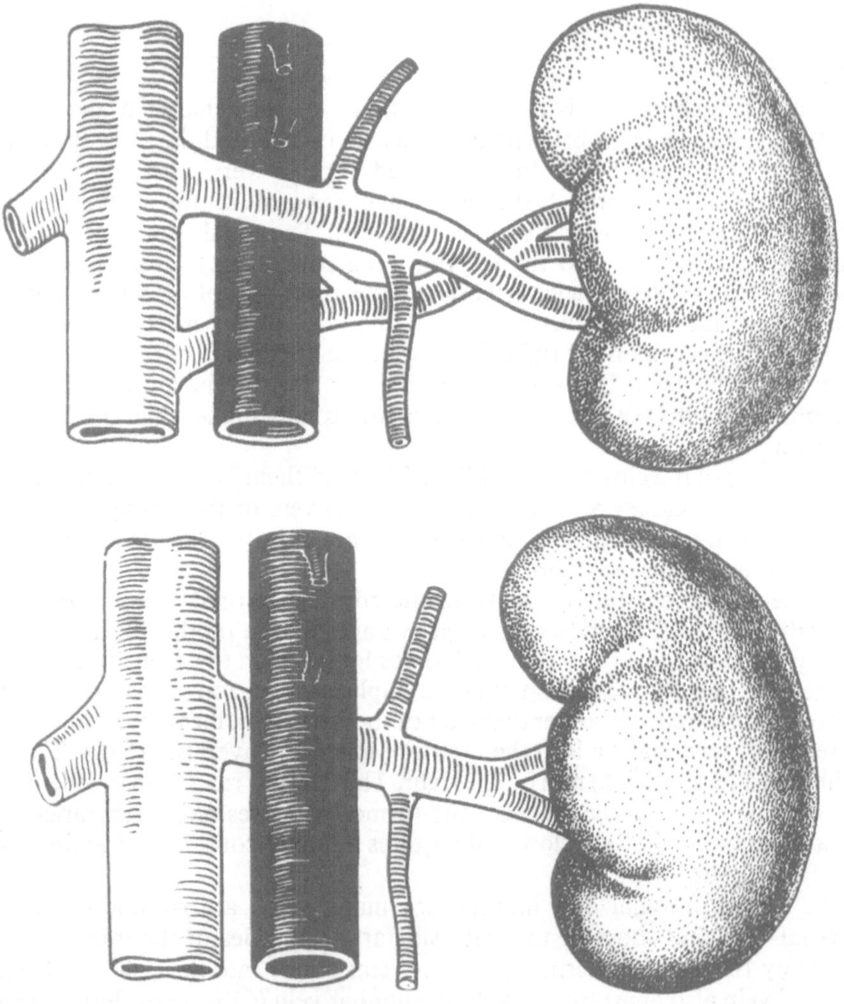

Figure 13.1 Variations of the renal vein. **A**: Circumaortic venous ring; **B**: retroaortic renal vein

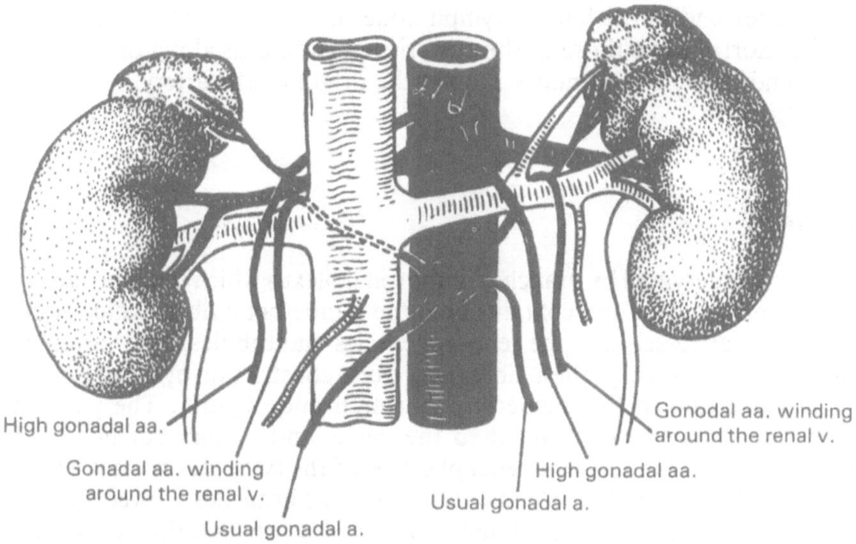

Figure 13.2 Gonadal arteries winding the renal vein

Relation between the components of the renal pedicle

In the medial part of the pedicle the renal vein is always in front of the artery, while in the lateral part variations in the renal vessels are common so that their topographical relationships vary accordingly. Three types may be recognized. In the first type (61%) the renal vein and artery and the pelvis are arranged in order from front backwards; in the second type (24%), the anteroposterior order is the artery, the vein and the pelvis; other types are uncommon, amounting to 15%.

The height of a normal renal pedicle is 2–2.5 cm. If an accessory renal artery arising from the abdominal aorta is present, the height of the pedicle may increase by one-third, rarely by two-thirds, of the height of the vertebral body in about four-fifths of cases. These are unfavourable for the ligation of the renal pedicle in nephrectomy.

Lymphatics of the kidney

The lymphatics of the kidney comprise two groups. The superficial group drains the renal capsule, and connects with the deep group at the hilum. The deep group winds round the renal tubules and drains the parenchyma of the organ. The lymphatics of the anterior portion of the right kidney course along the anterior aspect of the renal vein, crossing the inferior vena cava, and end in the lumbar lymph nodes between the abdominal aorta and the inferior vena cava or in front of the abdominal aorta. The lymphatics of the posterior portion pass along the right renal artery transversely or obliquely to end in the lumbar nodes behind the inferior vena cava. The lymphatics of the anterior portion of the left kidney end in the lumbar lymph nodes in front and to the left of the abdominal aorta, while those of the posterior portion pass along the left renal artery to end in the lymph nodes around the origin of the artery.

Nerves of the kidney

The kidney is innervated by branches of the renal plexus which is mainly derived from the coeliac plexus and contains both the sympathetic fibres which supply mainly the renal vessels and the renal corpuscles and tubules. It is vasomotor in function. Stimulation of these fibres may cause constriction of the vessels and result in a decrease in the glomerular filtration and oliguria. The parasympathetic fibres may be distributed to the pelvis and ureter, but not to the parenchyma of the kidney. The renal plexuses of the two sides are not entirely symmetrical, but are similar in constitution, i.e. the branches derived from the coeliac plexus are at first located above the renal artery and then collect into two to four thick nerves near the kidney to anastomose with other renal rami from the splanchnic nerves and the aortic plexus to form a reticular plexus around the renal artery to be distributed with its branches. There are no thick nerves either in front of the renal vein or behind the renal pelvis. The renal plexus and its branches surrounding the renal artery may be well recognized after careful dissection (Figure 13.3).

At present all of the nerves to the kidney have to be cut in renal transplantation. According to the regulation of renal vessels by the renal plexus it is

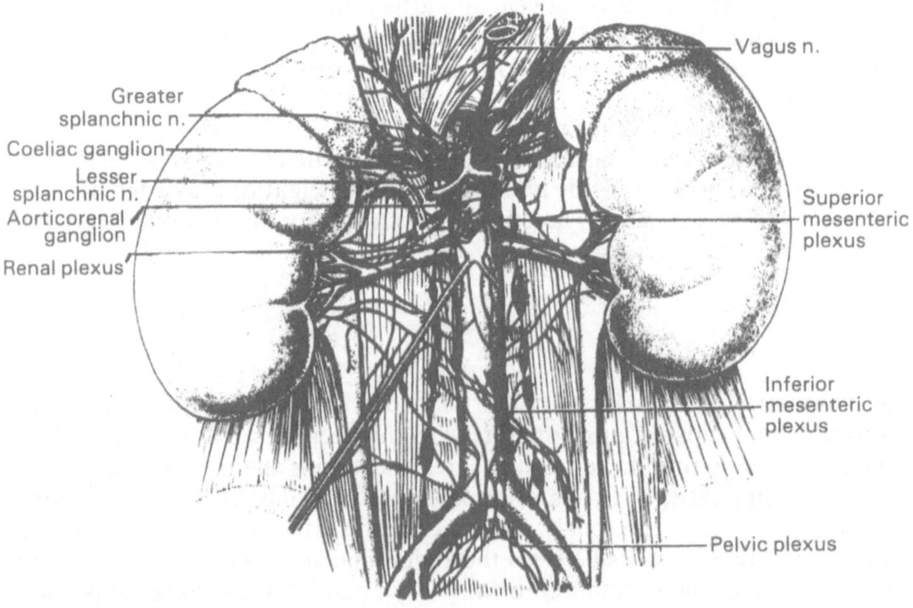

Figure 13.3 Renal plexus

conceivable that in renal transplantation, in addition to the anastomosis of vessels, suturing of the severed nerves may contribute to the recovery and maintenance of the normal function of the donor kidney.

Blood supply of the ureter

The arteries of the ureter are usually four or five in number on either side. The artery of its upper part arises from the renal artery, that of the middle part from the abdominal aorta or the testicular (or ovarian) artery, and that of the lower part from the inferior vesical (or uterine) artery. The diameters of these arteries are relatively small (Figure 13.4). Each of these arteries divides into an ascending and a descending branch in the connective tissue around the ureter, and anastomoses with adjacent similar branches. Secondary branches are given off to the wall of the ureter. These anastomose with one another to form a meshwork around the ureter, from which arise the tertiary branches to supply the muscular layer and the mucous membrane. Owing to the above characteristics of the blood supply of the ureter, the adipose tissue over the hilum of the kidney and the connective tissue around the ureter must be protected carefully during the removal of the donor kidney to avoid injury to these arteries. The blood supply of the lower part of the ureter of the donee must also be carefully guarded in ureteroureteral anastomosis, that is, the free segment of the ureter should be made as short as possible and it is not necessary to strip off the ureter from the extraperitoneal tissue.

Iliac vessels

Common iliac artery

The common iliac artery usually arises from the abdominal aorta on the left side of the body of the fourth lumbar vertebra. It passes downwards and laterally, and divides at the level of the fifth lumbar vertebra or the lumbosacral intervertebral disc (88%) into the external and internal iliac arteries. The length of the common iliac artery averages 4.8 (2.3–8.3) cm on the left, and 4.4 (1.9–7.8) cm on the right. Its outer diameter just above the bifurcation averages 11.8 (7.0–19.5) mm on the left, and 12.4 (7.0–18.0) mm on the right. The bifurcation of the common iliac artery may be found as high as the upper part of the fourth lumbar vertebra, or as low as the lower part of the first sacral vertebra. The points of bifurcation of both sides are not at the same level in 63% of cases. Those in which the left point is lower than the right amount to 51%, while the reverse occurs in 12%. The level of the bifurcation of the common iliac artery bears a close relation to its length, as well as that of the internal iliac artery. Since the site of bifurcation of the left common iliac artery is lower, the left common iliac artery is longer, while the left internal iliac artery becomes shorter. The point of bifurcation of the right common iliac artery is higher, so that the right common iliac artery becomes shorter and the right internal iliac artery longer.

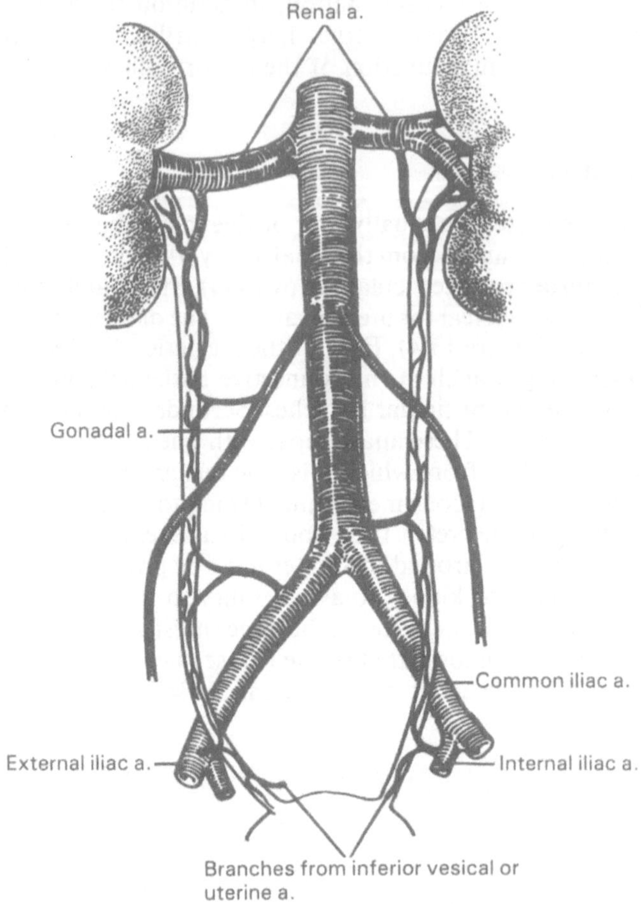

Figure 13.4 Blood supply of the ureter

Internal iliac artery

The internal iliac artery passes obliquely downwards and medially into the pelvis. In most cases it divides into an anterior and a posterior trunk at the upper margin of the greater sciatic foramen. From these are given off branches to the pelvic viscera and the wall of the pelvis (Figure 13.5). The length from its origin to the bifurcation averages 4.1 (1.5–8.2) mm on the left, and 4.3 (1.4–8.4) mm on the right. The right internal iliac artery is slightly longer than that of the left. The outer diameter at the origin averages 7.0 (4.5–12.5) mm on the left, and 7.3 (4.8–11.5) mm on the right and that just above its bifurcation averages 7.7 (5.0–12.5) mm on the left, and 7.73 (5.0–11.5) mm on the right. The angle between the internal and external iliac arteries is commonly less than 45°. Since most of the internal iliac arteries enter obliquely into the pelvis and are provided with an appropriate length, and their outer diameter is similar to that of the renal artery, the internal iliac artery, during renal transplantation, may be cut just above its lower end to anastomose end-to-end with the renal artery. However, in some cases (15%), the angle between the internal and external iliac arteries is larger than 45°, so that the internal iliac artery enters the pelvis vertically and its trunk is short, fixed and deeply located. This adds difficulty to the isolation during transplantation. Moreover, since the iliolumbar artery or one of its branches distributed to the pelvic wall usually comes from the stem of the internal iliac artery (63%), from which the lateral sacral artery may also be directly given off (5%), care must be taken when the internal iliac artery is isolated, to avoid injury to these branches.

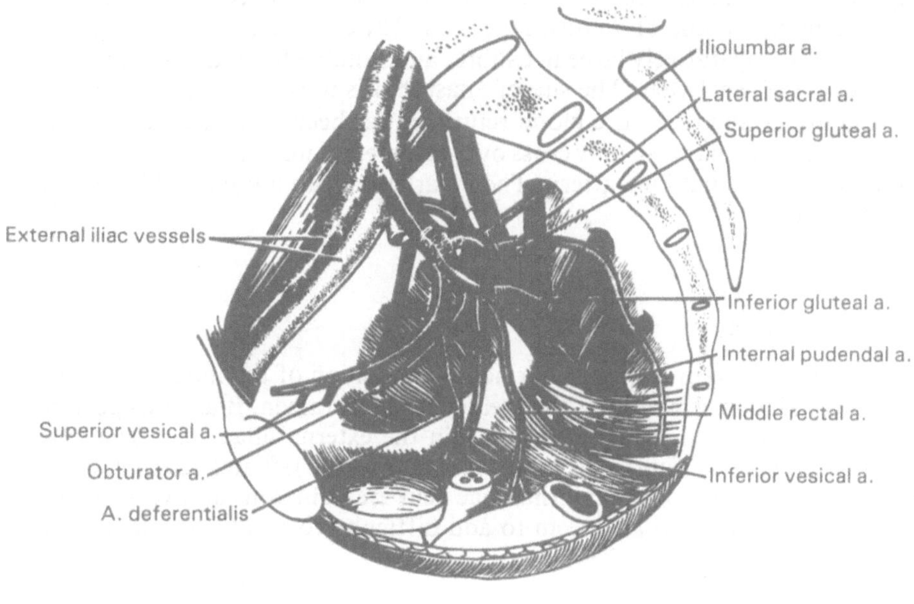

Figure 13.5 Internal iliac artery

External iliac artery

The external iliac artery passes downwards along the medial border of the psoas major to the mid-point of the inguinal ligament, where it passes through the vascular compartment (lacuna vasorum) to enter the thigh to function as the femoral artery. Its average length is 10.6 cm on the left and 11.3 cm on the right. The right artery is slightly longer than the left. The outer diameter at its origin averages 7.6 (4.5–11.5) mm on the left and 7.7 (5.0–12.0) mm on the right. The position of the external iliac artery is constant, its calibre being relatively large. In case of multiple renal arteries one of them may be used for end-to-side anastomosis with the external iliac artery.

External iliac vein

The external iliac vein accompanies the artery along the pelvic brim, and it unites mostly with the internal iliac vein to form the common iliac vein below the bifurcation of the common iliac artery and behind the internal iliac artery. The right external iliac vein lies at first medial to the artery. As it passes upward it inclines gradually to the back of the artery. The left iliac vein lies on the medial side of the artery in its whole course. The outer diameter near the confluence averages 13.2 mm on the left and 13.7 mm on the right. There are frequently valves in the external iliac vein (accounting for 17% on the left side and 28% on the right). The distance from the free edge of the valve to the origin of the common iliac vein averages 23.2 mm on the left and 14.5 mm on the right. The length of the valve measured from its free edge to the attached margin averages 10.5 mm on the left and 11.2 mm on the right. The external iliac vein is constant in position, comparatively large in calibre, and suitable for end-to-side anastomosis with the renal vein. The site of anastomosis must be kept off the valve to avoid injury and to ensure blood return. It has been reported that in a few cases the external iliac vein may cross over the internal iliac artery or lie posterolateral to the external iliac artery. These variations are unfavourable to renal transplantation.

Internal iliac vein

The internal iliac vein is usually formed by the union of the intrapelvic tributaries near the upper margin of the greater sciatic foramen. It ascends posteromedial to the corresponding artery to join the external iliac vein. The outer diameter near the confluence averages 11.1 mm on the left and 12.0 mm on the right. The tributaries of the internal iliac vein are numerous and vary greatly. They are deeply located and seem to add difficulty to renal transplantation.

Common iliac vein

The common iliac vein is formed by the union of the external and internal iliac veins. The site of confluence is at the same level as the bifurcation of the common iliac artery in 7%, or is higher than it in 3% or lower in 90%. The distance between them averages 3.0 cm on the left and 3.2 cm on the right. The right common iliac vein lies at first behind its fellow artery, then ascends almost vertically to the front and right side of the body of the fifth lumbar vertebra and lateral to the common iliac artery and finally unites with the left common iliac vein to form the inferior vena cava. The left common iliac vein is longer than the right and is at first situated on the medial side of the common iliac artery. It then ascends obliquely toward the median line to the back of the right common iliac artery to join the right common iliac vein.

The common iliac vein is large in calibre and constant in position. It can be used for the anastomosis of the renal artery with the common iliac artery. In case of end-to-end anastomosis of the renal artery with the internal iliac artery the renal vein can also be anastomosed with the common iliac vein. Since the position of the commencement of the common iliac vein is usually relatively low, the anastomotic part of the renal artery will not be too tortuous and upward after operation. When the right kidney is transplanted to the left iliac fossa it is difficult to make use of the left common iliac vein, because it is too deep to be conveniently operated on (Figure 13.6).

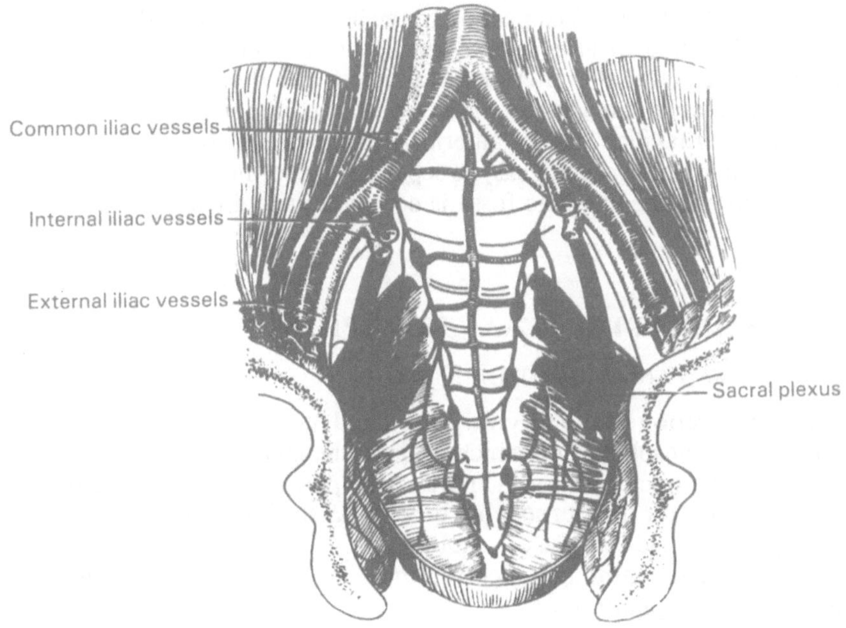

Figure 13.6 Iliac vessels

Topographical relations of the iliac vessels

On both sides and the back of the common iliac artery, there are four to six common iliac lymph nodes. On both sides and in front of the external iliac artery are the external iliac nodes (8–10 in number). Around the internal iliac artery and vein there is a group of internal iliac nodes. All of the afferent and efferent vessels of these nodes are located at the upper and lower extremities of the nodes, and pass along either side or the surface of the iliac vessels. In renal transplantation the lymphatic vessels which surround the nodes must be ligated carefully or electrocoagulated to avoid postoperative lymphatic fistula.

The common iliac artery is surrounded by the common iliac plexus, which is formed by the branches from the abdominal aortic plexus and the third and fourth lumbar splanchnic nerves. This plexus continues downward as the internal and external iliac plexuses. From the superior hypogastric plexus, which lies at the end of the abdominal aorta and its bifurcation, are given off the left and right hypogastric nerves. The hypogastric nerve may be single or be represented by two or three longitudinal branches running on the medial side of the internal iliac artery. It also sends off some branches to the internal iliac plexus. Some thick branches of these nerves can be clearly identified. Whether it is possible to anastomose the renal plexus with the internal iliac or hypogastric plexus during a renal transplantation requires experimental study.

The bifurcation of the right common iliac artery is crossed by the ureter. The right common iliac artery or the internal and external iliac arteries are usually crossed in front by the terminal portion of the ileum. Sometimes the vermiform appendix crosses these arteries to enter the pelvis. The left common iliac artery is crossed anteriorly by the inferior rectal artery and the ureter. The sigmoid colon and its mesocolon usually also cross the common iliac artery or the internal and external iliac arteries anteriorly to enter the pelvis. As the sigmoid colon and its mesocolon are not easy to separate, the technique of transplanting the right kidney to the left iliac fossa is comparatively difficult.

INFANTILE AND FETAL RENAL TRANSPLANTATION

ZHOU CHANGMAN AND LIU MUZHI

With the prolongation of the survival period and increment in the survival rate following renal transplantation which leads to the increasing demand for performance of such operation on the part of the patient, shortage of supply of cadaverous kidney for this purpose has become particularly prominent recently. In order to open a wide source of renal donors, investigation has been carried out in various fields, among which the more rapid and successful has been infantile renal transplantation.

Renal transplantation to an adult recipient using child kidneys was first adopted in 1966 by Kuss and his colleagues whose first report concerned the transplant of a 6-year-old child's kidneys to a 30-year-old woman, who survived for 4 months but died of septicaemia. This was followed by many reports in China and elsewhere. The Beijing Friendship Hospital succeeded for the first time in 1980 in renal transplantation from a 7-month-old infant to an adult. To solve the problem of renal donors, infantile kidneys have now more frequently been made use of in renal transplantation. It has been reported recently that the youngest organ successfully used as a transplant to an adult was that of a 4½-month-old infant. Investigations in embryology, histology and physiology, as well as clinical observations of premature infants, reveal that kidneys of the fetus above 34 weeks of fetal age have completely developed structures and are provided with proper physiological functions. It follows that a fetus of advanced development can be used as a donor in future renal transplantation.

Due to the small size and minute calibre of the vessels, the surgical manoeuvres involved in renal transplantation using child and infantile kidneys are quite different from those employing adult organs. It needs the help of microsurgical techniques for the anastomosis of minute vessels, this being particularly so in case of anastomosing fetal renal and accessory renal vessels. The operative methods of infantile renal transplantation to adult recipients, depending upon the conditions of the donors as well as the recipient, are as follows:

Block transplant of both kidneys

This is generally adopted for small infantile and fetal donors. The aorta of the donor is to be anastomosed end-to-end to the internal iliac artery of the recipient or to the external iliac artery side-to-end, and an end-to-side anastomosis is to be carried out between the inferior vena cava of the donor and the external iliac vein of the recipient (Figure 13.7). Both of the kidneys of the donor are stabilized in the right iliac fossa of the recipient or even in the right hypogastrium in case of a child recipient. The abdominal aorta and the inferior vena cava of the donor are anastomosed to the corresponding vessels of the recipient side-to-end, the mode of management of the ureters being similar to that of the adult. The data for reference purposes relevant to the vessels and ureters of the donor in child or fetal bi-kidney transplantation are as shown in Tables 13.1 and 13.2.

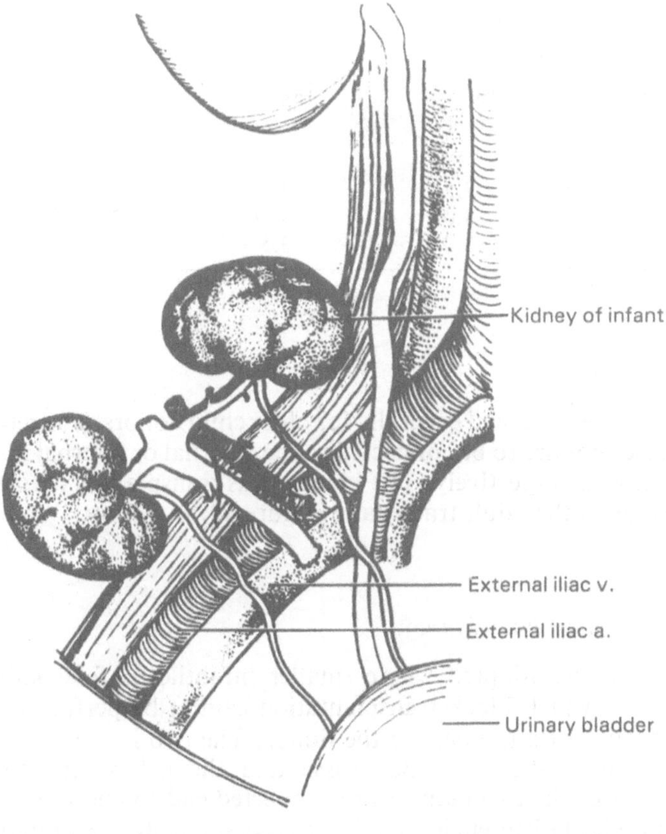

Figure 13.7 Bi-kidney block transplantation from infantile donor to an adult

Table 13.1 The external diameter of large abdominal vessels of infants and fetus (mm)

	Infant (1.5 years)		*Fetus (8 months)*	
	Upper pole of kidney	*Lower pole of kidney*	*Upper pole of kidney*	*Lower pole of kidney*
External diameter of abdominal aorta	7.0	7.0	5.0	5.0
External diameter of inferior vena cava	9.0	9.0	5.5	5.5

Table 13.2 Dimensions of the kidney and ureter of infants and fetus (mm)

	Infant (1.5 years)		*Fetus (8 months)*	
	Left	*Right*	*Left*	*Right*
Kidney				
length	63	68	38	35
width	34	38	16	16
thickness	32	27	14	18
Length of ureter	140	140	65	65
External diameter of ureter				
upper	2.5	3.0	3.0	3.0
middle	3.0	3.8	2.5	2.5
lower	3.0	3.5	2.5	2.5

Mono-kidney transplant

This method has been adopted generally for older child donors. The renal artery and vein of the donor are to be connected to the external or internal iliac artery and vein side-to-end respectively. The kidney thus transplanted is fixed in the iliac fossa just as in the adult transplant (Figure 13.8).

Separate transplant of both kidneys

This method is to be adopted where smaller infantile or fetal kidneys are used as donors in which block transplantation cannot be performed for the sake of blood vessels on the part of the donor. The two kidneys to be transplanted are fixed in the right iliac fossa and the pelvis separately. The arteries and veins of the two kidneys are connected end-to-end to the external iliac artery and vein at different levels. The ureters are treated separately (Figure 13.9).

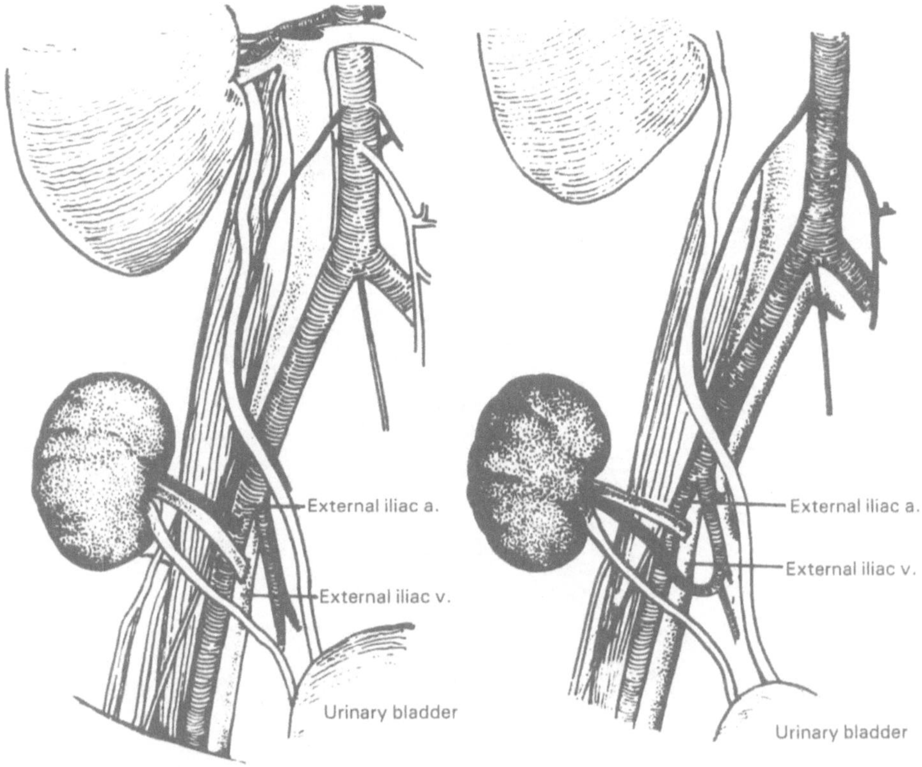

Figure 13.8 Mono-kidney transplantation from child donor to an adult

Data for reference purposes reflecting age difference on the renal vessels of infant and fetus are shown in Table 13.3.

Table 13.3 Data of renal vessels of infant and fetus (mm)

	Infant (1.5 years)		*Fetus (8 months)*	
	Left	*Right*	*Left*	*Right*
Renal artery				
length	28	43	8.0	13
calibre	3.2	3.0	1.3	1.3
Renal vein				
length	45	28	25	10
calibre	8.0	7.0	2.5	2.5

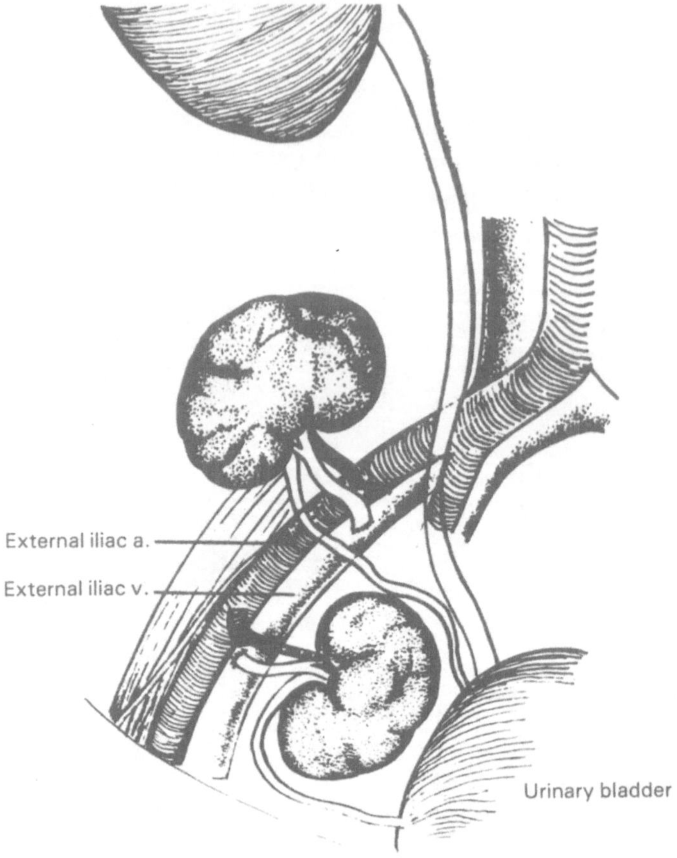

Figure 13.9 Separate transplantation of both kidneys from the infantile donor to an adult

Both the infant and fetus have variations in their accessory renal arteries. These arteries are often destined to supply a renal or secondary renal segment. Accordingly they ought not to be cut carelessly during operation, and if any of them is severed, it must be anastomosed before local ischaemia of the kidney transplanted occurs. The external diameter of the accessory renal artery of an 8-month-old fetus is about 0.5 mm and that of a 1½-year-old small baby would be 0.7–1.0 mm.

TRANSPLANTATION OF THYROID AND PARATHYROID GLANDS

XU DACHUAN AND ZHONG SHIZHEN

The incidence of damage to the parathyroid gland resulting from thyroidectomy is about 0.5–1.0%, according to clinical statistics. It is difficult to treat parathyroid damage because non-vascularized parathyroid glands have short survival periods after transplantation.

Parathyroid glands obtain their rich blood supply either from the inferior thyroid artery or the anastomotic arteries between the superior and inferior thyroid arteries. As the arterial branches to the parathyroid gland are minute and situated within the thyroid capsule, it is quite difficult to carry out a separate vascularized parathyroid transplantation. In consequence it is the total transplantation of the thyroid gland together with the parathyroid that has been done in clinical practice and has gained good results. With regard to the selection of donors, Sterling and Goldsmith (1954) considered that the chief cells of the parathyroid gland begin to be active around 10 years of age, which is thought to be the optimal period for transplantation. However, Chen Guorui and others (1981) succeeded in using as donors the parathyroid glands of 6–7-month-old fetuses in six cases of clinical transplantation. They reported that the parathyroid glands of a 5-month-old fetus were already well developed and that the concentration of serum calcium was 11–13 mg/100 ml, which proved that the parathyroid gland was then very active in function. Therefore, we introduce with emphasis some applied anatomical data about the use of fetus or neonates as donors.

Blood vessels of the thyroid gland

Arteries of the thyroid gland

The thyroid gland has a rich blood supply from the posterior and inferior thyroid arteries. In about 10% of cases there is an additional blood supply from the thyroidea ima. Moreover, fine branches from the neighbouring oesophageal and bronchial arteries are also available. All of these arteries form an extensive anastomosis in the gland.

(1) The superior thyroid artery arises mostly (48%) from the anterior wall of the bifurcation of the common carotid artery. It may come from the external (21%) on the left side and 42% on the right and common carotid artery (31%) on the left side and 10% on the right.

The distance from the origin of the superior thyroid artery, which arises from the external carotid, to the bifurcation of the common carotid artery averages 2.1 mm on the left and 3.1 mm on the right, while the distance from the superior thyroid artery, which arises from the common carotid artery, to the bifurcation of the common carotid averages 3.1 mm on the left and 2.0 mm on the right.

The superior thyroid artery presents a curvature facing anteromedially at its commencement. It then descends anteromedially and gives off, on the way, the superior laryngeal and sternocleidomastoid arteries. At the upper extremity of the lateral lobe of the thyroid gland the main trunk of the superior thyroid artery usually divides into two terminals, the anterior and posterior branches, which run along the anterosuperior and posterior borders of the lateral lobe respectively and are finally distributed to the gland.

The length from the origin of the superior thyroid artery to the upper extremity of the lateral lobe of the thyroid gland in a 7–9-month-old fetus averages 14.5 mm, and the outer diameter of the artery at its commencement averages 1.1 mm with a minimum of 0.8 mm.

(2) The inferior thyroid artery arises mostly from the thyrocervical trunk (90%). The artery may come from other sources such as the subclavian, vertebral and common carotid arteries in 6%. However, it may be absent in 4% of cases. The inferior thyroid artery courses obliquely behind the sympathetic trunk (70%) to enter the lower pole of the thyroid. Nevertheless, it may pass in front of the trunk (28%) or between the two divisions of the trunk (2%). On the way the artery gives off muscular branches to the neighbouring muscles, the inferior laryngeal artery and the bronchial artery. After entering the gland it divides into the inferior and ascending branches which are distributed to the parathyroid glands and the posteroinferior part of the thyroid.

The topographical relations between the inferior thyroid artery and the recurrent laryngeal nerve are complicated and may be classified into three patterns: (1) the branches of the artery interdigitate with those of the nerve in 50%, (2) the artery runs entirely anterior to the nerve in 34%, and (3) the artery passes posterior to the nerve in 7%. The outer diameter of the inferior thyroid artery is smaller than that of the superior thyroid artery, being 0.7–1.2 mm in a 7–9-month-old fetus. However, it is a little longer than the superior thyroid artery.

Veins of the thyroid gland

Veins of the thyroid gland come from the venous network, which is situated between the fascial sheath and the fibrous capsule of the thyroid gland and forms two or three pairs of thyroid veins.

(1) The superior thyroid vein, usually single, begins by tributaries at the upper extremity of the lateral lobe of the thyroid gland. It is in company with and lateral to the artery. About one-third of the superior thyroid vein join the veins of the pharynx and larynx before ending into the internal jugular vein. However, most of them end directly into it. The superior thyroid vein is a little longer than the artery but their outer diameters are nearly equal.

(2) The middle thyroid vein usually arises from the junction between the middle and lower thirds of the thyroid gland and crosses over the common carotid artery to end into the internal jugular vein through its anterolateral wall. The incidence of the vein is about 50%. The left vein is usually single, but the right vein may be single in 83%, double in 11%, and triple in 6%. The middle thyroid vein of the fetus is very short, averaging 6.0 mm in length, and its outer diameter averages 1.1 mm.

(3) The inferior thyroid vein arises from the lower pole of the lateral lobe of the thyroid gland. It is single in 79% of cases. However, the left and right veins may join into one in the anteroinferior aspect of the gland in 18%, while the plexiform type accounts for only 3%.

The inferior thyroid veins empty into the right and left innominate veins (80%), the right and left internal jugular veins (18%) and the vertebral veins (2%). Their outer diameter and length average 1.0 and 19.5 mm respectively.

Outer diameters of the common and external carotid arteries and the internal jugular vein

In a 7–9-month-old fetus the outer diameter of the common carotid artery measured at the level of 2 cm below its bifurcation averages 3.4 mm, and that of the commencement of the external carotid artery and of the internal jugular vein at the same level are 2.3 and 4.0 mm respectively.

Dimensions of the thyroid gland

In a 7–9-month-old fetus the average length from the upper to the lower pole of the lateral lobe of the thyroid gland is 18 mm. The mediolateral breadth and the anteroposterior thickness of the lateral lobe measured at its middle portion are 10 and 8.9 mm respectively.

Applied anatomy of the donor area

There are two types of vascular pedicle of the thyroid gland to be chosen for operation. One of these is composed of the superior thyroid vessels connected with the carotid vessels, and the other consists of the pan-thyroid vessels in combination with the carotid and innominate vessels. Although the calibres of both pedicles are large enough for anastomosis, it would still be better to operate under the surgical microscope in taking the materials from the donor and the anastomosis of the vessels. By this method injury to the blood vessels and tissues can be avoided.

If the vascular pedicle of the first type is to be adopted, the lateral lobe of the thyroid gland on either side can be chosen as the donor, because there is not any obvious anatomical difference between the two sides. If that of the second type is adopted, the right lobe is preferable to the left, because the right common carotid and subclavian arteries arise from a common trunk, the innominate artery, while the left common carotid and subclavian arteries arise from the aortic arch separately.

In taking the vascular pedicle the levels of the origins of the superior and inferior thyroid arteries and those of the terminations of their corresponding veins should be noted. The length of the thyroid vessels measured from their origin or termination should be kept appropriately in order to ensure the circulation of the thyroid gland. Since some of the superior thyroid arteries may arise from the external carotid artery 2–5 mm above the bifurcation of the common carotid artery, the external carotid artery should be ligated well above the origin of the superior thyroid artery.

The incidence of the middle thyroid vein is about 50%. In order to ensure the venous return of the thyroid gland the middle thyroid vein, if present, should always be anastomosed. If the vascular pedicle of the second type is adopted the medial half of the right clavicle should be excised to expose in full the innominate vessels. The inferior thyroid veins should be preserved as far as possible in dissecting the innominate vein which is to be cut near its entrance into the superior vena cava. After the anterior scalenus muscle has been cut, at the point lateral to the origin of the thyrocervical trunk (corresponding to the lateral border of the anterior scalenus muscle), ligate and cut the subclavian, the vertebral and the internal thoracic arteries and all of the branches of the thyrocervical trunk except the inferior thyroid artery. The right vagus nerve is severed and extracted from the carotid sheath.

In freeing the thyroid gland its capsule and the connective tissue, especially that on the posterior border of the lateral lobe, should be included so as to ensure the intactness of the parathyroid glands. According to a report made by Chiu Zhiming, in 16% of cases the parathyroid glands are buried in the connective tissue outside the thyroid capsule near the superior and inferior extremities of the lateral lobe.

Comparison between the two types of vascular pedicle

Though both types have been used clinically and have achieved good results, in regard to the blood supply of the parathyroid glands the second type is more preferable, because the blood supply of the parathyroid glands mainly comes from the inferior thyroid artery as well as the anastomosis between it and the superior thyroid artery. Moreover, the calibres of the innominate vessels (the calibres of the innominate artery and vein of a 7-month-old fetus are 4.3–5.5 and 5.5–7.2 mm respectively) are larger than those of the carotid vessels, and this allows easier manipulation.

Applied anatomy of the recipient area

The inguinal region is an ideal recipient area because of its concealed position, loose subcutaneous tissue and sufficient room for holding the small transplanted mass from fetal or neonatal donors. In the inguinal region there are the profunda femoris vessels, the medial and lateral circumflex vessels and the greater saphenous vein. Any of these can be moved to the superficial layer and be anastomosed with the vessels of the transplanted mass. The outer diameter of the lateral circumflex artery averages 5.4 mm and the accompanying vein is a little wider. The vein of the transplanted mass can also be anastomosed with the proximal end of the greater saphenous vein. The calibres of these vessels in the inguinal region approximate those of the donor's. The vessels available in the recipient area are so numerous that they make the operation flexible (Figure 13.10).

TRANSPLANTATION OF THE PANCREAS

XU DACHUAN AND ZHONG SHIZHEN

Since insulin was discovered 60 years ago it has played an important role in the treatment of diabetes mellitus. However, it cannot effect a radical cure for diabetes as well as for the prevention of vascular complications, so that

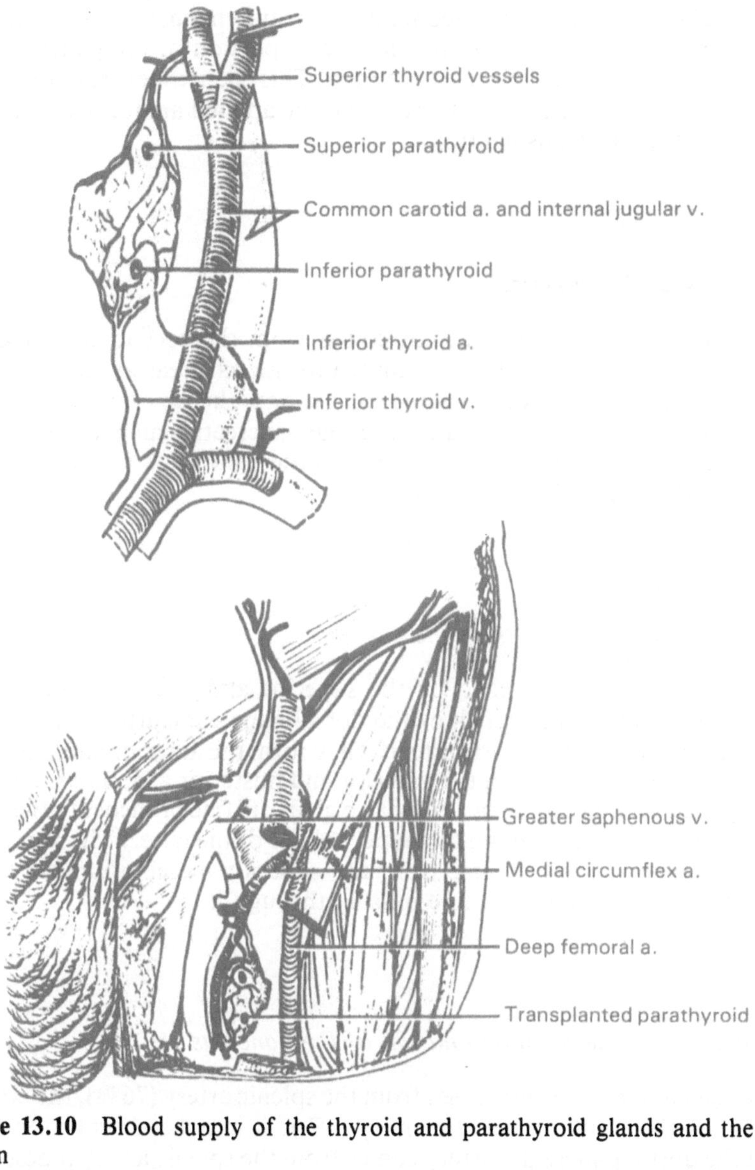

Figure 13.10 Blood supply of the thyroid and parathyroid glands and the inguinal region

transplantation of the pancreas has been widely noted. Since clinical transplantation of the pancreas was first carried out by Kelly in 1966 various procedures have been reported. Owing to the strong rejection as a result of duodenal graft, the transplantation of pancreas and duodenum in total was refuted in the main. It is found that more pancreatic islets are distributed in the tail of the pancreas. Experiments and clinical practice have also proved that only the tail of the pancreas transplanted to the recipient is enough to maintain the normal level of insulin. In view of the utmost difficulty in managing the exocrine of the pancreas, it turns to be one of the important problems in pancreatic transplantation. The prenatal fetus, neonatal fetus and neonates have become candidates for the donor, because the endocrine portion of the pancreas has become mature ahead of the exocrine function. This chapter covers data on the segmental transplantation of the pancreas and the applied anatomy of fetus or neonates in relation to transplantion.

Arterial supply of the pancreas

The rich blood supply of the pancreas comes from the coeliac and superior mesenteric arteries. The branches distributed to the pancreas as shown in the specimen of the arterial cast of the adult pancreas are the superior and inferior pancreaticoduodenal, the dorsal pancreatic, the pancreatica magna, the caudal pancreatic and inferior pancreatic arteries and the pancreatic branches of the splenic artery (Figure 13.11).

Blood supply of the head of the pancreas

The head of pancreas is supplied by the superior and inferior pancreaticoduodenal arteries, the right branch of the dorsal pancreatic artery and several twigs from the superior mesenteric artery. They form the anterior and posterior pancreaticoduodenal arcades on the anterior and posterior aspects of the head respectively. The common hepatic artery also gives off fine branches to the head of the pancreas as it courses along the upper border of the latter. The abnormal hepatic and cystic arteries arising from the superior mesenteric artery also supply some twigs to the head while passing through it.

Blood supply of the neck, body and tail of the pancreas

(1) The dorsal pancreatic artery arises from the splenic artery (76%), the coeliac artery (9%) or the common hepatic artery (6%). It may be absent in 9%.

When the dorsal pancreatic artery comes from the splenic artery it descends behind the pancreas, reaching the neck or the body of the pancreas and then divides into the right and left branches. The right branch anastomoses with the pancreaticoduodenal arcade, and is distributed to the head and uncinate process of the pancreas, while the left one passes along the dorsoinferior part of the body of pancreas and anastomoses, in the substance of the pancreas, with the arteria pancreatica magna and the caudal pancreatic artery to form the inferior (or transverse) pancreatic artery. Sometimes the dorsal pancreatic artery gives off branches to the transverse colon and the mesocolon.

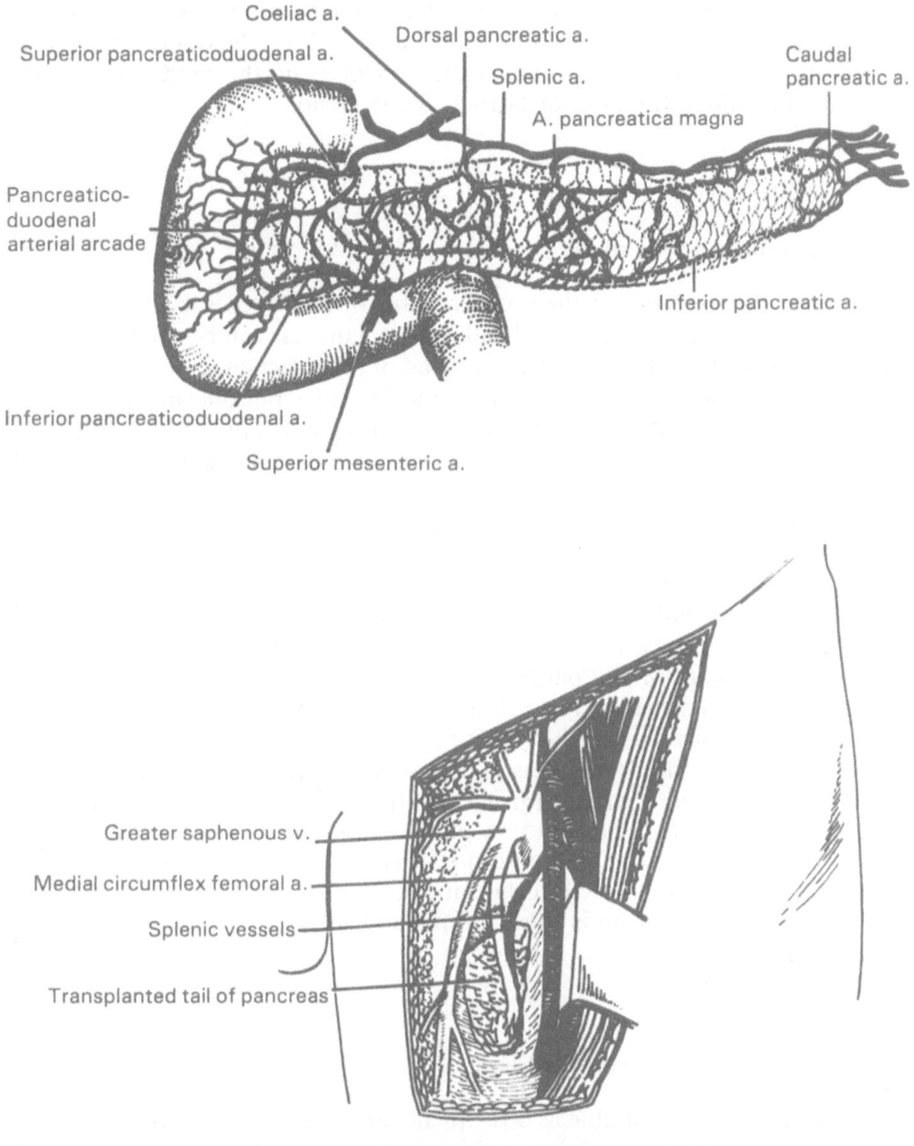

Figure 13.11 Blood supply of the pancreas and the inguinal recipient area

(2) The arteria pancreatica magna is a comparatively large branch of the splenic artery, the incidence of which is 94%. It runs parallel to the pancreatic duct to anastomose with the left branch of the dorsal and caudal pancreatic arteries.

(3) The caudal pancreatic artery is quite a large branch arising from the splenic artery near the tail of the pancreas. It is single in 88% of cases, double in 9%, and absent in only 3%. It arises from the splenic artery or its inferior division in 84% and 8% respectively, and from the gastroepiploic artery in 8%.

(4) The inferior pancreatic artery is smaller and is formed, as clearly shown in the cast specimen, by the union of the left branch of the dorsal pancreatic artery with a large branch of a. pancreatica magna and the caudal pancreatic artery. It runs along the inferior border of the gland.

Applied anatomy of the donors

As a donor, the pancreas of the prenatal fetus or neonates is easily obtained. The tail and the body, but not the head, of the pancreas can be used for transplantation. Since the duodenum and the head of the pancreas are closely related in embryonic origin, blood supply, lymphatic drainage, bile duct and pancreatic duct, they may be regarded as a structurally inseparable unit and should not be obstinately divided, so as to avoid discord of the anatomical and physiological integrity.

The body and tail of the pancreas may be considered as another structural unit. The vascular pedicle is formed by the splenic artery and vein. Though some of the dorsal pancreatic arteries (17%) do not arise from the splenic artery, they anastomose freely with the branches of a. pancreatica magna and the caudal and inferior pancreatic arteries to form a rich arterial network in the substance of the tail and body of the pancreas to ensure the blood supply. The outer diameter of the splenic artery in a 6–8-month-old fetus averages 1.8 and 2.2 mm before and after birth respectively. The outer diameter of the splenic vein is greater than that of the artery. Vessels with such calibre are easy to anastomose and add no difficulty to microsurgical operations. The length of the body plus the tail averages 28 mm in a 6–8-month-old fetus and 37 mm in a neonate. Owing to the small size of the donor it need not be transplanted into the body cavity of the donee. It can be buried in the subcutaneous tissue without local bulge and tension. The operation is fairly simple and safe.

Applied anatomy of the recipient area

The inguinal region is suitable as a recipient site for the transplantation of the pancreas because of its concealed position and ability to hold the transplanted mass and the rich loose tissue it contains. The superficial epigastric, superficial circumflex and superficial external pudendal vessels in this region, provided with a calibre of more than 0.8 mm, can be regarded as the vascular pedicle for anastomosis in the recipient area. If the splenic vessels of the donor area are larger than the superficial vessels in the inguinal region of the recipient, so that no appropriate vessels for vascular anastomosis can be found in the superficial layer of this region, the lateral circumflex femoral artery may be dissected and taken to the superficial layer for anastomosis. The calibre of the stem of the lateral circumflex femoral artery is 5.4 mm. It can be used alternatively with its narrower branches.

TRANSPLANTATION OF THE SUPRARENAL GLAND

XU DACHUAN AND ZHONG SHIZHEN

Both homologous and autologous suprarenal glands can be used for transplantation. Autologous transplantation is generally used in hyperadrenalism such as Cushing's disease or chromaffinoma, and partial adrenalectomy is the treatment for hyperadrenalism. However, excessive resection of the adrenal gland may lead to hypoadrenalism. Therefore, part of the excised adrenal gland should be transplanted to the inguinal subcutaneous tissue in order to observe the efficacy of the operation. If hyperadrenalism remains, resection of the transplanted gland outside the abdominal cavity can be done without the risk of overresection of the gland. Homologous transplantation of the adrenal gland is used for the treatment of hypoadrenalism (Addison's disease).

Vessels of the suprarenal gland

Arteries of the suprarenal gland

The suprarenal gland possesses a rich blood supply. In addition to the superior, middle and inferior suprarenal arteries from the inferior phrenic artery, the abdominal aorta and the renal artery respectively, it receives many fine branches from the nearby gonadal, coeliac, superior ureteral and superior mesenteric arteries. The calibres of these branches are less than 0.3 mm in diameter when seen with the naked eye (Figure. 13.12).

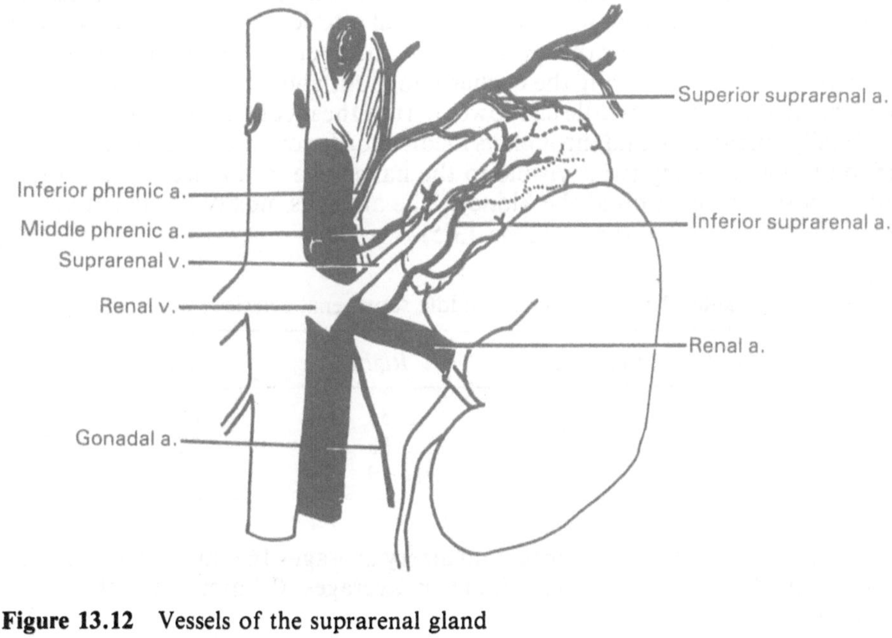

Figure 13.12 Vessels of the suprarenal gland

(1) The superior suprarenal arteries are the small and short branches distributed to the medial and upper borders of the suprarenal gland by the inferior phrenic artery.

The incidence of the superior suprarenal arteries is 97% on the right and 100% on the left. The calibres of these arteries are nearly equal, being generally less than 0.5 mm. The superior suprarenal arteries average 7 and 6.5 in number on the right and left sides respectively. Before entering the gland these arteries ramify into many twigs. Thus the number of branches to the parenchyma of the gland may increase to dozens on each side. They nourish the posterior and posteromedial aspects of the gland.

The length of the inferior phrenic artery from its origin to the most distal branch is 58 mm on the right and 44 mm on the left. The outer diameter measured at its commencement is 1.5 mm on the right and 1.7 mm on the left.

(2) The middle suprarenal artery arises mostly from the abdominal aorta, and a few of them come from the inferior phrenic or coeliac artery. Details about its origin are given in the Table 13.4.

Table 13.4 Origins of the middle suprarenal artery (%)

Origins	*Right*	*Left*
Abdominal aorta	68	74
Inferior phrenic artery	23	9
Coeliac artery	6	8
Absent	3	9

Most of the middle suprarenal arteries arise from the abdominal aorta at its anterolateral wall between the coeliac and renal arteries, while a few come from the abdominal aorta below the level of the renal artery. The middle suprarenal artery runs laterally, piercing the coeliac ganglion, and crossing the crus of the diaphragm to reach the middle and lower part of the medial border of the gland, and finally enters the gland through its medial border or anterior aspect. It gives off, on the way, many twigs visible to the naked eye to the nearby structures and adipose capsule around the kidney. The artery is mostly single but varies in number from one to three (Table 13.5).

Table 13.5 Number of middle suprarenal arteries (%)

Number of arteries	*Right*	*Left*
1	55	69
2	36	22
3	9	9

The length of the middle suprarenal artery averages 16 mm on the right and 15 mm on the left. Its outer diameter averages 0.7 mm on either side (Table 13.6).

Table 13.6 Outer diameter of the middle suprarenal artery (%)

Outer diameter (mm)	*Right*	*Left*
0.3–0.5	33	36
0.6–1.0	50	48
1.1–1.5	17	16

(3) The inferior suprarenal artery frequently arises from the upper wall of the renal artery or its division. The distance from the origin of the artery to that of the renal artery is 11 mm on the right and 17 mm on the left. The length of the renal artery from its origin to the hilum of the kidney is 42 mm on the right and 49 mm on the left. The artery is mostly double but varies in number from one to three (Table 13.7).

Table 13.7 Number of inferior suprarenal arteries (%)

Number of arteries	*Right*	*Left*
1	40	32
2	44	45
3	16	23

In regard to its origin, the inferior suprarenal artery stems mostly from the renal artery (Table 13.8).

Table 13.8 Origin of the inferior suprarenal artery (%)

Origin	*Right*	*Left*
Renal artery	77	83
Accessory renal artery	11	7
Gonadal artery	7	5
Inferior phrenic artery	5	5

The inferior suprarenal artery is one of the major choices in the donor site because of its definite length and large calibre. After arising from the upper border of the renal artery, it frequently runs in an acute angle with the renal artery, and enters the suprarenal gland through its renal surface to supply the lower half of the gland. It is 15 mm and 10 mm in length on the right and left side respectively. Its outer diameter averages 0.8 mm on either side (Table 13.9).

The superior, middle and inferior suprarenal arteries form a rich vascular network within the capsule of the suprarenal gland, especially behind its posterior surface. The arteries also communicate with those in the adipose capsule around the kidney, forming extensive anastomoses visible to the naked eye.

Table 13.9 Outer diameter of the inferior suprarenal artery (%)

Outer diameter (mm)	*Right*	*Left*
0.3–0.5	36	37
0.6–1.0	43	47
1.1–1.7	21	16

Veins of the suprarenal gland

Most of the suprarenal veins are drained by a large central vein via the hilum of the gland, while a few of them communicate with those of the adipose capsule of the kidney.

(1) The left suprarenal vein commences at the hilum of the gland. It receives the left inferior phrenic vein coming from the superomedial part of the gland and then descends over the lower part of the anterior surface of the gland to end in the left renal vein with an acute angle (about 45–80°). The left suprarenal vein averages 21 mm in length and the renal vein from the termination of the suprarenal vein to the inferior vena cava averages 23 mm. The outer diameter of the suprarenal vein at its termination into the renal vein is 41 mm.

(2) The right suprarenal vein is single in 94% of cases and double in 6%. Its outer diameter averages 2.9 mm. Its length and sites of termination are listed in Table 13.10.

Table 13.10 Termination and length of the right suprarenal vein

	Inferior vena cava	*Right accessory hepatic vein*	*Right renal vein*
Percentage	50	39	11
Length (mm)	6.9	5.0	14.3

Applied anatomy

Donor site

Topographical relation of the suprarenal gland

The suprarenal gland is deeply seated in the retroperitoneal space and has a complex topographical relation. The anterior surface of the left suprarenal gland is related to the splenic artery and vein and a part of the pancreas. Medial to it is the abdominal aorta. The left coeliac ganglion is behind the middle and lower parts of the gland; thus the left suprarenal gland is easy to expose. The anterior surface of the right suprarenal gland is in contact with the posterior border of the liver. Its posterior surface is related to the diaphragm. The right coeliac ganglion and the inferior vena cava are anteromedial to it. The vena cava usually covers the large portion, or even the whole, of the gland. Owing to its deep position and complex relation with neighbouring structures it seems likely that the right suprarenal gland will add much more difficulty to the operation.

Applied anatomy of the suprarenal vessels

Suprarenal arteries The superior, middle and inferior suprarenal arteries can theoretically be used for vascular anastomosis, yet judging from the topographical relations the inferior suprarenal artery is the only ideal one. Though the superior suprarenal arteries arise regularly from the inferior diaphragmatic artery and assume a constant position and course, and the inferior diaphragmatic artery has quite a large calibre, they are not suitable for vascular anastomosis, owing to the deep position of the inferior diaphragmatic artery.

The middle suprarenal arteries are constant in their origin and course, their diameters being more than 0.3 mm, mostly 0.6–1.0 mm. They generally pierce the coeliac ganglion, and the length between their emergence from the ganglion to the gland is too short to be used for anastomosis. Only those of the middle suprarenal arteries that originate from the inferior diaphragmatic artery of the renal artery (24% on the right and 9% on the left) do not pierce the coeliac ganglion and can be used directly for anastomosing with the inferior diaphragmatic artery (Figure 13.13).

The inferior suprarenal artery is ideal for anastomosis because of its considerable length and outer diameter and ease of exposure. It can usually be found during operation by following the renal artery along its upper border laterally. The inferior suprarenal artery arises from the renal artery about 11 mm lateral to the abdominal aorta. In case of its absence from the renal artery it can be searched for from the accessory renal artery, the gonadal artery or the inferior phrenic artery of the lower origin. The renal artery and vein can be used for anastomosis in case a prenatal fetus or newborn infant is chosen as the donor.

Suprarenal veins The right suprarenal vein is rather short, about 7 mm in length. It ends mostly in the right posterior wall of the inferior vena cava or in the accessory hepatic vein. Owing to its deep position and complex relation it is not easy to anastomose. Thus the right suprarenal gland is unsuitable for transplantation. Since the left suprarenal vein is constant in termination and course, and has a sufficient length and outer diameter, it is ideal for anastomosis. The inferior diaphragmatic vein, which terminates in the left suprarenal vein, should be ligated and severed.

Recipient site

The inguinal region is of choice due to its concealed position and rich connective tissue, which is loose, and it is easy to hold the tissue graft. The superficial epigastric, the superficial circumflex iliac and the external pudendal vessels in

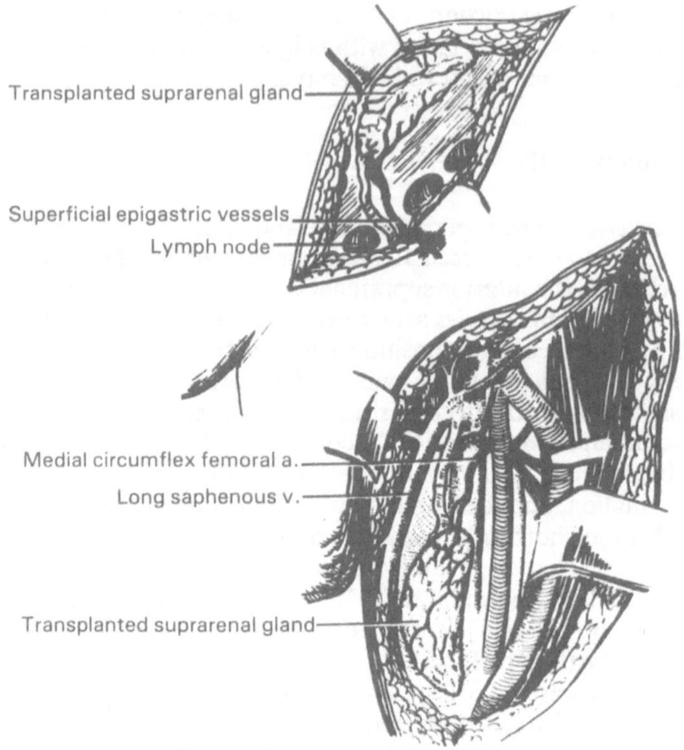

Figure 13.13 Diagram showing the suprarenal gland being transplanted to the inguinal region

the region have calibres over 0.8 mm, which approximates that of those vessels of the donor area. They are fit for anastomosis. Where the donor area has large vessels it is advisable to use the deeper branches of the femoral vessels to match. If the veins of the donor area are much larger than the superficial epigastric, the superficial circumflex iliac and the external pudendal veins, they may be connected to those venous trunks ending into the greater saphenous vein or to the lateral circumflex femoral vein. In a word, there are many vessels in the recipient area ready to be chosen for anastomosis (Figure 13.13).

TRANSPLANTATION OF GONADS

XU DACHUAN AND LIU MUZHI

Clinical gonadal transplantation at present consists of two categories: homologous and autologous grafts. The ovary is often used for homologous allotransplantation. Bilateral ovariectomy due to various causes frequently leads to serious endocrine disturbance which, in addition to hormonal therapy, can be treated with gonadal transplantation. Winston (1974) and Cohen (1976) both succeeded in vascularized ovarian transplantation in rabbit and sheep respectively. In 1979 Zhu Jiakai successfully carried out ovarian allotransplantation clinically.

The testicular graft is often used in those patients suffering from cryptorchidism whose intra-abdominal testes can be transferred to the scrotum by means of vascular anastomosis. Owing to the short vascular pedicle of the high intra-abdominal cryptorchid testes, the one-stage transference of the testis with spermatic vascular pedicle or cryptorchidopexy by stages used to lead to ischaemia of the testis, because of the excessive traction of the pedicle. The incidence of testicular atrophy has been up to 50%. The vascularized testicular transplantation consists of anastomosis of the spermatic vessels with the inferior epigastric or other superficial vessels in the inguinal region, the success rate of which is high.

Vessels of the gonads

Gonadal arteries

The artery of the male gonad is the testicular artery, and that of the female is the ovarian artery. There is no obvious difference between them in respect to their origin, number and abdominal course.

Gonadal arteries originate from the abdominal aorta in 87%, from the renal artery in 11%, and from the accessory renal or other arteries in 2%. Most of the gonadal arteries spring from the anterolateral wall of the abdominal aorta below the level of the renal artery, pass obliquely downward and laterally or curve upward at first and then descend laterally and downward, coursing below or behind the renal vein. A few of them come from the aorta at or above the level of the renal artery, passing in front of the renal vein. The gonadal arteries descend in front of the psoas major muscle and on the way give off fine branches to the suprarenal gland, the adipose capsule of the kidney, the ureter, the iliolumbar lymph nodes and the retroperitoneal tissues. The right gonadal artery passes in front of or behind the inferior vena cava in 82% and 9% respectively, and bears no relation to it in 9%. The gonadal artery is single in 86%, double in 12% and triple in 2%.

The ovarian artery crosses the upper part of the external iliac artery at the pelvic brim, enters the pelvic cavity and then runs between the two layers of the suspensory ligament of the ovary. It lies below the uterine tube, and gives off, in the mesovarium, three to five twigs to the ovary and fine branches to the Fallopian tube. The ovarian artery averages 189 mm in length, and the outer diameter of its commencement averages 0.95 (0.6–1.5) mm.

The testicular artery runs in front of the genitofemoral nerve and the lower segment of the external iliac artery, getting into the abdominal ring of the inguinal canal in company with the spermatic cord. It gives off twigs to the cord and its coverings and in the upper extremity of the testis, a medial and a lateral branch to the testis. The average length of the artery is 327 mm and the outer diameter of its commencement averages 1.1 (0.6–1.8) mm.

Gonadal veins

The ovarian veins, after emerging from the hilum ovarium, form a venous plexus in the mesovarium which communicates freely with the uterovaginal plexus, etc. They ascend between the two layers of the suspensory ligament of the ovary and unite to form two veins at the attachment of the suspensory ligament to the pelvis, which combine into a single one at a level 2–3 cm above the pelvic brim. This accompanies the corresponding artery and crosses the external iliac artery, assuming a course similar to that of the testicular vein. The length of the ovarian vein averages 122 mm on the right and 179 mm on the left. The outer diameter averages 4.8 mm. The testicular veins are formed by the confluence of small veins from the testis and epididymis. They ascend in front of the ductus deferens and wind around the testicular artery. These small veins anastomose freely to form the pampiniform plexus. At the superficial inguinal ring the veins of the plexus are drained by three or four veins, which pass through the inguinal canal to enter the abdomen via the deep inguinal ring and coalesce into two veins. The latter unite into a single vein 1–3 cm above the deep inguinal ring, and run upwards in front of the psoas major and the ureter in company with the testicular artery. At its termination the outer diameter of the vein averages 3.6 mm, and its length averages 320 mm on the right and 334 mm on the left.

The gonadal vein is single in 91% and double in 9%. All of the left gonadal veins end in the left renal vein, and the right ones end in the inferior vena cava (72%) and in the right renal vein (28%).

Applied anatomy of the donor

The ovary lies in the ovarian fossa, formed by the internal and external iliac arteries. In taking the ovary the mesovarium should be incised near the broad ligament. The ovarian ligament, the tubal branches of the ovarian artery and the ovarian branches of the uterine artery should also be cut and ligated. After making a longitudinal incision of the mesovarium, the ovarian artery and veins can be found. The vascular pedicle can be taken above the union of the ovarian veins, which usually takes its place 2–3 cm above the pelvic brim.

The vascular pedicle of the abdominal cryptorchid testis should be taken near the origin of the artery and the termination of the vein because of its high position and short vascular pedicle. Most of the testicular arteries arise from the abdominal aorta below the level of the origin of the renal artery, and a few of them arise from the aorta above the level of the renal artery or directly from the renal artery. The distance between the origin of the testicular artery and the bifurcation of the aorta into the external and internal iliac arteries averages 75 mm. The testicular artery can be found in front of the psoas major, where it is easily exposed. After the artery has been found it can be traced upward to its origin, where it is cut with its accompanying vein at the same level.

Applied anatomy of the recipient area

The inguinal region and the lateral part of the breast (lower margin of the pectoralis major) are the ideal recipient areas for ovary transplantation. These two places lie concealed and provided with abundant loose subcutaneous tissue, suitable for holding the transplanted tissues. Of the superficial epigastric, the

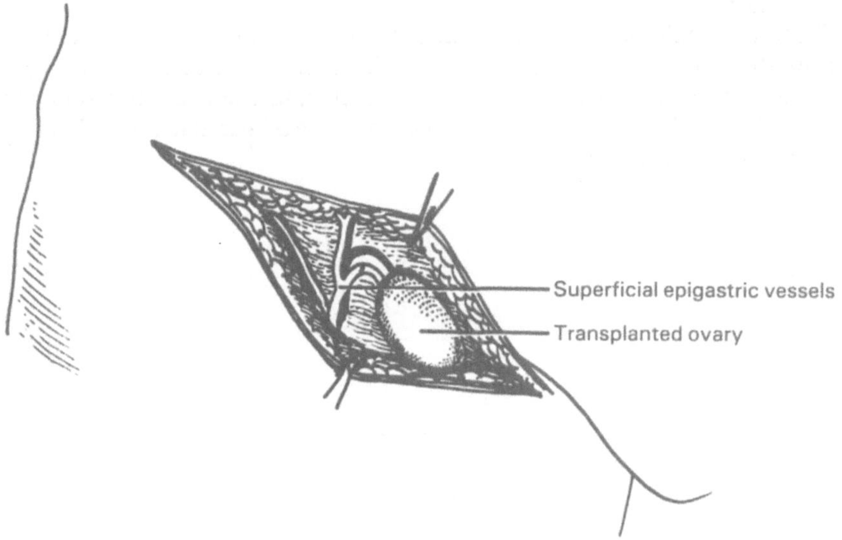

Figure 13.14 Diagram showing the ovary being transplanted to the inguinal region

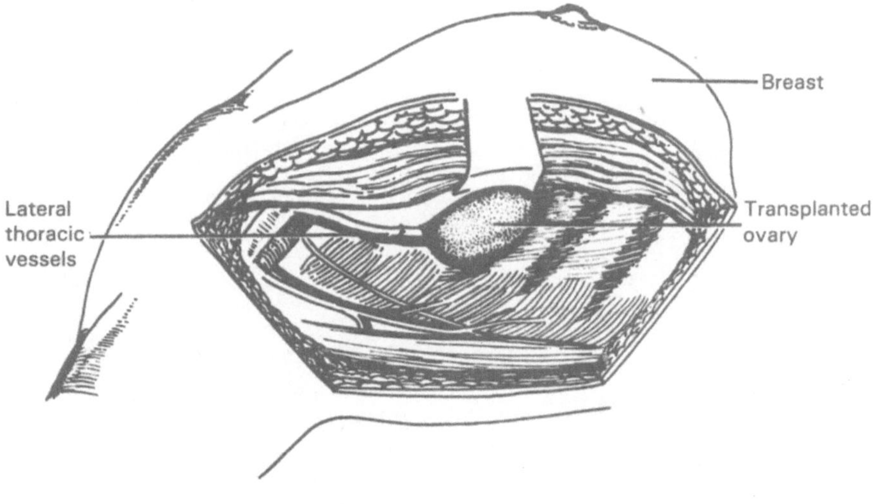

Figure 13.15 Diagram showing the ovary being transplanted lateral to the breast

superficial circumflex iliac and the superficial external pudendal vessels, the superficial epigastric vessels are first choice for ovary transplantation because the outer diameter is about 1.0 mm and approximates that of the donor artery (Figure 13.14). If there is a great disparity between the calibres of the vein of the donor and that of the superficial epigastric vein, the donor vein can be anastomosed with those draining into the greater saphenous vein. The lateral thoracic vessels in the lateral part of the breast are constant and provided with an outer diameter of 1.5 mm or so and the accompanying vein possesses a greater calibre.

The testis should be transplanted into the scrotum if possible, because it will promote the normal growth of the testis. The recipient area has many vessels available, such as the inferior epigastric vessels and the deep and superficial vessels of the inguinal region which can be made use of alternatively. This would add convenience to the operation.

Bibliography

Albert, P. W. R. M. The blood supply of the incus and the head and neck of stapes. *J. Laryngol.*, **79**, 964; 1965

Alday, E. S. and Goldsmith, H. S. Surgical technic for omental lengthening based on arterial anatomy. *Surg. Gynecol. Obst.*, **135**, 103; 1972

Alper, B. J. *et al.* Circle of Willis in cerebral vascular disorders. *Arch. Neurol.*, **8**, 398; 1963

Alpert, B. S. *et al.* Replacement of damaged arteries and veins with vein grafts when replanting crushed amputated fingers. *Plast. Reconstruct. Surg.*, **61**, 17; 1978

Andresov, P. I. Blood supply of mobilized intestine used for artificial esophagus. *A. Med. Assoc. Arch. Surg.*, **73**, 917; 1956

Anson, B. J. and Donaldson, J. A. *Surgical Anatomy of the Temporal Bone and Ear*, 2nd edn., pp. 37–41. W. B. Saunders, Philadelphia, 1973

Anson, B. J. and Winch, T. R. Vascular channels in the auditory ossicles in man. *Ann. Otol. Rhinol. Laryngol.*, **83**, 142; 1974

Azuma, H. *et al.* Treatment of chronic osteomyelitis by transplantation of autogenous omentum with microvascular anastomosis. *Acta. Orthop. Scand.*, **47**, 271; 1976

Bai Shuling. Microsurgical anatomy of the posterior leg flap. I. Direct cutaneous artery type. *Guangdong Anat. Bull.*, **4**, 8; 1932

Bai Shuling. Microsurgical anatomy of the posterior leg flap. II. Reticular type of arterial trunk. *Guangdong Anat. Bull.*, **13**, 13; 1982

Ballantyne, J. and Groves, J. *Scott-Brown's Disease of the Ear, Nose and Throat*, 4th edn. The ear, pp. 865–906. Butterworths, London, 1979

Baudet, J. *et al.* Successful clinical transfer of two free thoracodorsal axillary flaps. *Plast. Reconstruct. Surgery.*, **58**, 680; 1976

Bergland, R. M. *et al.* Anatomical variation in the pituitary gland and adjacent structures in 225 human autopsy cases. *Neurosurgery*, **28**, 93; 1968

Blunt, M. J. The blood supply of the facial nerve. *J. Anat.*, **88**, 520; 1954

Brockis, J. G. The blood supply of the flexor tendons of the fingers in man. *J. Bone Jt. Surg.*, **35A**, 141; 1953

Brown, R. G. *et al.* The omentum in facial reconstruction. *Br. J. Plast. Surg.*, **21**, 58; 1978

Buncke, H. J. *et al.* Thumb replacement: great toe transplantation by microvascular anastomosis. *Br. J. Plast. Surg.*, **26**, 194; 1973

Cabanie, H. *et al.* Anatomical bases of the thoracodorsal axillary flap with respect to its transfer by means of microvascular surgery. *Anat. Clin.*, **2**, 65; 1980

Chao Zhifu, Liu Dingyi *et al.* Treatment of chyluria with microsurgery. *Chin. J. Surg.*, **19**, 659; 1981

Chater, N. *et al.* Microvascular bypass surgery, part I: anatomical studies. *J. Neurosurg.*, **44**, 712; 1976

Chen Bing, Zhan Youhua *et al.* Anastomosis of thoracic duct with internal jugular vein for ascites due to late hepatic cirrhosis; report of 8 cases. *Chin. J. Surg.*, **19**, 530; 1981

Chen Eryu, He Gwangtsi *et al.* The vessels of the skin flaps at groin region. I. The macro-microanatomy of the superficial circumflex iliac vessels. *Acta Anat. Sinica*, **12**, 337; 1981

Chen Eryu, He Gwantsi *et al.* The vessels of the skin flaps at groin region. II. The macro-microanatomy of the superficial epigastric vessels. *Acata Anat. Sinica*, **13**, 113; 1982

Chen Eryu, Zhang Shuzhen *et al.* Observation of the superior masenteric artery in Chinese adult. *Acta Anat. Sinica*, **9**, 138; 1966

Chen Guorui, Lin Yongjie *et al.* Allotransplantation of parathyroid glands with vascular anastomosis: report of 6 cases. *Chin. J. Surg.*, **19**, 470; 1981

Chen Yaoliang, Shen Zhongwen *et al.* The blood supply of the fibula (the anatomical study of free vascularized fibular graft). *Acta Anat. Sinica*, **12**, 13; 1981

Chen Yiwei and Lin Hongyi. Preliminary study of dural venous sinus of the Chinese. *Acta Anat. Sinicia*, **2,** 65; 1957
Chen Yuanzhi. Microsurgical anatomy of the transverse colon. *Guandong Anat. Bull.*, **4,** 41; 1982
Chen Zhongwei and Wang Yan: 'Hand reconstruction' by autotransplantation of toes. *Chin. J. Surg.*, **19,** 7; 1981
Chen Zhongwei, Yan Dongyue and Zhan Disheng. *Microsurgery. Shanghai Science Publishing House, China, 1978*
Chen Zhongwei, Yu Zhongjia et al. A new treatment for congential tibial pseudoarthrosis - free fibula graft with microvascular anastomosis: a preliminary report of 12 cases. *Chin. J. Surg.*, **17,** 147; 1979
Chan Zhongwei, Chien Y. C. *et al.* Salvage of the forearm following complete traumatic amputation: report of a case. *Chin. Med. J.*, **82,** 632; 1963
Chen Zihua, Zhong Shizhen *et al.*, Applied anatomy of the veins of the head and face. *Guangdong Anat. Bull.*, **3,** 76; 1981
Cheng Gengli, He Gwangtsi *et al.* The arteries of the dorsalis pedis flap. *Acta Anat. Sinica*, **11,** 225; 1980
Cheng Xuxi, Lu Jiaze *et al.* Free dorsal pedis flap transplantation in repair of deep electric injury. *Chin. J. Surg.*, **18,** 136; 1980
Cobbett, J. R. Free digital transfer. *J. Bone Jt. Surg.*, **51B,** 677; 1979
Dai Hengru and Yao Jiaqing. On the formation of the superficial volar arch in Chinese. *Acta Anat. Sinica*, **3,** 15; 1958
Daviel, R. K. *et al.* Neurovascular free flaps: a preliminary report. *Plast. Reconstruct. Surg.*, **56,** 13; 1975
Das, A. C. *et al.* The occipital sinus. *J. Neurosurg.*, **33,** 307; 1970
Das, S. K. The size of the human omentum and methods of lengthening it for transplantation. *Br. J. Plast. Surg.*, **29,** 170; 1976
Dasgupta, G. and Kacher, S. J. Congenital abnormalities in the occisular chain in routine tympanotomy operation. *Eye Ear Nose Throat J.*, **53,** 362; 1974
Dass, R. *et al.* Human stapes and its variations. II. Footplate. *J. Laryngol. Otol.*, **80,** 471; 1966
Department of Anatomy, Ningxia Medical College. The distributive pattern of omental artery and their clinical significance. *Natl. Med. J. China*, **57,** 486; 1977
Dichiro, G. and Nelson, B. The volume of the sella turcia. *Am. J. Roentgenol. Radiol.*, **87,** 989; 1962
Dolwans, S. M. *et al.* The upper arm flap. *J. Microsurg.*, **1,** 162; 1979
Donaghy, R. M. P. What's new in surgery. *Surg. Gynecol. Obstet.*, **134,** 269; 1972
Dong Yiru, Lia Youjun *et al.* Transplantation of free omental flaps to the brain surface by microvascular technique for cerebral ischemic stroke. *Chin. J. Surg.*, **20,** 8; 1982
Doubilet, H. *et al.* The anatomy of peri-esophageal vagi. *Ann. Surg.*, **127,** 128; 1948
Doyle, P. J. *et al.* Results of surgical section and repair of the recurrent laryngeal. *Laryngoscope*, **77,** 1245; 1967
Duport, C. and Menard, Y. Transposition of the greater omentum for reconstruction of the chest wall. *JPRS*, **49,** 263; 1972
Durcan, D. J. *et al.* Bifurcation of the facial nerve. *Arch. Otolaryngol.*, **86,** 619; 1967
Edwards, E. A. Organization of the small arteries of the hand and digits. *Am. J. Surg.*, **99,** 837; 1960
ENT Department of Shanghai Sixth People's Hospital. Repair of recurrent laryngeal nerve in the treatment of vocal cord paralysis. *Chin. J. Otorhinolaryngol.*, **14,** 42; 1978
Eüchi Otomo. Anterior choroidal artery. *Arch. Neurol.*, **13,** 656; 1956
Feidberg, S. R. *et al.* Use of microscopic technique in neurosurgery. *Surg. Clin. N. Am.*, **56,** 781; 1976
Frank, S., Harris, M. D. *et al.* Anatomy of the cavernous sinus - a microsurgical study. *J. Neurosurg.*, **45,** 169; 1976
Fujino, T. Microvascular surgery in reconstructive plastic surgery. *Keio J. Med.*, **23,** 137; 1974
Gao Longyuan. Anatomical study of the marginal arterial arch of colon. *Acta Anat. Sinica*, **11,** 23; 1980
Georges, E. *et al.* Geniculate neuralgia and audio-vestibular disturbances due to compression of the intermediate and eighth nerves by the postero-inferior cerebellar artery. *Surg. Neurol.*, **13,** 147; 1980
Goldsmith, H. S. *et al.* Omental transposition of brain of stroke patients. *Stroke*, **10,** 471; 1979

Goodyear, H. M. Ophthalmic condition referable to diseases of the paranasal sinuses. *Arch. Otolaryngol.*, **48**, 202; 1948

Guo Fen. Observation on the blood supply of fibula. *Chin. J. Surg.*, **16**, 347; 1978

Guo Liankui and Luo Shudong. Aponeurosis palmaris and palmar fascial spaces. *Chin. J. Surg.*, **18**, 256; 1980

Hale, A. R. *et al.* The arteriovenous anastomoses and blood vessels of the human finger. *Medicine (Balt)*, **39**, 191; 1960

Han Yongjian, Zhang Keju *et al.* The measurements of the auditory ossicles. *Jiepouxue Tongbao*, **000**, 000; 1982a

Han Yongjian, Zhang Kaju *et al.* A study of the microsurgical anatomy of the auditory ossicles. I. Form and malformation of the auditory ossicles. *Guangdong Anat. Bull.*, **4**, 37; 1982b

Han Yongjian, Zhang Keju *et al.* A study of the microsurgical anatomy of the auditory ossicles. II. Arteries supply of the auditory ossicles. *Guangdong Anat. Bull.*, **4**, 40; 1982c

Harii, K. and Ohmori, K. Successful clinical transfer of ten free flaps by microvascular anastomoses. *Plast. Reconstruct. Surg.*, **53**, 259; 1973

Harii, K. and Ohmori, S. The use of the gastroepiploic vessels as recipient or donor vessels in the free transfer of composite flaps by microvascular anastomoses. *Plast. Reconstruct. Surg.*, **52**, 541; 1973

Harii, K. *et al.* Free gracilis muscle transplantation, with microneurovascular anastomoses for the treatment of facial paralysis. *Plast. Reconstruct. Surg.*, **57**, 133; 1976

Harii, k. *et al.* Microvascular free skin flap transfer. *Clin. Plast. Surg.*, **5**, 239; 1978

Hayren, S. S. *et al.* The ophthalmic artery. I. Origin and intra-cranial and intra-canalicular course. *Br. J. Ophthalmol.*, **46**, 65; 1962

Hill, L. *et al.* The tensor fasciae latae myocutaneous free flap. *Plast. Reconstruct. Surg.*, **61**, 517; 1978

Hoffmann, H. H. and Kuntz, A. Vagus nervo components. *Anat. Rec.*, **127**, 551; 1957

Hoffmann, H. H. and Schaitzlein, H. N. The number of nerve fibers in the vagus nerve of man. *Anat. Rec.*, **139**, 429; 1960

Holbach, K. H. *et al.* Superficial temporal-middle cerebral artery anastomosis for internal carotid occlusion. *Acta Neurochirurgica*, **37**, 201; 1977

Hollinshead, W. H. *Anatomy for Surgeons*, 2nd edn, vol. 2. Harper and Row, New York and London, 1971

Hollingshead, W. H. *Anatomy for Surgeons*, 2nd edn, vol. 1. Harper and Row, New York and London, 1968

Hough, J. V. D. Congenital malformations of the middle ear. *Arch. Otolaryngol.*, **78**, 355; 1963

Hough, J. V. D. Malformations and anatomical variations seen in middle ear during operation of the stapes. *Laryngoscope*, **67**, 1337; 1958

Hu Bincheng, Jiang Junben *et al.* Surgical anatomy of the free lateral thoracic flap. *Chin. J. Surg.*, **19**, 479; 1981

Hu Renzhao. Regional anatomy of internal iliac artery and its application in renal transplantation. *Chin. J. Surg.*, **18**, 160; 1980

Huang Gongkang *et al.* Microvascular free iliac bone transfer based on the deep circumflex iliac vessels. *J. Microsurg.*, **2**, 113; 1980

Huang Gongkang, Liu Zongzhao *et al.* Revascularized free transfer of iliac bone with anastomosis of deep circumflex iliac vessels. *Chin. J. Surg.*, **20**, 23; 1982

Huang Ying, Shi Enjuan *et al.* Observation, measurement and microdissection of the sural nerve. *Chin. Anat. Bull.*, **4**, 82; 1981

Huber, J. F. The arterial network supplying the dorsum of the foot. *Anat. Rec.*, **80**, 373; 1941

Ikuta, Y. Autotransplant of omentum to cover large denudation of the scalp: case report. *Plast. Reconstruct. Surg.*, **55**, 490; 1975

Jacobson, J. H. and Suarez, E. L. Microsurgery in anastomosis of small vessels. *Surg. Forum*, **11**, 243; 1960

Jackson, R. G. Anatomy of vague nerves in the region of the lower esophagus and the stomach. *Anat. Rec.*, **103**, 1; 1949

Jiang Shuxue, Li Ji *et al.* Microsurgical anatomy of the medial arm flap. *J. Zhongguo Med. Coll.*, **10**(6), 1; 1981

Jiang Shuying and Ying Ruqing. Transplantation of free omental flaps by microvascular anastomosis report of 10 cases. *Chin. J. Surg.*, **19**, 421; 1981

Jin Jiamin, Zhang Tingoai *et al.* Anatomy of the blood vessels in extra and intracranial arterial anastomosis. 2. The measurement and distribution of the posterior temporal arteries of the middle cerebral artery. *Acta Anat. Sinica*, **13**, 15; 1982

Kaplan, H. A. Collateral circulation of the brain. *Neurology*, **11**(2), 9; 1960

Kinnaert, P. Anatomical variations of the cervical portion of the thoracic duct in man. *J. Anat.*, **115**, 45; 1973

Kinnman, J. Surgical aspects of the anatomy of the spheroidal sinuses and the sella turcica. *J. Anat.*, **124**, 541; 1977

Kletter, G. *et al.* Importance of the histologic structure of the superficial temporal artery for the function of extra-intracranial bypass. In: *Microsurgery for Stroke*. Springer-Verlag, New York, 1976

Koos, W. T. *et al. Clinical Microneurosurgery*. Georg Thieme, Stuttgart, 1976

Kuo Fen. Observation on the blood supply of fibula. *Chin. J. Surg.*, **16**, 347; 1978

Lai Bingyao, Xie Jialun *et al.* Preliminary report on the repairing of muscle levator ani with muscle glataeus maximus in the treatment of fecal incontinence after congenital anal atresia operation. *Chin. J. Ped. Surg.*, **1**, 229; 1980

Lanz, W. *Praktische Anatomie*. 1 Band, Teil B. New York, 1979

Li Fuzhuang, Wang Yongxian *et al.* Anatomy of blood vessels of groin flap. *Acta Acad. Med. Sichuan*, **11**, 200; 1980

Li Ji, Hao Xianchun *et al.* Microsurgical anatomy of the anterior leg flap. *Guangdong Anat. Bull.*, **4**, 17; 1982

Li Ji, Jiang Shuxue *et al.* A vascular study of skin flap of forearm. *J. Zhongguo Med. Coll.*, **10**, 1; 1981

Li Ji, Jiang Shuxue *et al.* Vascularization of the tensor fasciae latae myocutaneous free flap. *Acta Anat. Sinica*, **12**, 235; 1981

Li Ji, Jiang Shuxue *et al.* Microsurgical anatomy of the lateral arm flap. *J. Zhongguo Med. Coll.*, **10**(6), 1; 1981

Li Shufen, Liu Xuejun *et al.* Anatomical studies on the blood vessels in extra-intracranial arterial anastomosis. 1. Distribution of superficial temporal artery and occipital artery on the scalp and their measurement. *Acta Anat. Sinica*, **12**, 382; 1981

Li Xuguang and Zheng Silu. An observation of the arterial system of the Chinese brain: IV. The intracranial portion of the vertebral arteries and the basilar artery. *Acta Anat. Sinica*, **13**, 1; 1982

Lin Yaochen, Li Daihua *et al.* The types of the sural anastomotic nerve. *Acta Anat. Sinica*, **5**, 357; 1962

Ling Tong, Wang Xueli *et al.* Clinical significance of dorsalis pedis vessels in thumb reconstruction and flap graft. *Chin. J. Surg.*, **19**, 297; 1981

Liu Jingfang, Wang Zengzhi *et al.* Intracranial transposition of pedicled omentum in the management of ischemic cerebrevascular diseases (a report of 6 cases). *Chin. J. Nerv. Ment. Dis.*, **6**, 321; 1980

Liu Muzhi. Method of injection and dissection of human lymphatic system. *Chin. Anat. Bull.*, **2**(4), 64; 1965

Liu Muzhi. Microsurgical anatomy of the lymphatic system of the upper limb. *Microsurgery*, **2**, 152; 1979

Liu Muzhi and Zhong Shizhen. The microsurgical anatomy of the superficial lymphatic systems of the lower limbs. *Microsurgery*, **2**, 85; 1979

Liu Muzhi and Zhong Shizhen. Microsurgical anatomy of the deep lymph vessels of the lower limb. *Microsurgery*, **5**(1–2), 14; 1982

Liu Muzhi and Zhong Shizhen. Microsurgical anatomy of the lymph vessels of the male genital organs. *Microsurgery*, **5**(1–2), 26; 1982

Liu Muzhi and Zhong Shizhen. Microsurgical anatomy of the lymph vessels of the female external pudendal. *Microsurgery*, **5**(1–2), 30; 1982

Liu Muzhi and Zhong Shizhen. Microsurgical anatomy of the lymph nodes of the groin. *Microsurgery*, **5**(1–2), 22; 1982

Liu Muzhi, Zhong Shizhen *et al.* Morphological study of the submandibular lymph nodes. *Guangdong Anat. Bull.*, **3**, 110; 1981

Liu Muzhi, Zhong Shizhen *et al.* Microsurgical anatomy of the cervical part of the thoracic duct. *Guangdong Anat. Bull.*, **4**, 29; 1982

Liu Zhengjin and Zhong Shizhen. Sciatic nerve in relation to the piriform muscle in adult Chinese. *Acta Anat. Sinica*, **5**, 351; 1962

Liu Zhengjin and Zhong Shizhen. Anatomy of the oesophageal opening of the diaphragma. *Chin. J. Surg.*, **12**, 452; 1964
Liu Zhengjin and Zhong Shizhen. The observation of the sheath of the musculus rectus abdominis. *Acta Anat. Sinica*, **8**, 568; 1965
Liu Zhengjin and Zhong Shizhen. Observations on the external carotid artery and its branches. *Chin. Anat. Bull.*, **2**, 13; 1965
Lu Fan and Lei Xiaohuan. The vagus distribution of the stomach of China. *Chin. Anat. Bull.*, **4**, 65; 1981
Ma Fu, Zhong Shizhen *et al.* Observations on the facial artery (in the face portion). *Guangdong Anat. Bull.*, **1**, 30;1979
Meniscalco, J. E. Microanatomy of the optic canal.*J. Neurosurg.*, **48**, 402; 1978
Mao Zengrong. Dia Arterien der hirnbasis und ihre Verzweigungen. *Acta Anat. Sinica*, **3**, 103; 1958
Mao Zengrong, Huang Ying *et al.* Microsurgical anatomy of the gracilis and their blood vessels and nerves. *Acad J. Second Mil. Med. Coll.*, PLA 1.18, 1980
McCrow, J. B. *et al.* The versatile gastrocnemius flap. *Plast. Reconstruct. Surg.*, **62**, 15; 1979
McCrow, J. B. *et al.* Clinical definition of independent myocutaneous vascular territories. *Plast. Reconstruct. Surg.*, **60**, 341; 1977
McLean, D. H. and Buncke, H. J. Autotransplant of omentum to a large scalp defect, with microsurgica revascularization. *Plast. Reconstruct. Surg.*, **49**, 268; 1972
Miao Hua, Yin Zhengyin *et al.* Blood supply of the anterior part of the iliac crest. *Acta Anat. Sinica*, **12**, 376; 1981
Michels, N. A. *Blood Supply and Anatomy of the Upper Abdominal Organs*. Pitman, London, 1955
Millesi, I. E. *et al.* The interfascicular nerve grafting of the median and ulnar nerves. *J. Bone Jt. Surg.*, **54**, 727; 1972
Mo Jingguo and Li Zhikun. A primary observation of omentum of China. *Microsurgery*, **3**, 83; 1980
Nager, G. I. and Nager, M. The arteries of the human middle ear with particular regard to the blood supply of the auditory ossicles. *Ann Otol. Rhinol. Laryngol.*, **62**, 923; 1953
Naidich, T. P. The normal anterior inferior cerebellar artery. *Radiology*, **119**, 355; 1976
Nylen, C. O. The otomicroscope and microsurgery 1921–1971. *Acta Otolaryngol.*, **73**, 453; 1972
O'Brien, M. *Microvascular Reconstructive Surgery*. Churchill Livingstone, London, 1977
Ohmori, K. and Harii, K. Free dosalis pedis flap to the hand with microneurovascular anastomoses. *Plast. Reconstruct. Surg.*, **58**, 546; 1976
Panllus, W. E. *et al.* Microsurgical exposure of the petrous portion of the carotid artery. *J. Neurosurg.*, **47**, 713; 1977
Parese, D. M. Superficial veins of the brain from a surgical point of view. *J. Neurosurg.*, **17**, 402; 1960
Permutter, D. *et al.* Microsurgical anatomy of the anterior cerebral-anterior communicating-recurrent artery complex. *J. Neurosurg.*, **45**, 259; 1976
Perritt, R. A. *Recent advances in corneal surgery*. Am. Acad. Ophthalmol. Otolaryngol. Course No. 28, 1950
Proctor, B. The development of the middle ear spaces and their surgical significance. *J. Laryngol. Otol.*, **78**, 631; 1964
Qiu Zhimin and Zou Ningsheng. The blood vessels of thyroid gland. *Acta Anat. Sinica*, **11**, 357; 1980
Qiu Zhimin and Zou Ningsheng. The external branch of superior laryngeal nerve and recurrent laryngeal nerve. *Acta Anat. Sinica*, **12**, 33; 1981
Qiu Zhimin and Zou Ningsheng. The surgical anatomy of the parathyroid gland. *Acta Anat. Sinica*, **12**, 28; 1981
Qu Riying, Ren Guobao *et al.* Transplantation of rib with intact periosteum and vascular pedicle. *Chin. J. Orth.*, **1**, 204; 1981
Ren Wende and Sun Ningjia. Anastomosis of the superficial artery with middle cerebral artery in treating ischemic cerebrovascular disease - report of 60 cases. *Chin. J. Neurol. Psychiatry*, **14**, 90; 1981
Renn, W. H. and Rhoton, A. L. Microsurgical anatomy of the sellar region. *J. Neurosurg.*, **43**, 288; 1975
Rhoton, A. L. Anatomy of saccular aneurysm. *Surg. Neurol.*, **14**, 59; 1980
Rhoton, A. and Robert, B. Microsurgical anatomy of the jugular foramen. *J. Neurosurg.*, **42**, 541; 1975

Saeki, N. and Rhoton, A. L. Microsurgical anatomy of the upper basilar artery and the posterior circle of Willis. *J. Neurosurg.*, **46**, 563; 1977
Seidenberg, B. *et al.* Immedite reconstruction of the cervical esophagus by revascularized isolated jejunal segment. *Ann. Surg.*, **149**, 162; 1959
Shanghai Sixth People's Hospital. The free muscle transplantation, a case report. *Chin. J. Med.*, **55**, 562; 1975
Sheng Zuyao, Wang Shuhuan *et al.* Omental axial flap: A new technique for free skin flap. *Chin. J. Surg.*, **17**, 151; 1979
Silber, S. J. *Microsurgery*. Williams & Wilkins, Baltimore, 1979
Smith, J. W. Microsurgery of peripheral nerve. *Plast. Reconstruct. Surg.*, **33**, 318; 1964
Smith, P. I. *et al.* The anatomical basis of the groin flap. *Plast. Reconstruct. Surg.*, **49**, 41; 1972
Song Enxu and Wang Xueli. Anatomy and clinical significance of fibular nutrient foramen. *Natl. Med. J. China*, **59**, 261; 1979
Staphen, J. H. *et al.* Microvascular relations of the trigeminal nerve (an anatomy study with clinical correlation). *J. Neurosurg.*, **52**, 381; 1980
Stenbens, W. E. *Pathology of the Cerebral Blood Vessels*. CV Mosby Co., New York, 1972
Sterling, J. A. and Goldsnaith, R. Total transplantation of thyroid gland using vascular anastomosis. *Surgery*, **35**, 624; 1954
Sunderland, S. *Nerves and Nerve Injuries*, 2nd edn. Livingstone, Edinburgh and London, 1978
Tang Zhuwu, Sun Tingkui *et al.* The metrical feature and distribution of the muscular branches in the upper extremity. *Acta Anat. Sinica*, **6**, 95; 1963
Tang Zhuwu, Sun Tingkui *et al.* The metrical features and distribution of the muscular branches in the lower extremity. *Acta Anat. Sinica*, **6**, 310; 1963
Tang Yangquan, Chen Yiran *et al.* Selective vagotomy and hemigastrectomy for duodenal ulcer. *Chin. J. Surg.*, **18**, 13; 1980
Tao Jinzhun, Zhang Yanfeng *et al.* Free gracilis muscle transplantation for postpoliomyelitic paralysis of gluteus medius. *Chin. J. Orthop.*, **1**, 109; 1981
Tao Yongson, Zhong Shizhen *et al.* An applied anatomical study of the rectus femoris. *Guangdong Anat. Bull.*, **2**(2), 37; 1980
Tao Yongson and Zhong Shizhen. An applied anatomical study on the lateral circumflex femoral vessels. *Guangdong Anat. Bull.*, **2**, 33; 1980
Tao Yongson, Zhong Shizhen *et al.* Microsurgical anatomy of the pectoralis major. *Guangdong Anat. Bull.*, **3**, 36; 1981
Tao Yongson, Zhong Shizhen *et al.* Microsurgical anatomy of the brachioradialis. *Guangdong Anat. Bull.*, **3**, 173; 1981
Tao Yongson, Zhong Shizhen *et al.* Microsurgical anatomy of the extensor carpi radialis. *Guangdong Anat. Bull.*, **3**, 176; 1981
Tao Yongson, Zhong Shizhen *et al.* Microsurgical anatomy of the biceps femoris. *Guangdong Anat. Bull.*, **3**, 47; 1981
Tao Yongson, Zhong Shizhen *et al.* Microsurgical anatomy of the semitendinosus. *Guangdong Anat. Bull.*, **3**, 52; 1981
Tao Yongson, Zhong Shizhen *et al.* Microsurgical anatomy of the semimembranosus. *Guangdong Anat. Bull.*, **3**, 56; 1981
Tao Yongson and Zhong Shizhen. An applied anatomical study of the gastrocnemius replacement quadriceps femoris by hemifree transfer. *Jiepouxue Tongbao*, **4**, 231; 1981
Tao Yongson and Zhong Shizhen. An assessment of the anatomy of the small intestine for the replacement of the esophagus. *Acta Anat. Sinica*, **12**, 225, 1981
Tao Yongson and Zhong Shizhen. An applied anatomical study on vasa circumflexa femoris lateralis, ractus femoris and tensor fasciae latae. Acta Anat. Sinica, **13**, 8; 1982
Taylor G. I. *et al.* The free vascularized bone graft. *Plast. Reconstruct. Surgery.*, **55**, 533; 1975
Taylor, G. I. and Ham, J. The free vascularized nerve graft. *Plast. Reconstruct. Surg.*, **57**, 413; 1976
Taylor, G. I. and Daniel, R. K. The free flap: composite tissue transfer by vascular anastomoses. *Austral. N.Z. J. Surg.*, **43**, 1; 1973
Taylor, G. I. *et al.* The anatomy of several free flap donor sites. *Plast. Reconstruct. Surg.*, **56**, 243; 1975
Taylor, G. I. *et al.* One-stage repair of compound leg defects with free vascularized flap of groin skin and iliac bone. *Plast. Reconstruct. Surg.*, **61**, 494; 1978

Taylor, G. I. *et al.* Superiority of the deep circumflex iliac vessels as the supply for free groin flaps - Clinical work. *Plast Reconstruct. Surg.*, **64**, 745; 1979

Thompson, N. Autogenous free grafts of skeletal muscle. *Plast. Reconstruct. Surg.*, **48**, 11; 1971

Tian Zhongrui and Wang Peiying. The measurements of the auditory ossicles and the reconstruction of the ossicular chain. *Chin. J. Otorhinolaryngol.*, **14**, 1; 1979

Toel, J. M. *et al. Cerebrovascular Disorders*, 2nd edn. McGraw-Hill, New York, 1974

Tsung Jenho, Liu Wenyao *et al.* Anastomosis of extracranial arteries in obliterative cerebral vascular diseases. *Chin. J. Sur.*, **16**, 19; 1978

Wallace, J. G. *et al.* Reconstruction of hemifacial atrophy with a free flap of omentum. *Br. J. Plast. Surg.*, **23**, 15; 1979

Walters, W. *et al.* Anatomic distribution of the vagus nerves at lower end of the esophagus: relation to gastric neurectomy for ulcer. *Arch. Surg.*, **55**, 400; 1947

Wan Liming and Zhang Dachuan. The observation and measurement of the region of the sella turcica. *J. Anhui Med. Coll.*, **16**, 24; 1981

Wang Zhongcheng, Xue Qingcheng *et al.* Progress of neurosurgery in China during the past 15 years. *Chin. J. Neurol. Psychiatry*, **12**, 129; 1979

Wang Zhongcheng, Yang Jiongda *et al.* Extracranial and intracranial arterial anastomosis in the treatment of cerebral ischemia. *Chin. J. Neurol. Psychiatry*, **11**, 20; 1978

Wang Qihua, Lin Zhenyan *et al.* The applied anatomical study of rectus abdominis. *Guangdong Anat. Bull.*, **3**, 184; 1981a

Wang Qihua, Lin Zhenyan *et al.* The applied anatomical study of tensor fasciae latae. *Guangdong Anat. Bull.*, **3**, 186; 1981b

Wang Qihua, Lin Zhenyan *et al.* Microsurgical anatomy of the blood supply of vagus nerve. *Guangdong Anat. Bull.*, **4**, 32; 1982

Wang Qihua, Lin Zhenyan *et al.* The microsurgical anatomy of the recurrent laryngeal nerve. *Guangdong Anat. Bull.*, **3**, 17; 1981c

Wang Qihua, Xiao Shangying *et al.* The applied anatomical study of ???????????. *Bull.*, **3**, 59; 1981d

Wang Qihua, Xiao Shangying *et al.* The applied anatomical study of gracilis. *Guangdong Anat. Bull.*, **3**, 188; 1981e

Wang Qihua, Xiao Shangying *et al.* Applied anatomical study of the sartorius. *Guangdong Anat. Bull.*, **4**, 34; 1982

Wang Xizeng, Zhou Zhiyao *et al.* Multiple renal vessels reconstruction in renal transplantation. *Chin. Urol.*, **2**, 217; 1981

Weathery, H. J. The artery of the index finger. *Anat. Rec.*, **122**, 57; 1955

Webster, J. C. The intratemporal nerve. *Ear Nose Throat J.*, **57**, 251; 1978

Wei Baolin and Wang Xueli. An applied anatomical study of the sural nerve. *Guangdong Anat. Bull.*, **3**, 25; 1981

Wei Jianing, Wang Shuhuan *et al.* Peripheral nerve repair of the upper limb: An analysis of 87 cases. *Chin. J. Surg.*, **19**, 3; 1981

Wei Linyu, Li Zhixin *et al.* Study of the nutrient foramen of rib and principles of its clinical use. *J. Harbin Med. Coll.*, **2**, 69; 1981

Weiland, A. T. and Daniel, R. K. Microvascular anastomoses for bone grafts in the treatment of massive defects in bone. *J. Bone Jt. Surg.*, **61A**, 98; 1979

Williams, P. L. and Warwick, R. *Gray's Anatomy*, 36th edn. Churchill Livingstone, London and New York, 1980

William, W. *et al.* Conservation of major leg arteries when used as recipient supply for a free flap. *Plast. Reconstruct. Surg.*, **63**, 317; 1979

Wu Jinbao, Cheng Xinheng *et al.* The distribution of arteries supplying the dorsum and sole of the foot. *Acta Anat. Sinica*, **11**, 13; 1980

Wu Jinbao, Fan Lengyan *et al.* Diaphyseal nutrient foramina and artery of tibia and fibula. *Acta Anat. Sinica.*, **11**, 234; 1980

Wu Jinbao, Fan Lengyan *et al.* The diaphyseal nutrient foramina and the nutrient arteries of radius and ulna in the Chinese. *Acta Anat. Sinica*, **12**, 1; 1981

Wu Renxiu. Microsurgical anatomy of proximal branches of the femoral artery of the children. *Guangdong Anat. Bull.*, **3**, 75; 1981

Wu Xianyou. Roentgenological study of sella turcica in normals. *Chin. J. Radiol.*, **10**, 316; 1965

Wu Yongmu. A study of the ribs and their blood supply. *Guangdong Anat. Bull.*, **3**, 191; 1981

Wu Yongmu and Ding Xunzhao. The peroneal artery and its relation to the blood supply of fibula in 100 Chinese adults. *Acta Anat. Sinica*, **12**, 20; 1981

Xiong Shuming, Ding Yongshan *et al*. The blood supply and nerve innervation of the rectus femoral muscle. *Acta Anat. Sinica*, **12**, 121; 1981

Xiong Shuming, Zhang Shenggui *et al*. The blood supply and nerve innervation of the gracilis muscle. *Acta Anat. Sinica*, **12**, 129; 1981

Xu Dachuan, Zhong Shizhen *et al*. An anatomical study of the thyroid gland and parathyroid glands transplantation with fetus or newborn as donor. *Microsurgery*, **4**, 100; 1981a

Xu Dachuan, Zhong Shizhen *et al*. Microsurgical anatomy of the transplantation of the suprarenal gland. *Microsurgery*, **4**, 94; 1981b

Xu Dachuan, Zhong Shizhen *et al*. An anatomical study of the pancreas transplantation with fetus or newborn as donor. *Chin. J. Organ Transplant.*, **3**, 33; 1982

Xu Dachuan, Zhong Shizhen *et al*. Microsurgical anatomy of the transplantation of gonad. *Guandong Anat. Bull.*, **4**, 25; 1982

Xu Enduo, Chen Jun *et al*. Surgical anatomy of the blood vessels of feet. *Chin. J. Orthop.*, **1**, 240; 1981

Xu Enduo, Han Ziyu *et al*. Surgical anatomy of the superficial temporal vessels and their branches. *Guandong Anat. Bull.*, **4**, 20; 1982

Xu Rongnan, Cai Zhongpei *et al*. Highly selective vagotomy: early results in 27 cases. *Chin. J. Surg.*, **18**, 15; 1980

Xue Xingwe, Li Zhixin *et al*. An anatomical observation of microvascular anastomoses concerning transplantation of fibula. *J. Harbin Med. Coll.*, **1**, 77; 1979

Yang Chunlin, Xu Shijia *et al*. The types of the thoracic duct. *Acta Anat. Sinica*, **12**, 360; 1981

Yang Dongyue, Gu Yudong *et al*. The thumb reconstruction by second digital free transfer: report of 40 cases. *Chin. J. Surg.*, **15**, 13; 1977

Yang Dongyue, Gu Yudong *et al*. Transfer of a 40 cm long skin flap. *Chin. J. Surg.*, **17**, 167; 1979

Yang Dongyue, Gu Yudong *et al*. Management of vascular problems in microsurgery. *Chin. J. Surg.*, **19**, 131; 1981

Yang Guofang, Chen Baoju *et al*. Forearm free skin flap transplantation. *Natl. Med. J. China*, **61**, 139; 1981

Yang Zengnian, Shi Haoran *et al*. Free transplantation of lateral thoracic axillary flap in burns. *Chin. J. Surg.*, **20**, 236; 1982

Yasargil, M. G. *Microsurgery*. Georg Thieme Verlag, Stuttgart, 1969

Yasargil, M. G. *et al*. Microneurosurgical arterial reconstruction. *Surgery*, **67**, 221; 1970

Yu Guozhong and Zhu Jiakai. Application of omentum in the miscrosurgery. *Microsurgery*, **2**, 9; 1979

Yu Guozhong and Zhu Jiakai. The clinical application of the omentum by microvascular anastomoses technique. *Microsurgery*, **3**, 87; 1980

Yu Guozhong, Zhu Jiakai *et al*. The diameter and thickness of the omental vessels. *Microsurgery*, **3**, 100; 1980

Yu Huiyuan *et al*. Transplantation of children's kidneys into adult recipients. *Chin. J. Organ Transplant.*, **2**, 1; 1981

Yu Shoumin and Zheng Guande. Variations in the tendons of the insertion of the abductor pollicis longus and extensor pollicis brevis. *Acta Anat. Sinica*, **2**, 352; 1957

Yu Tianlin, Liu Defu *et al*. The use of double renal transplants from newborn to adult recipients. *Chin. J. Organ Transplant.*, **3**, 53; 1982

Yu Zhe, Li Ruixiang *et al*. The blood vessels and nerves of musculus gracili. *Acta Acad. Med. Sichuan*, **11**, 295; 1980

Zang Renho *et al*. Anastomosis of extracranial and intracranial arteries in obliterative cerebral vascular diseases. *Chin. J. Surg.*, **16**, 19; 1978

Zeng Silu and Li Xuguang. An observation of the arterial system of Chinese brain. I. The extracerebral arteries. *Acta Anat. Sinica*, **8**, 259; 1965

Zeng Silu and Li Xuguang. An observation of the arterial system of Chinese brain. III. The cerebellar arteries. *Acta Anat. Sinica*, **12**, 113; 1981

Zeng Silu and Yuan Longqing. An observation of the arterial system of Chinese brain. II. The arteries of the corpus striatum, thalamus and internal capsule. *Acta Anat. Sinica*, **9**, 258; 1966

Zhao Minxue, Chan Muxun *et al*. On the number and distribution of the perforating branches of the peroneal artery. *Acta Anat. Sinica*, **2**, 125; 1957

Zhao Weipang and Shen Jlali. Treatment of chyluria by anastomosis of lymphatic vessels with veins in inguinal region and on dorsum of foot. *Chin. J. Surg.*, **19**, 157; 1981
Zhang Cheng, Tan Ziti *et al.* Microsurgical total resection of pituitary tumor through fronto-sphenoidal approach. *Chin. J. Neurol. Psychiatry*, **14**, 197; 1981
Zhang Cheng, Zhang Shuchen *et al.* Extra-intracranial arterial anastomosis in the treatment of cerebral ishemic diseases. *Chin. J. Neurol. Psychiatry*, **14**, 86; 1981
Zhang Chenli, Mao Zhengrong *et al.* Microsurgical anatomy of the vessels and nerves of rectus femoris. *Chin. Anat. Bull.*, **4**, 74; 1981
Zhang Disheng, Huang Oulin *et al.* Free jejunum graft for esophageal reconstruction by microvascular anastomosis: report of 7 cases. *Chin. J. Surg.*, **17**, 154; 1979
Zhang Disheng, Wang Wei *et al.* Preliminary report of experimental homologous free transfer of great omentum in dogs. *Chin. J. Organ Transplant.*, **2**, 86; 1981
Zhang Dongming, Zhang Chenli *et al.* A study on gastrocenemius myocutaneous vessels and nerves. *Acad. J. Second Mil. Coll. PLA*, **2**, 170; 1981
Zhang Lifu, Li Futian *et al.* Middle meningeal artery-middle cerebral artery anastomosis (a case report). *Chin. J. Neurol. Psychiatry*, **6**, 141; 1980
Zhang Weilong. An observation of the extrarenal veins in Chinese. *J. Bethune Med. Coll.*, **6**, 9; 1980
Zhang Weilong. Microanatomy of the middle cerebral artery. *Acta Anat. Sinica*, **12**, 366; 1981
Zhang Weilong. Microsurgical anatomy of cortical branches of middle cerebral artery. *Chin. J. Surg.*, **20**, 126; 1982
Zhang Weilong and Dai Guilin. The extra-renal arteries. *Acta Anat. Sinica*, **6**, 350; 1963
Zhang Weilong and Dai Guilin. Regional anatomy of the pararenal arteries. *Chin. Anat. Bull.*, **2**, 32; 1965
Zhang Zhaowu *et al.* Microsurgical repair of urethra using vermiform appendix: report of 2 cases. *Chin. J. Urol.*, **2**, 132; 1981
Zhen Deru, Wu Xuetao *et al.* Study on the nutrient vessels and nerve of the gracilis muscle. *Acta Acad. Med. Wuhan*, **9**, 21; 1980
Zhong Shizhen. Observation on the intracranial portion of the vertebral arteries and the vasilar artery and their main branches. *Acta. Anat. Sinica*, **3**, 177; 1958
Zhong Shizhen. The relation between advance of the microsurgery and the applied anatomy. *Guangdong Anat. Bull.*, **2**, 1; 1980
Zhong Shizhen and Liu Zhengjin. Observation on the inferior mesenteric artery and its branches. *Acta Anat. Sinica*, **7**, 428; 1964
Zhong Shizhen and Liu Zhengjin. Observation on the internal iliac artery and its main branches. *Acta Anat. Sinica*, **7**, 173; 1964
Zhong Shizhen and Liu Zhengjin. The origin of the obturator artery and other blood vessels related to the femoral ring. *Acta Anat. Sinica*, **7**, 181; 1964
Zhong Shizhen and Liu Zhengjin. Variations of the muscles of foot. *Chin. Anat. Bull.*, **1**, 151; 1964
Zhong Shizhen and Liu Zhengjin. Surface anatomy of the sciatic nerve in the gluteal region. *Med. J. PLA*, **3**, 252; 1966
Zhong Shizhen and Tao Yongsen. An anatomical study on the reconstruction of the urethra by appendix transplantation. *Chin. J. Urol.*, **2**, 129; 1981
Zhong Shizhen and Tao Yongson. The applied anatomy of the scrotal skin flap: a new donor site of free skin flap. *Chin. Anat. Bull.*, **4**, 228; 1981
Zhong Shizhen, He Gwangtsi *et al.* The patterns and variations of the tendons on dorsum of the hand. *Acta Anat. Sinica*, **8**, 71; 1965
Zhong Shizhen, Liu Muzhi *et al.* A study of the microsurgical anatomy of the median nerve. *Acta Anat. Sinica*, **11**, 337; 1980
Zhong Shizhen, Liu Muzhi *et al.* A study of the microsurgical anatomy of the ulnar nerve. *Acta Anat. Sinica*, **12**, 346; 1981a
Zhong Shizhen, Liu Muzhi *et al.* A study of the microsurgical anatomy of the radial nerve. *Guangdong Anat. Bull.*, **3**, 165; 1981b
Zhong Shizhen, Liu Muzhi *et al.* The patterns of blood supply of the skin flap and their applied anatomy. *Microsurg.*, **4**, 13; 1981c
Zhong Shizhen, Liu Muzhi *et al.* On the applied anatomical study of the microsurgery – a review. *J. Microsurg.*, **9**, 13; 1982a
Zhong Shizhen, Ma Fu *et al.* Surgical anatomy of the blood vessels relation to extraintracranial arterial anastomosis. *Chin. J. Neurol. Psychiatry*, **14**, 156; 1981d

Zhong Shizhen, Sun Bo *et al.* The flaps pedicled by the vessels of intramuscular space: a new type of free skin flaps. *Guangdong Anat. Bull.*, **4**, 1; 1982c

Zhong Shizhen, Sun Bo *et al.* The applied anatomy on the scapula transplantation by microvascular anastomosis. *Chin. Appl. Anat.*, **1**, 3; 1983

Zhong Shizhen, Tao Yongson *et al.* Observations on the superficial temporal artery and its branches. *Guangdong Anat. Bull.*, **1**, 36; 1979

Zhong Shizhen, Tao Yongson *et al.* An anatomical study on skin flaps supplied by the vessels of intramuscular septa. *Acta Anat. Sinica*, **13**, 230; 1982b

Zhou Jiabao and Dai Xianglin. Microsurgical anatomy of the optic canal. *Chin. Anat. Bull.*, **4**, 212; 1981

Zhou Zhangman. A study of microsurgical anatomy on the sciatic nerve. *Acta 1st Mil. Med. Coll. PLA*, **2**, 233; 1982

Zhu Jiakai. The method of interfoscicular suture of peripheral nerves. *Microsurgery*, **1**, 64; 1979

Zhu Jiakai and Wang Chengda. Long term results of interfascicular nerve grafting: analysis of 8 cases. *Chin. J. Surg.*, **17**, 47; 1979

Zhu Jiakai and Yu Guozhong. Lymphaticovenous anastomosis treated obstructive lymphoedema of the limbs. *Chin. J. Surg.*, **18**, 416; 1980

Zhu Jiakai and Yu Guozhong. Anatomy, physiology and clinical application of the omentum. *Microsurgery*, **3**, 93; 1980

Zhu Jiakai, Wang Chengda *et al.* Heterotransplantation by microvascular anastomosis. *Microsurgery*, **3**, 200; 1980

Zhu Shenxiu, Lu Shibi *et al.* Free inguinal skin flap transfer: report of 19 cases. *Chin. J. Surg.*, **17**, 163; 1979

Zhu Shengxiu, Lu Shibi *et al.* Transfer of free gracilis flap: report of 7 cases. *Chin. J. Surg.*, **19**, 143; 1981

Zhu Shenxiu, Zhang Boxun *et al.* Transplantation of free musculocutaneous flap of extensor digitorum brevis for the restoration of functions of thenar muscles and adductor pollicis. *Acta Postgrad. Med. Coll. PLA*, **2**, 26; 1981

Zhu Tailai, Tan Junsheng *et al.* Vagus innervation of lower oesophagus and stomach: an anatomical study on 100 cadavers. *Chin. J. Surg.*, **18**, 4; 1980

Zhu Yu and Wang Baochun. A regional anatomy on the recurrent laryngeal nerve in cervical region. *Chin. Anat. Bull.*, **4**, 90, 1981

Zuo Caijie. The patterns and surface projection of the superficial volar arch in Chinese. *Acta Anat. Sinica*, **7**, 409; 1964

Index